Polycystic Ovary Syndrome

Polycystic Ovary Syndrome

Editors

Gautam N Allahbadia

MD, DNB, FNAMS, FCPS, DGO, DFP, FICMU, FICOG
Scientific Director
The Prince Aly Khan Hospital IVF Center and The Aesculap Academy-Asia
Pacific Center For Minimally Invasive Surgery, Training and Research,
Mazgaon, Mumbai, India

Medical Director
Rotunda – The Center For Human Reproduction
Bandra, Mumbai, India

Rina Agrawal

MD, DGO, MRCOG, PhD
Deputy Medical Director
Centre for Reproductive Medicine,
London, UK

Editorial Assistant

Rubina Merchant

PhD
Embryologist
Rotunda – The Center for Human Reproduction, Bandra, Mumbai, India

ANSHAN

First published in 2007 by

Anshan Ltd
6 Newlands Road
Tunbridge Wells
Kent.
TN4 9AT. UK

Tel: +44 (0) 1892 557767
Fax: +44 (0) 1892 530358

e-mail: info@anshan.co.uk
www.anshan.co.uk

ISBN–13: 978 1 904798 74 3

Whilst the advice and information in this book are believed to be true and accurate at the date of going to press, neither the author(s) not the publisher can accept any legal responsibility or liability for any errors or omissions that may be made. In particular, (but without limiting the generality of the preceding disclaimer) every effort has been made to check drug dosages; however it is still possible that errors have been missed. Furthermore, dosage schedules are constantly being revised and new side-effects recognized. For these reasons the reader is strongly urged to consult the drug companies' printed instructions before administering any of the drugs recommended in this book.

British Library Cataloguing in Publication Data
A catalogue record for this book is available from the British Library

Copy Editor : Rubina Merchant
Cover Design: Terry Griffiths

Typeset, printed and bound by Replika Press, India.

This book is dedicated to our children
Akanksha, Ranveer and Sharan

Contents

Pathophysiology of PCOS and its Consequences

Impaired Glucose Metabolism and Insulin Resistance

Obesity

Hyperandrogenemia

Dyslipidemia

Risk of Cardiovascular Disease

Surgical Treatment   **415**

Pregnancy and Polycystic Ovary Syndrome   **431**

Foreword

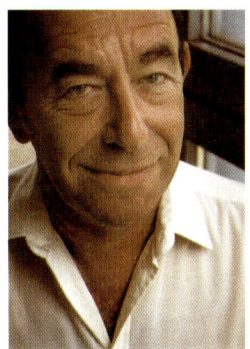

When Stein and Leventhal first described the Polycystic Ovary Syndrome (PCOS) in 1935, I doubt whether they would have believed that thousands of researchers throughout the world would still be trying to unravel its mysteries more than 70 years later. This syndrome is the most prevalent female endocrinopathy with the commonest association with anovulatory infertility. Yet, after all this time, controversy still rages even regarding the very definition of the syndrome, not to mention the best way to treat it.

One of the fascinations of PCOS is that, it is no longer just a gynecological curiosity, but a syndrome in its full blown form that can affect almost every organ in the female body from the hypothalamus to the hair follicles and the pituitary to the pancreas, from adolescence to menopause. As a consequence, many medical disciplines are now involved in the investigation of the syndrome, from diabetologists to dermatologists and from epidemiologists to endocrinologists.

The heterogeneity of the presentation of the syndrome and the diversity of its manifestations and long-term consequences are almost matched by the treatment options that have been proposed and theories regarding the pathogenesis of the syndrome. The geneticists are having a hard time trying to explain the etiology, while the clinicians are debating the worth of insulin lowering agents and the plethora of infertility treatments available. Putting all this together, and making some sense of it, is a mammoth task. The editors of this comprehensive book, Gautam N Allahbadia and Rina Agrawal, are thus to be heartily congratulated for assembling a team of international experts from almost every country in the world, to state their case. It is a stimulating volume that is truly thought-provoking and comprehensive, and will surely encourage further research until we finally have all the answers.

Roy Homburg

Preface

Landmarked in the Hall of Disorders as a multifaceted, heterogeneous syndrome with widespread systemic manifestations that enmesh the body in debilitating and life-threatening long-term health consequences, the Polycystic Ovary Syndrome (PCOS), ironically, still remains a pathophysiological and molecular enigma. It is perhaps, the most common endocrinopathy that poses a continuing challenge to treating clinicians, and one that has engaged researchers in an endless strive to unravel the pathophysiology of the disorder and formulate specific therapeutic approaches. While therapy has advanced from the use of controlled ovarian hyperstimulation and GnRH agonists to promote ovulation induction, laparoscopic ovarian drilling, laparoscopic ovarian multi-needle intervention (LOMNI), depending on the indication, to the current use of insulin sensitizing drugs like metformin, pioglitazone and rosiglitazone, and aromatase inhibitors to treat the biochemical manifestations of the syndrome, explorative research into the genetics of the syndrome is still gaining ground. Attempts to identify candidate genes involved in steroidogenesis, steroid hormone effects, GnRH-a regulation and action, insulin regulation and action and adipose tissue metabolism, have culminated in the belief that PCOS is a polygenic trait that involves the interaction of susceptible and protective variants under environmental influence. Hence, a search for candidate genes that regulate every step of the metabolic and reproductive pathway, to provide clues to solving the genomic puzzle and give a clearer idea of the pathophysiology of the syndrome, is imperative. Where does this leave us? Still searching for a way out of the complex labyrinth of possibilities for articulate answers!

Systematically taking the reader through the history and evolution of PCOS, the prevalence, diagnosis, genetics and pathophysiology of the syndrome and the cascade of symptoms it triggers, the current modes of therapy, the long-term health consequences, and the lifestyle modifications it demands, this concise compilation intends to give the reader a panoramic, updated, more coherent and sound view of the syndrome we know as PCOS. It thus serves to reach out to all gynecologists, reproductive physicians, support personnel working in IVF/ICSI units, researchers, and patients groping for the right knowledge in the field. Since the book highlights definitions, classifications and treatment algorithms, it will also be useful to students and postgraduates in the field. The list of most commonly asked questions with appropriate answers, that concludes each chapter in the book, serves to bring the most frequent doubts on a common platform to help expand and elaborate difficult practice problems.

The content and layout style of the chapters speak immensely of the intellectual finesse and the academic and clinical experience of the contributors who cherish international acclaim for their contributions in the field. We are grateful to the authors for contributing to an endless effort to disseminate updated knowledge and research to fight the malice of a disease that continues to befuddle treating clinicians and distort the mindscape of patients who suffer the plight. We do hope we have been successful in our attempt to impart medically useful knowledge and fulfill the intended purpose of this monograph.

Gautam N Allahbadia   **Rina Agrawal**

List of Contributors

Michel Abou Abdallah MD
Reproductive Endocrinologist
Division of Reproductive Endocrinology and
Infertility
Rizk Hospital
Beirut
Lebanon

Mohamed A Aboulghar MD
Cairo University – Department of
Obstetrics and Gynecology
The Egyptian IVF-ET Center
Cairo
Egypt

Malek Mansour Aghssa MD
Infertility Specialist
Assistant Professor of Obstetrics and Gynecology
Vali Asr Reproductive Research Center
Tehran Medical Sciences University
Tehran
Iran

Rina Agrawal MD, DGO, MRCOG, PhD
Deputy Medical Director
Centre for Reproductive Medicine
London
UK

Jairam K Aithal MD, DM (Cardiology)
Consultant Cardiologist
Dr LH Hiranandani Hospital
Powai, Mumbai
India

Richard Ajayi MRCOG, FWACS
Consultant Gynecologist and Director
The Assisted Conception Unit
The Bridge Clinic Limited
Victoria Island
Lagos, Nigeria
Africa

Gautam N Allahbadia MD, DNB, FNAMS, FCPS,
DGO, DFP, FICMU, FICOG
Scientific Director
The Prince Aly Khan Hospital IVF Center and
The Aesculap Academy-Asia Pacific Center For
Minimally Invasive Surgery, Training & Research,
Mazgaon, Mumbai
Medical Director
Rotunda – The Center For Human Reproduction
Bandra (W), Mumbai
India

Lawrence S Amesse MD, PhD
Associate Professor
Director, Division of Reproductive Endocrinology
and Infertility, Department of Obstetrics and
Gynecology
Wright State University Boonshoft School of
Medicine
Dayton, Ohio
USA

Teresa-Pfaff Amesse MD
Assistant Professor
Department of Pathology and Department of
Neuroscience, Cell Biology and Physiology
Wright State University Boonshoft School of
Medicine
Dayton, Ohio
USA

Aydin Arici MD
Professor and Director
Section of Reproductive Endocrinology and
Infertility
Yale University School of Medicine
Department of Obstetrics, Gynecology, and
Reproductive Sciences
Cedar Street
New Haven
USA

Sulbha Arora MD, DNB
Clinical Associate
Prince Aly Khan Hospital IVF Center
Aesculap Academy - Asia Pacific Center for
Minimally Invasive Surgery, Training & Research
Mazagaon, Mumbai
India

Paolo Giovanni Artini MD
Department of Reproductive Medicine and Child
Development
Division of Gynecology and Obstetrics
University of Pisa, Pisa
Italy

Hedie Asheghan MD
Infertility Specialist
Senior Obstetrician and Gynecologist
Department of Obstetrics and Gynecology
Day General Hospital
Tehran
Iran

Cem S Atabekoglu MD
Associate Professor
Division of Reproductive Endocrinology
Department of Obstetric and Gynecology
Ankara University School of Medicine
Ankara
Turkey

Johnny Awwad MD
Associate Professor
Obstetrician/Gynecologist
Department of Obstetrics and Gynecology
Division of Reproductive Endocrinology and
Infertility
American University of Beirut Medical Center
American University Hospital
Beirut
Lebanon

Samuel Hernandez Ayup MD
Co-Director
Professor of Reproductive Endocrinology and
Infertility
Instituto para el Estudio de la Concepción Humana
(IECH)
Monterrey, NL
México CP

Maryam Bagheri MSc
Senior Coordinator
Vai Asr Reproductive Research Center
Emam Khomini Hospital
Tehran
Iran

Marina Baldi PhD
Genetist-Technical Director
Consultorio di Genetica
Genoma Laboratory
Rome
Italy

Socorro Benavides MD
Reproduction and Genetics Clinic
Angeles del Pedregal Hospital
Mexico

M Benkhalifa PhD
Laboratory Director
ATL R&D
Reproductive Biology and Genetics Laboratory
France

Murat Berkkanoglu MD
Consultant Gynecologist and Obstetrician, IVF
Practitioner
Antalya IVF
Antalya
Turkey

Alexandra Bermúdez MD
Scientific Director
Specialist in Obstetrics, Gynecology, Reproductive
Medicine
CONCIBE Reproducción Asistida
Colonia Lomas de Chapultepec
Mexico City
Mexico

Galia Biran MD
IVF unit
Wolfson Medical Center
Holon
Israel

Andrea Borini MD
Gynecologist, Director
Tecnobios Procreazione, Center for Reproductive
Health
Via Dante Bologna
Italy

Gurkan Bozdag MD
Obstetrician and Gynecologist, Specialist in
Infertility and
Reproductive Medicine
Department of Obstetrics and Gynecology
Reproductive Biology and Infertility Unit
Hacettepe University, School of Medicine
Sihhiye, Ankara
Turkey

Rudi Campo MD
Gynecologist and Specialist In Reproductive
Medicine
Leuven Institute for Fertility and Embryology
Tiensevest, Leuven
Belgium

Howard J Carp MBBS, FRCOG
Department of Obstetrics and Gynecology
Sheba Medical Center, Tel Hashomer
University of Tel Aviv
Tel Aviv
Israel

Donatella Caserta MD, PhD
Professor
Department Gynecological Sciences and
Perinatology
University La Sapienza
S Andrea Hospital, Rome
Italy

Robert F Casper MD, FRCS(C)
Professor, Division of Reproductive Sciences
Department of Obstetrics and Gynecology
The University of Toronto
Senior Scientist
Samuel Lunenfeld Research Institute
Mount Sinai Hospital, Toronto
Ontario
USA

Hasim Cemal MD
Consultant Gynecologist and Obstetrician, IVF
Practitioner
Antalya IVF
Antalya
Turkey

Julio Chanona MD
Associate
Specialist in Obstetrics, Gynecology, Reproductive
Medicine
Instituto Mexicano De Infertilidad
Centro Medico Puerta De Hierro
Boulevard Puerta De Hierro
Zapopan, Jalisco
Mexico

Luciana Chessa MD, PhD
Professor
Faculty of Medicine
Clinical Genetics Unit
University La Sapienza
S Andrea Hospital, Rome
Italy

Francesca Cristello MD
Department of Reproductive Medicine and Child
Development
Division of Gynecology and Obstetrics
University of Pisa, Pisa
Italy

Sandra Cubillos
Biologist, Embryologist., IVF Laboratory Director
CONCIBE Reproducción Asistida
Colonia Lomas de Chapultepec
Mexico City
Mexico

Silvio Cuneo MD
Medical Director
Specialist in Obstetrics, Gynecology, Reproductive
Medicine
CONCIBE Reproducción Asistida
Colonia Lomas de Chapultepec
Mexico City
Mexico

Preeti Dabadghao MD
Assistant Professor
Department of Endocrinology
Sanjay Gandhi Postgraduate Institute of Medical
Sciences
Raebareli Road, Lucknow
India

Erbil Dogan MD
Assistant Professor
Department of Obstetrics and Gynecology
Division of Reproductive Medicine and Infertility
Dokuz Eylul University School of Medicine
Dokuz Eylul University, Izmir
Turkey

Ibrahim Esinler MD
Obstetrician and Gynecologist
Specialist in Infertility and Reproductive Medicine
Department of Obstetrics and Gynecology
Division of Reproductive Medicine and Infertility
Baskent University School of Medicine
Ankara
Turkey

Dov Feldberg MD
Professor
Vice Chairman
Department of Obstetrics and Gynecology
Rabin Medical Center and
Tel-Aviv University School of Medicine
Israel

Francesco Fiorentino PhD
Technical Director
Genoma Lab, Rome
Italy

Richard Fleming MD
Honorary Professor Reproductive Medicine
University Department Obstetrics and Gynaecology
Division of Developmental Medicine
University of Glasgow
Glasgow Royal Infirmary
Glasgow, Scotland
UK

Yair Frenkel MD
Senior Physician
Department of Obstetrics and Gynecology
Physician in Charge, Menopause service
Sheba Medical Center
Sheba Medical Center, Tel Hashomer
Israel

Martha García MD
Associate
Specialist in Obstetrics, Gynecology, Reproductive
Medicine
Instituto Mexicano De Infertilidad
Centro Medico Puerta De Hierro
Boulevard Puerta De Hierro
Zapopan, Jalisco
Mexico

Tarek A Gelbaya MRCOG, MD
Specialist Registrar Obstetrics & Gynaecology
Royal Albert Edward Infirmary
Wigan Lane
Wigan
Lancashire
UK

Andrea Riccardo Genazzani MD, PhD
Professor
Director of the Department of Obstetrics and
Gynecology
Department of Reproductive Medicine and Child
Development
Division of Gynecology and Obstetrics,
University of Pisa, Pisa
Italy

Charles J Glueck MD
Medical Director
The Jewish Hospital, Cholesterol Center
Alliance Hospitals
Cholesterol Center
Cincinnati, Ohio
USA

Carlos Ortega-González MD
Assistant Professor
Department of Endocrinology
Instituto Nacional de Perinatología
Colonia Lomas Virreyes
México, DF
México

José Sepúlveda González MD, PhD
Medical Director
Instituto para el Estudio de la Concepción Humana
(IECH)
Monterrey, NL
México. CP

Stephan Gordts MD
Gynecologist and Specialist In Reproductive
Medicine
Leuven Institute for Fertility and Embryology
Tiensevest, Leuven
Belgium

Sylvie Gordts Jr MD
Gynecologist and Specialist In Reproductive
Medicine
Leuven Institute for Fertility and Embryology
Tiensevest, Leuven
Belgium

Bulent Gulekli MD
Head, Professor in Obstetrics and Gynecology
Department of Obstetrics and Gynecology
Division of Reproductive Medicine and Infertility
Dokuz Eylul University School of Medicine
Dokuz Eylul University, Izmir
Turkey

Alfonso Javier Gutiérrez MD
Reproduction and Genetics Clinic
Angeles del Pedregal Hospital
Mexico

Alfonso Javier Nájar Gutiérrez MD
Medical Director
Reproduction and Genetics Clinic
Angeles del Pedregal Hospital
Mexico

Roberto Santos Halliscak MD
Co-Director
Professor of Reproductive Endocrinology and
Infertility, IECH
Instituto para el Estudio de la Concepción Humana
(IECH)
Monterrey, NL
México CP

Roger Hart MD FRANZCOG MRCOG
Senior Lecturer in Obstetrics and Gynaecology
UWA School of Women's and Infants' Health
University of Western Australia
King Edward Memorial Hospital
Subiaco, Perth
Australia

Roy Homburg MD
Professor of Reproductive Medicine
Department of Obstetrics and Gynecology
VU University Medical Centre
Amsterdam
The Netherlands
Emma Neiman Chair
Obstetric Investigation at the Sackler School of
Medicine
Tel Aviv University
Israel

Hesham Al-Inany MD
Faculty of Medicine
Cairo University and The Egyptian IVF-ET Center
Cairo
Egypt

Mete Isikoglu MD
Consultant Gynecologist and Obstetrician, IVF
Practitioner
Antalya IVF
Antalya
Turkey

Ariel Jaffa MD
Department of Obstetrics and Gynecologic
Lis Maternity Hospital, Tel-Aviv Sourasky Medical
Center
Sackler Faculty of Medicine
Tel Aviv University, Tel Aviv
Israel

Hashim Jamal MD
Obstetrician and Gynecologist
Antalya IVF
Antalya
Turkey

Seyed Mehdi Kalantar PhD
Associate Professor
Yazd Clinical and Research Center for Infertility
Shahid Sadoughi University of Medical Sciences
Bouali Ave, Safayeh, Yazd
Iran

Evanthia Diamanti-Kandarakis MD, PhD
Associate Professor
Athens University School of Medicine
Laiko General Hospital
Athens
Greece

Shahin Khazali MD
Specialist Registrar in Obstetrics and Gynecology
Department of Obstetrics and Gynecology
John Radcliff Hospital
Oxford
UK

AV Ganesh Kumar MD, DNB (Internal Med), DNB
(Cardiology), DM
(cardiology)
Consultant Interventional Cardiologist
Dr LH Hiranandani Hospital
Powai, Mumbai
India

Richard S. Legro MD
Professor
Department of Obstetrics and Gynecology
Pennsylvania State University
M.S. Hershey Medical Center
College of Medicine
Hershey, Pennsylvania
USA

David Levran MD
Director, IVF Unit
Department of Obstetrics and Gynecology
Wolfson Medical Center
Holon
Israel

Ronit Machtinger MD
IVF Unit, Division of Obstetrics and Gynecology
The Chaim Sheba Medical Center
Tel-Hashomer, and
Sackler School of Medicine
Tel Aviv University, Tel Aviv
Israel

Sharon Maslovitz MD
Department of Obstetrics and Gynecology
Lis Maternity Hospital
Tel Aviv Sourasky Medical Center
Tel-Aviv
Israel

Landaverde Molina María Mercedes MD
Reproduction and Genetics Clinic
Angeles del Pedregal Hospital
Mexico

Yashodhara Mhatre MD
Consultant
Center For Human Reproduction
Dr L H Hiranandani Hospital
Hiranandani Gardens
Powai
Mumbai

Mohamed FM Mitwally MD
Clinical Assistant Professor & Fellow
Division of Reproductive Endocrinology and
Infertility
Department of Obstetrics and Gynecology
Wayne State University
University Ob/Gyn, Inc.
Detroit, Michigan
USA

Patrizia Monteleone MD
Department of Reproductive Medicine and Child
Development
Division of Gynecology and Obstetrics
University of Pisa, Pisa
Italy

María Lidia Arenas-Montezco MD
Professor of Reproductive Endocrinology and
Infertility
Coordinator of Operative Room
Instituto para el Estudio de la Concepción Humana
(IECH)
Monterrey, NL
México. CP

Massimo Moscarini MD, PhD
Professor and Perinatology Director
Department Gynecological Sciences and
Sterility Fertility Unit
University La Sapienza
S Andrea Hospital, Rome
Italy

Pritesh Naik MD, DNB, MRCOG
Consultant Gynecologist and Endoscopic Surgeon
Suvarna General Hospital
Mumbai
Visiting Endoscopic Surgeon
Haria Hospital, Vapi– Gujarat
Rotunda Centres of Assisted Reproduction,
Mumbai, Gorakhpur and Jalandhar
India

Suresh Nair MMED, FRCOG (UK)
Consultant Obstetrician & Gynecologist
Gynecology Consultants Clinic & Surgery
Division of Minimal Access Endoscopic Surgery
Reproductive Endocrinology;
Infertility and Assisted Reproductive Techniques
Consultant, Mount Elizabeth Fertility Centre
Visiting Consultant
National University Hospital
Mt Elizabeth Medical Centre
Mt Elizabeth Hospital
Singapore

Luciano G Nardo MD
Department of Reproductive Medicine
St Mary's Hospital
Whitworth Park
Manchester
United Kingdom

Sergio Oehninger MD, PhD
Professor and Vice-Chair, Department of Obstetrics
and Gynecology and
Professor of Urology
Director, Division of Reproductive Endocrinology
and Infertility
The Jones Institute for Reproductive Medicine;
Eastern Virginia Medical School
Norfolk, Virginia
USA

Adegbite Ogunmokun FWACS
West African College of Surgeons
Edmunds Crescent
Yaba, Lagos, Nigeria
Africa

Kemal Ozgur MD
Clinic Director
Consultant Gynecologist and Obstetrician, IVF
Practitioner
Antalya IVF
Antalya
Turkey

Muralidhar V Pai MD
Professor and Head
Department of Obstetrics & Gynecology
Melaka Manipal Medical College
Malaysia

Adalberto Parra MD
Head
Department of Endocrinology
Instituto Nacional de Perinatología
Colonia Lomas Virreyes
México, DF
México

Hernán E Lara Peñaloza PhD
Professor
Dept. Biochemistry and Molecular Biology
Faculty of Chemistry and Pharemaceutical Sciences
Santiago, Chile
South America

Teresa Sir-Petermann MD
Professor
Faculty of Medicine Universidad de Chile
Santiago, Chile
South America

Luca Dal Prato MD
Gynecologist
Tecnobios Procreazione, Center for Reproductive
Health
Via Dante Bologna
Italy

Patrick Puttemans MD
Gynecologist and Specialist In Reproductive
Medicine
Leuven Institute for Fertility and Embryology
Tiensevest, Leuven
Belgium

Amir Ravhon MD
IVF Unit, Department of Obstetrics and
Gynecology
Wolfson Medical Center, Holon
Sackler Faculty of Medicine, Tel Aviv University
Tel Aviv
Israel

Victor Alfonso Batiza Resendiz MD, PhD
Professor of Obstetrics and Gynecology EMIS-
ITESM
Mexican Board Professor of Obstetrics and
Gynecology
Director of Research
Medical Coordinator
Professor of Reproductive Endocrinology and
Infertility, IECH
Instituto para el Estudio de la Concepción Humana
(IECH)
Monterrey NL
México. CP

Luis Ruvalcaba MD
Medical Director
Specialist in Obstetrics, Gynecology, Reproductive
Medicine
Instituto Mexicano De Infertilidad
Centro Medico Puerta De Hierro
Boulevard Puerta De Hierro
Zapopan, Jalisco
Mexico

Marzieh Salehi MD
Assistant Professor of Medicine
Division of Endocrinology
University of Cincinnati
The Jewish Hospital, Cholesterol Center
Alliance Hospitals
Cincinnati, Ohio
USA

Naveed Sattar MBChB, PhD, FRCPath, FRCP
(Glasgow)
Professor of Metabolic Medicine
BHF Glasgow Cardiovascular Research Centre
Departments of Obstetrics and Clinical
Biochemistry and
Honorary Consultant in Clinical Biochemistry
Department of Clinical Biochemistry
University of Glasgow
Glasgow Royal Infirmary
Glasgow, Scotland,
UK

Daniel S Seidman MD
Associate Professor
Director, R & D Unit
Department of Obstetrics and Gynecology
The Chaim Sheba Medical Center
Tel-Hashomer
Sackler Faculty of Medicine
Tel-Aviv University, Tel Aviv
Israel

Mohammad Hasan Sheikhha MD, PhD
Assistant Professor
Genetic and Biotechnology Lab.
Yazd Research and Clinical Center for IVF
Yazd Medical Science University
BoAli Avenue, Safayeh, Yazd
Iran

Pablo Diaz Spindola MD
Medical Director
Reproductive and Endocrinology Medicine
Instituto para el Estudio de la Concepción Humana
(IECH)
Monterrey, NL
México CP

Laurel A Stadtmauer MD, PhD
Assistant Professor of Obstetrics and Gynecology
Eastern Virginia Medical School
The Jones Institute for Reproductive Medicine
Norfolk, Virginia
USA

András Szilágyi MD, PhD
Professor of Obstetrics and Gynecology
Department of Obstetrics and Gynecology
Faculty of Medicine
University of Pecs
Hungary

Patricia Tambucho MD
The Jones Institute for Reproductive Medicine
Eastern Virginia Medical School
Norfolk, Virginia
USA

Maria Rosaria Parisen Toldin MD
Department of Reproductive Medicine and Child
Development
Division of Gynecology and Obstetrics
University of Pisa, Pisa
Italy

Pedro Galache Vega MD
Professor of Obstetrics and Gynecology EMIS-
ITESM
Co-Director
Professor of Reproductive Endocrinology and
Infertility, IECH
Instituto para el Estudio de la Concepción Humana
(IECH)
Monterrey, NL
México CP

Jim X Wang MPH, PhD
Research Fellow
Research Centre for Reproductive Health
Department of Obstetrics and Gynaecology
University of Adelaide, Woodville, SA
Australia

Sawaek Weerakiet MD
Associate Professor and
Division Director of Reproductive Endocrinology
Department of Obstetrics and Gynecology
Faculty of Medicine
Ramathibodi Hospital, Bangkok
Thailand

Ariel Weissman MD
IVF Unit, Department of Obstetrics and Gynecology
Wolfson Medical Center
Holon
Israel

Hakan Yarali MD
Professor
Obstetrician and Gynecologist, Specialist in
Infertility and
Reproductive Medicine
Department of Obstetrics and Gynecology
 Reproductive Biology and Infertility Unit
Hacettepe University, School of Medicine,
Sihhiye, Ankara,
Turkey

Hulusi B Zeyneloglu MD
Professor
Obstetrician and Gynecologist,
Specialist in Infertility and Reproductive Medicine
Department of Obstetrics and Gynecology
Division of Reproductive Medicine and Infertility
Baskent University School of Medicine,
Ankara,
Turkey

History and Origins of PCOS

1
Early Origins of Polycystic Ovary Syndrome

Sulbha Arora, Gautam N Allahbadia

Summary

There is increasing evidence to support a major genetic basis for Polycystic Ovary Syndrome, (PCOS) since it is strongly familial. Though a single gene is largely considered to be responsible for PCOS and the search is ongoing, most investigators believe that several clustering genes could perhaps be responsible and environmental factors, such as diet and exercise could undoubtedly influence the clinical and biochemical presentation of the syndrome. Results from recent animal experiments along with supporting clinical evidence, point to the development of PCOS as a linear process with an origin prior to adolescence. Recent studies have shown that PCOS can originate during puberty or much earlier, during the first and second trimesters of pregnancy. Animal models developed in adult female rhesus monkeys, as well as in ewes, have helped to study the effects of excess androgen exposure during prenatal life. When the female offsprings such born, grow to adulthood, they demonstrate many of the phenotypic as well as biochemical features typically seen in human adults suffering from PCOS. This points to excess in-utero androgen exposure as being a likely cause of the origin of the syndrome. It has been further postulated that the cause of this hyperandrogenism is fetal rather than maternal. Other researchers have pointed to fetal growth retardation as a causative factor. A defined developmental origin for PCOS holds great promise for specific clinical interventions, the possibility of eliminating the expression of the adult phenotype, and improvement of the constellation of metabolic derangements associated with it.

Introduction

Polycystic Ovary Syndrome (PCOS) is the most common, yet complex, endocrine disorder affecting women in their reproductive years. Its complexity stems from its typical heterogeneity (Table 1.1) and unknown etiology.[1]

There is increasing evidence to support a major genetic basis for PCOS, since the syndrome is strongly familial.[2,3] Support for a single gene for PCOS remains and the search is ongoing, but most investigators believe that there are several, perhaps clustering, genes responsible[4] and the clinical and biochemical presentation is undoubtedly influenced by additional environmental factors such as, diet and exercise.[5] Considering the complex interaction of various factors on the PCOS phenotype, a single developmental factor seems unlikely. Results from recent animal experiments along with supporting clinical evidence suggest that the development

Table 1.1   Important disorders of reproduction, metabolism and general health that are manifest in women with polycystic ovaries: their combination and degree of expression are highly variable between individuals, including first degree relatives

Reproductive disorders
    Polycystic ovaries
    Hyperandrogenism (hirsutism, acne, androgenic alopecia)
    Anovulation (amenorrhea, oligomenorrhea)
    Hypersecretion of LH
    Increased risk of early miscarriage

Metabolic disorders
    Hyperinsulinemia and insulin resistance
    Impaired pancreatic β-cell insulin secretion and type 2 diabetes
    Obesity (including preferential abdominal adiposity)
    Hyperlipidemia

Disorders of general health
    Increased cardiovascular disease risk factors
    Endometrial cancer

of PCOS could be a linear process that perhaps originates prior to adolescence (the current clinical perception of age of onset of the disorder). Superimposed on this are interacting genetic and environmental factors that may alter the phenotypic expression of PCOS during adult life, particularly the susceptibility to anovulation.[6,7]

PCOS can originate during puberty or much earlier during the first and second trimesters of pregnancy, according to the research conducted by David Abbott, Ph.D., of the Wisconsin National Primate Center at the University of Wisconsin-Madison. By developing a rhesus monkey model for PCOS, Abbott and his colleagues have shown that the disease may arise in humans due to excess androgen levels during critical developmental periods.[1]

Dr Michael Davies, senior research fellow at the Research Centre in Reproductive Health at the University of Adelaide, Australia, told the 21st annual conference of the European Society of Human Reproduction and Embryology[8]: "Our research suggests that, during pregnancy and birth, there are several different factors working through different pathways that are implicated in the overlapping and varying symptoms of PCOS that emerge in the offspring's later life. Existing research has already established links between fetal growth restriction, postnatal growth and metabolic disorders such as diabetes in adulthood. The idea that events in very early life can have an enduring, complex and important influence on subsequent disease is referred to as developmental programming, and this research theme has been applied to PCOS recently. Different studies have produced conflicting evidence that shows that large babies grow to become heavier adults with polycystic ovaries, but that the most severe symptoms of PCOS are associated with growth restriction as a fetus."

Clinical Discussion

Effects of in utero androgen excess

Many clinical and biochemical features of PCOS are found in adult female rhesus monkeys, exposed in utero to levels of testosterone equivalent to those found in male fetuses. They particularly exhibit hypersecretion of luteinizing hormone (LH), abnormal insulin secretion or action and, in obese hyperinsulinemic individuals, hyperandrogenic anovulation.[9,10] Padmanabhan[11] and Robinson[12] verified these findings in separate studies on pregnant ewes by exposing them to large doses of testosterone and demonstrating increased LH secretion and abnormal ovarian cycles in the female offspring. Enlarged ovaries with multiple medium-sized antral follicles developed in the prenatally androgenized females of these species.

However, any maternal source of excess androgen production is unlikely to affect the human female fetus. McClamrock and Adashi[13] have shown that even pregnant women with extremely high circulating levels of testosterone (due, for example, to an ovarian thecoma) are unlikely to have a virilized female child.[13] The high circulating levels of sex hormone-binding globulin (SHBG) and efficient placental metabolism, provide an effective barrier against maternal androgens reaching the fetal circulation. Thus, it is difficult to imagine that hyperandrogenism is passed across the placenta from a mother with PCOS to a previously unaffected daughter, unless placental function is compromised by circumstances such as placental aromatase deficiency, stress or inadequate diet.

More likely sources of excess prenatal androgen production are the hyperandrogenic fetal ovary,[14,15] the hyperandrogenic adrenal cortex,[16] or both. Adrenal androgens may be used as a substrate for ovarian androgen production, as noted by Barnes et al.[16] who showed that patients with 21-hydroxylase deficiency and adrenal hyperandrogenism, also showed evidence of polycystic ovaries and excess ovarian androgen production. Fetal and adult ovaries are both capable of converting steroid precursors, including adrenal dehydroepiandrosterone sulphate, to potent androgens and then to estrogen.[17,18]

Androgens produced during differentiation are potent gene transcription factors and induce other critical transcription factors (such as *c-fos*) that interact with their own receptors in many fetal tissues, permanently enhancing gene expression (including increased serine phosphorylation of the cAMP response element).[19] Fetal androgen excess in human females therefore, seems to simultaneously reprogram multiple organ systems that will later manifest the heterogenous phenotype of PCOS. Herman et al.[20] have illustrated the subtle but permanent effects that androgen reprogramming can exert on female physiology, and have not found virilization of female genitalia to occur in women with PCOS.

Genetic basis for ovarian hyperandrogenism

Biochemical evidence of hyperandrogenism is the most consistent feature of both, women with PCOS, as well as prenatally androgenized female rhesus monkeys.[21,22] Although it has been shown by Azziz et al.[23] that the adrenal gland may contribute to the high circulating levels of testosterone, other studies have concluded that the major source of excess androgens is the ovary.[24–26]

Gilling-Smith have shown that cultured human theca cells from polycystic ovaries produce 20 times more androstenedione than similar cells from normal ovaries.[27] Recent studies by Wickenheisser et al.[28] have confirmed this, and also shown an increased mRNA expression of many of the steroidogenic enzymes.[28]

These findings in cultured human theca cells prompted the consideration of genes encoding steroidogenic enzymes as candidate loci in the etiology of PCOS. A pentanucleotide repeat polymorphism was identified in the *CYP11a* promoter region. Gharani et al.[29] have found evidence linking variants at the *CYP11a* locus with hyperandrogenism in women with PCOS.[29] Though this is unlikely to be the sole cause of PCOS, it may contribute to the excess androgen production, and support the view that there is a genetically determined abnormality of ovarian function. Abnormal ovarian follicular development may lead to abnormal theca cell function. Recent studies by Urbanek et al.[30,31] implying the role of the follistatin gene in the etiology of the syndrome, remain unconfirmed.[30,31] However, such studies reinforce the possibility that abnormal ovarian folliculogenesis may indeed be the key ovarian abnormality.

Witchel et al.[32] have shown in their study that the *G972R* variant of the *IRS1* gene might represent a modifier locus among women who are heterozygous carriers of *CYP21* mutations, potentially increasing their risk of developing adrenal androgen excess in PCOS.[32] They have found approximately 33% of their patients with premature pubarche or adolescent hyperandrogenism to be heterozygous carriers of *CYP21* mutations, compared to 6% of the control population. However, this *IRS1* variant and *CYP21* mutations seem to play a limited role in the development of PCOS in the population studied.

Familial clustering of PCOS occurs in a pattern suggestive of autosomal dominant inheritance. However, to date, none of the candidate gene loci, investigated by mutation analysis, linkage, and case-control association studies, have been consistently demonstrated to be associated with

PCOS. These loci include *CYP17*, *CYP11A*, *CYP19*, insulin receptor, insulin, follistatin, caplain-10, and gonadotropin releasing hormone (GnRH) receptor.[4,29,33–37]

Affected or unaffected status may be difficult to determine on the basis of clinical manifestations because asymptomatic sisters of affected women can have biochemical evidence of hyperandrogenemia,[22] making traditional linkage analysis difficult to perform. The search for the PCOS gene has also been hampered by the extreme phenotypic heterogeneity, even within a single family, and the lack of a male phenotype. Several loci presumably contribute to the phenotype, and one such locus is the *CYP21* gene. Because the majority of the obligate carriers of the *CYP21* mutations are asymptomatic despite mildly elevated androgen concentrations, other factors must promote development of hyperandrogenic symptoms.

Prenatal androgen exposure as a cause of abnormal LH secretion

Anovulatory PCOS women have high serum levels of LH, represented by increased LH pulse amplitude as well as frequency. This feature is also seen in prenatally androgenized rhesus monkeys and ewes, suggesting that in utero exposure to androgens may permanently diminish hormonal negative feedback on the hypothalamic-pituitary axis, thereby stimulating androgen hypersecretion. Elevated serum LH levels in women with hyperandrogenemia due to 21-hydroxylase deficiency, a classical cause of adrenal hyperandrogenism, provide indirect evidence for such in utero programming in humans.[24] Recent data suggest that impaired negative feedback on LH secretion is mediated by either estradiol or progesterone in women with PCOS, prenatally androgenized female rhesus monkeys and prenatally androgenized ewes.[12,38,39] However, the mechanism for this LH hypersecretion is not entirely clear.

Origin of insulin resistance

Anovulatory women with PCOS are relatively hyperinsulinemic and more insulin resistant than weight-matched control subjects.[40] Intrinsic abnormalities in post-receptor insulin signaling and abnormal insulin secretion have been implicated.[26,40,41] Eisner et al.[10] have shown that early in utero exposure to androgen excess in female rhesus monkeys leads to an impairment in insulin secretion, whereas a similar exposure late in gestation, causes an impairment in insulin action.[10] The key question is whether these impairments represent a primary defect in the insulin-signaling pathway (or in the β cell), or whether they reflect the abnormal androgen environment. The former argument is supported by three recent reports, which have implicated polymorphisms in the insulin receptor gene and genes involved in insulin secretion in women with PCOS.[30,37,42] However, other studies have shown that weight loss in obese women with PCOS significantly improved insulin sensitivity.[41] This finding supports the fact that body fat distribution is a major determinant of insulin insensitivity in PCOS. Abbott et al.[1] have hypothesized that the hyperandrogenemic endocrine environment during prenatal life and puberty has a profound effect on body fat distribution, predisposing to insulin resistance.[1] Their hypothesis is supported by data from prenatally androgenized rhesus monkeys that selectively deposit fat intra-abdominally and exhibit insulin resistance.[1]

Effect of fetal growth rate in utero

In a study by Davies et al, maternal weight in late pregnancy, birth weight and placental weight were examined in relation to the symptoms of PCOS. Compared with their counterparts, young women without a diagnosis of PCOS but with irregular periods were heavier at birth, with larger placentas, and they tended to have mothers who were heavier in late pregnancy. In contrast, women with an existing diagnosis of PCOS tended to have smaller placentas and birth weights that were, on an average, 196 g lighter than women without PCOS.

Their data suggest that different developmental

pathways are implicated in the overlapping symptoms of PCOS. One pathway may be mediated by high maternal weight in late pregnancy, which is linked to irregular periods in the daughter, and possibly obesity and weight-related reproduction problems. A second pathway may involve reduced placental and fetal growth, which is linked to the more severe symptoms of PCOS in the daughter, usually resulting in an early clinical diagnosis of the syndrome. A fetus that has been affected by restricted growth is more likely to have problems with insulin metabolism in later life due to an underlying metabolic derangement.

In another study by Ibanez et al.[43] birth weight SD scores were found to be lower in premature pubarchal girls than in controls, and particularly so, in those girls who showed hyperinsulinemia and subsequently developed ovarian hyperandrogenism.

PCOS and puberty

Despite the original description of PCOS by Stein and Leventhal[44] in 1935, it was not until 1976 that Huffman[45] reported a series of adolescent girls with polycystic ovaries and hyper-androgenism. After that, it was postulated that PCOS is a disorder that begins at menarche and whose characteristics are not changed by age.[46] Adolescents with PCOS have clinical, hormonal, and ultrasonographic features comparable to those of adult women with PCOS.[47–49] However, a clear distinction must be made between PCOS and polycystic ovaries (PCO) in adolescents, because the latter is a normal developmental finding. Multicystic ovaries containing more than six cysts with a diameter greater than 4 mm dispersed throughout the ovary occur in normal girls during pubertal development.[50] This is believed to be the ovarian response to the normal nocturnal pulsatile secretion of gonadotropin during puberty. This ovarian state is transitory and reversible because it is not present in adults and becomes less and less frequent as adolescents begin to ovulate regularly.[51] Thus, the confusing description of cystic ovaries in childhood as

polycystic should be abandoned and replaced with the term multicystic ovaries.

Anovulation or irregular menses, which is one of the two diagnostic criteria of PCOS, is a very common finding in normal adolescents during the first few postmenarche years. The establishment of regular ovulatory cycles is a slow process. Apter and colleagues[52] demonstrated that 85% of the menstrual cycles are anovulatory during the first menarcheal year, 59% during the third year, and 25% during the sixth year. These investigators and others found that serum testosterone, androstenedione, and LH levels were higher in adolescents with anovulatory cycles than in those with ovulatory cycles.[51–53] Thus, the distinction between pubertal physiologic anovulation and pathologic anovulation may create a diagnostic dilemma. On the other hand, some investigators would argue that oligomenorrhea in adolescents is not a stage in the physiologic maturation of the hypothalamic pituitary-ovarian axis but an early sign of PCOS associated with subfertility.[54] Therefore, hyperandrogenism may be the most robust diagnostic criteria in this age group. In fact, in a 13-year longitudinal study, serum testosterone and androstenedione concentrations during adolescence were preserved into adulthood and were reflected in fertility patterns during the third decade of life, higher serum androgen concentrations being associated with decreased fertility.[55] Furthermore, adolescent girls with hyperandrogenism have neuroendocrine features comparable to adult women with PCOS. Compared with normal pubertal girls, adolescents with hyperandrogenism have an increased number of LH pulses, higher mean 24-hour LH concentrations, increased LH:FSH ratio, and higher concentrations of 17-hydroxyprogesterone.[47,48,52,56,57]

Both, normal puberty and PCOS are common in hyperpulsatile gonadotropin secretion, hyperactive ovarian and adrenal androgen production, insulin resistance or hyperinsulinemia, with the consequent low insulin-like growth factor binding protein-1 (IGF-BP1) and low sex hormone-binding globulin (SHBG).[58–60] Because of the shared features of the two conditions, it has been hypothesized that puberty triggers PCOS in predisposed girls.[58]

In summary, there is a consensus that PCOS, not infrequently, begins during adolescence. The similarities between PCOS and normal puberty would suggest that PCOS is an exaggerated or hyperstimulated form of puberty. However, it remains unknown whether puberty triggers PCOS in predisposed individuals or unravels it. It is tempting to speculate that increasing insulin and insulin-like growth factor-1 (IGF-1) concentrations during puberty may play a role. This however, would not explain why the condition persists into adulthood in only a few women, and what the genetic/environmental modulators could be. Also, the relationship of physiologic adolescent anovulation with PCOS remains in debate and must be better investigated.

Adolescent PCOS and premature pubarche

It is proposed that premature pubarche might be an early marker of future PCOS.[47,61] Premature pubarche refers to the appearance of pubic hair or axillary hair before 8 years of age in girls without other signs of puberty.[62,63] The precise cause of premature pubarche is not known. Generally, it has been attributed to the early maturation of the zona reticularis, which leads to an increase in adrenal androgens to levels usually seen in early puberty. This early activation could be mediated through marked weight gain and resultant hyperinsulinemia.[64] It is also proposed that an increase in androgen biosynthesis might be caused by the preferential hyperphosphorylation of the enzyme P450c17 because of an activating mutation of the kinase responsible for the serine/threonine phosphorylation of the enzyme.[64,65] With the exclusion of virilizing congenital adrenal hyperplasia and androgen secreting tumors from diagnostic consideration, premature adrenarche reflecting premature adrenal maturation is the most common cause of premature pubarche.

Ibanez et al.[66,67] have shown that girls initially evaluated for premature pubarche showed signs and symptoms of functional ovarian hyperandrogenism on re-evaluation during mid-adolescent years. They found that 45% of the girls had oligomenorrhea and higher basal concentrations of 17-hydroxyprogesterone, androstenedione and testosterone on follow-up. Because of such findings, it has been proposed that premature pubarche may herald the future development of PCOS. However, this is not seen in all girls with premature adrenarche. Well-controlled prospective longitudinal studies are required to determine the proportion of girls who will develop PCOS and the risk factors.

Girls with premature pubarche are reported to have hyperinsulinemia, low sex hormone binding globulin, and low IGFBP-1 levels.[68–71] The question has been raised whether hyperinsulinemia in girls with premature pubarche is a marker for the future development of PCOS. Obesity and hyperinsulinemia in girls with premature adrenarche could be risk factors for development of hyperandrogenism. Total body adiposity and abdominal adiposity are major determinants of insulin sensitivity in girls. Richard et al.[72] studied the natural history of insulin resistance, obesity, acanthosis nigricans, and hyperandrogenism in 4-to-8-year-old girls. They found that the syndrome invariably began with the onset of obesity. In this very hyperinsulinemic group, all the subjects then developed acanthosis nigricans, which is a marker of hyperinsulinemia. Hyperinsulinemia occurred before hyperandrogenemia, which developed only after the age of menarche. Therefore, in this group, the pubertal increase in LH was required for the development of hyperandrogenism. Remer et al.[64] found that a change in body mass index (BMI) is an important physiologic regulator of adrenarche. A unifying hypothesis that could potentially link premature adrenarche and PCOS is that, hyperinsulinemia (whether through weight gain, or because of inherent defects in insulin action) stimulates both adrenal and ovarian cytochrome P450c17 activity. This would explain the progression to PCOS in girls with premature adrenarche at the time of pubertal gonadotropin activation.

Conclusion

Although PCOS is a complex, heterogenous disorder, most of the clinical and biochemical features can be explained on the basis of a developmental disorder of ovarian androgen production. This fetal and adolescent androgen excess programs the hypothalamic-pituitary control of LH, enhances visceral fat distribution, thus predisposing to insulin resistance and anovulation, and causes the clinical features of hyperandrogenism in adulthood. Interacting with this underlying process are other secondary genetic, environmental and dietary factors, which modify the final phenotype and produce the heterogenous nature of the syndrome. Thus, a defined developmental origin for PCOS holds great promise for specific clinical interventions, the possibility of eliminating the expression of the adult phenotype, and improvement in the constellation of metabolic derangements associated with it.

References

1. Abbott DH, Dumesic DA, Franks S. Developmental origin of polycystic ovary syndrome – a hypothesis. *J Endocrinol* 2002; 174: 1–5.

2. Franks S, Gharani N, Waterworth D, Batty S, White D, Williamson R, McCarthy M. The genetic basis of polycystic ovary syndrome. *Hum Reprod* 1997; 12: 2641–2648.

3. Legro RS, Spielman R, Urbanek M, Driscoll D, Strauss JF, Dunaif A. Phenotype and genotype in polycystic ovary syndrome. *Recent Progress in Hormone Research* 1998a; 53: 217–256.

4. Urbanek M, Legro RS, Driscoll DA, et al. Thirty-seven candidate genes for polycystic ovary syndrome: strongest evidence for linkage is with follistatin. *PNAS* 1999; 96: 8573–8578.

5. Huber-Buchholz MM, Carey DG, Norman RJ. Restoration of reproductive potential by lifestyle modification in obese polycystic ovary syndrome: role of insulin sensitivity and luteinizing hormone. *J Clin Endocrinol Metab* 1999; 84: 1470–1474.

6. White DW, Leigh A, Wilson C, Donaldson A, Franks S. Gonadotrophin and gonadal steroid response to a single dose of a long-acting agonist of gonadotrophin-releasing hormone in ovulatory and anovulatory women with polycystic ovary syndrome. *Clin Endocrinol* 1995; 42: 475–481.

7. Chang PL, Lindheim SR, Lowre C, et al. Normal ovulatory women with polycystic ovaries have hyperandrogenic pituitary-ovarian responses to gonadotropin-releasing hormone-agonist testing. *J Clin Endocrinol Metab* 2000; 85: 995–1000.

8. European Society for Human Reproduction and Embryology annual meeting in Copenhagen presented June 22, 2005.

9. Abbott DH, Dumesic DA, Eisner JR, Colman RJ, Kemnitz JW. Insights into the development of PCOS from studies of prenatally androgenized female rhesus monkeys. *Trends Endocrinol Metab* 1998; 9: 62–67.

10. Eisner JR, Dumesic DA, Kemnitz JW, Abbott DH. Timing of prenatal androgen excess determines differential impairment in insulin secretion and action in adult female rhesus monkeys. *J Clin Endocrinol Metab* 2000; 85: 1206–1210.

11. Padmanabhan V, Evans N, Taylor JA, Robinson JE. Prenatal exposure to androgens leads to the development of cystic ovaries in the sheep. *Bio Reprod* 1998; 56 (suppl): 194.

12. Robinson JE, Forsdike RA, Taylor JA. *In utero* exposure of female lambs to testosterone reduces the sensitivity of the gonadotropin-releasing hormone neuronal network to inhibition by progesterone. *Endocrinol* 1999; 140: 5797–5805.

13. McClamrock HD, Adashi EY. Gestational hyperandrogenism. *Fertil Steril* 1992; 57: 257–274.

14. Barbieri RL, Saltzman DH, Torday JS, Randall RW, Frigoletto FD, Ryan KJ. Elevated concentrations of the beta-subunit of human chorionic gonadotropin and testosterone in the amniotic fluid of gestations of diabetic mothers. *Am J Obstet Gynecol* 1986; 154: 1039–1043.

15. Beck-Peccoz P, Padmanabhan V, Baggiani AM, et al. Maturation of hypothalamic-pituitary-gonadal function in normal human fetuses: circulating levels of gonadotropins, their common alpha-subunit and free testosterone, and discrepancy between immunological and biological activities of circulating follicle-stimulating hormone. *J Clin Endocrinol Metab* 1991; 73: 525–532.

16. Barnes RB, Rosenfield RL, Ehrmann DA, Cara JF, Cutler L, Levitsky LL, Rosenthal IM. Ovarian hyperandrogenism as a result of congenital adrenal virilizing disorders: evidence for perinatal

masculinization of neuroendocrine function in women. *J Clin Endocrinol Metab* 1994; 79: 1328–1333.

17. Payne AH, Jaffe RB. Androgen formation from pregnenolone sulfate by the human fetal ovary. *J Clin Endocrinol Metab* 1974; 39: 300–304.

18. Bonser J, Walker J, Purohit A, Reed MJ, Potter BV, Willis DS, Franks S, Mason HD. Human granulosa cells are the site of sulphatase activity and are able to utilize dehydroepiandrosterone sulphate as a precursor for oestradiol production. *J Endocrinol* 2000; 167: 465–471.

19. Auger AP, Hexter DP, McCarthy MM. Sex difference in the phosphorylation of camp response element binding protein (CREB) in neonatal rat brain. *Brain Research* 2001; 890: 110–117.

20. Herman RA, Jones B, Mann DR, Wallen K. Timing of prenatal androgen exposure: anatomical and endocrine effects on juvenile male and female rhesus monkeys. *Hormones and Behaviour* 2000; 38: 52–66.

21. Franks S. The ubiquitous polycystic ovary. *J Endocrinol* 1991; 129: 317–319.

22. Legro RS, Driscoll D, Strauss JF III, Fox J, Dunaif A. Evidence for a genetic basis for hyperandrogenemia in polycystic ovary syndrome. *PNAS* 1998b; 95: 14956–14960.

23. Azziz R, Rittmaster RS, Fox LM, Bradley EL Jr, Potter HD, Boots LR. Role of the ovary in the adrenal androgen excess of hyperandrogenic women. *Fertil Steril* 1998; 69: 851–859.

24. Ehrmann DA, Barnes RB, Rosenfield RL. Polycystic ovary syndrome as a form of functional ovarian hyperandrogenism due to dysregulation of androgen secretion. *Endocrine Reviews* 1995; 16: 322–353.

25. Gilling-Smith C, Story H, Rogers V, Franks S. Evidence for a primary abnormality of thecal cell steroidogenesis in the polycystic ovary syndrome. *Clin Endocrinol* 1997; 47: 93–99.

26. Eisner JR, Barnett MA, Dumesic DA, Abbott DH. Ovarian hyperandrogenism in adult female rhesus monkeys exposed to prenatal androgen excess. *Fertil Steril* 2002; 77: 167–172.

27. Gilling-Smith C, Willis DS, Beard RW, Franks S. Hypersecretion of androstenedione by isolated theca cells from polycystic ovaries. *J Clin Endocrinol Metab* 1994; 79: 1158–1165.

28. Wickenheisser JK, Quinn PG, Nelson VL, Legro RS, Strauss JF, McAllister JM. Differential activity of the cytochrome P450c17 alpha-hydroxylase and steroidogenic acute regulatory protein gene promoters in normal and polycystic ovary syndrome

theca cells. *J Clin Endocrinol Metab* 2000; 85: 2304–2311.

29. Gharani N, Gharani N, Waterworth DM, et al. Association of the steroid synthesis gene *CYP11a* with polycystic ovary syndrome and hyperandrogenism. *Hum Molec Genet* 1997; 6: 397–402.

30. Urbanek M, Legro RS, Driscoll D, Strauss JF, Dunaif A, Spielman RS. Searching for the polycystic ovary syndrome genes. *J Ped Endocrinol* 2000a; 13 (supp 5): 1311–1313.

31. Urbanek M, Wu X, Vicekery KR, et al. Allelic variants of the follistatin gene in polycystic ovary syndrome. *J Clin Endocrinol Metab* 2000b; 85: 4455–4461.

32. Witchel SF, Kahsar-Miller M, Aston CE, White C, Azziz R. Prevalence of *CYP21* mutations and *IRS1* variant among women with polycystic ovary syndrome and adrenal androgen excess. *Fertil Steril* 2005; 83: 371–375.

33. Calvo RM, Villuendas G, Sancho J et al. Role of the follistatin gene in women with polycystic ovary syndrome. *Fertil Steril* 2001; 75: 1020–1023.

34. Talbot JA, Bicknell EJ, Rajkhowa M et al. Molecular scanning of the insulin receptor gene in women with polycystic ovarian syndrome. *J Clin Endocrinol Metab* 1996; 81: 1979–1983.

35. Cohen DP, Stein EM, Li Z et al. Molecular analysis of the gonadotropin-releasing hormone receptor in patients with polycystic ovary syndrome. *Fertil Steril* 1999; 72: 360–363.

36. Gharani N, Waterworth DM, Williamson R, et al. 5' polymorphism of the CYP17 gene is not associated with serum testosterone levels in women with polycystic ovaries. *J Clin Endocrinol Metab* 1996; 81: 4174.

37. Waterworth DM, Bennett ST, Gharani N, et al. Linkage and association of insulin gene VNTR regulatory polymorphism with polycystic ovary syndrome. *Lancet* 1997; 349: 986–990.

38. Eagleson CA, Gingrich MB, Pastor CL, Arora TK, Burt CM, Evans WS, Marshall JC. Polycystic ovary syndrome: evidence that flutamide restores sensitivity of the gonadotropin-releasing hormone pulse generator to inhibition by estradiol and progesterone. *J Clin Endocrinol Metab* 2000; 85: 4047–4052.

39. Steiner RA, Clifton DK, Spies HG, Resko JA. Sexual differentiation and feedback control of luteinizing hormone secretion in the rhesus monkey. *Biology of Reproduction* 1976; 15: 206–212.

40. Dunaif A. Insulin resistance and the polycystic

ovarian syndrome: mechanism and implications for pathogenesis. *Endocrine Reviews* 1997; 18: 774–800.

41. Holte J, Bergh T, Berne C, Wide L, Lithell H. Restored insulin sensitivity but persistently increased early insulin secretion after weight loss in obese women with polycystic ovary syndrome. *J Clin Endocrinol Metab* 1995; 80: 2586–2593.

42. Tucci S, Futterweit W, Concepcion ES, Greenberg DA, Villanueva R, Davies TF, Tomer Y. Evidence for association of polycystic ovary syndrome in Caucasian women with a marker at the insulin receptor gene locus. *J Clin Endocrinol Metab* 2001; 86: 446–449.

43. Ibanez L, de Zegher F, Potau N. Premature pubarche, ovarian hyperandrogenism, hyperinsulinism and the polycystic ovary syndrome: from a complex constellation to a simple sequence of prenatal onset. *J Endocrinol Invest* 1998; 21(9): 558–66.

44. Stein IF, Leventhal ML. Amenorrhea associated with bilateral polycystic ovaries. *Am J Obstet Gynecol* 1935; 29: 81–191.

45. Huffman JW. Polycystic ovaries in young girls. Proceedings of the III International Symposium on Pediatric and Adolescent Gynecology, Lausanne, Switzerland, 1976; 193–206.

46. Yen SSC. The polycystic ovary syndrome. *Clin Endocrinol* 1980; 12: 177–181.

47. Rosenfield RL, Ghai K, Ehrmann DA, et al. Diagnosis of the polycystic ovary syndrome in adolescence: comparison of adolescent and adult hyperandrogenism. *J Pediatr Endocrinol Metab* 2000; 13: 1285–1289.

48. Veldhius JD, Pincus SM, Garcia-Rudaz MC, et al. Disruption of the joint synchrony of luteinizing hormone, testosterone, and androstenedione secretion in adolescents with polycystic ovarian syndrome. *J Clin Endocrinol Metab* 2001; 86: 72–79.

49. Gulekli B, Turhan NO, Senoz S, et al. Endocrinological, ultrasonographic and clinical findings in adolescent and adult polycystic ovary patients: A comparative study. *Gynecol Endocrinol* 1993; 7: 273–277.

50. Stanhope R, Adams J, Jacobs HS, et al. Ovarian ultrasound assessment in normal children, idiopathic precocious puberty and during low dose pulsatile GnRH therapy of hypogonadotrophic hypogonadism. *Arch Dis Child* 1985; 60: 116–119.

51. Venturoli S, Porcu E, Fabbri R, et al. Menstrual irregularities in adolescents. Hormonal pattern and ovarian morphology. *Hormone Res* 1986; 24: 269–279.

52. Apter D. Endocrine and metabolic abnormalities in adolescents with PCOS-like condition: Consequences for adult reproduction. *Trends in Endocrinol Metab* 1998; 9: 58–61.

53. Venturoli S, Porcu E, Fabbri R et al. Postmenarcheal evolution of endocrine pattern and ovarian aspects in adolescents with menstrual irregularities. *Fertil Steril* 1987; 48: 78–85.

54. van Hooff MH, Voorhorst FJ, Kaptein MB, et al. Endocrine features of polycystic ovary syndrome in a random population sample of 14–16 year old adolescents. *Hum Reprod* 1999; 14: 2223–2229.

55. Apter D, Vihko R. Endocrine determinants of fertility: Serum androgen concentrations during follow-up of adolescents into the third decade of life. *J Clin Endocrinol Metab* 1990; 71: 970–974.

56. Taylor AE. The gonadotropic axis in hyperandrogenic adolescents. *J Pediatr Endocrinol Metab* 2000; 13: 1281–1284.

57. Apter D, Butzow T, Laughlin GA, et al. Accelerated 24-hour luteinizing hormone pulsatile activity in adolescent girls with ovarian hyperandrogenism: Relevance to the developmental phase of polycystic ovarian syndrome. *J Clin Endocrinol Metab* 1994; 79: 119–125.

58. Nobels F, Dewailly D. Puberty and polycystic ovarian syndrome: the insulin/insulin-like growth factor I hypothesis. *Fertil Steril* 1992; 58: 655–666.

59. Apter D, Butzow T, Laughlin GA, et al. Metabolic features of polycystic ovary syndrome are found in adolescent girls with hyperandrogenism. *J Clin Endocrinol Metab* 1995; 80: 2966–2973.

60. Ibanez L, Potau N, Georgopoulos N, et al. Growth hormone, insulin-like growth factor-I axis, and insulin secretion in hyperandrogenic adolescents. *Fertil Steril* 1995; 64: 1113–1119.

61. Ibanez L, Dimartino-Nardi J, Potau N, et al. Premature adrenarche-normal variant or forerunner of adult disease? *Endocrine Rev* 2000; 21: 671–696.

62. Saenger P, Reiter EO. Premature adrenarche: a normal variant of puberty? *J Clin Endocrinol Metab* 1992; 74: 236–238.

63. Ghizzoni L, Mastorakos G, Vottero A. Adrenal hyperandrogenism in children. *J Clin Endocrinol Metab* 1999; 84: 4431–4435.

64. Remer T, Manz F. Role of nutritional status in the regulation of adrenarche. *J Clin Endocrinol Metab* 1999; 84: 3936–3944.

65. Zhang LH, Rodriguez H, Ohno S, et al. Serine phosphorylation of human P450c17 increases 17,20-lyase activity: implications for adrenarche and the polycystic ovary syndrome. *Proc Natl Acad Sci USA* 1995; 92: 10619–10623.

66. Ibanez L, Potau N, Virdis R, et al. Postpubertal outcome in girls diagnosed of premature pubarche during childhood increased frequency of functional ovarian hyperandrogenism. *J Clin Endocrinol Metab* 1993; 76: 1599–1603.

67. Ibanez L, Potau N, Zampolli M, et al. Girls diagnosed with premature pubarche show an exaggerated ovarian androgen synthesis from the early stages of puberty: evidence from gonadotropin-releasing hormone agonist testing. *Fertil Steril* 1997; 67: 849–855.

68. DiMartino-Nardi J. Insulin resistance in prepubertal African-American and Hispanic girls with premature adrenarche: A risk factor for polycystic ovary syndrome. *Trends in Endocrinol Metab* 1998; 9: 78–82.

69. Oppenheimer E, Linder B, DiMartino-Nardi J. Decreased insulin sensitivity prepubertal girls with premature adrenarche and acanthosis nigricans. *J Clin Endocrinol Metab* 1995; 80: 614–618.

70. Vuguin P, Linder B, Rosenfeld RG, et al. The roles of insulin sensitivity, insulin-like growth factor I (IGF-I), and IGF-binding protein-1 and –3 in the hyperandrogenism of African-American and Caribbean Hispanic girls with premature adrenarche. *J Clin Endocrinol Metab* 1999; 84: 2037–2042.

71. Ibanez L, Potau N, Zampolli M, et al. Hyperinsulinemia and decreased insulin-like growth factor-binding protein-1 are common features in prepubertal and pubertal girls with a history of premature pubarche. *J Clin Endocrinol Metab* 1997; 82: 2283–2288.

72. Richards GE, Cavallo A, Meyer WJ, et al. Obesity, acanthosis nigricans, insulin resistance and hyperandrogenemia: Pediatric perspective and natural history. *J Pediatr* 1985; 107: 893–897.

Prevalence and Diagnosis

2

Definitions, Prevalence and Symptoms of Polycystic Ovaries and the Polycystic Ovary Syndrome

Roger Hart

Summary

Polycystic Ovary Syndrome (PCOS) is the commonest endocrine disorder of women in their reproductive years. Polycystic ovaries *per se* are present in 22% of randomly selected women. The prevalence of PCOS in selected populations is between 5 and 14% depending upon the population being studied. The implications for women with this condition are substantial as they are at an increased risk of obesity, have a markedly increased risk of diabetes and death after a myocardial event. A recent consensus has led to the formulation of unifying diagnostic criteria for the definition of PCOS. These criteria rely on the presence of two of the following symptoms; oligo/anovulation, clinical or biochemical evidence of hyperandrogenism and the presence of polycystic ovaries.

It is clear that some women have a genetic or environmental predisposition to PCOS, but do not demonstrate all the features of PCOS, however, upon gaining weight, particularly with a truncal distribution, the phenotype of PCOS may be manifest. Consequently, women may oscillate between expressing and then subsequently losing the features of PCOS throughout their lives.

Introduction

The Polycystic ovary syndrome was first described by Stein and Leventhal at the time of laparotomy in 1935 and was characterized by symptoms of excessive androgenisation, such as hirsutism and acne, and obesity in addition to infertility in the presence of bilateral polycystic ovaries (PCO). These ovaries were described as being enlarged, having a markedly thickened tunica albuginea with hyperplasia of the theca interna cells.[1]

Though Polycystic ovary syndrome is the commonest endocrine disturbance affecting women of reproductive age,[2] great debate still exists about its definition and pathogenesis. It is a condition that may not require medical treatment as the symptoms may be ameliorated by simply employing lifestyle measures such as weight loss,[3] however, current medical treatments consist of the use of insulin sensitizing agents,[4] aromatase inhibitors[5] and antiandrogens in conjunction with the oral contraceptive pill, with the occasional addition of an insulin sensitizing agent[6] or occasionally, the use of laparoscopic surgery.[7]

Prior to the development of ultrasonography, the diagnosis of Polycystic ovary syndrome was made by laparotomy and the clincal appearance of the Stein-Leventhal syndrome. Of 12,160 laparotomies conducted in women of reproductive age, Vara and Niemineva[8] reported that polycystic ovaries were present in 1.4% of cases. Fortunately, the advent of high resolution ultrasonography provided for a non-invasive technique to assess the size of the ovary and its morphology.

The term 'polycystic ovaries' is a description purely of ovarian morphology, which may be derived from observation at the time of ultrasound examination, intraoperative examination at laparoscopy, laparotomy or Caesarean section, or derived from a pathological examination after oophorectomy or post-mortem. In contrast, the term 'Polycystic ovary syndrome' describes a collection of clinical and/or biochemical findings, which may or may not include the appearance of polycystic ovaries, as will be described.

At a consensus meeting in Rotterdam in 2003, leading experts in the field of reproductive medicine agreed upon an international definition for the Polycystic ovary syndrome (PCOS).[9,10] It is now accepted that the ultrasound morphological features to diagnose polycystic ovaries require the presence of 12 or more follicles in each ovary, each measuring 2–9 mm in diameter, and/or increased ovarian volume (>10 ml). The subjective appearance of an increased follicle count, distribution, stromal volume or echogenicity, is not included in the definition of ESHRE/ASRM consensus, 2003. Previous ultrasound criteria defined a polycystic ovary as one, which when viewed via the transabdominal route, contains at least 10 follicles (between 2–8 mm in size) arranged peripherally around a dense core of ovarian stroma in one plane or scattered throughout an increased amount of stroma.[11] These criteria were adopted by many studies, which have used ultrasound scanning to detect polycystic ovaries.

The histopathological criteria for the description of polycystic ovaries have been defined as the observation of an increased numbers of follicles, hypertrophy and luteinization of the inner theca cell layer, and a thickened ovarian tunica.[12] Polycystic and normal ovaries appear to differ fundamentally with regard to early follicular development as assessed by histopathological analysis.[13] Hence, it is believed that an ovarian abnormality exists in women with polycystic ovaries. The authors suggest that an increased density of small preantral follicles in polycystic ovaries could result from an increased population of germ cells in the fetal ovary or from a decreased rate of loss of oocytes during late gestation, childhood, and puberty.[13] This follicular appearance would therefore, appear to have it origins early in life and possibly in-utero due to either a genetic predisposition, the maternal environment, or more likely, a combination of both.[14]

A good correlation appears to exist between the histopathological diagnosis of polycystic ovaries and the ultrasound appearance of polycystic ovaries.[15,16] Vaginal ultrasonography offers greater ultrasound resolution hence, it would be expected that this would increase the detection rate of polycystic ovaries, although this is reportedly not the case.[17]

Although polycystic ovaries (PCO) *per se*, appear to have no longterm implications for the patient,[18] they represent a risk factor for the development of ovarian hyperstimulation syndrome (OHSS).[19] Potentially, women with PCO may have an improved outcome when undergoing in vitro fertilization (IVF) treatment if they do not suffer the consequences of OHSS. Generally, women with polycystic ovaries without the symptoms of PCOS produce more follicles, oocytes and embryos and have an 80% greater chance of having a live birth, than matched women with normal ovaries, despite similar fertilization, cleavage and miscarriage rates.[20] Indeed, the appearance of polycystic ovaries in women attempting to conceive naturally has been shown to have no significant impact on fertility if they have no symptoms of PCOS.[18]

The definition of the Polycystic ovary syndrome (PCOS) in the past has been controversial, and until recently, there has been a marked difference in opinion between Europe, where it was generally expected that an ultrasound scan was required to confirm the presence of polycystic ovaries to meet the diagnostic criteria, and the North American and Australian view, where the widley held belief was that it is not essential for the diagnosis.

The background to the development of a consensus

To facilitate international collaboration and interpretation of clinical trials, an internationally agreed definition for PCOS for clinical use was essential. Prior to the recent consensus meeting, there were two disparate views.

The European view

PCOS was defined as a syndrome where there are polycystic ovaries on ultrasound examination in conjunction with some of the following features; signs, symptoms or biochemical evidence of androgen excess (acne, hirsutism or alopecia), obesity, oligomenorrhea or amenorrhea and raised luteinizing hormone (LH).[21]

The North American view

The generally accepted opinion in North America for the diagnosis of PCOS was based on the NIH/ NICHHD conference criteria at a consensus meeting in 1990. The definition relied on a combination of oligomenorrhea or amenorrhea and clinical or biochemical evidence of hyperandrogenemia, in the absence of non-classical adrenal hyperplasia, hyperprolactinemia and thyroid dysfunction.[22] Hence, the diagnosis did not require the ultrasound appearance of polycystic ovaries.

In view of these differing definitions of a very common medical condition, an internationally agreed upon definition was essential.

The International Consensus

(The Rotterdam ESHRE/ASRM sponsored consensus workshop group, May 2003)[9,10,23] (Table 2.1)

At a recent joint ASRM/ESHRE consensus meeting, an updated definition of PCOS,

Table 2.1   Revised 2003 ESHRE/ASRM Criteria for the Diagnosis of Polycystic Ovary Syndrome

Presence of 2 of the following 3 criteria:

1. Oligo/anovulation
2. Clinical/or biochemical evidence of hyperandrogenism
3. Polycystic ovaries on ultrasound examination

Exclusion of late onset congenital adrenal hyperplasia, androgen secreting tumours and Cushing's syndrome was required for elevated androgens and exclusion of thyroid disorder and elevated prolactin for oligo/anovulation.

encompassing a description of the morphology of the polycystic ovary was proposed. It was agreed that since the original 1990 NIH consensus meeting, it was recognized that hyperandrogenic women with regular cycles may be part of the syndrome (See Table 2.1). It was emphasised that PCOS is also a diagnosis of exclusion, and to establish the diagnosis of PCOS, it was important to exclude other disorders with a similar clinical presentation. These disorders included congenital adrenal hyperplasia, Cushing's syndrome and androgen secreting tumours. Exclusion of 21-hydroxylase deficient non-classic adrenal hyperplasia (NCAH) can be performed using a basal morning 17-hydroxyprogesterone level, with cut-off values ranging between 2 and 3 ng/ml.[24] Cushing's syndrome can be excluded by the measurement of a 24 urinary cortisol reading below 300 nmol/24 h, or inadequate suppression of early morning serum cortisol by dexamethasone administered the previous night.[25] The routine exclusion of thyroid related disorders and measurement of serum prolactin in women undergoing screening for PCOS was encouraged.

Ultrasound assessment of the ovaries should be performed on cycle days 3, 4 or 5, preferably using a vaginal ultrasound probe. Women with either oligomenorrhea or amenorrhea should have the examination performed at random, or on days 3, 4 or 5 after a progestin induced withdrawal bleed. The presence of 12 or more follicles measuring 2–9 mm in diameter and/or increased ovarian volume (>10 cm^3), on either vaginal or abdominal ultrasound, was proposed as the criteria fulfilling sufficient specificity and sensitivity to define polycystic ovaries. Ovarian volume is calculated from the formula for a prolate ellipsoid (0.5 × length × width × thickness). If at the time of ultrasound assessment, there is a follicle greater than 10 mm in diameter, the scan should be repeated at a time of ovarian quiescence in order to calculate the volume and area. The presence of a single polycystic ovary is sufficient to provide the diagnosis. The distribution of follicles and the description of the stroma are not required in the diagnosis. Increased stromal echogenicity, and/or stromal volume are specific to polycystic ovaries, but it has been shown that the measurement of the ovarian volume (or area) is a good surrogate for the quantification of the stroma in clinical practice. This description does not apply if the woman is taking the oral contraceptive pill. If there is evidence of a dominant follicle or a corpus luteum on ultrasound examination, the scan should be repeated in the following cycle. It is advised that regularly menstruating women should have their ultrasound examination performed between the third and fifth day of their menstrual cycle.[9,10]

The primary clinical indicator of androgen excess was perceived as the presence of hirsutism, although it was acknowledged that there was a paucity of data on the normal range for different populations, and that, the assessment of hirsutism was highly subjective, that few clinicians used standardised scoring methods, and that many women had undergone treatment for hirsutism prior to endocrinological assessment. Acne was also felt to be a good indicator of androgen excess. The limitations of the measurement of circulating androgen levels was highlighted by the group, due to the limitations of some of the assays, lack of normative data, wide variability in the normal population, and the fact that androgens may be suppressed even after the discontinuation of hormonal treatment. However, it was felt that the measurement of free testosterone, or the free androgen index, were the more sensitive methods of assessing hyperandrogenemia[9,10] (Table 2.1).

The consensus group advised that the presence of an elevated luteinizing hormone (LH) was not mandatory for the definition of PCOS, despite raised LH being a frequent finding in women with PCOS.[26] The consensus group acknowledged that there was speculation that high endogenous LH levels may have detrimental effects on oocyte maturity, fertilization, pregnancy and miscarriage rates.

The consensus group acknowledged that women with PCOS were at a markedly increased risk of type 2 diabetes, and potential candidates for cardiovascular disease in later life. In view of the high prevalence of insulin resistance[27] and impaired glucose tolerance amongst obese women with PCOS,[28] the consensus group advised that an oral glucose tolerance test and a metabolic screen be performed for obese women with PCOS.[9,10,28]

Clinical Discussion

Prevalence of PCOS

As with any chronic condition in medicine, an accurate population based prevalence of PCOS is difficult, as the prevalence is influenced by the population being studied. In addition, all methods of volunteer recruitment in a study are prone to selection bias, and indeed, also to the differing diagnostic criteria that, used in the past, have made the interpretation of the prevalence of PCOS problematic.

The incidental finding of polycystic ovaries at the time of ultrasound examination is a relatively frequent finding, occuring in up to 33% of the women,[29] although most studies report an incidence around 22% in randomly selected women[30–35] (Table 2.2). However, in women with symptoms consistent with the PCOS, the incidence is much more frequent (Tables 2.3 and 2.4). In a study of 173 women, the ultrasonographic appearance of polycystic ovaries occured in 92% of the women with hirsutism and regular menstrual cycles, 87% of the women with oligomenorrhea, 57% of anovulatory women and 26% of the women with amenorrhea.[11] Of the women diagnosed with polycystic ovaries on ultrasound examination, up to 25% will be asymptomatic, and of the women with evidence of hyperandrogenism and regular menstrual cycles, only 50% will have polycystic

Table 2.2 The prevalence of polycystic ovaries in the general population

Authors	Polson et al. (1988)[30]	Tayob et al. (1990)[35]	Clayton et al. (1992)[31]	Farquhar et al. (1994b)[32]	Bostis et al. (1995)[33]	Cresswell et al. (1997)[34]
	Volunteers recruited from clinical and secretarial staff at St. Mary's Hospital, London	Volunteers using a low dose combined OCP, recruited from routine clinics at the Margaret Pyke centre and the Royal Free Hospital, London	Volunteers born between 1952–1969 recruited from a list of a Group Practice in Harrow, London, by random postal invitation	Volunteers recruited from two electoral rolls in Auckland NZ, by random postal invitation	Volunteers recruited from women presenting to an outpatient clinic for routine Pap smear	Volunteers born between and 1953 recruited from Jessop Hospital, Sheffield, by invitation and personal interview.
Study population	n = 257	n = 120	n = 190	n = 183	n = 1078	n = 235
Response rate	Unknown	Unknown	18%	16%	Unknown	68%
Age range	18–36 years	18–30 years mean 24 years	18–36 years	18–45 years mean 33 years	17–40 years	40–42 years
Prevalence (%)	22	22	22	21	17	21
95% CI	17–27%	14–30%	16–28%	14–27%	14–19%	16–26%

From Balen and Michelmore. What is polycystic ovary syndrome? Are national views important? Hum Reprod, 2002; 17, (9): 2219-27. © *European Society of Human Reproduction and Embryology. Reproduced with permission of Oxford Univeristy Press / Human Reproduction.*

Table 2.3   Clinical symptoms and signs in women with PCOS pre-ESHRE/ASRM revised definition

	Percentage frequency of symptom or sign			
	Balen *et al.* (1995)[40] $n = 1741$ (%)	Franks (1989)[55] $n = 300$ (%)	Goldzieher *et al.* (1981)[57] $n = 1079$ (%)	No. of cases[a]
Menstrual cycle disturbance				
Oligomenorrhea	47	52	29	547
Amenorrhea	19	28	51	640
Hirsutism	66.2	64	69	819
Obesity	38	35	41	600
Acne	35	27	–	–
Alopecia	6	3	–	–
Acanthosis nigricans	3	<1	–	–
Infertility (primary/secondary)	20	42	74	596

[a]In the Goldzieher study, clinical details were not available for the entire group of 1079 women, thus the number of cases which were used to determine the frequency of each symptom is stated.
From Balen and Michelmore. What is polycystic ovary syndrome? Are national views important? Hum Reprod, 2002; **17**, (9): 2219–27. © *European Society of Human Reproduction and Embryology. Reproduced with permission of Oxford Univeristy Press/Human Reproduction.*

Table 2.4   Frequency of clinical symptoms and signs in women with and without polycystic ovaries

	Percentage frequency									
	Polson *et al.* (1988)[30]		Clayton *et al.* (1992)[31]		Farquhar *et al.* (1994b)[32]		Bostis *et al.* (1995)[33]		Cresswell *et al.* (1997)[35]	
	PCO $n = 33$	Normal $n = 116$	PCO $n = 43$	Normal $n = 165$	PCO $n = 39$	Normal $n = 144$	PCO $n = 183$	Normal $n = 823$	PCO $n = 49$	Normal $n = 186$
Menstrual cycle disturbance (%)	76	1	29	27	46	20	80	–	41	27
Hirsutism (%)	–	–	14	2	23	4	40	10	14	2
Obesity (%)	–	–	33	29	23	19	41	10	35	48
Infertility primary/ secondary (%)	–	–	12	10	26	11	–	–	16	15

From Balen and Michelmore. What is polycystic ovary syndrome? Are national views important? Hum Reprod, 2002; **17**, (9): 2219–27. © *European Society of Human Reproduction and Embryology. Reproduced with permission of Oxford Univeristy Press/Human Reproduction.*

ovaries on ultrasound assessment. Of those who had regular menstrual cycles but were anovulatory, polycystic ovaries were present in 91% of cases consistent with the findings of Adams et al.[11]

In an unselected group of women attending a pre-employment medical appointment, Knochenhauer et al.[36] observed elevated androgens in 4.7% of the women.

Prevalence of PCOS using the Recent Consensus Definition of PCOS

There have been two studies that have addressed the incidence of PCO on ultrasound examination since the publication of the revised consensus statement of the ultrasound definition of PCO in 2004. The prevalence of PCO on ultrasound examination was 23% in partners of azoospermic men in an Australian population,[37] 32% in a heterosexual sub-fertile population of women in London and 80% in a lesbian population of women attending for donor insemination treatment at the same clinic.[39] The prevalence of PCOS has only been assessed by one study.[38] This group reported PCOS with a prevalence of 14% in the heterosexual subfertile population and 32% in lesbian women. An American prevalence study of women attending a pre-employment medical assessment, that unfortunately did not include an ultrasound assessment, demonstrated that 8.0% of the Black women and 4.8% of the White women had features of PCOS.[39] This study however, underestimates the prevalence of PCOS in this population, as women with biochemical evidence of hyperandrogenemia, in addition to those women with ultrasound evidence of PCO, were not included.

Symptomatic presentation of the polycystic ovary syndrome

Menstrual disturbance

In the largest series of women with PCOS, Balen et al.[40] reported that of the 1871 women with at least one symptom of PCOS, using the previous European definition of PCOS, approximately 50% of the patients had oligomenorrhea, 30% had a regular menstrual cycle, and 20% were amenorrheic. Indeed, menstrual disturbance is so common, and PCOS is so frequent that the occurrence of oligomenorrhea may be explained by PCOS in approximately 85–90% of women,[41] and as many as 30–40% of amenorrheic patients have PCOS.[41] The deposition of adipose tissue increases the likelihood of anovulation in women with PCOS due to increased insulin resistance

and in addition, due to increased peripheral aromatisation of androgens in the adipose tissue.[42] Indeed, weight loss has consistently been shown to restore ovulation and regular cycles.[3]

Obesity

The occurrence of obesity in PCOS is relatively common, with more than 50% being overweight (BMI >25 kg/m^2) or obese (BMI >27 kg/m^2).[43] The weight distribution is classically with a central deposition of fat in the truncal region and manifest in an increased waist/hip ratio.[44] The increased weight of women with PCOS has been linked to an increased risk of type 2 diabetes, with up to 30% of obese PCOS women having impaired glucose tolerance and 7.5% likely to develop frank diabetes by their forties.[28] The central deposition of fat is a marker of the metabolic syndrome, which is defined differently by different groups; however, there is universal agreement that central fat deposition is a marker of the metabolic syndrome.[45] It is either defined as a waist/hip ratio in excess of 85, or a waist circumference greater than or equal to 80 cm.[45–48] The central deposition of adipose tissue and the resultant insulin resistance is believed to be a significant factor leading to the seven-fold increased risk of death after a myocardial infarction in women with PCOS.[49] For the motivated patient, several authors have demonstrated the significant beneficial effects that can be derived from weight reduction with regard to menstrual cycle frequency, ovulatory disorder and insulin resistance.[50–54]

Acne

Acne is an inflammatory disorder of the hair follicle and its associated sebaceous and apocrine gland, and often, the serum androgen levels are not elevated. It is present in up to one third of the women with PCOS.[40,55]

Hirsutism

Hirsutism is the growth of terminal hair on the

body of a woman, in the same pattern as in an adult male. It is recognized that hirsutism is in part, ethnically determined, being commoner in women with dark skin.[56] The cause of hirsutism is androgen action upon the hair follicle, particularly the local action of dihydrotestosterone. Particular manifestations are the occurrence of excess facial hair on the chest between the breasts and on the lower abdomen. Knochenhauer et al.[36] in 1998, reported that Ferriman-Gallwey hirsutism scores of atleast 6, 8, and 10 occurred in an unselected female population with a prevalence of 8%, 2.8% and 1.6% respectively in White women and 7.1%, 6.1% and 2.1% respectively in Black women. In women with a diagnosis of PCOS, the incidence can be as much as 70%.[57] Weight loss as a strategy to reduce hirsutism has been demonstrated to be effective by several authors.[50,58]

Androgenic alopecia

Androgenic alopecia is a progressive pattern of hair loss of scalp terminal hair, which is a common finding in men, and occurs in less than 10% of women with PCOS, although this symptom is probably under-reported.[55] A genetic expression of a predisposition to baldness and an associated increase in circulating androgens are required in order to present with alopecia hence, all women with an excess of circulating androgens will not suffer from androgenic alopecia. In a study of women with androgenic alopecia, two-thirds had polycystic ovaries on ultrasound examination, 20% also complained of hirsutism, and surprisingly, most of the women with alopecia had androgen levels within the normal range.[59]

Acanthosis nigricans

Acanthosis nigricans is a mucocutaneous eruption that occurs most frequently in the axillae, skin flexures and the nape of the neck. It is manifest by increased pigmentation and papillomatosis. It is a marker associated with insulin resistance and compensatory increased insulin secretion.[60] It occurs in 1–3% of the women with PCOS and may be a more frequent finding in adolescent girls with PCOS.[40,55]

The natural history of PCOS

The first manifestation of PCOS may be an early adrenarche with an early appearance of pubic hair.[61] It is increasingly being recognized that oligomenorrhea in adolescence may be one of the first manifestations of PCOS.[62–64] Although PCOS is not diagnosed until 2–3 years after menarche, it is believed that its origins lie in childhood or fetal life, as excess androgen exposure to animals in-utero produces PCOS like features.[14,65–67] Due to the family clustering of cases of PCOS, it is believed that there is a genetic predisposition to PCOS, whereby, genomic variants act under the influence of environmental factors.[68] The severity of hyperinsulinemia that is manifest in adulthood in over 50% of normal weight women with PCOS,[27] is influenced by both genetic and environmental factors, particularly obesity. It is believed that although a woman may have the predisposition to PCOS, whether genetic or environmental, it is the development of insulin resistance due to the deposition of adipose tissue that leads to the expression of the phenotype of PCOS. Hence, it is possible for a woman to have PCOS and then with weight loss, lose some of the features PCOS, and consequently, not express the PCOS phenotype.[50–54]

As discussed, the central deposition of fat in women with PCOS, predisposes these women to a markedly increased chance of developing type 2 diabetes[28,69] and possibly, cardiovascular disease in later life, although the evidence for cardiovascular disease is disputed.[49,70,71] In addition, women with PCOS are believed to be at an increased risk of developing endometrial cancer.[72]

Conclusion

PCOS is the commonest endocrine disorder of women in their reproductive years. The implications for women with this condition are substantial as they are at an increased risk of obesity, have a markedly increased risk of diabetes and death after a myocardial event. A recent consensus has led to the formulation of unifying diagnostic criteria for the definition of PCOS. These criteria rely on the presence of two of the following; oligo/anovulation, clinical or biochemical evidence of hyperandrogenism and the presence of polycystic ovaries.

References

1. Leventhal ML. The Stein-Leventhal syndrome. *Am J Obstet Gynecol* 1958; 76(4): 825–838.

2. Hart R, Hickey M, Franks S. Definitions, prevalence and symptoms of polycystic ovaries and polycystic ovary syndrome. *Best Pract Res Clin Obstet Gynaecol* 2004; 18(5): 671–683.

3. Norman RJ, Davies MJ, Lord J, Moran LJ. The role of lifestyle modification in polycystic ovary syndrome. *Trends Endocrinol Metab* 2002; 13(6): 251–257.

4. Harborne L, Fleming R, Lyall H, Norman J, Sattar N. Descriptive review of the evidence for the use of metformin in polycystic ovary syndrome. *Lancet.* 2003; 361(9372): 1894–1901.

5. Mitwally MF, Casper RF. Single-dose administration of an aromatase inhibitor for ovarian stimulation. *Fertil Steril* 2005; 83(1): 229–231.

6. Ibanez L, de Zegher F. Flutamide-metformin plus ethinylestradiol-drospirenone for lipolysis and antiatherogenesis in young women with ovarian hyperandrogenism: the key role of metformin at the start and after more than one year of therapy. *J Clin Endocrinol Metab* 2005; 90(1): 39–43.

7. Hart R, Magos A. Polycystic Ovarian Syndrome. *Seminars in Laparoscopic Surgery* 1997; 4: 210–218.

8. Yara P, Niemineva K. Small-cystic degeneration of ovaries as an incidental finding in gynecological laparotomies. *Acta Obstet Gynecol Scand* 1951; 31(1): 94–107.

9. ESHRE/ASRM. ESHRE/ASRM Rotterdam Consensus Meeting Revised 2003 consensus on diagnostic criteria and long-term health risks related to polycystic ovary syndrome (PCOS). *Hum Reprod* 2004; 19(1): 41–47.

10. ESHRE/ASRM. Revised 2003 consensus on diagnostic criteria and long-term health risks related to polycystic ovary syndrome. *Fertil Steril* 2004; 81(1): 19–25.

11. Adams J, Polson DW, Franks S. Prevalence of polycystic ovaries in women with anovulation and idiopathic hirsutism. *Br Med J (Clin Res Ed)* 1986; 293(6543): 355–359.

12. Balen A, Michelmore K. What is polycystic ovary syndrome? Are national views important? *Hum Reprod* 2002; 17(9): 2219–2227.

13. Webber LJ, Stubbs S, Stark J, Trew GH, Margara R, Hardy K, et al. Formation and early development of follicles in the polycystic ovary. *Lancet* 2003; 362(9389): 1017–1021.

14. Abbott DH, Dumesic DA, Franks S. Developmental origin of polycystic ovary syndrome – a hypothesis. *J Endocrinol* 2002; 174(1): 1–5.

15. Saxton DW, Farquhar CM, Rae T, Beard RW, Anderson MC, Wadsworth J. Accuracy of ultrasound measurements of female pelvic organs. *Br J Obstet Gynaecol* 1990; 97(8): 695–699.

16. Faddy MJ. Follicle dynamics during ovarian ageing. *Mol Cell Endocrinol* 2000; 163(1–2): 43–48.

17. Farquhar CM, Birdsall M, Manning P, Mitchell JM. Transabdominal versus transvaginal ultrasound in the diagnosis of polycystic ovaries in a population of randomly selected women. *Ultrasound Obstet Gynecol* 1994a; 4(1): 54–59.

18. Hassan MA, Killick SR. Ultrasound diagnosis of polycystic ovaries in women who have no symptoms of polycystic ovary syndrome is not associated with subfecundity or subfertility. *Fertil Steril* 2003; 80(4): 966–975.

19. MacDougall MJ, Tan SL, Jacobs HS. In-vitro fertilization and the ovarian hyperstimulation syndrome. *Hum Reprod* 1992; 7(5): 597–600.

20. Engmann L, Maconochie N, Sladkevicius P, Bekir J, Campbell S, Tan SL. The outcome of in-vitro fertilization treatment in women with sonographic evidence of polycystic ovarian morphology. *Hum Reprod* 1999; 14(1): 167–171.

21. Balen A. Pathogenesis of polycystic ovary syndrome – the enigma unravels? *The Lancet* 1999; 354: 966–967.

22. Zawadzki J, Dunaif A. Diagnostic criteria for polycystic ovary syndrome: towards a rational approach. In: Dunaif A, Givens J, Haseltine F, Merriam G, editors. *Polycystic Ovarian Syndrome* Boston: Blackwells, 1992: 377–384.

23. Revised 2003 consensus on diagnostic criteria and long-term health risks related to polycystic ovary syndrome (PCOS). *Hum Reprod* 2004; 19(1): 41–47.

24. Azziz R, Hincapie LA, Knochenhauer ES, Dewailly D, Fox L, Boots LR. Screening for 21-hydroxylase-deficient nonclassic adrenal hyperplasia among hyperandrogenic women: a prospective study. *Fertil Steril* 1999; 72(5): 915–925.

25. Eddy RL, Jones AL, Gilliland PF, Ibarra JD, Jr., Thompson JQ, MacMurry JF, Jr. Cushing's

syndrome: a prospective study of diagnostic methods. *Am J Med* 1973; 55(5): 621–630.

26. Fauser BC, Pache TD, Lamberts SW, Hop WC, de Jong FH, Dahl KD. Serum bioactive and immunoreactive luteinizing hormone and follicle-stimulating hormone levels in women with cycle abnormalities, with or without polycystic ovarian disease. *J Clin Endocrinol Metab* 1991; 73(4): 811–817.

27. Chang RJ, Nakamura RM, Judd HL, Kaplan SA. Insulin resistance in nonobese patients with polycystic ovarian disease. *J Clin Endocrinol Metab* 1983; 57(2): 356–359.

28. Legro RS, Kunselman AR, Dodson WC, Dunaif A. Prevalence and predictors of risk for type 2 diabetes mellitus and impaired glucose tolerance in polycystic ovary syndrome: a prospective, controlled study in 254 affected women. *J Clin Endocrinol Metab* 1999 Jan; 84(1): 165–169.

29. Michelmore KF, Balen AH, Dunger DB, Vessey MP. Polycystic ovaries and associated clinical and biochemical features in young women. *Clin Endocrinol (Oxf)* 1999; 51(6): 779–786.

30. Polson DW, Adams J, Wadsworth J, Franks S. Polycystic ovaries – a common finding in normal women. *Lancet* 1988; 1(8590): 870–872.

31. Clayton RN, Ogden V, Hodgkinson J, Worswick L, Rodin DA, Dyer S, et al. How common are polycystic ovaries in normal women and what is their significance for the fertility of the population? *Clin Endocrinol (Oxf)* 1992; 37(2): 127–134.

32. Farquhar CM, Birdsall M, Manning P, Mitchell JM, France JT. The prevalence of polycystic ovaries on ultrasound scanning in a population of randomly selected women. *Aust N Z J Obstet Gynaecol* 1994b; 34(1): 67–72.

33. Botsis D, Kassanos D, Pyrgiotis E, Zourlas PA. Sonographic incidence of polycystic ovaries in a gynecological population. *Ultrasound Obstet Gynecol* 1995; 6(3): 182–185.

34. Cresswell JL, Barker DJ, Osmond C, Egger P, Phillips DI, Fraser RB. Fetal growth, length of gestation, and polycystic ovaries in adult life. *Lancet* 1997; 350(9085): 1131–1135.

35. Tayob Y, Robinson G, Adams J, Nye M, Whitelaw N, Shaw R, et al. Ultrasound Appearance of the ovaries during the pill-free interval. *Br. J. Family Planning* 1990; 16: 94–96.

36. Knochenhauer ES, Key TJ, Kahsar-Miller M, Waggoner W, Boots LR, Azziz R. Prevalence of the polycystic ovary syndrome in unselected black and white women of the southeastern United States: a prospective study. *J Clin Endocrinol Metab* 1998; 83(9): 3078–3082.

37. Lowe P, Kovacs G, Howlett D. Incidence of polycystic ovaries and polycystic ovary syndrome amongst women in Melbourne, Australia. *Aust N Z J Obstet Gynaecol* 2005; 45(1): 17–19.

38. Agrawal R, Sharma S, Bekir J, Conway G, Bailey J, Balen AH, et al. Prevalence of polycystic ovaries and polycystic ovary syndrome in lesbian women compared with heterosexual women. *Fertil Steril* 2004; 82(5): 1352–1357.

39. Azziz R, Woods KS, Reyna R, Key TJ, Knochenhauer ES, Yildiz BO. The prevalence and features of the polycystic ovary syndrome in an unselected population. *J Clin Endocrinol Metab* 2004; 89(6): 2745–2749.

40. Balen AH, Conway GS, Kaltsas G, Techatrasak K, Manning PJ, West C, et al. Polycystic ovary syndrome: the spectrum of the disorder in 1741 patients. *Hum Reprod* 1995; 10(8): 2107–2111.

41. Carmina E, Lobo R. Do hyperandrogenic women with normal menses have polycystic ovary syndrome? *Fertil Steril* 1999; 71: 319–322.

42. Goldzieher JW, Green JA. The polycystic ovary. I. Clinical and histologic features. *J Clin Endocrinol Metab* 1962; 22: 325–338.

43. Gambineri A, Pelusi C, Vicennati V, Pagotto U, Pasquali R. Obesity and the polycystic ovary syndrome. *Int J Obes Relat Metab Disord* 2002; 26(7): 883–896.

44. Rebuffe-Scrive M, Cullberg G, Lundberg PA, Lindstedt G, Bjorntorp P. Anthropometric variables and metabolism in polycystic ovarian disease. *Horm Metab Res* 1989; 21(7): 391–397.

45. Eckel RH, Grundy SM, Zimmet PZ. The metabolic syndrome. *Lancet* 2005; 365(9468): 1415–1428.

46. Balkau B, MA C. Comment on the provisional report from the WHO consultation. European Group for the Study of Insulin Resistance (EGIR). *Diabet Med* 1999; 16: 442–443.

47. Expert Panel on Detection E, And Treatment of High Blood Cholesterol In Adults. Executive Summary of The Third Report of The National Cholesterol Education Program (NCEP) Expert Panel on Detection, Evaluation, And Treatment of High Blood Cholesterol In Adults (Adult Treatment Panel III). *JAMA* 2001; 285: 2486–2497.

48. Alberti K, Zimmet PZ. Definition, diagnosis and classification of diabetes mellitus and its complications. Part1 diagnosis and classification of diabetes mellitus provisional report of a WHO consultation. *Diabet Med* 1998; 15: 539–553.

49. Dahlgren E, Janson PO, Johansson S, Lapidus L, Oden A. Polycystic ovary syndrome and risk for myocardial infarction. Evaluated from a risk factor

model based on a prospective population study of women. *Acta Obstet Gynecol Scand* 1992; 71(8): 599–604.

50. Kiddy DS, Hamilton-Fairley D, Bush A, Short F, Anyaoku V, Reed MJ, et al. Improvement in endocrine and ovarian function during dietary treatment of obese women with polycystic ovary syndrome. *Clin Endocrinol (Oxf)* 1992; 36(1): 105–111.

51. Norman RJ, Noakes M, Wu R, Davies MJ, Moran L, Wang JX. Improving reproductive performance in overweight/obese women with effective weight management. *Hum Reprod Update* 2004; 10(3): 267–280.

52. Crosignani PG, Colombo M, Vegetti W, Somigliana E, Gessati A, Ragni G. Overweight and obese anovulatory patients with polycystic ovaries: parallel improvements in anthropometric indices, ovarian physiology and fertility rate induced by diet. *Hum Reprod* 2003; 18(9): 1928–1932.

53. Clark AM, Thornley B, Tomlinson L, Galletley C, Norman RJ. Weight loss in obese infertile women results in improvement in reproductive outcome for all forms of fertility treatment. *Hum Reprod* 1998; 13(6): 1502–1505.

54. Hoeger KM, Kochman L, Wixom N, Craig K, Miller RK, Guzick DS. A randomized, 48-week, placebo-controlled trial of intensive lifestyle modification and/or metformin therapy in overweight women with polycystic ovary syndrome: a pilot study. *Fertil Steril* 2004; 82(2): 421–429.

55. Franks S. Polycystic ovary syndrome: a changing perspective. *Clin Endocrinol (Oxf)* 1989; 31(1): 87–120.

56. Carmina E, Koyama T, Chang L, Stanczyk FZ, Lobo RA. Does ethnicity influence the prevalence of adrenal hyperandrogenism and insulin resistance in polycystic ovary syndrome? *Am J Obstet Gynecol* 1992; 167(6): 1807–1812.

57. Goldzieher JW. Polycystic ovarian disease. *Fertil Steril* 1981; 35(4): 371–394.

58. Piacquadio DJ, Rad FS, Spellman MC, Hollenbach KA. Obesity and female androgenic alopecia: a cause and an effect? *J Am Acad Dermatol* 1994; 30(6): 1028–1030.

59. Cela E, Robertson C, Rush K, Kousta E, White DM, Wilson H, et al. Prevalence of polycystic ovaries in women with androgenic alopecia. *Eur J Endocrinol* 2003; 149(5): 439–442.

60. Schwartz RA. Acanthosis nigricans. *J Am Acad Dermatol* 1994; 31(1): 1–19; quiz 20–22.

61. Lucky AW, Rosenfield RL, McGuire J, Rudy S, Helke J. Adrenal androgen hyperresponsiveness to adrenocorticotropin in women with acne and/or hirsutism: adrenal enzyme defects and exaggerated adrenarche. *J Clin Endocrinol Metab* 1986; 62(5): 840–848.

62. van Hooff MH, Voorhorst FJ, Kaptein MB, Hirasing RA, Koppenaal C, Schoemaker J. Predictive value of menstrual cycle pattern, body mass index, hormone levels and polycystic ovaries at age 15 years for oligo-amenorrhoea at age 18 years. *Hum Reprod* 2004; 19(2): 383–392.

63. van Hooff MH, Voorhorst FJ, Kaptein MB, Hirasing RA, Koppenaal C, Schoemaker J. Endocrine features of polycystic ovary syndrome in a random population sample of 14–16 year old adolescents. *Hum Reprod* 1999; 14(9): 2223–2229.

64. Ibanez L, Potau N, Marcos MV, De Zegher F. Adrenal hyperandrogenism in adolescent girls with a history of low birthweight and precocious pubarche. *Clin Endocrinol (Oxf)* 2000; 53(4): 523–527.

65. Abbott DH, Barnett DK, Bruns CM, Dumesic DA. Androgen excess fetal programming of female reproduction: a developmental aetiology for polycystic ovary syndrome? *Hum Reprod Update* 2005; 11(4): 357–374.

66. Robinson JE, Birch RA, Taylor JA, Foster DL, Padmanabhan V. In utero programming of sexually differentiated gonadotrophin releasing hormone (GnRH) secretion. *Domest Anim Endocrinol* 2002; 23(1–2): 43–52.

67. Short RV. Sexual differentiation of the brain of the sheep: effects of prenatal implantation of androgen. Film: general discussion. *Ciba Found Symp* 1978; (62): 257–269.

68. Diamanti-Kandarakis E, Piperi C. Genetics of polycystic ovary syndrome: searching for the way out of the labyrinth. *Hum Reprod Update* 2005; 11(6): 631–643.

69. Norman RJ, Masters L, Milner CR, Wang JX, Davies MJ. Relative risk of conversion from normoglycaemia to impaired glucose tolerance or non-insulin dependent diabetes mellitus in polycystic ovarian syndrome. *Hum Reprod* 2001; 16(9): 1995–1998.

70. Pierpoint T, McKeigue PM, Isaacs AJ, Wild SH, Jacobs HS. Mortality of women with polycystic ovary syndrome at long-term follow-up. *J Clin Epidemiol* 1998 1; 51(7): 581–586.

71. Wild RA. Long-term health consequences of PCOS. *Hum Reprod Update* 2002; 8(3): 231–241.

72. Hardiman P, Pillay OC, Atiomo W. Polycystic ovary syndrome and endometrial carcinoma. *Lancet* 2003; 361(9371): 1810–1812.

Frequently Asked Questions

1.   What is the current definition of PCOS?

It is the presence of 2 of the following 3 conditions:

1.   Oligo/anovulation
2.   Clinical/or biochemical evidence of hyperandrogenism
3.   Polycystic ovaries on ultrasound examination

after the exclusion of late onset congenital adrenal hyperplasia, androgen secreting tumours and Cushing's syndrome in women with elevated androgens, and exclusion of thyroid disorder and elevated prolactin in women with oligo/anovulation.

2.   Does a woman with a genetic or environmental predisposition to PCOS always express the phenotype of PCOS?

No. It is possible for a woman to express the phenotype of PCOS only if her gains weight mainly truncal obesity, and if her insulin resistance is increased. However, if she loses weight and reduces her insulin resistance, good evidence exists that her menstrual cycles may normalize and her elevated serum androgen levels may decrease; she may not therefore, qualify for a diagnosis of PCOS.

3.   Should a vaginal ultrasound examination be performed to confirm a polycystic appearance of the ovaries?

Not necessarily. The vaginal ultrasound examination is preferred as it offers greater ultrasound resolution, although the morphological appearance of the ovaries in slim women is easily determined via an abdominal examination and indeed, evidence exists that it is just as effective in distinguishing the appearance of polycystic ovaries. In overweight women, the vaginal route of examination is to be preferred, if possible.

3

Diagnostic Criteria in Polycystic Ovary Syndrome

Mohammad Hasan Sheikhha, Seyed Mehdi Kalantar

Summary

Polycystic Ovary Syndrome (PCOS) reflects multiple potential etiologies and variable clinical presentations. It is clearly a heterogeneous syndrome, and current proposed diagnostic criteria include a number of disorders with similar phenotypes but radically different etiologies. The lack of well-defined diagnostic criteria poses a dilemma to many clinicians in the diagnosis of PCOS and seriously delays the analysis of the genetics, etiology, clinical associations of the syndrome and the therapy to follow. There is no universally accepted clinical definition for PCOS. In this chapter, the most acceptable diagnostic criteria of PCOS will be discussed.

Introduction

Polycystic ovary syndrome affects 4% to 12% of women of reproductive age.[1–3] Despite its frequency, PCOS is still difficult to diagnose in endocrinology, gynecology and reproductive medicine. Since the first description of PCOS by Stein and Leventhal (1935),[4] the etiology of this syndrome is still speculative while its pathophysiology appears to be both multifactorial and polygenic. There is considerable heterogeneity in the signs and symptoms amongst women with PCOS, and these may change over time for an individual.[5,6] In fact, considering persistent anovulation as the hallmark of PCOS with a variety of etiologies and clinical manifestations is far more useful. PCOS should be defined by the exclusion of related disorders, such as Cushing's syndrome, hyperprolactinemia, thyroid dysfunction, androgen-producing tumours and nonclassical adrenal hyperplasia.[7,8]

Further identification of specific causes, and exclusion of the multiple phenocopies that make up PCOS, will assist its diagnosis.[9]

Clinical Discussion

PCOS includes a variety of potential signs and symptoms, including oligo-ovulation, biochemical or clinical hyperandrogenism, polycystic ovaries, and hyperinsulinemia, but no single diagnostic criterion is recommended for the diagnosis of PCOS. In addition, PCOS is associated with an increased risk of type 2 diabetes and cardiovascular events. Insulin resistance and elevated serum luteinizing hormone (LH) levels are also common features in PCOS.[10–12] Among different criteria, hyperandrogenemia, specifically elevated bioavailable testosterone, and the recognition of oligo-ovulation are academically conducive in the diagnosis. Diagnostic criteria in PCOS are at crossroads between consensus-based guidelines and evidence-based guidelines.

Many support a combination of hyperandrogenemia and oligo-ovulation as diagnostic criteria in the absence of known causes, while many others use ovarian morphology to identify and diagnose the syndrome.[9] To help solving this issue, the Rotterdam consensus conference proposed to include the ultrasonographic (USG) follicle count as a new diagnostic criterion, in addition to hyperandrogenism and oligo-anovulation.[13] Unfortunately, its assessment does not offer enough trustworthiness worldwide.[14] Some publications confirm the unreliability of the USG images with the help of magnetic resonance images (MRI).[15]

Overall, the three recommended criteria are: (1) oligomenorrhea, (2) any form of hyperandrogenemia, either clinical (hirsutism and acne), or endocrine (the hormonal diagnosis of high androgen levels), and (3) the ultrasound picture of polycystic ovaries. These are the major three criteria, but in order to make the diagnosis it would be necessary to fulfil only two out of three criteria. This makes PCOS a heterogeneous disorder.[13] Normal ovulatory women with polycystic ovaries (PCO), who exhibit only the ovarian morphology, are not considered to have PCOS. A subgroup of these women may, however, have subtle abnormalities resembling PCOS.

Oligomenorrhea

Oligomenorrhea or dysfunctional bleeding is a frequently early and dominant symptom of the anovulatory component of PCOS. Menstrual irregularity in PCOS is chronic and can be manifested in several different ways. Irregular menstruation due to anovulation is perhaps the most common. Some women with PCOS have long-lasting amenorrhea associated with endometrial atrophy. Some women have regular cycles at first and experience menstrual irregularity in association with weight gain, while sometimes, the onset of PCOS is peripubertal. In fact, there is strong evidence of a peripubertal onset of PCOS and this has been used as a diagnostic criterion.[16]

Infertility and PCOS

Infertility was included in the original description of PCOS by Stein and Leventhal.[4] The prevalence of infertility, caused mainly by anovulation in PCOS women varies between 35% and 94%.[17] According to one retrospective study, however, women with PCOS are as likely to have children as healthy women, although often, after infertility treatment.[18] Some studies have also described an increased miscarriage rate in PCOS, the mechanism of which is inadequately understood. It has been suggested that high follicular phase concentrations of LH have a harmful effect on conception rates and may cause miscarriage.[19,20]

Hyperandrogenism

Hyperandrogenism is the second essential characteristic of PCOS. Clinically, the most common sign of hyperandrogenism in PCOS women is hirsutism, which can be defined as the growth of coarse hair on a woman in a male pattern (upper lip, chin, chest, upper abdomen and back). This must be distinguished from hypertrichosis that involves a more uniform, whole body distribution of fine hair. The prevalence of hirsutism in PCOS women varies between 17% and 83%. Another common sign of hyperandrogenism is acne, which is related to hyperandrogenism. Thus, an adolescent female with moderate to severe acne should be investigated for PCOS. Furthermore, the progress or persistence of acne into adulthood is unusual and should raise awareness. It has also been shown that hyperandrogenism may be related to overt signs of virilization, i.e. male pattern balding, alopecia, increased muscle mass, a deepening voice or clitoromegaly, but these signs partly resolve before menopause in women with PCOS. These women tend to acquire more regular menstrual cycles with increasing age (40 years and above).[6]

Gonadotropin secretion

An inappropriate gonadotropin secretion is associated with the classic form of PCOS.

Compared with the follicular phase of the normal menstrual cycle, women with PCOS exhibit an unreasonably high LH secretion with comparatively constant low follicle stimulating hormone (FSH) secretion. Therefore, an elevated LH/FSH-ratio of 2–3:1 is commonly used to indicate abnormal gonadotropin secretion. The prevalence of increased serum LH in PCOS ranges from 30% to 90%.[21,22]

Ultrasonographic finding of PCOS

In clinical practice, ultrasonography has replaced the histologic evaluation of PCO and many parameters have been used for its definition. The most reliable ultrasound definition of PCO was that of Adams and colleagues[23] which was published as a seminal paper and has most often been quoted in the literature on PCOS. Their criteria were as follows; the presence of either at least 10 follicles (usually between 2–8 mm in diameter) distributed uniformly around the ovarian periphery with an increased amount of stroma, or (less commonly) multiple small cysts 2–4 mm in diameter distributed throughout abundant stroma.[23] The combination of multiple follicles and an increased amount of stroma contribute to the overall increase in the ovarian size. Interestingly, the ovarian volume may sometimes be within the normal range in a considerable proportion of women with all other morphological criteria for PCOS.[24] The Adams criteria was revised over time and according to the most updated available literature, the criteria that fulfill satisfactory specificity and sensitivity to define PCO include atleast one of the following: either 12 or more follicles measuring 2–9 mm in diameter, or increased ovarian volume (> 10 cm^3). Three-dimensional and Doppler ultrasound studies may be useful research tools, but are not required to define PCOS.[25] The follicular cysts in the ovaries of PCOS women do not mature completely and few granulosa cells are present in these arrested follicles.

It has been proposed that increased ovarian stroma is the most valuable diagnostic criterion for PCO to differentiate it from multifollicular ovaries (MFO).[21,26] MFO are usually detected in women with hypogonadotrophic amenorrhea, without increased stroma and packed by 6 or more follicles 4–10 mm in diameter.

Overall, the USG findings are not sufficient for the diagnosis of PCOS. In fact, the typical USG findings of PCO are demonstrated in 8% to 25% of normal women.[26,27] This USG picture can also be found in 14% of the women on oral contraceptives.[28]

Anti-Mullerian hormone

Anti-Mullerian hormone (AMH) measurement in the serum could be a replacement for antral follicle count in the diagnostic criteria of PCOS. In circumstances where accurate USG data are not available, AMH estimation could be used instead of the follicle count as a diagnostic criterion.[14]

Obesity

Although there are no controlled systematic studies to determine the exact prevalence of obesity, most investigators have found that 30–50% of PCOS women are obese with a tendency for an increased waist-hip ratio, or abdominal obesity. They exhibit significantly increased glucose and plasma insulin levels during an oral glucose tolerance test (OGTT) compared with obese control women.[17]

Insulin resistance

The association between glucose intolerance and hyperandrogenism was first described in a case by Archard and Thiers.[29] Recent insights into the pathophysiology of PCOS have shown insulin resistance (IR) to play a considerable role.[30] Upper-body obesity is a key component of the insulin resistance syndrome (IRS).[31]

Acanthosis nigricans is a grey-brown velvety discoloration of the skin caused by hyperkeratosis and papillomatosis, usually in the areas of neck, axillae, groin and under the breast. This condition is often associated with glucose intolerance and hyperandrogenism.[32]

Genetics of PCOS

Despite the completion of the Human Genome Project, many of the genes, which are involved in female infertility still remain unknown. The genetics of common disorders causing female infertility have received lesser attention than have many rare gynecological disorders. The cause of PCOS is not fully understood, but genetics may be a factor. Many studies have suggested a dominant mode of inheritance for PCOS[33] but genetic studies have not as yet concluded the pattern of inheritance.[34] There are apparent problems, which make genetic studies of PCOS difficult to perform. The heterogeneity and lack of universally acceptable clinical or biochemical diagnostic criteria have been discussed. PCOS is a disorder, which primarily affects women of reproductive age and it is therefore, difficult to perform studies in more than one generation. There is no commonly accepted male phenotype. Male pattern premature balding has been demonstrated in male relatives in familial PCOS studies.

A relation between PCOS and the X chromosome has been demonstrated. Some cases of PCOS may represent an intermediate condition in a spectrum that extends from the presence of streak gonads typical of Turners syndrome to the normal ovary. The concept is that at least some cases of PCOS may be due to X chromosomal factors causing an abnormal follicular apparatus.[35] Increased androgen secretion and insulin resistance persist in cultured theca cells and skin fibroblasts respectively, from women with PCOS, suggesting that these are intrinsic, presumably genetic defects. Studies have indicated a genetic susceptibility to PCOS. Polycystic ovaries and hyperandrogenemia are present in 50% of sisters of affected women. Genetic analysis of candidate genes have been performed. Both linkage and association studies have suggested that PCOS can be explained by the interaction of a small number of key genes with environmental, and particularly, nutritional factors. The steroid synthesis gene CYP11a, coding for P450 cholesterol side chain cleavage and the insulin gene regulatory region may be involved. Hyperandrogenemia is genetically determined and the result of familial studies indicates that hyperandrogenism clusters as a dominant genetic trait.[36] However, it is unlikely that the hyperandrogenemia of PCOS is principally determined by polymorphisms or mutations in the genes encoding a single steroidogenic enzyme activity, such as CYP17 or CYP11a.[37–40] Also, an increase in mRNA abundance corresponding to the genes of aldehyde dehydrogenase-6 and retinol dehydrogenase-2, both of which increase the expression of 17α-hydroxylase, has been found in PCOS.[41]

As we are unable to exclude an autosomal or X-linked dominant mode of inheritance, the inheritance of PCOS is probably more complex, similar to that of type 2 diabetes mellitus, or cardiovascular disease. However, a positive family history as a risk factor for the development of PCOS appears to be the most informative. Furthermore, environmental factors alter the clinical and biochemical presentation in women with a genetic predisposition to PCOS.

Conclusion

Much has been learned about the pathophysiology of PCOS since its first description in 1935.[4] Yet, despite a better understanding of the disease itself (and the passage of nearly 70 years), it still lacks specific diagnostic criteria making identification of patients with the disorder difficult. With an appreciation of the role that IR plays in PCOS, proper identification has become more important than ever before. There are several other disease states that may present in much the same way as PCOS, and evaluation to rule out these is crucial to apply appropriate management options. Further research into updated diagnostic criteria for the definition of PCOS and proper identification of patients with the disorder is needed.

References

1. Knochenhauer ES, Key TJ, Kahsar-Miller M, Waggoner W, Boots LR, Azziz R. Prevalence of the polycystic ovary syndrome in unselected black and white women of the southeastern United States: a prospective study. *J Clin Endocrinol Metab* 1998; 83: 3078–3082.

2. Farah L, Lazenby AJ, Boots LR, Azziz R. Prevalence of polycystic ovary syndrome in women seeking treatment from community electrologists. Alabama Professional Electrology Association Study Group. *J Reprod Med* 1999; 44: 870–874.

3. Hahn S, Tan S, Elsenbruch S, Quadbeck B, Herrmarnn BL, Mann K, Janssen OE. Clinical and biochemical characterization of women with polycystic ovary syndrome in North Rhine-Westphalia. *Horm Metab Res* 2005; 37(7): 438–444.

4. Stein IF, Leventhal ML. Amenorrhea associated with bilateral polycystic ovaries. *Am J Obstet Gynecol* 1935; 29: 181.

5. Balen AH, Dunger D. Pubertal maturation of the internal genitalia. *Ultrasound Obstet Gynecol* 1995; 6: 164–165.

6. Elting MW, Korsen TJM, Rekers-Mombarg LTM, Schoemaker J. Women with polycystic ovary syndrome gain regular menstrual cycles when ageing. *Hum Reprod* 2000; 15: 24–28.

7. Zawadzki JA, Dunaif A. Diagnostic criteria for polycystic ovary syndrome: towards a rational approach. In: Dunaif A, Givens JR, Haseltine FP, Merriam GR. (eds), Polycystic Ovary Syndrome. Blackwell Scientific, Boston, 1992; pp. 377–384.

8. Lane DE. Polycystic ovary syndrome and its differential diagnosis. *Obstet Gynecol Surv* 2006; 61(2): 125–135.

9. Legro RS. Diagnostic criteria in polycystic ovary syndrome. *Semin Reprod Med* 2003; 21(3): 267–275.

10. Ehrmann DA, Barnes RB, Rosenfield RL, Cavaghan MK, Imperial J. Prevalence of impaired glucose tolerance and diabetes in women with polycystic ovary syndrome. *Diabetes Care* 1999; 22: 141–146.

11. Legro RS, Kunselman AR, Dodson WC, Dunaif A. Prevalence and predictors of risk for type 2 diabetes mellitus and impaired glucose tolerance in polycystic ovary syndrome: a prospective, controlled study in 254 affected women. *J Clin Endocrinol Metab* 1999; 84: 165–169.

12. Pfeifer SM. Polycystic ovary syndrome in adolescent girls. *Semin Pediatr Surg* 2005; 14(2): 111–117.

13. The Rotterdam ESHRE/ASRM-Sponsored PCOS consensus workshop group. Revised 2003 consensus on diagnostic criteria and long-term health risks related to polycystic ovary syndrome (PCOS). *Hum Reprod* 2004; 19(1): 41–47.

14. Pigny P, Jonard S, Robert Y, Dewailly D. Serum Anti-Mullerian hormone as a surrogate for antral follicle count for definition of the polycystic ovary syndrome. *J Clin endocrinol metab* 2005; [Epub ahead of print] 10.1210/jc. 2005–2076.

15. Kimura I, Togashi K, Kawakami S, Nakano Y, Takakura K, Mori T, Konishi J. Polycystic ovaries: implications of diagnosis with MR imaging. *Radiology* 1996; 201: 549.

16. Chakrabarty S, Miller BT, Collins TJ, Nagamani M. Ovarian dysfunction in peripubertal hyperinsulinemia. *J Soc Gynecol Investig* 2006; 13(2): 122–129.

17. Franks S. Polycystic ovary syndrome. *N Engl J Med* 1995; 333: 853–861.

18. Dahlgren E, Johansson S, Lindstedt G, Knutsson F, Oden A, Janson PO et al. Women with polycystic ovary syndrome wedge resected in 1956 to 1965: a long-term follow-up focusing on natural history and circulating hormones. *Fertil Steril* 1992; 57: 505–513.

19. Homburg R, Armar NA, Eshel A, Adams J, Jacobs HS. Influence of serum luteinising hormone concentrations on ovulation, conception, and early pregnancy loss in polycystic ovary syndrome. BMJ 1988; 297: 1024–1026.

20. Balen AH, Tan SL, McDougall J, Jacobs HS. Miscarriage rates following IVF are increased in women with PCO and reduced pituitary desisitization with buserelin. *Hum Reprod* 1993; 8: 959–964.

21. Conway GS, Honour JW, Jacobs HS. Heterogeneity of the polycystic ovary syndrome: clinical, endocrine and ultrasound features in 556 patients. *Clin Endocrinol (Oxf)* 1989; 30: 459–470.

22. Franks S. Polycystic ovary syndrome: a changing perspective. *Clin Endocrinol (Oxf)* 1989; 31: 87–120.

23. Adams J, Franks S, Polson DW, Mason HD, Abdulwahid N, Tucker M, et al. Multifollicular ovaries: clinical and endocrine features and response to pulsatile gonadotropin releasing hormone. *Lancet* 1985; 2(8469–70): 1375–1379.

24. Pache TD, Hop WC, Wladimiroff JW, Schipper J, Fauser BC. How to discriminate between normal and polycystic ovaries. *Radiology* 1992; 17: 589–593.

25. Balen AH, Laven JS, Tan SL, Dewailly D. Ultrasound

assessment of the polycystic ovary: international consensus definitions. *Hum Reprod Update* 2003; 9(6): 505–514.

26. Polson DW, Adams J, Wadsworth J, Franks S. Polycystic ovaries – a common finding in normal women. *Lancet*. 1988; 1(8590): 870–872.

27. Farquhar CM, Birdsall M, Manning P, Mitchell JM, France JT. The prevalence of polycystic ovaries on ultrasound scanning in a population of randomly selected women. *Aust N Z Obstet Gynaecol* 1994; 34: 67–72.

28. Clayton RN, Ogden V, Hodgkinson J, Worswick L, Rodin DA, Dyer S, Meade TW. How common are polcystic ovaries in normal women and what is their significance for the fertility of the population? *Clin Endocrinol* 1992; 37: 127–134.

29. Archard C, Thiers J. Le virilisme pilaire et son association a I,insuffisance glycolytique (diabete des femmes a barbe). *Bul Acad Natl Med* 1921; 86: 51.

30. Sheehan MT. Polycystic ovarian syndrome: diagnosis and management. *Clin Med Res* 2004; 2(1): 13–27.

31. Expert Panel on Detection, Evaluation, and Treatment of High Blood Cholesterol in Adults. Executive Summary of The Third Report of The National Cholesterol Education Program (NCEP) Expert Panel on Detection, Evaluation, and Treatment of High Blood Cholesterol in Adults (Adult Treatment Panel III). *JAMA* 2001; 285: 2486–2497.

32 Charnvises K, Weerakiet S, Tingthanatikul Y, Wansumrith S, Chanprasertyothin S, Rojanasakul A. Acanthosis nigricans: clinical predictor of abnormal glucose tolerance in Asian women with polycystic ovary syndrome. *Gynecol Endocrinol* 2005; 21(3): 161–164.

33. Carey AH, Chan KL, Short F, White D, Williamson R, Franks S. Evidence for a single gene effect causing polycystic ovaries and male pattern baldness. *Clin Endocrinol* 1993; 38: 653–658.

34. Diamanti-Kandarakis E, Piperi C. Genetics of polycystic ovary syndrome: searching for the way out of the labyrinth. *Hum Reprod Update* 2005; 11(6): 631–643.

35. Hickey T, Chandy A, Norman RJ. The androgen receptor CAG repeat polymorphism and X-chromosome inactivation in Australian Caucasian women with infertility related to polycystic ovary syndrome. *J Clin Endocrinol Metab* 2002; 87(1): 161–165.

36. Legro RS, Spielman R, Urbanek M, Driscoll D, Strauss JF, Dunaif A. Phenotype and genotype in polycystic ovary syndrome. *Recent Prog Horm Res* 1998; 53: 217–256.

37. Gharani N, Waterworth DM, Williamson R and Franks S. Polymorphism of the CYP17 gene is not associated with serum testosterone levels in women with polycystic ovaries. *J Clin Endocrinol Metab* 1996; 81: 4174–4180.

38. Gharani N, Waterworth D, Batty S, White D, Gilling-Smith C, Conway G et al. Association of the steroid synthesis gene CYP11a with polycystic ovary syndrome and hyperandrogenism. *Hum Mol Genet* 1997; 3: 397–402.

39. Urbanek M, Legro RS, Driscoll DA, Azziz R, Ehrmann DA, Norman RJ et al. Thirty-seven candidate genes for polycystic ovary syndrome: strongest evidence for linkage is with follistatin. *Proc Natl Acad Sci USA* 1999; 96: 8573–8578.

40. SanMillan JL, Sancho J, Calvo RM, Escobar-Morreale HF. Role of the pentanucleotide (tttta)n polymorphism in the promoter of the CYP11a gene in the pathogenesis of hirsutism. *Fertil Steril* 2001; 75: 797–802.

41. Wood JR, Nelson VL, Ho C, Jansen E, Wang CY, Urbanek M et al. The molecular phenotype of polycystic ovary syndrome (PCOS) theca cells and new candidate PCOS genes defined by microarray analysis. *J Biol Chem* 2003; 278: 26380–26390.

4

Prevalence and Characteristics of the Metabolic Syndrome in Women with Polycystic Ovary Syndrome

Ronit Machtinger, Daniel S Seidman

Summary

Polycystic Ovary Syndrome (PCOS) is a syndrome of ovarian dysfunction that most likely represents a heterogeneous disorder. Metabolic abnormalities as insulin resistance, dyslipidemia and other components of the metabolic syndrome have been reported at a higher frequency among women with polycystic ovaries (PCO). The metabolic syndrome is also associated with an increased risk of development of type 2 diabetes and cardiovascular disease.

This chapter summarizes the characters of the metabolic syndrome and its association with PCO.

Introduction

Polycystic Ovary Syndrome (PCOS) affects 4% to 10% of women of reproductive age.[1,2,3] This condition of hyperandrogenism and polycystic ovarian morphology, most likely represents a heterogeneous disorder whose etiology is unknown.

Although originally considered a gynecological disorder, the phenomenon is associated with a wide range of endocrine and metabolic abnormalities. PCOS may also be accompanied with insulin resistance and cardiovascular risk factors including obesity, hypertension, dyslipidemia, hyperhomocysteinemia, increased intima media thickness and impaired vascular elasticity.[4] The combination of hyperinsulinemia (frequently associated with acanthosis nigricans), obesity, dyslipidemia [decreased high-density lipoprotein cholesterol (HDL-C) and hypertriglyceridemia], hypertension, and artherosclerosis are components of the metabolic syndrome (MBS) (Table 4.1). The metabolic syndrome is also associated with an increased risk of development of type 2 diabetes and cardiovascular disease.[5]

Clinical Discussion

Prevalence

Apridonidze et al.[5] reported that the prevalence of MBS in women with PCOS was 43%, nearly

Table 4.1   Components of the metabolic syndrome.

Hyperinsulinemia (frequently associated with acanthosis nigricans)

Obesity

Dyslipidemia [decreased high-density lipoprotein (HDL) cholesterol and hypertriglyceridemia]

Hypertension

Atherosclerosis

Increased risk of development of type 2 diabetes and cardiovascular disease

2-fold higher than in age-matched women in the general population. In the 20 to 29-year-old group, women with PCOS had a nearly 8-fold greater prevalence of MBS than women in the general population (44.8 *vs.* 5.9%, respectively). Women with PCOS aged 30–39 years had a nearly 4-fold increased prevalence of the MBS compared with similarly aged women in the general population. In this study, the prevalence of MBS was found to increase with age from 23% of PCOS women less than 20 years old to 45% of women aged 20–29 years, and then to 53% of PCOS women aged 30–39 years, representing a significant trend ($P < 0.001$). Women with MBS had significantly higher body mass index (BMI) values and tended to present more often with hirsutism and acanthosis nigricans than those lacking this condition.

Similar results were reported by Glueck et al.[6] who compared the rates of metabolic syndrome among 138 women with PCOS versus a control group of 1887 women. Metabolic syndrome was found in 46% of the women with PCOS versus 22.8% of the control group (p < 0.0001). In these women with PCO and MBS, there were abnormalities in the waist circumference (98%), high-density lipoprotein cholesterol (HDL-C) (95%), blood pressure (70%), triglycerides (56%), and glucose (11%).

Sam et al.[7] examined the prevalence of MBS among sisters of patients with PCOS. The study included 385 sisters of women with PCOS with the following reproductive phenotypes: sisters with PCOS (n = 51), sisters with hyperandrogenemia (HA) and regular menses (n = 38), unaffected sisters (n = 143), and unknown phenotypes (n = 153). They were compared with 125 control women of comparable age, body mass index, and ethnicity to women with PCOS. The main outcome measures included lipid and lipoprotein levels and prevalence of the metabolic syndrome. Sisters with PCOS and HA phenotypes had higher total (P < or = 0.001) and low-density lipoprotein cholesterol levels (P < or = 0.01) compared with unaffected sisters and control women. Triglyceride levels were elevated only in sisters with the PCOS phenotype (P < 0.05).

The prevalence of MBS was increased in sisters with the PCOS (n = 29) and HA (n = 17) phenotypes compared with unaffected sisters (n = 85) (P < 0.001 and P < 0.05, respectively).

Cardiovascular disease and PCOS

Although cardiovascular risk factors are more prevalent in women with PCOS, definitive evidence for an increased incidence of cardiovascular disease is lacking. Echocardiography, imaging of coronary and carotid arteries and assessments of both endothelial function and arterial stiffness have recently been employed to address this question.[8]

A significant majority of women with PCOS have multiple cardiovascular (CV) risk factors (Table 4.2) associated with insulin resistance, hypertension, dyslipidemia and central obesity, which is present in the majority of women with PCOS.[9] Retrospective long-term outcome studies have failed to demonstrate increased CV mortality among PCOS patients compared with control populations.[10, 11] Some limitations of these studies include poor documentation of clinical CV events, and a relatively young age of women at follow up.[9]

Table 4.2 Cardiovascular risk factors associated with polycystic ovary syndrome.

Insulin resistance
Central obesity
Hypertension
Dyslipidemia
Hyperhomocysteinemia
Increased intima media thickness
Impaired vascular elasticity

Recently, some studies examined the relationship between early predictors for early cardiovascular disease and PCOS. Structural markers such as carotid intima-media thickness, and functional markers including pulse wave velocity and brachial artery flow-mediated vasodilation, have been examined to determine whether women with PCOS have evidence of sub-clinical CV disease, compared with controls. Two studies on the evaluation of carotid intima-media thickness have demonstrated an increase in carotid disease only in older women with PCOS,[12,13] whereas another study suggested early CV disease in women aged younger than 35 yr.[14]

Meyer et al.[9] postulated that overweight women with PCOS have increased cardiovascular risk factors and evidence of early CVD potentially related to insulin resistance compared with weight-matched controls.

Insulin resistance, type 2 diabetes mellitus and PCOS

Women with PCOS are at increased (3–7 times) risk of developing type 2 diabetes.[11,15–18] It was previously assumed that women with PCOS have profound insulin resistance independent of obesity,[15,16] that is secondary to a unique, apparently genetic disorder of insulin action.[19–23] Insulin resistance and pancreatic β-cell dysfunction are major risk factors for the development of type 2 diabetes mellitus.[24–26] These abnormalities are also found in PCOS.[27–29] PCOS women would thus be predicted to be at an increased risk for type 2 diabetes mellitus.[15]

Norman et al.[30] followed 67 women with PCOS (54 with normal glucose tolerance and 13 with impaired glucose tolerance) for a mean of 6.2 years. In those with normal glucose tolerance at baseline, 17% developed impaired glucose tolerance or type 2 diabetes mellitus over time, while 54% of those with impaired glucose tolerance at baseline had progressed to type 2 diabetes mellitus. Further support for the high prevalence of abnormal glucose tolerance in PCOS is the 10-fold increased risk of developing gestational diabetes mellitus compared to the general population (baseline risk ~3%).[31]

The role of insulin sensitizers for preventing or delaying the onset of type 2 diabetes mellitus in PCOS patients is still unclear. The Diabetes Prevention Program[32] examined the effect of metformin or lifestyle modifications compared to placebo in obese patients (68% of whom were women) with impaired glucose tolerance. Metformin resulted in a 31% reduction in the development of type 2 diabetes mellitus over 2.8 years versus placebo, while lifestyle modifications reduced the risk to a greater extent (58%).[32] If metformin is used for the prevention of type 2 diabetes mellitus, it is unclear how long it should be continued, as the risk is lifelong and the effectiveness of this agent wanes after it is discontinued.[33]

Conclusion

Women with PCOS are at increased risk (nearly 2 fold) for the development of metabolic syndrome. Insulin resistance, type 2 diabetes mellitus and gestational diabetes are increased by 3–10 fold among women with PCOS. Cardiovascular risk factors too are more prevalent in women with PCOS, but there is no definitive evidence for an increased incidence of cardiovascular disease is this population. Early diagnosis and management of these risk factors may postpone, or even prevent, the onset of type 2 diabetes mellitus and coronary artery disease.

References

1. Chang RJ. A practical approach to the diagnosis of polycystic ovary syndrome. *Am J Obstet Gynecol* 2004; 191(3): 713–717.
2. Farah L, Lazenby AJ, Boots LR. Prevalence of polycystic ovary syndrome in women seeking treatment from community electrologists. Alabama Professional Electrology Association Study Group. *J Reprod Med* 1999; 44: 870–874.
3. Knochenhauer ES, Key TJ, Kahsar-Miller M, Waggoner W, Boots LR, Azziz R. Prevalence of the polycystic ovary syndrome in unselected black and white women of the southeastern United States: a prospective study. *J Clin Endocrinol Metab* 1998; 83(9): 3078–3082.
4. Lakhani K, Prelevic GM, Seifalian AM, Atiomo WU, Hardiman P. Polycystic ovary syndrome, diabetes and cardiovascular disease: risks and risk factors. *J Obstet Gynaecol* 2004; 24(6): 613–621.
5. Apridonidze T, Essah PA, Iuorno MJ, Nestler JE. Prevalence and characteristics of the metabolic

syndrome in women with polycystic ovary syndrome. *J Clin Endocrinol Metab* 2005; 90(4): 1929–1935.

6. Glueck CJ, Papanna R, Wang P, Goldenberg N, Sieve-Smith L. Incidence and treatment of metabolic syndrome in newly referred women with confirmed polycystic ovarian syndrome. *Metabolism* 2003; 52(7): 908–915.

7. Sam S, Legro RS, Bentley-Lewis R, Dunaif A. Dyslipidemia and metabolic syndrome in the sisters of women with polycystic ovary syndrome. *J Clin Endocrinol Metab* 2005; 90(8): 4797–4802.

8. Cussons AJ, Stuckey BG, Watts GF. Cardiovascular disease in the polycystic ovary syndrome: new insights and perspectives. *Atherosclerosis* 2006; 185(2): 227–239.

9. Meyer C, McGrath BP, Teede HJ. Overweight women with polycystic ovary syndrome have evidence of subclinical cardiovascular disease. *J Clin Endocrinol Metab* 2005; 90(10): 5711–5716.

10. Pierpoint T, McKeigue P, Isaacs A, Wild S, Jacobs H. Mortality of women with polycystic ovary syndrome at long-term follow-up. *J Clin Epidemiol* 1998; 51: 581–586.

11. Wild S, Pierpoint T, McKeigue P, Jacobs H. Cardiovascular disease in women with polycystic ovary syndrome at long-term follow-up: a retrospective cohort study. *Clin Endocrinol (Oxf.)* 2000; 52: 595–600.

12. Guzick D, Talbott E, Sutton-Tyrrell K, Herzog A, Kuller L, Wolfson S. Carotid atherosclerosis in women with polycystic ovary syndrome: initial results from a case control study. *Am J Obstet Gynecol* 1996; 174: 1224–1232.

13. Talbott E, Guzick D, Sutton-Tyrrell K, McHugh-Pemu P, Zborowski J, Remsberg K. Evidence for the association between polycystic ovary syndrome and premature carotid atherosclerosis in middle-aged women. *Arterioscler Thromb Vasc Biol* 2000; 20: 2414–2421.

14. Lakhani K, Hardiman P, Seifalian A. Intima-media thickness of elastic and muscular arteries in young women with polycystic ovaries. *Arteriosclerosis* 2004; 175: 353–359.

15. Legro RS, Kunselman AR, Dodson WC, Dunaif A. Prevalence and predictors of risk for type 2 diabetes mellitus and impaired glucose tolerance in polycystic ovary syndrome: a prospective, controlled study in 254 affected women, *J Clin Endocrinol Metab* 1999; 84: 165–169.

16. Dunaif A, Graf M, Mandeli J, Laumas V and Dobrjansky A. Characterization of groups of hyperandrogenic women with acanthosis nigricans, impaired glucose tolerance, and/or hyperinsulinemia. *J Clin Endocrinol Metab* 1987; 65: 499–507.

17. Dahlgren E, Johansson S, Lindstedt G. Women with polycystic ovary syndrome wedge resected in 1956 to 1965: a long-term follow-up focusing on natural history and circulating hormones. *Fertil Steril* 1992; l57: 505–513.

18. Ehrmann DA, Barnes RB, Rosenfield RL, Cavaghan MK, Imperial J. Prevalence of impaired glucose tolerance and diabetes in women with polycystic ovary syndrome. *Diabetes Care* 1999; 22: 141–146.

19. Dunaif A, Segal KR, Shelley DR, Green G, Dobrjansky A, Licholai T. Evidence for distinctive and intrinsic defects in insulin action in polycystic ovary syndrome. *Diabetes* 1992; 41: 1257–1266.

20. Ciaraldi TP, el-Roeiy A, Madar Z, Reichart D, Olefsky JM, Yen SSC. Cellular mechanisms of insulin resistance in polycystic ovarian syndrome. *J Clin Endocrinol Metab* 1992; 75: 577–583.

21. Dunaif A, Xia J, Book CB, Schenker E, Tang Z. Excessive insulin receptor serine phosphorylation in cultured fibroblasts and in skeletal muscle. A potential mechanism for insulin resistance in the polycystic ovary syndrome. *J Clin Invest* 1995; 96: 801–810.

22. Dunaif A. Insulin resistance and polycystic ovary syndrome: mechanisms and implications for pathogenesis. *Endocr Rev* 1997; 18: 774–800.

23. Ek I, Arner P, Bergqvist A, Carlstrom K, Wahrenberg H. Impaired adipocyte lipolysis in nonobese women with the polycystic ovary syndrome: a possible link to insulin resistance? *J Clin Endocrinol Metab* 1997; 82: 1147–1153.

24. Warram JH, Martin BC, Krolewski AS, Soeldner JS, Kahn CR. Slow glucose removal rate and hyperinsulinemia precede the development of type II diabetes in the offspring of diabetic parents. *Ann Intern Med* 1990; 113: 909–915.

25. Reaven GM. Banting lecture. Role of insulin resistance in human disease. *Diabetes* 1988; 37: 1595–1607.

26. Lillioja S, Mott D, Spraul M, et al. Insulin resistance and insulin secretory dysfunction as precursors of non-insulin-dependent diabetes mellitus. *N Engl J Med* 1993; 329: 1988–1992.

27. O'Meara NM, Blackman JD, Ehrmann DA, et al. Defects in beta-cell function in functional ovarian hyperandrogenism. *J Clin Endocrinol Metab* 1993; 76: 1241–1247.

28. Ehrmann DA, Sturis J, Byrne MM, Karrison T, Rosenfield RL, Polonsky KS. Insulin secretory

defects in polycystic ovary syndrome. Relationship to insulin sensitivity and family history of non-insulin-dependent diabetes mellitus. *J Clin Invest* 1995; 96: 520–527.

29. Dunaif A, Finegood DT. Beta-cell dysfunction independent of obesity, and glucose intolerance in the polycystic ovary syndrome. *J Clin Endocrinol Metab* 1996; 81: 942–947.

30. Norman RJ, Masters L, Milner CR, Wang JX, Davies MJ. Relative risk of conversion from normoglycaemia to impaired glucose tolerance or non-insulin dependent diabetes mellitus in polycystic ovarian syndrome. *Hum Reprod* 2001; 16(9): 1995–1998.

31. Glueck CJ, Wang P, Kobayashi S, Phillips H, Sieve-Smith L. Metformin therapy throughout pregnancy reduces the development of gestational diabetes in women with polycystic ovary syndrome. *Fertil Steril* 2002; 77: 520–525.

32. Knowler WC, Barrett-Connor E, Fowler SE, Hamman RF, Lachin JM, Walker EA, Nathan DM; Diabetes Prevention Program Research Group. Reduction in the incidence of type 2 diabetes with lifestyle intervention or metformin. *N Engl J Med* 2002; 346: 393–403.

33. Sheehan MT. Polycystic ovarian syndrome: diagnosis and management. *Clin Med Res* 2004; 2(1): 13–27.

5

The Importance of Diagnosing Polycystic Ovary Syndrome

Richard Ajayi, Adegbite Ogunmokun

Summary

Irvin Stein and Michael Leventhal in 1935[1] described an association between the presence of polycystic ovaries and signs of hirsutism and menstrual irregularity (eg, oligomenorrhea amenorrhea). Subsequently, after successful wedge resection of the ovaries in women diagnosed with Stein-Leventhal syndrome, menstrual cycles became regular and these patients were able to conceive. Consequently, a primary ovarian defect was thought to be the main culprit, and the disorder came to be known as polycystic ovarian disease or Stein-Leventhal disease. Further biochemical, clinical, and endocrinologic studies revealed an array of underlying abnormalities; hence, the condition is now referred to as polycystic ovary syndrome (PCOS).

Although seventy years have passed since the first description of the syndrome, its definition and diagnostic criteria are still controversial. Several hormonal assays have been widely used to support the diagnosis and are essential for the exclusion of specific disorders that can cause polycystic ovaries.

The late consequences of PCOS such as risk of infertility, cardiovascular disease, insulin resistance, diabetes mellitus and endometrial cancer, warrant an early and effective diagnosis of the syndrome to provide a basis for follow-up and institution of measures to prevent dangerous sequelae.

Rationale

Polycystic ovary syndrome is a heterogeneous disorder, varying from one extreme of classical symptoms of oligomenorrhea, hirsutism and obesity to the other extreme of complete absence of symptoms with only incidental findings of polycystic ovaries diagnosed on ultrasound scan or during laparoscopy.[2] Heterogeneity of the clinical and endocrine features has long been a confounding factor in the definition and investigation of PCOS. The condition onsets in the perimenarchal years, with young women of reproductive age most frequently seeking medical attention because of irregular menses, acne and hirsutism, but PCOS has a long prodrome with detectable abnormalities throughout the life cycle of affected women.[3] The condition is considered progressive with an increasing severity of symptoms and the onset of new clinical problems such as infertility, obesity, abnormal serum lipid levels, hyperinsulinemia, cardiovascular problems, endometrial hyperplasia or carcinoma as the years go by. The importance of early and clear diagnosis can therefore, not be overemphasised, so that a close watch is instituted as early as a diagnosis is made. This could prevent if possible, or recognise, the onset of complications early, so that their effects can be minimized by appropriate interventions.

Introduction

Polycystic ovary syndrome is one of the most common endocrinopathies in women of reproductive age, with wide range of clinical symptoms. According to the initial description of Stein and Leventhal 1935,[1] the diagnosis was based on the clinical features of oligo/amenorrhea, infertility, hirsutism and obesity in the presence of histologically verified polycystic ovaries (PCO) With the use of ultrasound scan nowadays, it is a lot easier to recognize PCO and this has been found to correlate well with histological findings.[4,5]

When any anovulatory state exists for a period of time, the ovaries tend to become polycystic.[6] However, 80–100% of women with PCOS have polycystic ovaries, which are defined as the presence of 10 or more small (2–8 mm) follicles scattered either around an echo dense thickened central stroma in each ovary giving the so called pearl necklace pattern on an ultrasound scan. Polycystic ovaries can also be present in other causes of androgen excess and in approximately 20–25% of regularly ovulating healthy women.[7,8]

There are many abnormalities, which may collectively produce the findings, which characterise PCOS as originally described, thereby leading to problems in diagnosis. In 1990, the National Institute of Health (NIH) proposed new diagnostic criteria for this disorder – hyper-androgenism and chronic anovulation, excluding other causes such as adult-onset congenital adrenal hyperplasia, hyperprolactinemia and androgen-secreting neoplasm.[9] Some authors believe that it is far more useful clinically to avoid the use of eponyms and even the term polycystic ovary syndrome or disease, and that it is better to consider this problem as one of persistent anovulation with a spectrum of etiologies and clinical manifestations that now include insulin resistance and hyperinsulinemia, as well as hyperandrogenism, of course excluding extragonadal androgen sources.[10] The baseline endocrinological and biochemical abnormalities are actually the determinants of the extent of the clinical manifestations.

Clinical Discussion

The importance of diagnosing PCOS can be examined with the following in mind. Firstly, it gives an opportunity to offer an explanation for the variety of seemingly unrelated symptoms a woman might present with. The three main symptoms that a woman with PCOS may present with include menstrual irregularities, infertility and symptoms associated with androgen excess like hirsutism, male pattern balding, and acne. Other symptoms include obesity, skin lesions like acanthosis nigricans, insulin resistance and type 2 diabetes mellitus.[3] Though patients may experience these symptoms to varying degrees, they are often severe enough to cause concern to the individual. Hence, arriving at a diagnosis that relate the symptoms to a clinical condition is bound to provide some comfort to the patient and make treatment decisions rational.

Also, a knowledge of the diagnosis would mean that all other medical conditions e.g. adrenal or ovarian androgen – secreting tumours, in which there is rapid progression of virilizing symptoms, and that may present in like manner with more sinister implications, have been ruled out.

A firm and convincing diagnosis will offer basis for counseling about the prognosis and allay fears. For example, cosmetic alterations of some PCOS symptoms like acne, excessive body hair, and unsightly raised black skin lesions like acanthosis nigricans, may affect body image and self esteem and can result in depression and withdrawal from social and career pursuits[3] with far reaching consequences, especially in adolescent girls. Education, support, counseling and early treatment may help young women cope with the physical and psychological aspects of PCOS.

PCOS is, in some cases, a familial disorder, but the genetic basis of the syndrome remains unclear. One study revealed evidence of an autosomal dominant mode of inheritance.[11,12] Full expression of the syndrome may require an insulin abnormality and a defect in androgen biosynthesis but no gene(s) has been identified. It has been reported that 40% of the sisters and 20% of the mothers of affected women have the syndrome to varying degrees.[13] In the light of this, once a family member has been diagnosed as having PCOS, there is a need to screen the other female members of the family in order to pick up other cases at the earliest stage.

Accurate diagnosis of PCOS also affords an institution of appropriate treatment. Because the primary cause of polycystic ovary syndrome is unknown, treatment is presently directed at the symptoms of the disorder. Few treatment approaches improve all aspects of the syndrome, and the patient's desire for fertility may preclude treatment despite the presence of symptoms.

Treatment goals should include maintaining a normal endometrium, antagonizing the actions of androgens on target tissues, reducing insulin resistance (when present) and correcting anovulation. The patient's desire for fertility is an important consideration because the available treatments, particularly those used to induce ovulation, have their own complications. Treatment, most of the time, is individualized based on symptoms, age, desirability or otherwise of pregnancy and the degree of androgen excess. Treatment is not aimed at providing a cure but at alleviating the symptoms. For example, the use of oral contraceptive pills (OCPs) is advocated in cycle control and alleviation of the features of androgen excess like acne and hirsutism.[3] For patients desiring conception, OCP is obviously not appropriate. Therefore, a multidisciplinary, co-operative approach is essential, considering the heterogeneous nature of the clinical presentation. Hence, referral to appropriate centers and specialists, depending on the presentation, is paramount in the management of PCOS. There may be a need for referral to dermatologists, diabetologists and assisted reproduction practitioners.

Women with PCOS are frequently referred for assisted conception treatment, either because of intractable anovulatory problems, or failure to conceive because of some other infertility factors. For infertility management, the diagnosis of PCOS imposes certain conditions on the practitioners to limit the possible complications thus presenting a distinct therapeutic challenge.

Induction of ovulation with clomiphene citrate will result in ovulation in 50–60% of cases, with a 20% risk of multiple gestation.[13] For patients who will require assisted reproduction following stimulation with gonadotropins, the specific risk of ovarian hyperstimulation syndrome (OHSS) with the drug regimen should be borne in mind and the patient closely monitored during treatment.[14] The response to gonadotrophin stimulation in women with PCOS often differs significantly from the norm, frequently exhibiting an initial slow response, followed by an 'explosive' development of a large numbers of follicles. In vitro fertilization (IVF) stimulation protocols should therefore, specifically address concerns surrounding polycystic ovaries.[14] Additional strategies might include early thresholds for coasting, as well as cryopreservation of all the embryos for future transfer in selected cases.

In vitro oocyte maturation (IVM) is a recent addition to assisted conception treatment and will be of great application in treating cases with PCOS as it will prevent the development of ovarian OHSS. In PCOS, it is thought that whilst the initial steps of folliculogenesis may be functional, the selection of a dominant follicle for ovulation does not always occur. The approach in IVM is either to minimally stimulate the patients with gonadotropins and then carry out egg retrieval before the follicles reach 14 mm diameter, or to carry out egg retrieval in non-stimulated cycles. Thereafter, the immature oocytes are cultured to maturity with special media for either conventional IVF or intracytoplasmic sperm injection (ICSI). Thus, the risk of OHSS is obviated.

There is evidence to suggest that a high luteinizing hormone (LH) level in PCOS patients is accompanied with reduced fertilization rates and increased miscarriage rates.[15] The pathogenic mechanism of this complication remains controversial, but it has been observed that there are a high percentage of immature forms with resultant poor egg quality among oocytes obtained following gonadotropin administration in PCOS patients.[16] These facts are essential in counseling patients with PCOS.

A firm diagnosis of PCOS also provides a basis for long-term follow-up in order to prevent or recognize early, the development of complications.

For example, approximately 25 to 30 percent of these women show impaired glucose tolerance by the age of 30, and 8 percent of the women with PCOS develop frank type 2 diabetes mellitus annually.[17]

Markers of premature coronary artery and cardiovascular disease are prevalent. Women with polycystic ovaries are observed to have more extensive coronary artery disease by angiography.[18] In two case-control studies, women in their forties had greater intima-media thickness of the carotid vessels and more atherogenic lipid profiles: increased total and low-density lipoprotein (LDL) cholesterol and triglyceride levels, and decreased high-density lipoprotein (HDL) cholesterol levels.[19–21]

Untreated polycystic ovary syndrome may be regarded as a disorder that progresses until the time of menopause and because of the increased risk for the development of cardiovascular disease and associated lipid abnormalities, affected women could benefit from measures to prevent cardiovascular disease and the other sequelae of long-standing hypertension and diabetes mellitus that are associated with the syndrome. All obese women with PCOS should be screened for abnormal glucose metabolism and dyslipidemia. The fasting lipoprotein profile should include total cholesterol, LDL cholesterol, HDL cholesterol and triglyceride measurements.[22] Advice on lifestyle modifications in the form of dietary control and exercise, leading to improvement in cardiovascular risks and insulin sensitivity, is mandatory.[3]

More importantly, the long-term effects of unopposed estrogen, place women with the syndrome at considerable risk for endometrial cancer, endometrial hyperplasia, and perhaps, breast cancer. The risk of endometrial cancer is three times higher in women with polycystic ovary syndrome than in normal women. In addition, small observational studies have suggested that chronic anovulation during the reproductive years is associated with a three to four times increased risk of breast cancer in the postmenopausal years.[23,24] Although there is no evidence that outcomes are improved, mammography and endometrial sampling to search for underlying estrogen-stimulated cancer should be considered in high-risk women with dysfunctional uterine bleeding.[25]

Conclusion

Knowledge gained over the past seventy years has carried PCOS beyond the realm of gynecology and infertility, and warrants heightened attention from physicians who will focus on the functional abnormalities that have serious long-term consequences. It is important to recognize that PCOS is an entity with a long lifespan, requiring "control" rather than "cure," and that therapies will change with the stage of life. A considerable armamentarium of therapies exists for the clinician using specialty referral for patients with PCOS.

References

1. Stein IL and Leventhal ML. Amenorrhea associated with bilateral polycystic ovaries. *Am J Obstet Gynecol* 1935; 29: 181–191.
2. Basu S, Amos N, Bhaumik J. Polycystic ovary syndrome: genetics and health consequences. In: Allahbadia GN, Das RB, Merchant R. editors. The Art and Science of Assisted Reproductive Techniques (ART). New Delhi: *Jaypee Brothers Medical Publishers* 2003: 154–161.
3. Richardson MR. Current perspectives in polycystic ovary syndrome. *J Am Fam Physician* 2003; 68(4): 697–704.
4. Saxton DW, Farquhar CM, Rae T, Beard RW, Anderson MC, Wadsworth J. Accuracy of Ultrasound measurement of female pelvic organs. *Br J Obstet Gynecol* 1990; 97: 695–699.
5. Takahashi K, Eda Y, Okada S, Abu-Musa A, Yoshino K, Kitao M. Morphological assessment of polycystic ovaraies using transvaginal ultrasound. *Human Reprod* 1993; 6: 844–849.
6. Mellisa H, Hunter and James J, Sterreh, Pharm D. Polysystic ovary syndrome. Its not just infertility. *J Am Fam Physicians* 2000; 62: 1679–1688.
7. Polson DW, Adams J, Wadsworth J, Franks S.

Polycystic ovaries – a common finding in normal women. *Lancet* 1988; 1 (8590): 870–872.

8. Clayton RN, Ogden V, Hodgkinson J, Worswick L, Rodin DA, Dyer S. et al. How common are polycystic ovaries in normal women and what is their significance for the fertility of the population? *Clin Endocrinol* 1992; 37: 127–134.

9. Zawadiki JK, Dunaif A. Diagnostic criteria for polycystic ovary syndrome: towards a rational approach. In Dunaif A, Givens JR, Haseltime FP, Merriam GR eds, Polycystic Ovary Syndrome. Oxford, England. *Blackwell Scientific* 1992: 377–384.

10. Sperof L and Fritz M.A – Anovulation and the polycystic ovary. In: Clinical Gynaecologic Endocrinology and Infertility 7th Edition. *Pub Lippincott Williams & Wilkings* USA, 2004: 465–498.

11. Cooper HE, Spellacy NN, Prem KA, Cohen WD. Hereditary factors in the Stein Leventhal syndrome. *Am J Obstet Gynecol* 1968; 100: 371–387.

12. Givens JR. Familial polycystic ovarian disease. *Endocrinol Metab Clin North Am* 1988; 17(4): 771–783.

13. Legro RS, Driscoll D, Strauss JF, Fox J, Dunaif A. Evidence for a genetic basis for hyperandrogenaemia in polycystic ovary syndrome. *Proc Natl Acad Sci* (USA) 1998; 95: 14956–14960.

14. Wang CG, Gemzell C. The use of human gonadotrophins for the induction of ovulation in women with polycystic ovarian disease. *Fertil Steril* 1980; 33: 479–486.

15. Nani JM. (2004) Polycystic Ovary Syndrome (PCOS): An update. In : Allhbadia GN, Das RB, Merchant R. editors. The Art and Science of Assisted Reproductive Techniques (ART). New Delhi: Jaypee Brothers Medical Publishers, 2003: 145–151.

16. Vollenhoven B, Clark S, Kovacs G, Burger H, Healy D. Prevalence of gestational diabetes mellitus in polycystic ovarian syndrome (PCOS) patients pregnant after ovulation induction with gonadotrophins. *Aust N Z J Obstet Gynaecol* 2000; 40 (1): 54–58.

17. Legro RS, Kinselman AR, Dodson WC, Dunarf A. Prevalence and predictors of risk for type 2 diabetes mellitus and impaired glucose tolerance in polycystic ovary syndrome: a prospective, controlled study in 254 affected women. *J. Clin Endocrinol Metab* 1999; 84: 165–169.

18. Birdsall MA, Farquhar CM, White HD. Association between polycystic ovaries and extent of coronary artery disease in women having cardiac catheterization. *Ann Intern Med* 1997; 126 (1): 32–35.

19. Guzick DS, Talbott EO, Sutton-Tyrrell K, Herzog HC, Kuller LH, Wolfson SK Jr. Carotid atherosclerosis in women with polycystic ovary syndrome: initial results from a case-control study. *Am J Obstet Gynecol* 1996 Apr; 174(4): 1224–1229.

20. Talbott E, Clerici A, Berga SL, Kuller L, Guzick D, Detre K, Daniels T, Engberg RA. Adverse lipid and coronary heart disease risk profiles in young women with polycystic ovary syndrome: results of a case-control study. *J Clin Epidemiol* 1998 May; 51(5): 415–422.

21. Cibula D, Cifkova R, Fanta M, Poledne R, Zivny J, Skibova J. Increased risk of non-insulin dependent diabetes mellitus, arterial hypertension and coronary artery disease in perimenopausal women with a history of the polycystic ovary syndrome. *Hum Reprod* 2000; 15(4): 785–789.

22. Barret M Schroeder. Practice Guidelines- ACOG releases guidelines on diagnoses and management of polycystic ovary syndrome. *J Am Acad of Fam Phy* 2003; 67(7).

23. Coulam CB, Annegers JF, Kranz JS. Chronic anovulation syndrome and associated neoplasia. *Obstet Gynecol* 1983; 61(4): 403–407.

24. Ron E, Lunenfeld B, Menczer J, Blumstein T, Katz L, Oelsner G et al. Cancer incidence in a cohort of infertile women. *Am J Epidemiol* 1987; 125: 780–790.

25. Wild RA. Hyperandrogenism: Implications for cardiovascular endometrial and breast disease. In: Adashi EY, Rock J.A, Rosenwaks Z. editors Reproductive Endocrinology Surgery and Technology. Philadephia: Lipincott-Ravens 1996; 1617.

Frequently Asked Questions

1. What is PCOS?

Polycystic ovary syndrome (PCOS), also known clinically as Stein-Leventhal syndrome, is an endocrine disorder that affects 5–10% of women. It occurs among all races and nationalities, is the most common hormonal disorder among women of reproductive age, and is a leading cause of infertility. The symptoms and severity of the syndrome vary greatly between women. While the causes are unknown, insulin resistance (often secondary to obesity) is heavily correlated with PCOS.

2. Why do women with PCOS have trouble with their menstrual cycle?

In women with PCOS, the ovary does not make all of the hormones it needs for any of the eggs to fully mature. They may start to grow and accumulate fluid but no one egg becomes large enough. Instead, some may remain as cysts. Since no egg matures and ovulation does not occur, the hormone progesterone is not made. Without progesterone, a woman's menstrual cycle is irregular or absent. Also, the cysts produce male hormones, which continue to prevent ovulation.

3. What is the role of weight reduction in PCOS management?

Weight reduction, which may be very difficult, is also very important. For those with polycystic ovaries who are overweight, weight loss can reduce insulin resistance, stimulate ovulation, and improve fertility rates. Insulin sensitizing medication like metformin may sometimes be effective in treating polycystic ovaries.

4. Why are estrogen levels normal in PCOS?

In normally fertile women, estrogen is made from the follicles. In this case, however, high insulin stimulates excess androgen production and the body converts the androgen into estrogen. In obese women, estrogen will also be stored in fat cells.

This constant estrogen level confuses the hypothalamus, which assumes that high estrogen levels are present because of a developing egg inside the follicle. The hypothalamus then sends signals to the pituitary to slow down the release of FSH. Without FSH, follicles fail to mature and rupture and hence, no ovulation.

5. Who is at risk for PCOS?

PCOS is hereditary and is more common among women of Mediterranean descent. It is also uncommon to develop PCOS later in life, although it can happen. Generally, a PCOS woman will begin to experience menstrual irregularities within 3-4 years after her menarche (first period). Women who are obese can be predisposed to PCOS because their fatty tissues produce estrogen, which can confuse the pituitary gland. Women who are diabetic, or who have a problem with their adrenal glands, thyroid gland, or pituitary gland, can develop symptoms of PCOS, but technically not have the condition. In some cases, PCO may coincide with these conditions.

6. What is the role of insulin in PCOS

It has recently been discovered that insulin resistance and polycystic ovary syndrome go hand-in-hand. Women with insulin resistance are either at risk for, or have been diagnosed with type 2 diabetes. Lowering insulin in women with polycystic ovary syndrome seems to help restore menstrual cycles and lower male hormone levels. Oral hypoglycemic agents used to treat type 2 diabetes are now being used to treat PCOS. Only about half the women diagnosed with PCO have insulin resistance, which means that the body does not respond properly to the insulin produced by the pancreas and therefore, insulin accumulates in the bloodstream resulting in hyperinsulinemia. In PCOS, hyperinsulinemia contributes to excess androgen production within the ovary, which causes follicular wasting and anovulation. The elevated androgen also contributes to common symptoms of PCOS like acne and hirsutism and male pattern body hair growth. Diet and exercise also help the body use insulin more efficiently and are therefore, important in the treatment of PCOS.

7. What is the origin of cysts in PCOS

First, women with PCOS usually have an increase in LH secretion from the pituitary. An elevated LH level promotes secretion of androgens from the ovaries. In turn, the increased androgen production causes wasting of the developing ovarian follicles and interferes with the production of a dominant follicle. Normally, an egg is released from the dominant follicle, but in PCOS, the follicles do not mature properly and instead, develop into ovarian cysts.

8. What are the long-term effects of the disease?

The long-term effects of polycystic ovary syndrome depend on the woman's condition and her response to treatment, but they may include:

- endometrial hyperplasia, or a build-up of cells that line the uterus, which increases her risk for cancer of the uterus
- heart disease, hypertension, ischaemic heart disease
- infertility
- insulin resistance, which can contribute to obesity and diabetes

9. What are the current treatment modalities for PCOS

Treatment of polycystic ovary syndrome has two distinct directions. Patients not desiring pregnancy at the time of treatment will be managed differently compared to patients actively seeking pregnancy.

For patients desiring pregnancy, there are several approaches. The more modern approach in younger patients involves the use of insulin sensitizing agents. These medications allow for a better response to the insulin in the circulation. Very frequently, the manifestations of PCOS will resolve. Many women begin to ovulate with a return of normal menses. Many clinics have been successful at achieving pregnancy by using insulin-sensitizing agents alone. These drugs are discontinued after achieving pregnancy. In some patients, ovulation induction using Clomid and subsequently gonadotropins may be required, however, because of the risk of ovarian hyperstimulation and multiple gestation associated with controlled ovarian hyperstimulation (COH), this approach is used as a secondary treatment.

Patients not seeking pregnancy are generally treated with oral contraceptive pills, which allow the endometrium to cycle normally (reducing the risks of endometrial cancer and hyperplasia), reduce acne, and reduce hair growth. Additional therapy may be required to decrease the androgenic effects of PCOS. Such agents include Finasteride (Proscar, Propecia), Reglan, and Spironolactone. Current trends to treat these patients with insulin sensitizing agents are gaining more popularity.

Insulin sensitizing agents include metformin (Glucophage) and rosiglitazone (Avandia).

Ovarian drilling can be performed at the time of laparoscopy. A laser fibre or electrosurgical needle is used to puncture the ovary 10–12 times. This treatment results in a dramatic lowering of male hormones within days. Studies have shown that up to 80% will benefit from such treatment. Many who failed to ovulate with letrozole or metformin therapy, will respond when rechallenged with these medications after ovarian drilling. The procedure may result in adhesion formation or ovarian failure if an inexperienced surgeon performs the procedure.

10. Does polycystic ovary syndrome (PCOS) change at menopause?

Researchers are looking at how male hormone levels change as women with PCOS grow older. They think that as women reach menopause, ovarian function changes and the menstrual cycle may become more normal. But even with falling male hormone levels, excessive hair growth continues, and male pattern baldness or thinning hair gets worse after menopause.

11. How does polycystic ovary syndrome (PCOS) affect a woman during pregnancy?

There appears to be a higher rate of miscarriage, gestational diabetes, pregnancy-induced high blood pressure, and premature delivery in women with PCOS. Researchers are studying how the medicine metformin prevents or reduces the chances of having these problems during pregnancy, in addition to looking at how the drug lowers male hormone levels and limits weight gain in women who are obese when they get pregnant.

6

Current Recommendations for the Follow-up of Patients Presenting with Symptomatic Polycystic Ovary Syndrome

Evanthia Diamanti-Kandarakis, Richard S Legro

Summary

Polycystic Ovary Syndrome (PCOS) is a common endocrine disorder with a variable clinical presentation. It is associated with cosmetic, reproductive and long-term metabolic abnormalities. Management of women with PCOS is a great challenge for clinical specialists, since the lack of a single clinical presentation is reflected on the lack of a single therapeutic approach. In this article, the main medical therapeutic options are presented. Lifestyle modification and weight reduction are the first steps of the therapeutic strategies used to modify the majority of the components of PCOS. Oral contraceptives and antiandrogens can treat the main classical symptoms like irregular menstrual bleeding, hirsutism and acne. Insulin sensitizing agents are discussed in detail for their beneficial effects on the reproductive and metabolic aspects and for their potential long-term ameliorating effect on cardiovascular dysfunction. However, due to the lack of large randomized controlled trials, their potential efficacy should be evaluated in long-term studies.

Introduction

Polycystic ovary syndrome (PCOS) is the most common reproductive endocrine disorder and the most frequent cause of chronic anovulation. It affects 5–10% of women of reproductive age.[1] It is often associated with a specific insulin resistance with consequent important metabolic abnormalities. This suggests that it is not only a reproductive disorder but also a metabolic one with long-term health consequences. This chapter will discuss the treatment of women with PCOS and will consider both, short term and long-term consequences of the syndrome.

Clinical Discussion

Lifestyle modification and obesity management

Whatever the priority in the mind or the body of a woman with PCOS, the first step should always include lifestyle modification and body weight normalization (Figure 6.1). Thirty to eighty per cent of women with PCOS are obese and overweight, which is associated with visceral adiposity as reflected by an increased waist circumference or waist to hip ratio. Increased intra-abdominal fat is found even in normal weight PCOS women. Studies indicate that changes in the lifestyle could improve insulin resistance, which in turn can prevent the development of diabetes in high-risk individuals without PCOS. Physical activity and especially weight loss, can reduce the incidence of type 2 diabetes by 58%, demonstrating a greater impact compared with the 31% reduction following metformin treatment.[3]

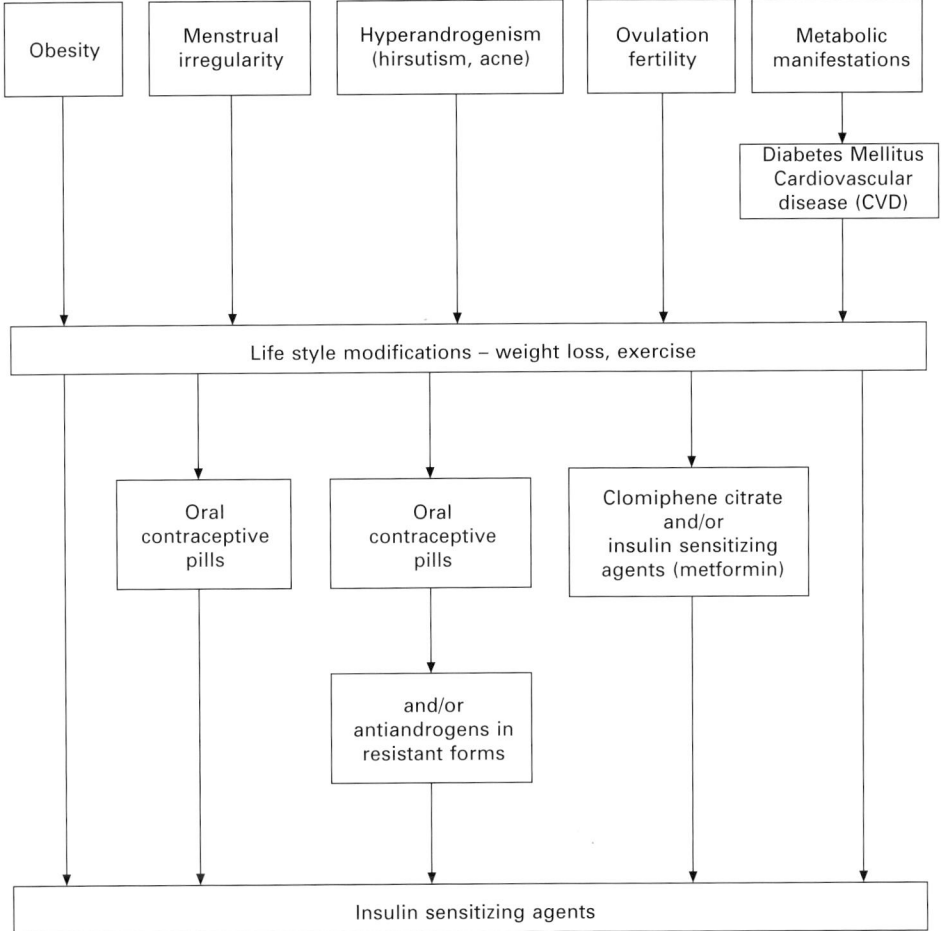

Figure 6.1   Management for PCOS women.

Therefore, the best initial management for overweight PCOS women is weight loss through lifestyle modification. Even when weight loss is modest, there is a significant reduction in visceral fat that improves metabolic alterations. Dietary modification, consisting of a hypocaloric diet (with ~500 kcal deficit per day), should be accompanied with moderate exercise (30 min day), reduction of psychosocial stressors, cessation of smoking and reduction of alcohol and caffeine consumption. Pharmacological treatments, including insulin-sensitizing agents, should be adopted as a second option reserved for women in whom weight loss was not successful. Weight loss has been shown to

improve both clinical and metabolic parameters in PCOS women.[4] Moreover, exercise by itself, such as regular walking, has been reported to reduce waist to hip ratio and homocysteine levels in overweight PCOS women.[5]

Long-term studies on lifestyle modification indicated improvement in fertility with modest weight loss (5–10% of the initial body weight). It has been shown that the combination of diet and exercise, restores ovulation in 23.8% of the women, increases pregnancy rates in 77.6% of the women and reduces miscarriage rates in 18% of the women compared to 75% in previously anovulatory women, within 6 months of weight reduction.[6] Recently, it has been reported that weight loss, whether with lifestyle modification or metformin therapy, might play the most significant role in restoring ovulation.[7] Lifestyle modification also improves psychological parameters including self-esteem, anxiety and mean depression scores in obese PCOS women.[8] Therefore, lifestyle changes should be the first aim in the management of obese PCOS women to improve their reproductive dysfunction, their metabolic disorders and their long-term metabolic health.

Apart from diet, a combination with pharmacological treatment, with metformin, or with weight reducing agents, has been used when required for further weight reduction. It has been reported that the combination of a low calorie diet with metformin treatment induced a greater reduction in body weight and visceral obesity in women with PCOS compared with a low calorie diet and placebo treatment.[9] Weight reducing agents have been shown to increase the effect of lifestyle modification in reducing the incidence of type 2 diabetes mellitus (T2DM) in obese patients,[10] and similar effects have been noted in women with PCOS. Sibutramine treatment alone, and in combination with ethinyl estradiol and cyproterone acetate in obese women with PCOS has been found to have positive effects on clinical and metabolic risk factors for cardiovascular disease (decrease in waist to hip ratio, blood pressure, triglycerides and insulin levels).[11] Furthermore, orlistat treatment in obese women with PCOS, induced a more significant weight reduction than metformin treatment. It also induced a reduction in testosterone levels, consistent with the reduction in testosterone levels in overweight women with PCOS after weight loss by dietary changes and exercise.[12] However, it is difficult to assess the long-term clinical efficiency of the medications because the literature is rather inconclusive (small number of patients and short-term studies).

Oral contraceptive pills

Combination oral contraceptive pills (OCPs) are the most common treatment for menstrual abnormalities and skin manifestations (hirsutism and acne) in PCOS women. They are used for symptomatic therapy, since they suppress androgen production. The progestin component of OCP primarily suppresses the circulating luteinizing hormone (LH) surge, leading to a decrease in ovarian androgen production. It also antagonizes to varying degrees, the 5 alpha-reductase and androgen receptor. The estrogen component stimulates hepatic sex hormone-binding globulin (SHBG) production, reducing the free fraction of testosterone levels. OCPs may also decrease adrenal androgen production by a negative feedback through the glucocorticoid receptor. It is theoretically preferable to select preparations containing a low dose of estrogen (<35 μg ethinyl estradiol) and a non-androgenic progestin, such as norgestimate, desogestrel or gestodene, or one with an anti-androgenic profile. Two progestins that meet this latter requirement are cyproterone acetate (CA) and drospirenone. Both these chemically related substances have antimineralocorticoid and antiandrogenic activity and when used in combination with ethinyl estradiol in an OCP, have shown beneficial effects in hyperandrogenic women.[13,14]

In conclusion, treatment with OCPs is an excellent choice for young women who do not desire to become pregnant and who do not have contra-indications to the pill (age, smoking, hypertension, vascular disease, etc.). The most important beneficial effects are the regulation of menstrual cycle, prevention of the development of endometrial carcinoma and the amelioration of moderate symptoms of androgen excess (acne, seborrhea and hirsutism). Disadvantages of the treatment may include the absence of improvement in the metabolic disorders of the syndrome, such as insulin sensitivity and glucose tolerance, and the reappearance of skin androgenic manifestations after discontinuation of treatment.

Antiandrogens

Women with PCOS who have severe hirsutism and acne, need additional treatment with antiandrogens, which block peripheral androgen action, since the suppression of androgen production with OCPs alone is usually modest. They are either androgen receptor blockers or 5-alpha-reductase inhibitors. In general, the degree of improvement depends more on the intrinsic sensitivity of hirsutism to the androgen block than on the dose or the particular antiandrogen used. Due to an increased risk of feminization of the male fetus, antiandrogens should be used with adequate contraception in women desiring pregnancy. The most broadly used substances are cyproterone acetate and spironolactone, whereas flutamide and finasteride are potent antiandrogens that can be used in certain resistant cases with appropriate contraception.

Cyproterone acetate (CA) is a potent progestin available in Europe and Canada, but not in the United States, as an OCP (2 mg CA and 35 μg ethinyl estradiol), or alone as a 10 mg and 50 mg tablet. It improves hirsutism and acne. Although the OCP with 2 mg CA is used and is effective in some women, usually greater doses, at least initially, are required to treat significant hirsutism. Side effects may include weight gain, edema, irregular uterine bleeding and rarely transient hepatotoxicity.

Spironolactone is an aldosterone antagonist used to treat hypertension. It also possesses moderate antiandrogenic properties when given in doses of 100–200 mg/day. Its effectiveness is related to the administrated dose. When women are severely hirsute or obese, a higher dose is needed in comparison with lean hirsute women.[15] It has been proposed to start with a dose of 25 or 50 mg twice a day with a progressive increment in the dose if there is no improvement. The most effective dose has been shown to be 200 mg/day for 3–6 months followed by progressively decreased doses (25–50 mg/day) to maintain the clinical results. In a recent meta-analysis, 100 mg spironolactone was found to be more effective in reducing hirsutism than 5 mg finasteride and 12.5 mg CA.[16] The most common side effects are menstrual irregularity due to progestin – like properties of the drug, polyurea and fatigue. Hyperkaliemia may rarely develop in patients who have been on a potassium-saving diuretic. In general, spironolactone should be used in combination with an OCP in an attempt to control abnormal uterine bleeding and to potentiate its antiandrogenic effect.

Flutamide is a potent nonsteroidal antiandrogen, widely used in the treatment of prostate cancer. It is also effectively used in the treatment of hirsutism. It seems that it reduces hair diameter more quickly than other antiandrogens. At the metabolic level, it improves the lipid profile reducing total and LDL cholesterol levels. However, whether it improves insulin resistance is still under debate.[17] It is effective in doses of 500 mg/day. Recent studies, investigating lower doses of 250 mg, 125 mg or even 62.5 mg, reported the same efficacy in reducing hirsutism as with the greater one, and with decreased side effects and cost.[18] In comparative studies, a dose of 250 mg for 6 months was more, or as effective as 100 mg/day-spironolactone treatment.[19] However, patients with more severe hyperandrogenism that includes alopecia, may respond better to flutamide than to spironolactone.[20] Side effects are mild and include the appearance of greenish urine, skin dryness, and liver enzyme abnormalities. Rarely, its use has caused fatal hepatocellular toxicity. Because of its potential hepatotoxicity, it should be given in the lowest therapeutic dose and liver transaminases should be monitored.

Finasteride is a potent inhibitor of skin 5 alpha-reductase, the enzyme that converts testosterone in dihydrotestosterone, the active androgen in the hair follicle. It is used in the treatment of benign prostate hypertrophy, while in lower doses, it is used in the treatment of male pattern baldness. Finasteride inhibits both type 1 and type 2 isoenzymes of 5 alpha-reductase, but its potency for skin manifestations is limited because it is less active against type 1 enzyme, which is the prominent isoenzyme in the pilosebaceous unit.

Finasteride is also effectively used in doses of 5 mg/day for the treatment of hirsutism in women.[21] Recently, it was found that the use of a low dose of 2.5 mg/day has an equivalent effect to the standard dose in improving hirsutism after 6 and 12 months treatment.[22] Nevertheless, it seems that it is somewhat less effective than the androgen receptor blockers. Finasteride has fewer side effects than other antiandrogens although feminization of a male fetus is a concern since type 2-5 alpha-reductase is responsible for masculinization. Therefore, finasteride might not be the most appropriate treatment for skin manifestations in PCOS women.

In conclusion, antiandrogens, despite different modalities of action and different effects on androgen levels, constitute a satisfactory alternative therapy for enhancing the clinical result of hyperandrogenism. There is some evidence of more pronounced improvement in skin manifestations using flutamide in low doses, or CA-estrogen combinations. Furthermore, although more investigation is needed, flutamide seems to have an additional beneficial effect on the lipid profile, body composition and metabolic parameters. Various combinations of antiandrogens with OCPs and sensitizing drugs have been used in order to decrease the prescribed doses and side effects and to increase the desired result.

GnRH analogues

Another option to suppress ovarian androgen production and to improve hirsutism is treatment with long-acting gonadotropin releasing hormone (GnRH) analogues. The administration of a GnRH agonist, by providing constant GnRH levels, reduces pituitary gonadotropin secretion and thereby, decreases ovarian estrogen and androgen secretion. However, add-back therapy with estrogen-progestin replacement or better, OCPs should be given to avoid vasomotor symptoms and loss of bone mineral density from estrogen deficiency. Given the serious side effects, such as hypoestrogenism and the high cost, this therapy is not widely used. Probably, it may be beneficial in severe forms of PCOS with ovarian hyperandrogenism, which do not respond to OCPs and antiandrogens.

Insulin sensitizing agents

It is well established that women with PCOS have metabolic abnormalities and are at an increased risk of cardiovascular disease (CVD) over time. Hyperinsulinemia/insulin resistance is strongly implicated in the pathophysiology of the syndrome and is present in approximately 70% of the women. This observation is of fundamental clinical significance because apart from intervention with lifestyle modification, pharmacological reduction of insulin levels appears to offer another challenge for these women. There are two groups of insulin-sensitizing drugs that have been used in the management of PCOS: metformin and thiazolidinediones.

Metformin, is a biguanide agent that has been used in the treatment of T2DM. Its mechanism of action is still not completely understood. It lowers blood glucose levels by significantly, reducing the hepatic glucose production and by increasing peripheral glucose utilization. Usually, treatment starts with a low dose, followed by a progressive dose increase (850 mg or 1000 mg, twice a day). Its most serious, but rare side effect, is lactic acidosis, which has been reported in individuals with renal deficiency, liver disease, heart and respiratory failure. However, in a recent comparative outcome study, lactic acidosis was not observed in type 2 diabetes patients receiving metformin.[23] The most common side effect is gastrointestinal disturbances, but this is rarely a cause to discontinue the drug. Metformin could also decrease folic acid and vitamin B12 absorption.

A number of studies, investigating the effect of metformin on insulin resistance in women with PCOS, have been published. Metformin, in a meta-analysis of 13 studies in women with PCOS, was shown to significantly reduce fasting insulin levels, even in this heterogeneous population.[24] There was a small reduction in fasting glucose levels and the lipid profile was also positively affected by metformin, but LDL-cholesterol was significantly reduced after metformin treatment. Furthermore, the meta-analysis showed that the effects of metformin are independent of body mass index (BMI) changes, or of fat distribution as assessed by waist-hip (W/H) ratio. Metformin reduces insulin levels and ovarian androgen secretion in obese and in non-obese women with PCOS, since intrinsic insulin resistance is associated with the disorder.[25] Secondarily, it seems that metformin has also a direct action on theca cells, decreasing the androgen production[26].

Various studies have shown that metformin has a significant effect on decreasing total testosterone, free testosterone and androstenedione concentrations, whereas its effect on the adrenal androgen dehydroepiandrosterone sulfate (DHEA-S) is unclear, and needs further investigation. Furthermore, although various studies have reported an increase in the SHBG levels, data from the meta-analysis do not provide evidence for increased and improved SHBG levels.[24] Nevertheless, long-term use of metformin in the meta-analysis did not influence the hirsutism score despite the improvement in hyperandrogenemia and menstrual cycle.[24] However, this finding is based on a small number of studies that lasted for 3 to 6 months in which a small number of patients was included. To evaluate the effect of the drug in hirsutism, perhaps it is necessary to conduct a treatment for at least 12 months, given the long period of the hair growth cycle. Noteworthy, is a recent well designed randomized controlled study that has reported a significant improvement in hirsutism with metformin treatment, despite the fact that it did not significantly reduce androgen levels.[27]

The use of metformin for improving menstrual cyclicity and ovulation induction in women with PCOS has become popular in the last few years (Figure 6.2). In a systematic review of 7 randomized-controlled trials, it has been shown that women on metformin treatment have a small improvement in ovulation rate that is, on an average, one additional ovulation every 5 months.[28] The Cochrane meta-analysis examined the effectiveness of metformin in spontaneous and clomiphene-induced ovulation.[24] Specifically, ovulation was achieved in 46% of the women

who received metformin alone (compared with 24% receiving placebo), and in 76% of those who received metformin in combination with CC (compared with 42% receiving CC alone). Pregnancy rates were difficult to interpret due to the small number of patients, the short follow up period and the study design. An additional meta-analysis showed similar results.[29]

It is uncertain whether metformin is superior to CC in inducing ovulation and pregnancy in PCOS women. Recently, a prospective parallel, randomized, double blind, controlled trial, compared CC with metformin as the first line treatment for ovulation induction in non-obese PCOS women.[30] This study reported that the ovulation rate was not different between the CC treated group and metformin treated one, whereas the pregnancy rate was significantly higher in the metformin treated group than in the CC treated group. Therefore, women who fail to ovulate following weight loss, may benefit from an insulin-lowering agent (Figure 6.2). It is also possible that not all types of PCOS will benefit from treatment, perhaps due to the heterogeneity of the syndrome.

Thiazolidinediones

They are a new group of insulin-sensitizing drugs used for the treatment of hyperglycemia in patients with type 2 diabetes. They act by enhancing glucose uptake in adipose and muscle tissues. In contrast to the effect observed by metformin, thiazolidinediones increase more peripheral glucose uptake and decrease hepatic glucose output. They improve insulin sensitivity and they not only decrease circulating insulin, but also the release of free fatty acids and tumor necrosis factor alpha (TNF-α) from adipose tissue. Side effects include small weight gain, fluid retention and hepatic dysfunction. In PCOS women, the therapeutic effect of drugs like metformin, is mediated by the reduction of hyperinsulinemia, insulin resistance and consequently, by the reduction of ovarian steroidogenesis.[31] An additional direct effect on the ovaries has also been reported.[32]

Troglitazone was the first of the

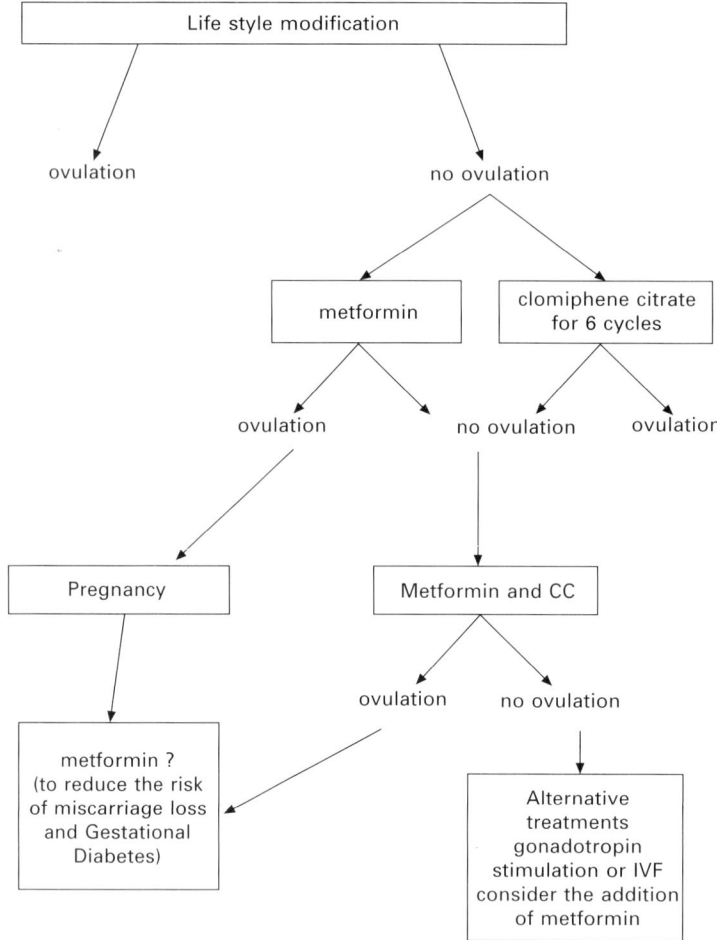

Figure 6.2   Induction of ovulation and pregnancy in PCOS women.

thiazolidinediones to become available for the treatment of insulin resistance diabetes, but was removed from the market due to hepatotoxicity. It has also been used in PCOS treatment and like metformin, its effect on insulin resistance, metabolic profile, hyperandrogenemia and ovulation has been investigated. A reduction in insulin levels, an improvement in glucose tolerance and a reduction in serum testosterone have been reported after its administration in obese women. The best data were obtained from a large, randomized, placebo-controlled study, where 305 moderately obese women received troglitazone in different doses (150, 300, 600 mg/day) or placebo. There was a dose dependent reduction in testosterone, an increase in SHBG levels, an improvement in hirsutism, menstrual cycle and an increase in ovulation rates in women who received troglitazone.[31] Those patients treated with 600 mg/day had a 60% ovulation rate compared to a 32% among the placebo group (and this placebo rate was greater than that traditionally noted in metformin trials) (Figure 6.3).

Unlike metformin, there was no significant change in any of the circulating lipids (serum cholesterol, LDL and HDL-cholesterol and triglycerides) during treatment in women with PCOS.[33] The other two thiazolidinediones, rosiglitazone and pioglitazone, have not demonstrated significant hepatotoxicity, and their

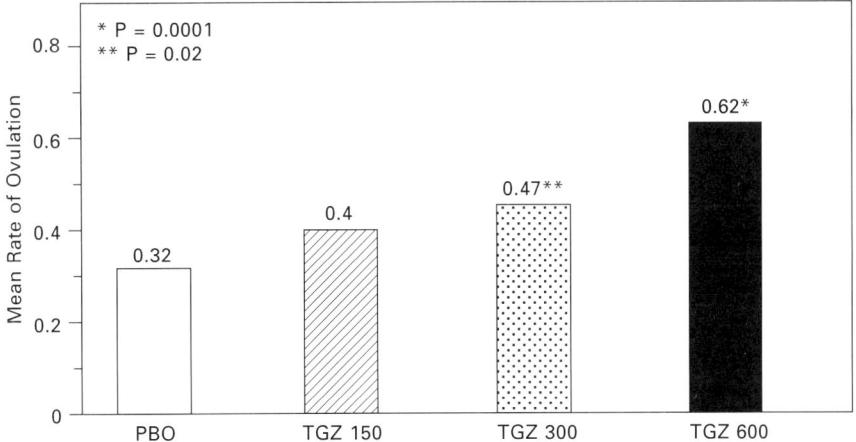

Figure 6.3   The mean rate of ovulation in patients with PCOS increased in a dose-related fashion with troglitazone (TGZ) treatment and was significantly different from placebo (PBO) for TGZ 300 mg/d and TGZ 600 mg/d groups, but not for TGZ 150 mg/d patients. Adapted from.[31]

administration has showed similar results in improving insulin sensitivity, reducing testosterone levels, improving the menstrual cycle and restoring ovulation.[34,35] Similar improvement has also been reported after rosiglitazone administration in obese PCOS women with severe insulin resistance and acanthosis nigricans.[36] In a recent study, the effectiveness of pioglitazone has been compared with metformin in obese PCOS women. It has been shown that pioglitazone is as effective as metformin in improving insulin sensitivity and hyperandrogenemia, despite an increase in weight, BMI and waist to hip ratio associated with pioglitazone.[37] In addition, studies have not found significant changes in lipid profile after treatment. Other cardiovascular risk factors have not been studied yet.

Obviously, large randomized control trials are needed to confirm their effect. There are two limitations in using these drugs. They can provoke a small weight gain (0.5-3.5 kg), which it is not suitable in already obese PCOS women and they are pregnancy category C drugs, which means that in animal studies, there has been fetal toxicity. This potential embryotoxicity could limit their use in women who desire pregnancy. Therefore, thiazolidinediones should be considered a second line treatment alternative to metformin, for the management of PCOS women with insulin resistance.

In conclusion, therapy with insulin sensitizing agents may offer a global therapeutic approach in obese and non-obese PCOS women. The most studied agent is metformin. Though it has little effect to date on skin manifestations of androgen excess, it may improve hyperandrogenemia, ovulatory dysfunction and infertility, as well as ameliorate the devastating long-term co-morbidities of the dysmetabolic syndrome. Since there are no data regarding its safety following long-term use, further investigations in large prospective studies are required.

Conclusions

- The management of PCOS women is a very complex issue since there is no established single therapy for all aspects of the syndrome.
- One of the major difficulties in medical management of PCOS is that there are no specific diagnostic parameters or characterized phenotypes, which could preclude the response to different therapeutic modalities, particularly regarding the efficacy of insulin sensitivity.
- It is indispensable to assess carefully the

predominant symptoms and the risk factors for metabolic disease in each woman and consequently, to individualize the treatment appropriately.

- The first line approach should be lifestyle modification including a hypocaloric diet and exercise with the aim of long-term weight control. Even a small weight loss can improve the metabolic and endocrine status in PCOS women.

- OCPs should be the treatment of choice if the predominant symptoms are menstrual irregularities, hirsutism and acne. It is preferred in young women who also require contraception.

- Antiandrogens may have more pronounced effects on clinical symptoms related to hypcrandrogenemia. It is suggested that flutamide may improve the lipid and metabolic profile too.

- Insulin sensitizing agents, such as metformin, seem to be the most promising therapy. They offer an etiological treatment for the underlying insulin resistance associated with the syndrome and improve insulin sensitivity, lipid profile, endothelial function, as well as menstrual cycle, frequency of ovulation and fertility in PCOS women.

- Metformin should be the treatment of choice in hyperinsulinemic obese or non-obese women who probably desire pregnancy and are at risk for heart disease and diabetes mellitus. However, large randomized controlled studies are needed to ascertain its safety throughout pregnancy and its efficacy in reducing long-term metabolic aberrations.

- Further research is also needed to identify the different phenotypes of the heterogeneous population of PCOS women in order to give specific medical treatment respective to the individual case.

This work was supported by the National Cooperative Program in Infertility Research (NCPIR) U54 HD34449, a GCRC grant MO1 RR 10732 to Pennsylvania State University and K24 HD01476 (to RSL)

References

1. Azziz R, Woods KS, Reyna R, Key TJ, Knochenhauer ES, Yildiz BO. The prevalence and features of the polycystic ovary syndrome in an unselected population. *J Clin Endocrinol Metab* 2004; 89(6): 2745–2749.

2. Ehrmann DA. Polycystic ovary syndrome. *N Engl J Med* 2005; 352(12): 1223–1236.

3. Knowler WC, Barrett-Connor E, Fowler SE, Hamman RF, Lachin JM, Walker EA, et al. Reduction in the incidence of type 2 diabetes with lifestyle intervention or metformin. *N Engl J Med* 2002 7; 346(6): 393–403.

4. Norman RJ, Noakes M, Wu R, Davies MJ, Moran L, Wang JX. Improving reproductive performance in overweight/obese women with effective weight management. *Hum Reprod Update* 2004; 10(3): 267–280.

5. Randeva HS, Lewandowski KC, Drzewoski J, Brooke-Wavell K, O'Callaghan C, Czupryniak L, et al. Exercise decreases plasma total homocysteine in overweight young women with polycystic ovary syndrome. *J Clin Endocrinol Metab* 2002; 87(10): 4496–4501.

6. Clark AM, Thornley B, Tomlinson L, Galletley C, Norman RJ. Weight loss in obese infertile women results in improvement in reproductive outcome for all forms of fertility treatment. *Hum Reprod* 1998; 13(6): 1502–1505.

7. Hoeger KM, Kochman L, Wixom N, Craig K, Miller RK, Guzick DS. A randomized, 48–week, placebo-controlled trial of intensive lifestyle modification and/or metformin therapy in overweight women with polycystic ovary syndrome: a pilot study. *Fertil Steril* 2004; 82(2): 421–429.

8. Galletly C, Clark A, Tomlinson L, Blaney F. Improved pregnancy rates for obese, infertile women following a group treatment program. An open pilot study. *Gen Hosp Psychiatry* 1996; 18(3): 192–195.

9. Pasquali R, Gambineri A, Biscotti D, Vicennati V, Gagliardi L, Colitta D, et al. Effect of long-term treatment with metformin added to hypocaloric diet on body composition, fat distribution, and androgen and insulin levels in abdominally obese women with and without the polycystic ovary syndrome. *J Clin Endocrinol Metab* 2000 Aug; 85(8): 2767–2774.

10. Torgerson JS, Hauptman J, Boldrin MN, Sjostrom L. XENical in the prevention of diabetes in obese subjects (XENDOS) study: a randomized study of orlistat as an adjunct to lifestyle changes for the

prevention of type 2 diabetes in obese patients. *Diabetes Care* 2004; 27(1): 155–161.

11. Sabuncu T, Harma M, Nazligul Y, Kilic F. Sibutramine has a positive effect on clinical and metabolic parameters in obese patients with polycystic ovary syndrome. *Fertil Steril* 2003; 80(5): 1199–1204.

12. Jayagopal V, Kilpatrick ES, Holding S, Jennings PE, Atkin SL. Orlistat is as beneficial as metformin in the treatment of polycystic ovarian syndrome. *J Clin Endocrinol Metab* 2005; 90(2): 729–733.

13. Falsetti L, Gambera A, Tisi G. Efficacy of the combination ethinyl oestradiol and cyproterone acetate on endocrine, clinical and ultrasonographic profile in polycystic ovarian syndrome. *Hum Reprod* 2001; 16(1): 36–42.

14. Guido M, Romualdi D, Giuliani M, Suriano R, Selvaggi L, Apa R, et al. Drospirenone for the treatment of hirsute women with polycystic ovary syndrome: a clinical, endocrinological, metabolic pilot study. *J Clin Endocrinol Metab* 2004; 89(6): 2817–2823.

15. Azziz R. The evaluation and management of hirsutism. *Obstet Gynecol* 2003; 101(5 Pt 1): 995–1007.

16. Farquhar C, Lee O, Toomath R, Jepson R. Spironolactone versus placebo or in combination with steroids for hirsutism and/or acne. *Cochrane Database Syst Rev* 2003 (4): CD000194.

17. Diamanti-Kandarakis E, Mitrakou A, Raptis S, Tolis G, Duleba AJ. The effect of a pure antiandrogen receptor blocker, flutamide, on the lipid profile in the polycystic ovary syndrome. *J Clin Endocrinol Metab* 1998; 83(8): 2699–2705.

18. Muderris II, Bayram F, Guven M.A prospective, randomized trial comparing flutamide (250 mg/d) and finasteride (5 mg/d) in the treatment of hirsutism. *Fertil Steril*, 2000; 73(5): 984–987.

19. Moghetti P, Tosi F, Tosti A, Negri C, Misciali C, Perrone F, et al. Comparison of spironolactone, flutamide, and finasteride efficacy in the treatment of hirsutism: a randomized, double blind, placebo-controlled trial. *J Clin Endocrinol Metab* 2000; 85(1): 89–94.

20. Cusan L, Dupont A, Gomez JL, Tremblay RR, Labrie F. Comparison of flutamide and spironolactone in the treatment of hirsutism: a randomized controlled trial. *Fertil Steril* 1994; 61(2): 281–287.

21. Wong IL, Morris RS, Chang L, Spahn MA, Stanczyk FZ, Lobo RA. A prospective randomized trial comparing finasteride to spironolactone in the treatment of hirsute women. *J Clin Endocrinol Metab* 1995; 80: 233–238.

22. Bayram F, Muderris, II, Guven M, Kelestimur F. Comparison of high-dose finasteride (5 mg/day) versus low-dose finasteride (2.5 mg/day) in the treatment of hirsutism. *Eur J Endocrinol* 2002; 147(4): 467–471.

23. Cryer DR, Nicholas SP, Henry DH, Mills DJ, Stadel BV. Comparative outcome study of metformin intervention versus conventional approach the COSMIC Approach Study. *Diabetes Care* 2005; 28(3): 539–543.

24. Lord JM, Flight IH, Norman RJ. Insulin-sensitising drugs (metformin, troglitazone, rosiglitazone, pioglitazone, D-chiro-inositol) for polycystic ovary syndrome. *Cochrane Database Syst Rev* 2003 (3): CD003053.

25. Nestler JE, Jakubowicz DJ. Lean women with polycystic ovary syndrome respond to insulin reduction with decreases in ovarian p 450c17 alpha activity and serum androgens. *J Clin Endocrinol Metab* 1997; 82(12): 4075–4079.

26. Attia GR, Rainey WE, Carr BR. Metformin directly inhibits androgen production in human thecal cells. *Fertil Steril* 2001; 76(3): 517–524.

27. Harborne L, Fleming R, Lyall H, Sattar N, Norman J. Metformin or antiandrogen in the treatment of hirsutism in polycystic ovary syndrome. *J Clin Endocrinol Metab* 2003; 88(9): 4116–4123.

28. Harborne L, Fleming R, Lyall H, Norman J, Sattar N. Descriptive review of the evidence for the use of metformin in polycystic ovary syndrome. *Lancet* 2003; 361 (9372): 1894–1901.

29. Kashyap S, Wells GA, Rosenwaks Z. Insulin-sensitizing agents as primary therapy for patients with polycystic ovarian syndrome. *Hum Reprod* 2004; 19(11): 2474–2483.

30. Palomba S, Orio F Jr, Falbo A, Manguso F, Russo T, Cascella T, et al. Prospective parallel randomized, double-blind double-dummy controlled clinical trial comparing clomiphene citrate and metformin as the first-line treatment for ovulation induction in nonobese anovulatory women with polycystic ovary syndrome. *J Clin Endocrinol Metab* 2005; 90 (7): 4068–4074.

31. Azziz R, Ehrmann D, Legro RS, Whitcomb RW, Hanley R, Fereshetian AG, et al. Troglitazone improves ovulation and hirsutism in the polycystic ovary syndrome: a multicenter, double blind, placebo-controlled trial. *J Clin Endocrinol Metab* 2001; 86(4): 1626–1632.

32. Mitwally MF, Witchel SF, Casper RF. Troglitazone: a possible modulator of ovarian steroidogenesis. *J Soc Gynecol Investig* 2002; 9(3): 163–7.

33. Legro RS, Azziz R, Ehrmann D, Fereshetian AG, O'Keefe M, Ghazzi MN. Minimal response of circulating lipids in women with polycystic ovary syndrome to improvement in insulin sensitivity with troglitazone. *J Clin Endocrinol Metab* 2003; 88(11): 5137–5144.

34. Belli SH, Graffigna MN, Oneto A, Otero P, Schurman L, Levalle OA. Effect of rosiglitazone on insulin resistance, growth factors, and reproductive disturbances in women with polycystic ovary syndrome. *Fertil Steril* 2004; 81(3): 624–629.

35. Brettenthaler N, De Geyter C, Huber PR, Keller U. Effect of the insulin sensitizer pioglitazone on insulin resistance, hyperandrogenism, and ovulatory dysfunction in women with polycystic ovary syndrome. *J Clin Endocrinol Metab* 2004; 89(8): 3835–3840.

36. Sepilian V, Nagamani M. Effects of rosiglitazone in obese women with polycystic ovary syndrome and severe insulin resistance. *J Clin Endocrinol Metab* 2005; 90(1): 60–65.

37. Ortega-Gonzalez C, Luna S, Hernandez L, Crespo G, Aguayo P, Arteaga-Troncoso G, et al. Responses of serum androgen and insulin resistance to metformin and pioglitazone in obese, insulin-resistant women with polycystic ovary syndrome. *J Clin Endocrinol Metab* 2005; 90(3): 1360–1365.

7

The Ultrasonographic Appearance of Polycystic Ovaries and Ovarian Hyperstimulation Syndrome

Sharon Maslovitz, Ariel Jaffa

Summary

The ability to perform an ultrasound scan and appropriately interpret its findings has become one of the fundamentals of contemporary gynecology. The clinical assessment of a patient is incomplete without sonographic evaluation of the morphology of the pelvic organs, their location, texture and blood flow. Ovarian hyperstimulation syndrome (OHSS) is an iatrogenic complication that arises following the use of drug regimens in assisted reproductive technology and which may culminate in life threatening complications unless timely diagnosis and intervention are ensued. Ultrasound plays a major role in the prevention, diagnosis and treatment of OHSS. Polycystic ovary syndrome (PCOS) is a common morphological-endocrine disorder, which may have long term complications if left undiagnosed and untreated. Since the polycystic ovary syndrome (PCOS) international consensus held at Rotterdam in 2003, ultrasound criteria are now included in the definition of this disease, thus, the importance of a thorough knowledge of the sonographic features of PCOS and OHSS cannot be over emphasized. This chapter describes the appearance of polycystic ovaries and OHSS in a simple and instructive manner.

Introduction

In 1935, Stein and Leventhal described amenorrhea associated with polycystic ovaries that could be visualized by laparotomy and confirmed by histology.[1] Further investigations revealed the biochemical alterations associated with the morphological appearance of "Stein-Leventhal syndrome". The endocrinologic and biochemical characteristics of polycystic ovary syndrome (PCOS) soon became the mainstay of diagnosis and included elevated luteinizing hormone (LH), normal follicle stimulating hormone (FSH), hyperandrogenemia (elevated testosterone, androstenedione and dehydroepiandrosterone [DHEA]) and insulin resistance with hyperinsulinemia.[2] The clinical features of the syndrome are diverse and include:

1. Hyperandrogenism [hirsutism,[3] acne,[4] oily skin and male pattern alopecia]
2. Anovulation, manifested as amenorrhea, oligomenorrhea or dysfunctional uterine bleeding[5]
3. Infertility[6]
4. Obesity[7]
5. Insulin resistance and hyperinsulinemia[5,8]
6. Increased risk for diabetes mellitus, endometrial cancer, ischemic heart disease and possibly, breast cancer[9,10]

The heterogeneity of the clinical, biochemical and morphological features of PCOS led to a myriad of diagnostic criteria and in 1990, a National Institute of Health (NIH)-sponsored conference recommended that the diagnosis be based on evidence of chronic anovulation and clinical or biochemical signs of hyperandrogenism in the absence of non-classical adrenal hyperplasia.[11] The diagnostic guidelines suggested by the conference did not include ultrasonographic findings of polycystic ovaries (PCOs) since the characteristic of PCOs appear when a state of anovulation persists, regardless of the reason. Various studies have demonstrated that 10–25% of normal women display the typical appearance of PCOs on sonographic imaging.[12–14] Since the 1990 PCOS conference, it became obvious that the syndrome encompasses a broader spectrum of signs and symptoms of ovarian dysfunction than those defined by the original diagnostic criteria. The Rotterdam consensus on diagnostic criteria for PCOS recently recognized that some women with the syndrome will have PCOs without clinical evidence of androgen excess, but will display signs of ovarian dysfunction and the characteristic ultrasonographic findings.[15] The refined definition by the Rotterdam consensus group includes, for the first time, a description of the ultrasound appearance of PCOS. Accordingly, PCOS is diagnosed when at least two of the following three features are present:

1. Oligo and/or anovulation
2. Clinical and/or biochemical hyperandrogenism
3. Polycystic appearance by an ultrasound scan

This chapter will define the sonographic appearance of PCOS and provide simple guidelines for the ultrasound examination of a woman suspected of having PCOS.

Clinical Discussion

Ultrasonographic features of polycystic ovaries

Background

The use of ultrasonography as a primary diagnostic method in the work-up of PCOS is now common practice although definitive criteria for identifying polycystic ovaries by ultrasound are still controversial. By and large, the characteristic sonographic features of PCOs are increased ovarian volume due to enhanced stromal volume and number of follicles (Fig. 7.1). Swanson et al.[16] were the first to sonographically describe PCOs by using high-resolution, real-time scanners in a transabdominal approach. The tiny follicles, so characteristic of PCOs, could not be detected by the older generation conventional contact static B-scanners. Swanson and his colleagues were able to detect multiple cysts ranging from 2-6 mm in diameter and arranged in the periphery of the ovary or throughout the parenchyma. The description by that group, however, lacked details on the number of follicles and the stromal characteristics. During the early 80's, ultrasound scans were performed in order to demonstrate the ovarian morphology of women known to have PCOS by endocrinologic findings or clinical symptoms, and not as a diagnostic tool.

In 1985, Adams et al.[17] published a state-of-

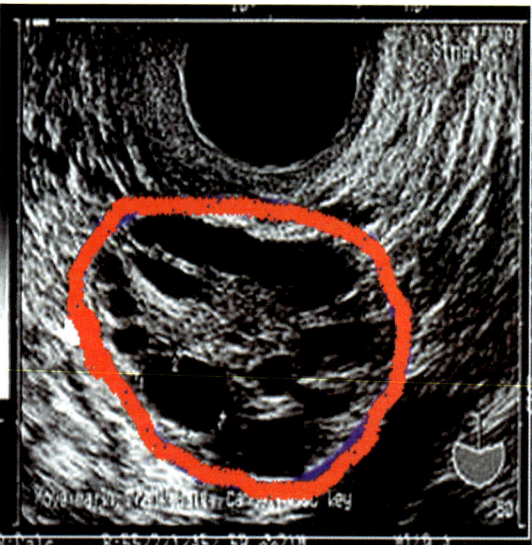

Figure 7.1 Polycystic ovary - the red circle outlines the ovary in which there are numerous small cysts (follicles) about 3–9 mm in diameter. The larger one at 8 o'clock measures 9 mm.

the-art paper aimed at defining the sonographic features of polycystic ovaries as at least 10 follicles (between 2-8 mm in diameter) seen in one plane around a thickened stromal component or throughout an enlarged ovary. The description was later referred to as the "Adam's criteria" and became the reference for many subsequent studies.[18] The sonographic finding of polycystic ovaries supported the diagnosis of the syndrome in symptomatic women, but it was not considered definitive for PCOS, nor was it obligatory for its validation.[12]

Transvaginal or transabdominal approach

The transvaginal approach has some advantages over the transabdominal approach, which are mainly related to greater resolution and a more precise demonstration of the ovarian structure. Some investigators have argued that the transvaginal approach is more sensitive in diagnosing PCOS compared with the transabdominal approach, especially with regard to the morphology and consistency of the stromal component. These advantages are more prominent in the obese patient in whom uniformly echogenous ovaries were often described with little added value to the diagnosis of PCOS. The proximity of the ovaries to the vaginal apex enables the use of high-frequency probes (> 6 MHz) with a better resolution in spite of less penetration. The same diagnostic guidelines apply to both transvaginal and transabdominal approaches for the diagnosis of PCOS.

The transvaginal approach is currently more popular in the diagnosis of PCOS, except for virgins and for women who refuse the vaginal probe. The contribution of three-dimensional (3D) ultrasound to the diagnosis of PCOS has yet to be defined, but its use has become widespread, mainly for calculating volumes.

The timing of the ultrasound scan

The optimal timing of the ultrasound scan to diagnose PCO is probably during the early follicular phase (days 1–3 of the menstrual cycle), but scheduling the examination during that specific period is not always practical since many women with PCOS are oligomenorrheic. Vigilance in timing the ultrasound scan is not mandatory in routine clinical practice, but it is highly recommended when reporting ovarian parameters in a study. Repeated scans are usually unnecessary and do not provide additional information.[19]

Guidelines for sonographic examination of polycystic ovaries

1. Identify each ovary. The left ovary may be more difficult to visualize due to the proximity of the sigmoid colon.
2. Measure the maximal length of each ovary in three planes (longitudinal, antero-posterior and transverse).
3. Determine the volume of each ovary. Many formulas have been proposed to calculate the ovarian volume but all have a similar validity in estimating the true volume. The most popular formula considers the ovary as having an elliptic shape so that the volume can be calculated by $\pi/6 * $ length $*$ width $*$ depth. Since $\pi/6$ roughly equals 0.5, the formula can be simplified to (length $*$ width $*$ depth)/2.[16,20] Nardo et al.[21] proposed two alternative formulas, the prolate spheroid formula and the spherical formula for ovarian volume measurement in PCOS, both with a good correlation with the 3D ultrasound measurement. The reference values for normal ovarian volume vary considerably between studies, with the range between 5.7 cm^3,[22] and 12.5 cm^3.[16] The cut-off points for defining polycystic ovaries also differ between studies: for example, Adams et al.[17] found the average volume of a PCO to be 14.6 $\pm$ 1.1 cm^3 while Fulghesu et al.[20] used 2 standard deviations above the mean (i.e., 13.2 cm^3). The conclusions of a recent joint ASRM/ESHRE international consensus meeting held in Rotterdam were published in 2003,[23] and

proposed an ovarian volume of 10 cm³ as the cut-off for PCO. The latter value stems from the integration of many studies and cannot be regarded as a prerequisite for the diagnosis of PCOS since, as the authors themselves note, not all polycystic ovaries will have a volume that high (Fig. 7.2).

4. Calculate the ovarian surface area by any one of three means:
   a   Length * width * π/4 – which is the formula for surface area of an ellipse
   b   Drawing the surface area by hand and calculating it
   c   Fitting an ellipse around the ovary and applying the formula to calculate the area of an ellipse [(length * width * depth)/2])

The surface area that delineates normal from polycystic ovaries is even less distinct. A cut-off of 7 cm² has been proposed,[20] although this parameter seems to be less valuable in the sonographic characterization of a polycystic ovary.

5. Use a stromal area/total area ratio cut-off of >0.34. This was found to be the most descriptive of PCO,[20] but measurements of the stromal area are not easily obtained and so this parameter is not routinely used.

6. Measure the uterus. The uterus is usually enlarged in women with PCOS due to continuous estrogen stimulation. Due to a wide range of ovarian/uterine area ratios, however, this parameter was abandoned and excluded from the Rotterdam consensus recommendations.

7. Note the follicle number and size, which play a critical role in the sonographic description of polycystic ovaries. The number of follicles should be determined for each ovary using two planes and counting from the inner to the outer margin in a longitudinal cross-section. The size and location of the follicles/cysts should be noted as well. There is a considerable disparity between different studies regarding the follicular size. For example, Adams et al.[17] reported the presence of at least 10 follicles between 2–8 mm in diameter arranged peripherally, while others suggested 15 follicles with a diameter of 2–10 mm as the criteria for PCOS (Fig. 7.3). Jonard et al.[24] found that a follicle number

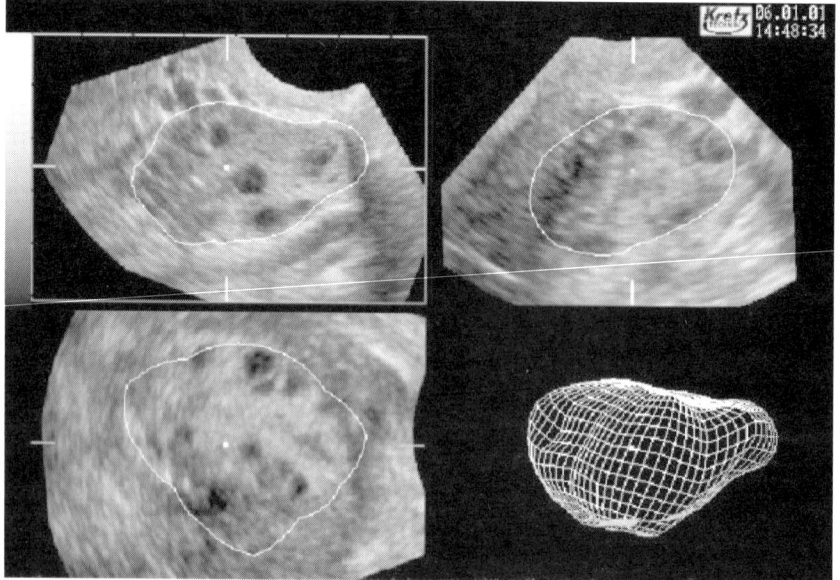

Figure 7.2   Ovarian volume calculation. Ovarian volume may be measured in the same way as endometrial volume through the manual delineation of the ovarian cortex.

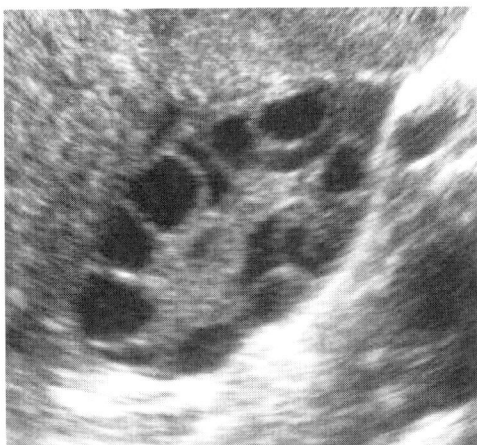

Figure 7.3 Polycystic ovary – note the "necklace" appearance of multiple follicles arranged around an echogenic stromal component.

per ovary (FNPO) >12 (ranging 2–9 mm in diameter) gave the best threshold for diagnosing PCOS (sensitivity 75%, specificity 99%). These findings were adopted by the consensus committee, which defined a polycystic ovary as one that contains at least 12 follicles, 2–9 mm in diameter.

8. Assess the stromal echogenicity. The stroma of polycystic ovaries is usually hyperechoic, but this feature depends largely on the ultrasound machine setting and the amount of fat tissue (Fig. 7.4). In an attempt to standardize the description of stromal echogenicity, it was suggested that it should be compared with the myometrial echogenicity: in normal ovaries, the echogenicity of the ovarian stromal tissue

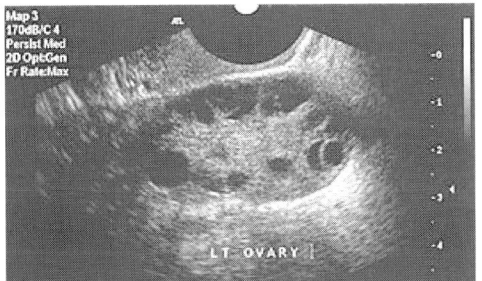

Figure 7.4 Polycystic ovary: note the abundant stromal portion.

is less than that of the myometrium.[25] Several groups have suggested various means for quantification of the stromal echogenicity, but since none has become common practice, subjective impression of the stromal appearance remains the most popular approach. The sensitivity and specificity of stromal echogenicity in the diagnosis of polycystic ovaries was found to be 90% and 94% respectively.

9. Take into account the stromal area and volume. The clinical significance of the stromal area stems from its correlation with 17-hydroxyprogesterone and androstenedione, as opposed to the follicular area, which does not correlate with the biochemical characteristics of PCOS.[26] Stromal volume calculated by 3-D ultrasonography correlates with androstenedione concentrations in women with PCOS[27] (Fig. 7.5). Since ovarian volume, as measured by 3-D ultrasound, correlates well with the clinical presentation of PCOS and given that the measurement of stromal volume is technically challenging, there is no need to assess stromal size in the routine diagnosis and description of PCOS.

10. Assess the vascular bed and blood flow within the ovarian stroma. Increased stromal blood flow [decreased resistance to flow (resistance index -RI), PI (pulsatility index)], correlates with the hormonal profile typical of PCOS and may predict ovarian response to hormonal stimulation in in vitro fertilization (IVF) treatment cycles.[28,29] Assessment of blood flow necessitates special expertise and equipment and is not considered mandatory in the primary diagnosis and description of a PCO.

Ultrasound assessment of PCO – International consensus definitions

The ASRM/ESHRE consensus committee on PCOS held in Rotterdam in 2003, agreed upon several key points in defining PCOS as follows:[23]

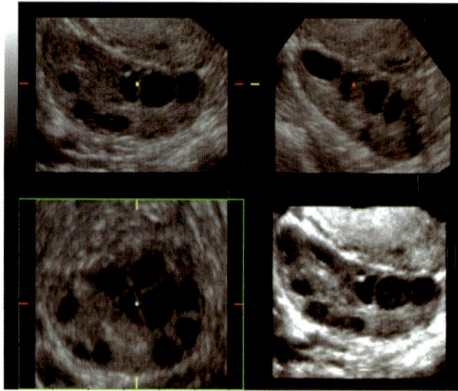

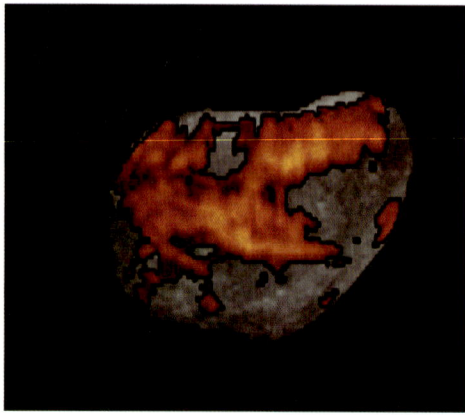

Figure 7.5 Polycystic ovaries. Three-dimensional sonography facilitates evaluation of the stromal component and allows the measurement of its echogenicity, its vascularity and its volume, which may be calculated by subtracting total follicular volume from total ovarian volume (a). Ovarian blood flow in PCOs is increased and associated with significantly higher three-dimensional indices of vascularity than ovaries with a normal appearance (b).

1. The PCO should have at least one of two features: either ≥12 follicles measuring 2–9 mm in diameter, or an increased ovarian volume (>10 cm^3). If there is evidence of a dominant follicle (>10 mm) or a corpus luteum, the scan should be repeated during the next cycle.

2. The subjective appearance of polycystic ovaries should not be substituted for this definition. The follicle distribution should be disregarded as should be the increase in stromal echogenicity and/or volume. Although the latter is specific to a PCO, it has been shown that measurement of the ovarian volume is a good surrogate for the quantification of the stroma in clinical practice.

3. Only one ovary fitting this definition, or the single occurrence of one of the above criteria, is sufficient to define the presence of a PCO. The presence of an abnormal cyst or ovarian asymmetry, which may suggest a homogeneous cyst, calls for further investigation.

4. This definition does not apply to women taking oral contraceptives since ovarian size is reduced, even though a polycystic appearance may persist.

5. A woman with a PCO in the absence of an ovulation disorder or hyperandrogenism ('asymptomatic PCO') should not yet be considered as having PCOS until more corroborative evidence is available.

6. In addition to its role in the definition of PCO, ultrasound is helpful in predicting fertility outcome in a patient with PCOS (i.e., response to clomiphene citrate, risk for ovarian hyperstimulation syndrome [OHSS], decision for in-vitro maturation of oocytes). It is well recognized that polycystic ovaries may be demonstrated in women undergoing ovarian stimulation for IVF in the absence of overt signs of PCOS.

7. The following technical recommendations should be observed:
   • State-of-the-art equipment is required and should be operated by appropriately trained personnel
   • Whenever possible, the transvaginal approach should be preferred, particularly in obese patients
   • Regularly menstruating women should be scanned in the early follicular phase (days 3–5)
   • Oligo/amenorrheic women should be scanned either at random, or between 3–5 days after progesterone-induced bleeding
   • If there is evidence of a dominant follicle (>10 mm) or a corpus luteum, the scan should be repeated during the next cycle.

- Calculation of the ovarian volume is performed using the simplified formula for a prolate ellipsoid (0.5 * length * width * thickness).
- Follicle number should be estimated both in longitudinal, transverse and antero-posterior cross-sections of the ovaries. Follicle size should be expressed as the mean diameter of all the diameters measured in the three sections.
- The usefulness of 3-D ultrasound, Doppler or magnetic resonance imaging (MRI) for the definition of PCO, has not been sufficiently established to date, and their use should be confined to research studies.

The ultrasound scan report should include the following information

1. Name and age of the patient
2. An identification number
3. Date of scan
4. Relation of date of scan to the menstrual cycle
5. Relevant treatment [e.g., gonadotropin releasing hormone (GnRH) agonists]
6. Type of scan (transabdominal/transvaginal)
7. Ovarian morphology (each ovary reported separately)
8. Ovarian volume (and area if relevant)
9. Number and size/range of cysts/follicles
10. Stromal echogenicity
11. Doppler studies
12. Uterine morphology, cross-sectional area and endometrial thickness

Ovarian Hyperstimulation Syndrome

Prevalence:

Ovarian hyperstimulation syndrome (OHSS) is a potentially lethal iatrogenic complication of induction of ovulation caused by almost every agent used for ovarian stimulation. OHSS has recently become more prevalent due to the widespread use of assisted reproduction technologies (ART) and the aggressive treatment protocols aimed at obtaining sufficient numbers of oocytes and embryos.[30] The severe form of OHSS is rare, with the reported prevalence ranging from 0.5% to 5% of stimulated ovarian cycles, but it is worth bearing in mind that OHSS is an iatrogenic complication of an elective treatment that has the potential for a fatal outcome with an estimated mortality rate of 1/450,000–500,000 patients.[31,32]

Clinical features: The cardinal features of OHSS include marked ovarian enlargement (Fig. 7.6) leading to an overproduction of ovarian hormones and vasoactive substances, including cytokines, angiotensin, and vascular endothelial growth factor, which contribute to an increase in capillary membrane permeability and acute third space fluid sequestration in the form of ascites, hydrothorax, and anasarca.[33] The clinical manifestations are a result of the increased capillary membrane permeability resulting in a loss of protein-rich fluid. A massive extracellular exudative fluid accumulation in addition to severe

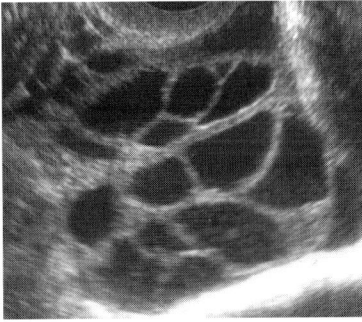

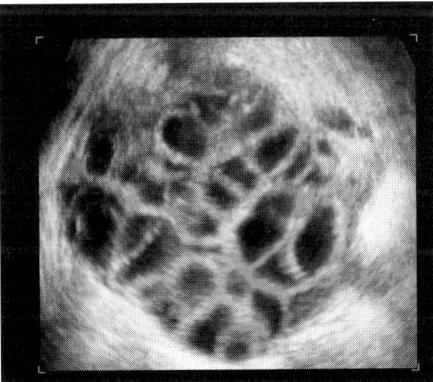

Figure 7.6   The multicystic appearance characteristic of ovarian hyperstimulation.

intravascular volume depletion and hemoconcentration eventually leads to multiple organ failure.

Risk factors:

There are multiple recognized risk factors for OHSS, including:

- Young age (<35 yrs)
- Low body weight
- Polycystic ovaries
- History of atopy or allergies
- Pregnancy
- High doses of exogenous gonadotropins
- High absolute or rapidly rising serum estradiol (E_2) levels
- Previous episodes of OHSS

Patients with ultrasonographic features of PCOS, demonstrated by the presence of ≥10 ovarian cysts <10 mm in size, were noted to have a higher incidence of OHSS,[32] thus pre-treatment ultrasound examination may assist in predicting the susceptibility for OHSS.

Classification:

Rabau et al.[34] were the first to suggest a classification of OHSS into mild, moderate and severe disease based on laboratory and clinical findings. Only moderate, severe and the recently proposed critical or life-threatening OHSS are clinically relevant, with the latter two being more commonly encountered by the intensive care unit physician (Table 7.1).

Complications:

The symptoms and signs of OHSS stem from increased vascular permeability and marked arterial dilation leading to fluid shifts from the intravascular to the extravascular space.[37] Fluid accumulation in the third space is considered as the cardinal event of OHSS, and not uncommonly, is the first indication of the disease, demonstrated by ascites on ultrasonographic evaluation. Massive accumulation of extravascular exudates can lead

to tense ascites, pleural or pericardial effusions, electrolyte derangements, oliguric renal failure, hemoconcentration, and hypovolemia with or without hypovolemic shock.[32] Severe ascites often accompany oliguria with decreased urinary sodium excretion and hyponatremia due to a low serum osmolality. The ovaries may enlarge (>12 cm) and pose potential hazards of rupture, hemorrhage or torsion and severe abdominal pain. Ultrasound examination of patients with OHSS usually reveals enlarged ovaries with numerous follicular cysts and ascites. Abdominal computed tomography can also be used to visualize ovarian enlargement and ascites in patients with OHSS.

Paracentesis: The management of ovarian hyperstimulation reflects its self-resolving nature and focuses on supportive measures aimed at minimizing the emergence of complications and relieving patients' discomfort.[38] Levin et al.[39] studied the beneficial effect of abdominal fluid removal by paracentesis on the urinary output and concluded that paracentesis increases urinary output and reduces blood urea nitrogen concentration in women with severe OHSS. Two theories were suggested to explain the mechanism by which paracentesis exerts its effect. One involves a direct decompression effect, which implies reduced intra-abdominal pressure (IAP) and thereby, enhanced splanchnic perfusion, including renal artery flow, consequently leading to augmented urine production. The other theory relates to the removal of harmful mediators from the peritoneal cavity, thus reversing the pathophysiology of the disease and leading to a cascade which culminates in improved hemodynamic status and urine production. Maslovitz et al.[40] assessed the Doppler ultrasound parameters, systolic/diastolic (S/D) ratio and resistance index (RI), before and after paracentesis of ascitic fluid in order to demonstrate alterations in renal arterial flow, which are temporarily associated with reduced IAP. The curves for IAP and S/D ratio as a function of the amount of fluid drained almost overlapped (Fig. 7.7). The decrement in both parameters was most marked during the drainage of the first two liters after which both curves flattened, reflecting that

Table 7.1 Different classifications of OHSS

Classification	Mild	Moderate	Severe	Critical
Rabau et al.[34]	**Grade I** Estrogen > 150 µg, Pregnanediol > 10 mg in 24h **Grade II** + Enlarged or palpable ovaries	**Grade III** Grade II + palpable cysts and distended abdomen **Grade IV** Grade III+ vomiting and diarrhea	**Grade V** Grade IV+ ascites and possibly hydrothorax	**Grade VI** Grade V + alterations in blood volume, viscosity and coagulation
Golan et al.[35]	**Grade I** Abdominal distension and discomfort **Grade II** Grade I + nausea or vomiting or diarrhea enlarged ovaries: 5–12 cm	**Grade III** Grade II with sonographic evidence of ascites	**Grade IV** Clinical evidence of ascites or hydrothorax or breathing difficulties	**Grade V** Grade IV and hemoconcentration, increased viscosity, coagulopathy and decreased renal perfusion
Navot et al.[36]			Enlarged ovaries Massive ascites Hydrothorax Hct > 45%, WBC > 15000 Oliguria, Cr > 1–1.5, Cr clearance > 50 ml/min, Liver dysfunction, Anasarca	Tense ascites Hct>55% WBC>25000 Cr>1.6 Cr clearance < 50 ml/min Renal failure Thromboembolism ARDS

Hct – hematocrit; WBC – White Blood Cells; Cr – Creatinine; ARDS – Adult Respiratory Distress Syndrome.

additional drainage had a minor effect on IAP. Moreover, there was no latency period between peritoneal decompression and lowered resistance to flow within the renal vasculature, an observation which further supports a direct causal relationship between decompression and renal flow rather than a cascade of processes reversing the pathophysiology and culminating in increased urine production. Although additional volume removal after the first 2000 ml had negligible effect on renal blood flow, it may be important in deferring the recurrence of symptoms. The authors suggested that the beneficial effect of paracentesis on urine production in OHSS is attributable to improved renal blood flow subsequent to immediate decompression.

Conclusion

Ultrasound examination in cases of OHSS assists the clinician in:

1. Predicting the susceptibility for OHSS prior to ovulation induction by demonstrating polycystic ovaries. This important information may affect decisions and alter treatment protocol in order to refrain from exaggerated stimulation of these susceptible ovaries.
2. Monitoring the individual's response to the stimulating agents during treatment. Repeated ultrasound examinations have become common practice as a method of monitoring

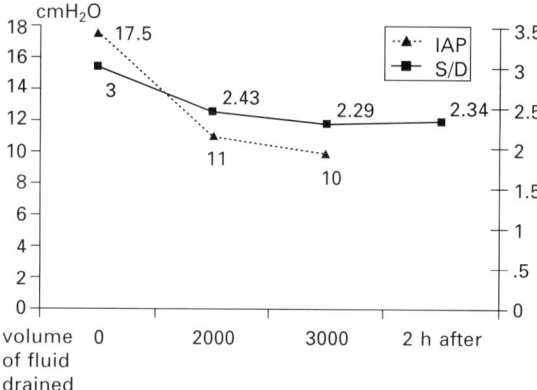

Figure 7.7 Intra-abdominal pressure (IAP) and systolic/diastolic (S/D) ratio as a function of amount of drained fluid during paracentesis. The dotted line drawn for IAP as a function of aspirate volume was very similar to the solid line drawn for the S/D ratio. There was no latency period between the reduced IAP and enhanced renal flow.

the number and size of developing follicles. Preventive measures, such as reduction in the dosage of induction agents or even suspending them for a few days (coasting), are based on ultrasound findings in conjugation with blood estradiol levels.

3. Detecting complications of ovarian hyperstimulation, such as torsion and ruptured cyst.

4. Classifying the severity of OHSS by measuring the size of the ovaries and detecting ascites.

5. Monitoring the effectiveness of treatment by observing reduced ovarian dimensions and decreased amounts of free peritoneal fluid.

6. Draining ascites under ultrasound guidance as an important treatment modality, leading to improved urine output and relieving the patient's discomfort.

References

1. Stein IF, Leventhal ML. Amenorrhea associated with bilateral polycystic ovaries. *Am J Obstet Gynecol* 1935; 29: 81–91.
2. Franks S. Polycystic ovary syndrome. *N Engl J Med* 1995; 333: 853–61.
3. Diamanti-Kandarakis E, Koulie CR, Bergiele AT, Filandra FA, Tsianateli TC, Spina GG, et al. A survey of the polycystic ovary syndrome in the Greek Island of Lesbos: a hormonal and metabolic profile. *J Clin Endocrinol Metab* 1999; 84: 4006–4011.
4. Slayden SM, Moran C, Sams WM, Boots LR Jr, Azziz R. Hyperandrogenemia in patients presenting with acne. *Fertil Steril* 2001; 75: 889–892.
5. Robinson S, Kiddy D, Gelding SV, Willis D, Niththyananthan R, Bush A, et al. The relationship of insulin insensitivity to menstrual pattern in women with hyperandrogenism and polycystic ovaries. *Clin Endocrinol (Oxf)* 1993; 39: 351–355.
6. Kousta E, White DM, Cela E, McCarthy MI, Franks S. The prevalence of polycystic ovaries in women with infertility. *Eur J Endocrinol* 2003; 149: 439–442.
7. Singh KB, Mahajan DK, Wortsman J. Effect of obesity on the clinical and hormonal characteristics of the polycystic ovary syndrome. *J Reprod Med* 1994; 39: 805–808.
8. Dunaif A, Graf M, Mandeli J, Laumas V, Dobrjansky A. Characterization of groups of hyperandrogenic women with acanthosis nigricans, impaired glucose tolerance, and/or hyperinsulinemia. *J Clin Endocrinol Metab* 1987; 65: 499–507.
9. Wild RA. Long-term health consequences of PCOS. *Hum Reprod Update* 2002; 8: 231–241.
10. Wild S, Pierpoint T, Jacobs H, McKeigue P. Long-term consequences of polycystic ovary syndrome: results of a 31 year follow-up study. *Hum Fertil (Camb)* 2000; 3: 101–105.
11. Zawadski JK, Dunaif A. Diagnostic criteria for polycystic ovary syndrome: towards a rational approach. In: Dunaif A, Givens JR, Haseltine F, editors. Polycystic ovary syndrome, Blackwell Scientific, Boston 1992: pp. 377–384.
12. Polson DW, Adams J, Wadsworth J, Franks S. Polycystic ovaries – a common finding in normal women. *Lancet* 1988; 1: 870–872.
13. Clayton RN, Ogden V, Hodgkinson J, Worswick L, Rodin DA, Dyer S, Meade TW. How common are polycystic ovaries in normal women and what is their significance for the fertility of the population? *Clin Endocrinol (Oxf)* 1992; 37: 127–134.
14. Farquhar CM, Birdsall M, Manning P, Mitchell JM, France JT. The prevalence of polycystic ovaries on ultrasound scanning in a population of randomly selected women. *Aust N Z J Obstet Gynaecol* 1994; 34: 67–72.
15. The Rotterdam ESHRE/ASRM-Sponsored PCOS Consensus Workshop Group. Revised 2003

consensus on diagnostic criteria and long-term health risks related to polycystic ovary syndrome. *Fertil Steril* 2004; 81: 19–25.

16. Swanson M, Sauerbrei EE, Cooperberg PL. Medical implications of ultrasonically detected polycystic ovaries. *J Clin Ultrasound* 1981; 9: 219–222.

17. Adams J, Franks S, Polson DW, Mason HD, Abdulwahid N, Tucker M, et al. Multifollicular ovaries: clinical and endocrine features and response to pulsatile gonadotropin releasing hormone. *Lancet* 1985; 2: 1375–1379.

18. Abdel Gadir A, Khatim MS, Mowafi RS, Alnaser HM, Muharib NS, Shaw RW. Implications of ultrasonically diagnosed polycystic ovaries. I. Correlations with basal hormonal profiles. *Hum Reprod* 1992; 7: 453–457.

19. Pache TD, Hop WC, Wladimiroff JW, Schipper J, Fauser BC. Transvaginal sonography and abnormal ovarian appearance in menstrual cycle disturbances. *Ultrasound Med Biol* 1991; 17: 589–593.

20. Fulghesu AM, Ciampelli M, Belosi C, Apa R, Pavone V, Lanzone A. A new ultrasound criterion for the diagnosis of polycystic ovary syndrome: the ovarian stroma/total area ratio. *Fertil Steril* 2001; 76: 326–331.

21. Nardo LG, Buckett WM, Khullar V. Determination of the best-fitting ultrasound formulaic method for ovarian volume measurement in women with polycystic ovary syndrome. *Fertil Steril* 2003; 79: 632–633.

22. Sample WF, Lippe BM, Gyepes MT. Gray-scale ultrasonography of the normal female pelvis. *Radiology* 1977; 125: 477–483.

23. Balen AH, Laven JS, Tan SL, Dewailly D. Ultrasound assessment of the polycystic ovary: international consensus definitions. *Hum Reprod Update* 2003; 9: 505–514.

24. Jonard S, Robert Y, Cortet-Rudelli C, Pigny P, Decanter C, Dewailly D. Ultrasound examination of polycystic ovaries: is it worth counting the follicles? *Hum Reprod* 2003; 18: 598–603.

25. Pache TD, Wladimiroff JW, Hop WC, Fauser BC. How to discriminate between normal and polycystic ovaries: transvaginal US study. *Radiology* 1992; 183: 421–423.

26. Dewailly D, Robert Y, Helin I, Ardaens Y, Thomas-Desrousseaux P, Lemaitre L, Fossati P. Ovarian stromal hypertrophy in hyperandrogenic women. *Clin Endocrinol (Oxf)* 1994; 41: 557–562.

27. Kyei-Mensah AA, LinTan S, Zaidi J, Jacobs HS. Relationship of ovarian stromal volume to serum androgen concentrations in patients with polycystic ovary syndrome. *Hum Reprod*, 1998; 13: 1437–1441.

28. Zaidi J, Barber J, Kyei-Mensah A, Bekir J, Campbell S, Tan SL. Relationship of ovarian stromal blood flow at the baseline ultrasound scan to subsequent follicular response in an in vitro fertilization program. *Obstet Gynecol* 1996; 88: 779–784.

29. Battaglia C, Artini PG, Salvatori M, Giulini S, Petraglia F, Maxia N, Volpe A. Ultrasonographic patterns of polycystic ovaries: color Doppler and hormonal correlations. *Ultrasound Obstet Gynecol* 1998; 11: 332–336.

30. Delvigne A, Rozenberg S. Review of clinical course and treatment of ovarian hyperstimulation syndrome (OHSS). *Hum Reprod Update* 2003; 9: 77–96.

31. Delvigne A, Rozenberg S. Epidemiology and prevention of ovarian hyperstimulation syndrome (OHSS): a review. *Hum Reprod Update* 2002; 8: 559–577.

32. Schenker JG, Weinstein D. Ovarian hyperstimulation syndrome: a current survey. *Fertil Steril* 1978; 30: 255–268.

33. The Practice Committee of the American Society for Reproductive Medicine. Ovarian hyperstimulation syndrome. *Fertil Steril* 2004; 82: S81–S86.

34. Rabau E, David A, Serr DM, Mashiach S, Lunenfeld B. Human menopausal gonadotropins for anovulation and sterility. *Am J Obstet Gynecol* 1967; 98: 92–98.

35. Golan A, Ron-el R, Herman A, Soffer Y, Weinraub Z, Caspi E Ovarian hyperstimulation syndrome: an update review. *Obstet Gynecol Surv* 1989; Jun; 44(6): 430–40.

36. Navot D, Bergh PA, Laufer N. Ovarian hyperstimulation syndrome in novel reproductive technologies: prevention and treatment. *Fertil Steril* 1992; 58(2): 249–61.

37. Semba S, Moriya T, Youssef EM, Sasano H. An autopsy case of ovarian hyperstimulation syndrome of massive pulmonary edema and pleural effusions. *Pathol Int* 2000; 50: 549–552.

38. Borenstein R, Elhalah U, Lunenfeld B, Schwartz ZS. Severe ovarian hyperstimulation syndrome: a reevaluated therapeutic approach. *Fertil Steril* 1989; 51: 791–795.

39. Levin I, Almog B, Avni A, Baram A, Lessing JB, Gamzu R. Effect of paracentesis of ascitic fluids on urinary output and blood indices in patients with severe ovarian hyperstimulation syndrome. *Fertil Steril* 2002; 77: 986–988.

40. Maslovitz S, Jaffa A, Eytan O, Wolman I, Many A, Lessing JB, Gamzu R. Renal blood flow alteration after paracentesis in women with ovarian hyperstimulation. *Obstet Gynecol* 2004; 104: 321–326.

8

Polycystic Ovary Syndrome – Clinical and Practical Issues

Hernán E Lara Peñaloza, Teresa Sir-Petermann

Summary

This work presents a review of polycystic ovary syndrome (PCOS), the most common cause of ovarian infertility in women. The etiology of PCOS is still uncertain; it is closely associated with insulin resistance, type 2 diabetes and obesity. In the last few years, this dysfunction has been evidenced, not only in women in their reproductive years, but also in prepubertal, or even younger girls. We discuss the physiopathology, etiopathogenia and practical evaluation of PCOS, and the therapeutic approach to PCOS in reproductive aged women and adolescents. The role of sympathetic activity and stress as an etiological factor is also discussed. We provide a succinct outline of the findings of our group in this area.

Introduction

General Concepts

Polycystic Ovary Syndrome (PCOS), also known as functional ovarian hyperandrogenism or chronic hyperandrogenic anovulation, is the most common cause of ovarian infertility with a 3% incidence in both adolescents and young adult women. PCOS is also present in 75% hirsute and in 10% premenopausal women. Although the etiology of PCOS is uncertain, it is closely associated with insulin resistance (IR) and type 2 diabetes, usually in the early stages. This syndrome could even arise during the prepubertal years or in a younger child.[1,2]

PCOS is a combination of anovulation, hyperandrogenism and hyperinsulinemia, usually accompanied by luteinizing hormone (LH) hypersecretion and by polycystic ovaries as observed by ultrasonography. The clinical manifestations of PCOS are heterogeneous and vary according to the patient's age. In general, they begin during perimenarche with menstrual alterations, mainly oligomenorrhea, hyperandrogenism and android obesity. PCOS is clinically difficult to diagnose during this time period because of the physiological changes in the somatotropic and reproductive axis that girls exhibit at this stage of their sexual development.[3] It should also be noted that recent studies state that PCOS may appear with premature menarche, precocious puberty and hyperinsulinism, which are associated with delayed intrauterine development and birth of small infants for gestational age (SGA)

The heterogeneity of the clinical manifestations of PCOS, makes it hard to define. In the last years, two definitions have been proposed: the presence of hyperandrogenism associated with chronic anovulation without any further specific cause of hypophysial or adrenal disease; and an ovarian dysfunction characterized by hyperandrogenism and morphology of a polycystic ovary.[4,5] PCOS is associated with numerous risks not only in reproduction, but also in metabolic and oncologic processes; this makes its diagnosis extremely important to initiate long-term preventive and therapeutic procedures. It is equally important not to overdiagnose the condition that might produce an emotional disturbance in patients. The reproductive risks associated with PCOS include dysfunctional metrorrhagia, infertility, a higher abortion rate in the first term of pregnancy, pregnancy induced hypertension, gestational diabetes, premature abortion and mortinates, a higher number of macrosomic infants or SGA. The oncological risks include an increased risk of endometrial, breast and ovarian cancer due to hyperestrogenism caused by the lack of cyclic progesterone. The metabolic risks include a higher incidence of type 2 diabetes, dyslipidemia, arterial hypertension and coronary cardiopathy as a result of chronic hyperinsulinemia.[6]

Physiopathology

The magnitude of complexity in the physiopathology of PCOS makes its etiology uncertain. Three kinds of inter-related alterations can be noticed: a neuroendocrine dysfunction characterized by increased luteinizing hormone (LH) secretion; a metabolic dysfunction characterized by insulin resistance and hyperinsulinemia, and a dysfunction of ovarian and adrenal steroidogenesis. This last dysfunction is strictly necessary to conform to the syndrome and consists of the hyperactivity of CYP17 enzyme (cytochrome P450), which has 17-hydroxylase and 17–20 lyase activity, and catalyzes the conversion of progesterone to 17αOH progesterone and then to androstenedione. This dysfunction has been suggested as exclusive to PCOS and could be a primary or secondary event to LH excess and/or insulin secretion. Insulin and LH increase in PCOS involves an overexpression of the enzyme, leading to a higher production of intraovarian androgens and chronic anovulation due to the inhibition of follicular development.[7] The gene for this enzyme has recently been determined and a possible dysfunction associated with PCOS has been proposed.

In addition, about 25% of PCOS patients exhibit adrenal androgen excess, expressed by a moderate dehydroepiandrosterone sulfate (DHEA-S) increase and a hyper-response to adrenocorticotropic hormone (ACTH). This phenomenon seems to be genetically determined and probably linked to an exaggerated activity of CYP17, and less probably, to other enzymatic dysfunctions. In any case, there would be a physiopathological inter-relation between the ovary and the adrenals in PCOS, the adrenal androgens acting as precursors of ovarian androgens and vice versa.[8]

The neuroendocrine dysfunction, characterized by increased LH secretion and a decreased FSH secretion, was one of the first PCOS descriptions. So far, it has not been determined whether it corresponds to a primary or secondary hypothalamic dysfunction due to high insulin levels, or to negative feedback by ovarian hormones. It has been established that the increased LH secretion in certain PCOS patients could be the expression of a hypothalamic dysfunction caused by "reprogramming" the gonadotropin releasing hormone (GnRH) pulse generator with a prenatal or prepubertal androgen exposure. In PCOS adolescents, an alteration of LH circadian secretion, an increased pulsatile LH secretion, a high LH/FSH ratio, and an increase in ovarian androgens compatible with an increment in 17-hydroxylase activity, has also been reported. Alterations in gonadotropin secretion can be manifested in a longitudinal way in pubertal girls with anovulation, particularly girls with premature pubarche; however, no intrinsic abnormalities have been found in the somatotropic axis growth hormone (GH)-insulin-like growth factor-1 (IGF-1), insulin-like growth factor binding protein 3 (IGF-BP$_3$) in these patients.[9]

On the other hand, hyperinsulinemia has been shown to decrease by lowering body weight, by ovarian wedge resection, fulguration of the ovary to reduce the ovarian secretory tissue and by the use of drugs, thus re-establishing ovarian cyclicity temporarily, which suggests that in some cases, the alterations in gonadotropic secretion would be secondary to the metabolic dysfunction, or to the abnormal negative feedback of ovarian hormones in which androgens play a preponderant role.[10,11]

In relation to the metabolic dysfunction in PCOS, most of these patients exhibit hyperinsulinemia, which can be considered a peripheral insulin resistance marker. Tissue sensitivity to the action of insulin, measured by various methods, is significantly reduced in obese and non-obese PCOS patients as compared with healthy controls with equal body mass index (BMI). The association between hyperinsulinemia and the increase in androgen biosynthesis in PCOS females is supported by numerous *in vivo* and *in vitro* studies. This led to the proposal that IR with compensatory hyperinsulinemia could lead to hyperandrogenemia through the stimulating effect of insulin on ovarian thecal cells and reticular cells of the adrenal gland. However, the effect of androgens on the genesis of hyperinsulinemia cannot be totally discarded. A recent study shows that androgens have a direct effect on the function of pancreatic islands, favoring insulin gene expression and secretion. In any case, the IR generating PCOS mechanism is unclear. A proposal has been forwarded that implies an alteration in post-receptor events in such patients. In PCOS, like in type 2 diabetes, IR would precede the decreased tolerance to glucose. Not all PCOS patients with IR develop glucose intolerance and type 2 diabetes, hence the coexistence of a β-pancreatic dysfunction, which could be conditioned either by the same IR generating defect, or by a pathological prenatal imprinting by the androgen effect on pancreatic islands, has been proposed. Thus, factors that regulate ovarian androgen secretion appear as potential inducers of the pathology.[12,13]

Etiopathogenia

The etiology of PCOS has not been clarified thus far and could include a combination of environmental and genetic factors.

Genetic basis

Although PCOS is a common dysfunction, it has been difficult to determine how it is inherited because of the absence of the male phenotype. However, in a family aggregation study, we determined that the male parents of PCOS females exhibited IR and type 2-diabetes more often than those of normal females, which suggests that at least the metabolic component of PCOS could basically be inherited through the father.

On the other hand, in order to determine the male involvement in the PCOS reproductive component, a study was carried out in brothers of PCOS females using the GnRH analogue (Lupron) test to evaluate the functionality of the reproductive axis. According to this recently published study, most brothers of PCOS females exhibited a Lupron response similar to that described for PCOS females, which suggests that the hyperactivity of P450c17 enzyme could also be present in males of PCOS families. From these two studies, it can be concluded that PCOS is not an exclusively female pathology, and that the male is also involved.[14,15]

Environmental factors

These could be ranked as those acting in postnatal life, such as obesity, stress, feeding and so on, and as those exerting an effect on prenatal life like intrauterine growth delay and prenatal androgen exposure (PAE). It has been proposed that PAE during fetal life in an experimental, accidental or pathological manner, could cause a series of changes in the reproductive axis and in the glucose homeostasis of the female fetus that could show up in postnatal life and that could be similar to those with PCOS.[16] Although PAE has been involved in PCOS development, it has not been determined whether a PCOS mother could be a source of fetal androgen excess. In congenital virilizing androgen hyperplasia, a classical PAE model, the origin of prenatal androgen excess could be the hyperandrogenic adrenal cortex of the same fetus, while in PCOS, the origin could be far more uncertain. We have recently been able to establish that pregnant PCOS women exhibit androgen levels significantly higher than those of normal pregnant females, which suggests the possibility that their child could be subjected to an abnormal steroidal condition during fetal life that could affect female as well as male fetuses.[17] Future studies will enable a long-term evaluation of prenatal androgen excess in male and female infants of pregnant PCOS women in order to determine whether PCOS should be treated during pregnancy to avoid excess androgen exposure during fetal life.

Stress as an etiological factor: Adrenergic stimulation and stress are other factors related with androgen secretion. Enhanced sympathetic and adrenal (SA) medullar activities are important links between defects in insulin action and the development of hypertension. The potential contribution of the sympathetic nervous system to the syndrome has been suggested in several studies and especially, because of the role of norepinephrine (NE) in enhancing androgens and progesterone secretion from the mammalian ovary including human.[18] This would explain the effectiveness of ovarian wedge resection or laparoscopic laser cauterization to increase ovulatory response in women with PCOS. Both procedures are likely to disrupt superior ovarian innervation. In addition, the tonic increase in sympathetic activity could be directly related to the changes in the sensitivity of the ovary and other tissues to adrenergic agonist and explain the multiple expression of PCOS as a metabolic disease. Many years ago, Semenova was the first to demonstrate that the ovary of patients with PCOS presented with an increased fluorescence to catecholamines, suggesting an increased activity of the sympathetic nerves. Our recent findings that biopsies of human ovaries release NE in vitro, and that this secretion is coupled to steroid production through the activation of the β-adrenoreceptor present on the ovarian secretory cells, strongly suggest that neural-mediated activation of ovarian steroid secretion influences on follicular development, could be the principal components in the development of the PCOS in humans.

To analyze the relation between chronic stress and the presence of PCOS, we have recently studied the depression and anxiety scores in patients with PCOS.[19] The Goldberg's 30-item General Health Questionnaire (GHQ-30) to measure anxiety, was significantly higher in patients than controls (10.4 ± 5.1 vs 4.8 ± 5.3, $p < 0.01$). The scores for GHQ-30 were similar to those obtained by Goldberg in his original study in England. The cut-off point used in our study[11,12] was chosen according to the results of the Chilean validation of the Spanish version. This higher cut-off also considered the emotional expressiveness of Latino American populations and the fact that in women, higher cut-off points seem to have a better discriminating capacity. The higher level of stress, not associated with depression in patients with PCOS, in addition to the incapacity to suppress the effect of dexamethasone and the increase in PCOS patients who secrete less urinary cortisol, strongly suggest that patients with PCOS presented a higher level of stress that could be causally related with an increased sympathetic tone.

Clinical Discussion

Practical evaluation of polycystic ovary syndrome

The PCOS diagnosis is based on a combination of irregular menstruation (oligomenorrhea or amenorrhea, mainly secondary type, and dysfunctional metrorrhagia with chronic anovulation); clinical hyperandrogenism (hirsutism, acne, seborrhea, and androgenic alopecia; virilization is rare), or biochemical hyperandrogenism (increase in circulating androgens in the absence of other specific causes for hypophysial or adrenal hyperandrogenism). Obesity is present in up to 60% of the patients and yet, it is not a part of the diagnostic criteria followed, since PCOS can occur independent of obesity.[20] According to NIH-NICHD consensus conference (1990), the definition of PCOS corresponds to a diagnosis made by excluding other pathologies like Cushing's syndrome, acromegaly, and congenital adrenal hyperplasia (CAH), that are normally associated with hyperandrogenism and chronic anovulation. However, the controversy persists, mainly in Europeans, over whether typical morphological changes should be included in the diagnosis, of PCOS, which led the ESHRE/ASRM consensus conference[5] to define it as a typical ovarian dysfunction characterized by hyperandrogenism and polycystic ovarian morphology. In relation to the latter, it should be noted that 21–23% of the female population in the fertile age produce PCOS-like echotomographic images (exhibiting multiple subcortical cystic images of 2-4 mm diameter associated with an increase in ovarian stroma), that 25% of them are asymptomatic, and that not all patients have PCOS-like echotomographic images, even when sophisticated computerized methods are used to measure ovarian stroma. It is important to emphasize that the PCOS diagnosis should be clinically stated and biochemically confirmed, echotomography being a quite an important co-adjuvant element, but not a diagnostic tool by itself. In relation to biochemical changes, total testosterone is discretely elevated only in 50% of the cases; because of this, determination of the free androgen index [Testosterone (nmol)/ (sexhormone binding globulin (SHBG) (nmol) × 100] and androstenedione concentration are useful to determine the presence of hyperandrogenemia. About 40–60% of the patients exhibit an elevated LH/FSH ratio (> than 3:1) but their normality does not discard the diagnosis. In addition, discrete elevations of DHEAS, prolactin and 17-OH progesterone can be observed in up to 40% of the cases. IR should be evaluated in all PCOS patients even in cases with normal body mass index because of its high prevalence; an oral glucose tolerance test (OGTT) including insulin measurement is used in the clinical routine. Basal insulinemia > 12.5 μU/ mL, greater than 100μU/mL at 60 min, greater than 160 μU/mL at 120 min, a glycemia/

insulinemia index <4.5 and a homeostasis model assessment-insulin resistance (HOMA – IR) value of 2.5 are suggestive of insulin resistance. The normality of basal insulinemia and of these indices does not discard the diagnosis of IR. In case IR is suspected, the study should be completed with a lipid profile.

The recommended scheme of study comprises of the following:

1. Studying hyperandrogenism with the determination of total testosterone, androstenedione, 17-hydroxyprogesterone, DHEAS, SHBG and the calculation of the free androgen index.
2. Further hormonal studies to determine other causes of oligo-ovulation, such as determination of LH, follicle stimulating hormone (FSH), thyroid stimulating hormone (TSH) and prolactin.
3. Evaluation of insulin resistance with a glucose tolerance test (75 grams of glucose), with glucose and insulin determination at times 0, 60, and 120 min (the full test is recommended) plus a lipid profile.
4. Gynecological echotomography.

Therapeutic approach to PCOS in reproductive age women

As mentioned above, PCOS is a frequent endocrine-metabolic dysfunction, characterized by chronic anovulation and hyperandrogenism affecting the reproductive function of young women and that is closely associated with IR, which plays a preponderant role in chronic anovulation and long-term metabolic consequences of the syndrome. PCOS treatment should therefore be directed to correct hyperandrogenism, chronic anovulation and the associated metabolic alterations. Whether the patient wants to get pregnant or not is a key issue in the preliminary selection of therapy. However, correcting the metabolic alterations should precede, or be associated with any therapeutic procedure. Since PCOS is an endocrine-metabolic dysfunction of doubtful spontaneous cure, treatment should start as early as possible, be long-lasting and adequate according to the clinical evolution of the syndrome and to the needs of each patient.

Any treatment of metabolic alterations involves correction of obesity and use of drugs to decrease hyperinsulinemia and/or to increase tissue sensitivity to insulin.

Obesity must be combatted first since this aggravates the decrease in SHBG, and alterations associated with IR and hyperinsulinemia, such as arterial hypertension, dyslipidemia and glucose intolerance. The treatment for obesity involves a change in lifestyle, that is, a balanced diet (diets with a low glycemic index are recommended) and regular physical exercise. In case of mild IR, or contraindications to the use of other drugs, orlistat should be added to the above-mentioned measures. This could have a beneficial action on body weight, lipid profile and sensitivity to insulin. The probable role of hyperinsulinemia in the pathogenesis of PCOS has promoted the use of drugs that lower insulin levels or increase insulin tissue sensitivity. Metformin and thiazolidinediones (glitazones), which could be potentially useful, have not been approved by the FDA for PCOS. Thus far, numerous clinical studies regarding metformin use in reproductive age women exist. This drug has proved to be useful in lowering circulating insulin levels, enhancing SHBG concentrations, and decreasing circulating androgen and LH concentrations. This could have a beneficial effect on hirsutism, appetite decrease and BMI, restoring ovarian cyclicity and ovulation. In PCOS, these effects could be due to metformin, which favors insulin signaling, enhances phosphorylation and the activity of insulin receptor substrate 2 (IRS-2) and, on the other hand, decreases the activity of the ovarian and adrenal enzyme CYP 17 (cytochrome P450C17). Besides, metformin could have two potential therapeutic applications during pregnancy: reducing premature abortions and decreasing the risk of gestational diabetes and prenatal androgenization.[21,22]

The *treatment of chronic anovulation* should begin with the management of obesity to lower plasma insulin levels, testosterone and LH, thus permitting a spontaneous restart of ovarian cyclicity and of ovulation. In obese and non-obese IR patients, an average metformin dose of 1500 mg, upto a maximum of 2000 mg, is recommended. In 4–6 months, up to 90% recovery of ovarian cyclicity is attained with an eight-fold increase in the ovulation rate. Patients unwilling to conceive and who have not yet had regular cycles by using metformin, can periodically use low doses of progestin. Low and progressive doses of clomiphene citrate (CC) (50–150 mg/day, 5th-9th days of the cycle) are recommended to initiate ovulation induction in patients who are eager to conceive but have so far been unsuccessful with the exclusive use of metformin. This treatment should not last longer than 6 consecutive months and metformin should be maintained. In patients who do not respond to CC, gonadotropins may be used; however, they are associated with other risks such as, ovarian hyperstimulation and multiple pregnancies, which could be reduced by the simultaneous use of metformin. In addition to the medical schemes, there are surgical procedures (ovarian wedge resection and laparoscopic fulguration of the ovarian surface with laser) that should be used only as the last alternative.

The *treatment of hyperandrogenism* can include an oral contraceptive pill (OCP) with low androgen progestins, such as desogestrel, gestodene, and drosperinone. These are quite useful to suppress LH secretion, decrease the ovarian synthesis of testosterone, increase plasma SHBG concentrations, decrease free androgens; and permit a regular desquamation of the endometrium, preventing the risk of endometrium hyperplasia. Possible IR aggravation, which is more likely with OCPs containing cyproterone acetate (CA), is one complication associated with the use of this drug. Drosperinone produces less weight gain and alteration in body composition than other contraceptives thus, it would be particularly appropriate for adolescents. Oral contraceptives can be used with some antiandrogens such as cyproterone acetate, spironolactone, flutamide or finasteride. The choice of antiandrogen depends on each particular case. The first two are quite effective in suppressing androgen levels, whereas flutamide and finasteride act as peripheral blockers of androgen action. When flutamide is used, monitoring liver function is essential because of the potential risk of liver damage. In addition, obese PCOS patients with IR usually have a concomitant fatty liver thus, obesity should be treated before using flutamide.

Similar to the use of contraceptives, GnRH analogues can equally be used to inhibit ovarian androgen production. However, they do not have a long-term cost-benefit effect better than the scheme mentioned above. Glucocorticoids, even at low doses, are not adequate for the treatment of hyperandrogenism in PCOS patients because of the adverse effects observed in 20% of patients.

The therapeutic approach to PCOS in adolescents begins during the prepubertal age for symptoms such as, hirsutism, acne, menstrual irregularities, android obesity, occasional acanthosis nigricans and dyslipidemia that can appear with a precocious pubarche. The clinical manifestations are polymorphic and hard to distinguish from the pubertal process itself. Thus, menstrual irregularities can be physiological until 2-3 years after menarche. During puberty, there is a physiological lowering of SHBG, which enhances the free androgen fraction and originates peripubertal acne. In addition, a physiological phenomenon of a decrease in insulin sensitivity mainly in Tanner stages 3 and 4 occurs, which is partially corrected at the end of puberty, without returning to the prepubertal values. All the above information permits the understanding of how difficult it may be to establish PCOS at this age. However, there are some guidelines for establishing the diagnosis of premature pubarche (pubic hair before 8 years), presence of android obesity, acanthosis nigricans, type 2 diabetes in first degree relatives, PCOS in mothers and sisters, and small for gestational age (SGA). From a therapeutic point of view, a differentiated scheme is suggested for PCOS adolescents according to the current physiological situation of the patient. In both the cases, the fundamental issue will be

IR treatment, with extreme care using non-pharmacological measures.

Metformin, or metformin associated with an antiandrogen such as flutamide in low doses (125–250 mg) or spironolactone, is suggested for perimenarche adolescents, while metformin associated with antiandrogens and oral contraceptives is the recommended scheme for postmenarche adolescents because of the potential risk of becoming pregnant.

Metformin has multiple beneficial effects—reproductive and metabolic in PCOS patients. It enhances the effect of hypocaloric diets in the metabolic control of PCOS as well as in improving the ovulation and pregnancy rates. In addition, it could have a potential beneficial effect during pregnancy.

Conclusions

The variety of evidence presented in this chapter strongly suggests that PCOS could have a genetic predisposition that may manifest itself even before menarche and that environmental factors during prenatal or postnatal life could lead to the clinical and biochemical expression of the syndrome in adult life. A chronic stress condition is related to changes in follicular development and increased disposition to PCOS. Due to the high prevalence of type 2 diabetes in women with this syndrome and their relatives, PCOS should be considered a marker of a family pathology, a pathway to type 2 diabetes and a public health problem. The knowledge of the mechanism underlying the syndrome, will improve the treatment of this pathology.

References

1. Abbott DH, Dumesic DA, Franks S. Developmental origin of polycystic ovary syndrome – a hypothesis. *J Endocrinol* 2002; 174: 1–5.
2. Apter D, Butzow T, Laughlin GA, Yen SS. Metabolic features of polycystic ovary syndrome are found in adolescent girls with hyperandrogenism. *J Clin Endocrinol Metab* 1995; 80(10): 2966–2673.
3. Chang RJ. A practical approach to the diagnosis of polycystic ovary syndrome. *Am J Obstet Gynecol* 2004; 191: 713–717.

4. Balen AH, Laven JS, Tan SL, Dewailly D. Ultrasound assessment of the polycystic ovary: international consensus definitions. *Hum Reprod Update* 2003; 9: 505–514.

5. Rotterdam ESHRE/ASRM-Sponsored PCOS consensus workshop group. Revised. 2003 consensus on diagnostic criteria and long-term health risks related to polycystic ovary syndrome (PCOS). *Hum Reprod* 2004; 19: 41–47.

6. Zawdaki JK, Dunaif A. Diagnostic criteria for polycystic ovary syndrome: towards a rationale approach. In: Polycystic Ovary Syndrome, editors. Dunaif A, Givens JR, Haseltine F, Merriam GR, Boston: *Blackwell Scientific* 1992: 377–384.

7. Nestler JE and Jakubowicz DJ. Decreases in ovarian cytochrome P450c17-alpha activity and serum free testosterone after reduction of insulin secretion in polycystic ovary syndrome. *N Engl J Med* 1996; 335: 617–623.

8. Rosenfield RL, Barnes RB, Cara JF, et al. Dysregulation of cytochrome P45017 as the cause of polycystic ovarian syndrome. *Fertil Steril* 1990; 53: 785–791.

9. Gonzalez F, Hatala DA, Speroff L. Adrenal and ovarian steroid hormone responses to gonadotropin-releasing hormone agonist treatment in polycystic ovary syndrome. *Am J Obstet Gynecol* 1991; 165: 535–545.

10. Salehi M, Bravo-Vera R, Sheikh A, Gouller A, Poretsky L Pathogenesis of polycystic ovary syndrome: what is the role of obesity? *Metabolism* 2004; 53: 358–376.

11. Pirwany I, Tulandi T. Laparoscopic treatment of polycystic ovaries: is it time to relinquish the procedure? *Fertil Steril* 2003; 80: 241–251.

12. Legro RS, Kunselman AR, Dodson WC, Dunaif A. Prevalence and predictors of risk for type 2 diabetes mellitus and impaired glucose tolerance in polycystic ovary syndrome: a prospective, controlled study in 254 affected women. *J Clin Endocrinol Metab* 1999; 84(1): 165–169.

13. Sir-Petermann T, Angel B Maliqueo M, Carvajal F, Santos JL, Pérez-Bravo F. Prevalence of type II diabetes mellitus and insulin resistance in parents of women with polycystic ovary syndrome. *Diabetologia* 2002; 45: 959–964.

14. Sir-Petermann T, Hitchsfeld C, Maliqueo M, Codner E, Echiburú B, Gacitúa R, et al. Birth weight in offspring of PCOS mothers. *Hum Reprod* 2005; 20: 2122–2126.

15. Sir Petermann T, Cartes A, Maliqueo M, Gutiérrez C, Toloza H, Echiburú B y Recabarren SE. Patterns of hormonal response to the gonadotrophin releasing hormone agonist leuprolide in brothers of women with polycystic ovary syndrome: a pilot study. *Hum Reprod* 2004; 19: 2742–2747.

16. Ibanez L, Potau N, Francois I, de Zegher F. Precocious pubarche, hyperinsulinism, and ovarian hyperandrogenism in girls: relation to reduced fetal growth. *J Clin Endocrinol Metab* 1998; 83(10): 3558–62.

17. Sir-Petermann T, Maliqueo M, Angel B, Lara HE, Pérez-Bravo F, Recabarren SE. Maternal serum androgens in pregnant women with polycystic ovary syndrome: possible implications in prenatal androgenization. *Hum Reprod* 2002; 17: 2573–2579.

18. Lara HE, Porcille A, Espinoza J, Romero C, Luza SM, Fuhrer J, et al. Release of norepinephrine from the human ovary: coupling to steroidogenic response. *Endocrine* 2001 15: 187–192.

19. Greiner M, Paredes A, Araya V and Lara HE. Role of Stress and Sympathetic Innervation in the Development of Polycystic Ovary Syndrome. *Endocrine* 2005; 28(3): out of press December 2005.

20. Dunaif A, Segal KR, Futterweit W, Dobrjansky A. Profound peripheral insulin resistance, independent of obesity, in polycystic ovary syndrome. *Diabetes* 1989; 38 (9): 1165–1174.

21. Costello MF, Eden JA. A systematic review of the reproductive system effects of metformin in patients with polycystic ovary syndrome. *Fertil Steril* 2003; 79: 1–13.

22. Glueck CJ, Wang P, Goldenberg N, Sieve-Smith L. Pregnancy outcomes among women with polycystic ovary syndrome treated with metformin. *Hum Reprod* 2002; 17: 2858–2864.

Genetics of PCOS

9

The Genetics of Polycystic Ovary Syndrome

Marina Baldi, M Benkhalifa, Luciana Chessa, Francesco Fiorentino, Donatella Caserta, Massimo Moscarini

Summary

Polycystic Ovary Syndrome (PCOS), the most common endocrine disorder of women of reproductive age, with an enigmatic pathophysiological and molecular basis, is commonly detected in women opting for assisted reproductive technology programs.[1] Furthermore, it is one of the most frequent causes of treatment failure and Ovarian hyperstimulation syndrome (OHSS) leading to cycle cancellation. PCOS is defined when at least two of the following three *features* (i) oligo-or anovulation, (ii) clinical and or/biochemical hyperandrogenism, or (iii) polycystic ovaries are present, after exclusion of other etiologies.[2] Nearly 45% to 50% sisters of PCOS patients have PCOS or hyperandrogenemia without anovulation, which is consistent with an autosomal dominant mode of inheritance.[3] It is likely that multiple genes and environmental factors contribute to the pathophysiology of PCOS and that no single gene mutation will be found that is both necessary and sufficient to cause the syndrome.[4] Different methodologies have been used to elucidate the complex polygenic origin of PCOS[1] and different genes have been suspected to play a key role in the PCOS pathology.[5] Genes involved in steroidogenesis, folliculogenesis and those involved in secretion and action of insulin or in other metabolic disorders have been suspected to be candidates for the pathogenesis of PCOS.[6]

Introduction

In human reproductive medicine, polycystic ovary syndrome (PCOS) is a common pathology characterized by irregular menstruation, anovulation, reduced spontaneous pregnancy rate, and hyperandrogenism, with or without insulin resistance.[7] It is possible that the ethnicity can affect the level of hyperandrogenism and insulin resistance.[8] It was reported in a cross-sectional analysis among a non-hospital population that the incidence of unexplained hyperandrogenic chronic anovulation in the United States population approaches 5%.[9] A survey of polycystic ovary syndrome in the Greek island, based on the hormonal and metabolic profiles, reported PCOS in nearly 7% of the women.[10] In 2000, a prospective study of Spanish women from an unselected group revealed a PCOS rate of 6.5%.[11]

An unbalanced luteinizing hormone (LH)/ follicle stimulating hormone (FSH) ratio was reported in many PCOS patients, but even if this ratio is increased over 2/1 or 2/3, this unbalanced ratio of gonadotropins is not a universal feature and not currently used for the differential diagnosis of PCOS.[2] In women of reproductive age, presenting with elevated gonadotropins and primary amenorrhea, a karyotype is indicated. The commonly observed karyotypes are 45, X (Turner's Syndrome), mosaic 46, XY cell lines and other sex chromosome abnormalities as well as Robertsonian and reciprocal translocations (autosome/autosome and/or autosome/gonosome) and deletions. In addition, deletion of chromosome X, mainly long (q) arm, can be observed with an increase risk of premature ovarian failure and fragile X syndrome. Other disorders as Kallman, Noonan syndromes or triplet repeat disorders can also be diagnosed also during the genome investigation.

Cytogenetic studies of PCOS patients failed to demonstrate specific or common chromosome disorders and abnormalities including cryptics. A specific gene analysis showed different altered patterns of expression, suggesting that genetic disorders in PCOS mainly affect the signal transduction pathways controlling a familial gene expression.[1] According to the literature, genetic investigation of PCOS shows the implication of androgen synthesis pathway and the role of insulin in the pathogenesis of the syndrome.

In PCOS, it is important to identify the rare cases of adrenal or ovarian tumors and evaluate the origin of the hyperandrogenism (adrenal versus ovarian) during the clinical *and* laboratory female evaluation. To investigate hyperandrogenism, the differential diagnosis includes Cushing syndrome, non-classical congenital adrenal hyperplasia, exogenous androgen use, rare forms of hyperprolactinemia, thyroid disease and finally, PCOS. Polycystic ovary syndrome is a large spectrum of disorders, and it is possible that ovulatory women with mild androgen excess and anovulatory women with polycystic ovaries (PCO) but without androgen excess may have variants of the classical syndrome of anovulation.[4]

For a better comprehension of the pathogenesis of the hyperandrogenism syndrome, some genes contributing to steroidogenesis were investigated. Androgen excess as well as hyperinsulinemia can suppress sex hormone binding globulin (SHBG), leading to a greater pool of bioavailable androgens. In patients with PCOS, an increase in 3-alpha hydroxy steroid dehydrogenase (HSD) and 17 alpha-hydroxylase/17, 20 lyase activities represents the main origin of hypersteroidogenesis

and androgen hypersecretion.[12,13] The copy numbers of cytochrome P450 17-hydroxylase/17, 20-desmolase (CYP17) and P450 cytochrome side chain cleavage (CYP11A), involved in cholesterol to pregnenolone transformation in the theca cells of PCOS women, are overexpressed.[13]

Clinical Discussion

An association between high serum testosterone level and a polymorphic sequence of a pentanucleotide (TTTTA)n repeat in the initiation code of 5'-locus of the CYP11A was reported in 1997.[14] Gene linkage analysis in 1999 showed a controversial correlation between CYP11A polymorphism and PCOS.[15] A complete elucidation of the (TTTTA)n polymorphism should be made for a better understanding of the CYP11A promoter polymorphism role in PCOS.[7]

In 1994[16] a single nucleotide polymorphism in the promoter region of CYP17 was reported. The author suspected that this polymorphism can be the cause of the increasing susceptibility to PCOS, but later,[17] it was published that 5'polymorphism of the CYP17 gene is not associated with serum testosterone levels in women with polycystic ovaries. In the year 2000,[18] an enhancement of CYP17 promoter in the theca cells of PCOS women compared to controls was reported.

In 1999 Escobar-Morseale et al.[19] reported a clear relation between cytochrome P450-21 hydroxylase enzyme (CYP21) deficiency in hirsute patients. A heterozygote mutation of CYP21 and PCOS was also reported by Witchel and Atson.[20] Hirsutism occurs when androgens stimulate the transformation of fine, unpigmented vellus hair to coarse, pigmented, thickened terminal hair. This is thought to be mediated by the intracellular actions of the enzyme 17-ketosteroid reductase, which converts androstenedione to testosterone, and 5 alpha-reductase, which converts testosterone to dihydrotestosterone.[21]

CYP21 is involved in cortisol synthesis and congenital adrenal hyperplasia. A possible CYP21 gene mutation or expression profile defect in the cytochrome P450-21 hydroxylase enzyme can be responsible for the hyperandrogenism syndrome in PCOS. A relative deficiency of the 21-hydroxylase enzyme in non-classical congenital adrenal hyperplasia (NC-CAH) can cause hirsutism or menstrual irregularity in females. Another gene, the glutathione S transferase gene (GST), has been suspected to be responsible for ovarian cysts. In 2004, a genetic polymorphism of GTS gene in association with susceptibility to polycystic ovaries in the South Indian women population was reported.[22]

Genes involved in gonadotropin (LH, FSH) regulation were investigated in PCOS patients because of the unbalanced ratio of LH/FSH. LH secretory abnormalities in PCOS appear to be the result of lack of cyclic progesterone production and androgen-induced resistance to the inhibitory effect of progesterone on LH secretion.[23] The mid-cycle LH surge initiates periovulation events and a pre-surge follicle development, and the absence of LH during the final stages of preovulatory maturation can result in anovulation. LH plays a key role in androgen production. A possible disorder in the LH gene or LH receptor gene may explain the deregulation observed in PCOS. Until today, there is no clear scientific data that shows any effect of gene disorder or polymorphism that clearly explains the contribution of a genomic disorder in the hyperandrogenemia syndrome.

In vivo, FSH stimulates the growth of follicles and granulosa cell differentiation. Granulosa cell growth requires other mitogenic factors such activin, insulin, insulin-like growth factor-II (IGF-II) and growth differentiation factor-9 (GDF-9) in addition to FSH. It is unclear whether FSH increases the expression of these and other growth factors/receptors.[24] More than the contribution to antral follicle growth, FSH plays an important role in granulosa cell differentiation to the preovulatory status, through an augmented expression of genes that code for the aromatase and LH receptors.[25]

Polymorphism of the follistatin gene was also investigated. Follistatin acts as an activin-binding protein and neutralizes the biological activity of activin. Activin plays a key role in FSH production and follicle maturation, and inhibits follicular androgen production. While the mitogenic action of activin is clear, the local function of inhibins are not well understood, but they may play a role in increasing LH-stimulated androgen synthesis from theca cells.[24] An excessive disorder of activin via a genetic/epigenetic deregulation of follistatin can reduce FSH secretion and follicle maturation and increase androgen production. There is no clear data demonstrating the relation between a follistatin gene defect and PCOS.[15,25]

Hyperinsulinemia and insulin resistance are observed in approximately 50–70% of women with PCOS, and nearly 25% of women with type 2 diabetes have PCOS.[26] Patients with insulin resistance also have severe ovarian hyperandrogenism and virilization.[27] The origin of insulin resistance in PCOS is not elucidated yet. A defect in insulin receptor autophosphorylation is present in about 50% of PCOS patients.[27] This disorder is characterized by an increase in serine phosphorylation, which inhibits the tyrosine kinase activity of the insulin receptor. The increase in serine phosphorylation of the insulin receptor appears to be the result of a serine kinase activity extrinsic to the receptor.[28]

In fibroblast cells of women with PCOS, insulin resistance is selective and inhibits the metabolic but not the mitogenic pathway of insulin signaling.[29] In skeletal muscle biopsies from obese PCOS patients, there is a significant decrease in insulin-stimulated activation of insulin receptor substrate-1-associated phosphatidylinositol 3-kinase activity.[4] An environmental factor may initiate insulin resistance and the consequent androgen excess. The hyperandrogenism of PCOS favours a central/visceral pattern of body fat distribution; other hormonal and genetic factors may also play a role.[30] Most women with stromal hyperthecosis have severe hyperinsulinemia, which may be the stimulus for excess stromal androgen production.[21]

A polymorphism in the variable number tandem repeat (VNTR) in the promoter region of the insulin gene can regulate its expression. In 1997, a relation and association between the class III allele at the insulin gene VNTR in the 5' region of the insulin gene and PCOS was observed.[31] Studies on the coding region of the insulin receptor gene in patients with PCOS showed a large number of silent polymorphisms. A majority of the observed polymorphisms have also been identified in normal patients. In 2002, a C/T single nucleotide polymorphism in the tyrosine kinase domain of the insulin receptor gene was reported.[32]

Nearly one third of the obese women with PCOS have impaired glucose tolerance and about 10% have type 2 diabetes mellitus. A similar prevalence of abnormal glucose tolerance is observed in adolescent women with PCOS. These disorders are associated with a high risk of cardiovascular disease.[4] In PCOS, lipid disorder is characterized by low high density lipoprotein (HDL) and HDL 2 cholesterol, high total and low density lipoprotein (LDL) cholesterol, high triglycerides and very low density lipoprotein (VLDL) cholesterol, with an increased risk for cardiovascular disease and atherosclerosis in women with hirsutism or PCO.[33]

To treat the metabolic abnormalities of PCOS, many approaches have been used; weight loss is effective in reducing the progression of diabetes. Fasting can significantly decrease the total cholesterol, LDL-cholesterol and triglycerides. Weight loss can affect a significant decrease in hyperandrogenism by decreasing the free circulating testosterone levels to nearly normal and increasing the sex hormone binding globulin (SHBG).[4] Metformin is used as the insulin sensitizing agent of choice in PCOS. It can reduce the total and/or free testosterone levels, weight, and improve the insulin response to glucose and total lipids. Oral contraception has recently been adopted as a treatment to favorably affect the metabolic parameters in PCOS.

Recent Advances and Conclusions

Assisted Reproductive Technlogy (ART) has now become an additional tool to obtain acceptable pregnacy rates. The outcome in terms of pregnancy and implantation rates between patients with PCOS and patients undergoing in vitro fertilization (IVF) for other indications is similar. But generally, in these patients, a smaller percentage of retrived oocytes are fertilized. Oocyte and embryo quality in women with PCOS is however, questionable as low fertilization rates and decreased embryo quality have been reported in some studies.[34] These observations can be explained by the previous unbalanced hormonal status, the low quality of the ovarian reserve and the effect of ovarian stimulation protocol on the cumulus and oocyte maturity. Moreover, we have to consider the risk of genetic or epigenetic disorders in oocytes and zygotes in PCOS patients undergoing ART. Increased numbers of oocytes available for insemination or intracytoplasmic sperm injection (ICSI) may compensate for decreased fertilization rates and embryo quality. On the other hand, the reduction in oocyte number to three may significantly reduce the fertilization and pregnancy rate, if not supported by individualized protocols. The solution in the future seems to be In vitro maturation (IVM) of oocytes, which offers the patient a treatment choice with a reduced risk of OHSS and a higher percentage of success due to the fact that in vitro maturation may guarantee a better controlled ovarian environment.

References

1. Diamanti-Kandarakis E and Piperi C. Genetics of polycystic ovary syndrome: searching for the way out of the labyrinth. *Hum Reprod Update* 2005; 11(6): 631–643.

2. Azziz R. PCOS: A diagnostic challenge. *RBM online* 2004; 8(6): 644–648.

3. Roldan B, San Millan JL, Escobar-Morreale F. Genetic basis of metabolic abnormalities in polycystic ovary syndrome: implication for therapy. *Am J Pharmacogenomics* 2004; 4(2): 93–107.

4. Barnes R. Polycystic ovary syndrome. In: Frontiers in reproductive endocrinology. A comprehensive review and update. Serono Symposia, Washington USA, 2005: 16–20.

5. Ben Slomo I. The polycystic ovary syndrome : what does insulin resistance have to do with it. *RBM Online* 2003; 6(36): 36–42.

6. Franks S, McCarthy M. Genetics of ovarian disorder:

Polycystic ovary syndrome. *Rev Endoc Metab Disord* 2004; 5(1): 69–76.

7. Fratantonio E, Vicari E, Pafumi C, Calogero A. Genetics of polycystic ovarian syndrome. *RBM Online* 2005; 10(6): 713–720.

8. Carmina E, Koyama T, Chang L, Stanczyk FZ, Lobo RA. Does ethnicity influence the prevalence of adrenal hyperandrogenism and insulin resistance in polycystic ovary syndrome? *Am J Obstet Gynecol* 1992; 167(6): 1807–1812.

9. Knochenhauer ES, Key TJ, Kahsar-Miller M, Waggoner W, Boots LR, Azziz R. Prevalence of the polycystic ovary syndrome in unselected black and white women of the southeastern United States: a prospective study. *J Clin Endocrinol Metab* 1998; 83(9): 3078–3082.

10. Diamanti-Kandarakis E, Kouli C, Bergiele A, Filandra F, Tsianateli T, et al. A survey of polycystic ovary syndrome in the Greek island of Lesbos: hormonal and metabolic profile. *J Clin Endocrinol Metab* 1999; 84: 4006–4011.

11. Asuncion M, Calvo RM, San Millan JL, Sancho J, Avila S, Escobar-Morreale HF. A prospective study of the prevalence of the polycystic ovary syndrome in unselected Caucasian women from Spain. *J Clin Endocrinol Metab* 2000; 85(7): 2434–2448.

12. Nelson VL, Legro RS, Strauss JF 3rd, McAllister JM. Augmented androgen production is a stable steroidogenic phenotype of propagated theca cells from polycystic ovaries. *Mol Endocrinol* 1999; 13(6): 946–957.

13. Nelson VL, Qin Kn KN, Rosenfield RL, Wood JR, Penning TM, Legro RS, Strauss JF 3rd, McAllister JM. The biochemical basis for increased testosterone production in theca cells propagated from patients with polycystic ovary syndrome. *J Clin Endocrinol Metab* 2001; 86(12): 5925–5933.

14. Gharani N, Waterworth DM, Batty S, White D, Gilling-Smith C, Conway GS, McCarthy M, Franks S, Williamson R. Association of the steroid synthesis gene CYP11a with polycystic ovary syndrome and hyperandrogenism. *Hum Mol Genet* 1997; 6(3): 397–402.

15. Urbanek M, Wu X, Vickery K, Kao L, Christenson L, Scheneyer A, et al. Allelic variants of the follistatin gene in polycystic ovary syndrome. *J Clin Endocrinol Metab* 2000; 85 4455–4461.

16. Carey AH, Waterworth D, Patel K, White D, Little J, Novelli P, Franks S, Williamson R. Polycystic ovaries and premature male pattern baldness are associated with one allele of the steroid metabolism gene CYP17. *Hum Mol Genet* 1994; 3(10): 1873–1876.

17. Gharani N, Waterworth DM, Williamson R, Franks S. 5′ polymorphism of the CYP17 gene is not associated with serum testosterone levels in women with polycystic ovaries. *J Clin Endocrinol Metab* 1996; 81(11): 4174.

18. Wickenheisser JK, Quinn PG, Nelson VL, Legro RS, Strauss JF 3rd, McAllister JM. Differential activity of the cytochrome P450 17alpha-hydroxylase and steroidogenic acute regulatory protein gene promoters in normal and polycystic ovary syndrome theca cells. *J Clin Endocrinol Metab* 2000; 85(6): 2304–2311.

19. Escobar-Morreale HF, San Millan JL, Smith RR, Sancho J, Witchel SF. The presence of the 21-hydroxylase deficiency carrier status in hirsute women: phenotype-genotype correlations. *Fertil Steril* 1999; 72(4): 629–638.

20. Witchel SF, Aston CE. The role of heterozygosity for CYP21 in the polycystic ovary syndrome. *J Pediatr Endocrinol Metab* 2000; 13 (5): 1315–1317.

21. Legro R. Etiology and management of hirsutism. In: Frontiers in reproductive endocrinology. A comprehensive review and update. Serono Symposia, Washington, USA 2005: 16–20.

22. Babu KA, Rao KL, Kanakavalli MK, Suryanarayana VV, Deenadayal M, Singh L.CYP1A1, GSTM1 and GSTT1 genetic polymorphism is associated with susceptibility to polycystic ovaries in South Indian women. *Reprod Biomed Online* 2004; 9(2): 194–200.

23. Ovalle F, Azziz R. Insulin resistance, polycystic ovary syndrome, and type 2 diabetes mellitus. *Fertil Steril* 2002; 77(6): 1095–1105.

24. Charles L, Jennifer D. Follicle Growth and Ovulation. In: Frontiers in Reproductive Endocrinology. A comprehensive review and update. Serono Symposia, Washington, USA 2005: 16–20.

25. Hirshfield AN. Development of follicles in the mammalian ovary. *Int Rev Cytol* 1991; 124: 43–101.

26. Peppard H, Marfori J, Iuorno M, Nestler J. Prevalence of polycystic ovary syndrome among premenopausal women with type 2 diabetes. *Care* 2001; 24(6): 1050–1052.

27. Dunaif A. Insulin resistance and the polycystic ovary syndrome: mechanism and implications for pathogenesis. *Endocr Rev* 1997 Dec; 18(6): 774–800.

28. Li M, Youngren JF, Dunaif A, Goldfine ID, Maddux BA, Zhang BB, Evans JL. Decreased insulin receptor (IR) autophosphorylation in fibroblasts from patients with PCOS: effects of serine kinase inhibitors and IR activators. *J Clin Endocrinol Metab* 2002; 87(9): 4088–4093.

29. Venkatesan AM, Dunaif A, Corbould A. Insulin resistance in polycystic ovary syndrome: progress and paradoxes. *Recent Prog Horm Res* 2001; 56: 295–308.

30. Holte J. Polycystic ovary syndrome and insulin resistance: thrifty gene struggling with over feeding and sedantary life style? *J Endocrinol Invest* 1998; 21(9): 589–601.

31. Waterworth D, Bennet S, Gharani N, McCarthy M, Hague S, Batty S, et al. Linkage and association of insulin VNTR regulatory polymorphism with polucystic ovary syndrome. *Lancet* 1997; 349: 986–990.

32. Siegel S, Futterweit W, Davies T, Concepcios E, Greenberg D, Villanueva R, Tomer Y. A C/T single nucleotide polymorphism at the tyrosine kinase domain of the insulin receptor gene associated with polycystic ovary syndrome. *Fertil Steril* 2002; 78, 1240–1243.

33. Wild RA. Long-term health consequences of PCOS. *Hum Reprod Update* 2002; 8(3): 231–241.

34. Fabregues F, Penarrubia J, Vidal E, Casals G, Vanrell JA, Balasch J. Oocyte quality in patients with severe ovarian hyperstimulation syndrome: a self-controlled clinical study. *Fertil Steril* 2004; 82(4): 827–833.

10

Familial Associations in Women with Polycystic Ovary Syndrome

Sulbha Arora, Gautam N Allahbadia

Summary

Polycystic Ovary Syndrome (PCOS), originally known as Stein-Leventhal syndrome, as we all know, after the doctors who first identified this disorder in 1935, is an endocrine disorder that affects 5–10% of women. It occurs in all races and nationalities, is the most common hormonal disorder among women of reproductive age, and is a leading cause of infertility. A family history of thyroid disease, diabetes, insulin resistance, or Syndrome X is often found in the immediate and extended biological family members of women with PCOS. The syndrome has a strong genetic component although, as with diabetes, environmental factors can affect the degree and nature of symptoms. Paternal transmission with PCOS occurs over 80% of the time when the father is affected with the gene. Males carrying the gene that causes PCOS in women, may have hypothyroidism, Syndrome X, diabetes (especially type 2), heart problems, poor lipid profile, inability to grow a full beard, or premature balding. Maternal transmission occurs approximately 45% of the time. Either parent can transmit the gene, without showing any symptoms of PCOS (in men, usually referred to as Metabolic Syndrome). Several recent lines of evidence suggest that women with PCOS may also be at an increased risk of having a personal or family history of ovarian cancer and breast cancer, especially since these women are hyperandrogenic and infertile, which are risk factors for breast and ovarian cancer, respectively.

Introduction

Polycystic Ovary Syndrome (PCOS) is a common and heterogeneous disorder of women of reproductive age, characterized by chronic anovulation and hyperandrogenism. The association of amenorrhea with bilateral polycystic ovaries was first described in 1935 by Stein and Leventhal[1] and was known for decades as the Stein-Leventhal Syndrome. The syndrome is present in 5–10% of women in the reproductive age group and is the commonest cause of anovulatory infertility. In the past, the clinical diagnosis rested on the triad of hirsutism, amenorrhea and obesity. Subsequently, it has been recognized that PCOS has an extremely heterogeneous clinical picture and is multifactorial in etiology.[2] In addition to the infertility issues associated with anovulation, these women are at risk for developing endometrial cancers usually at an earlier age and even premenopausally. For this endocrine disorder, there is an emerging picture of a strong familial component to PCOS with a phenotypic characteristic of hyperandrogenemia in sisters of affected individuals.

Insulin resistance and hyperinsulinemia are commonly exhibited in PCOS. Insulin resistance is now recognized as a major risk factor for the development of type 2 diabetes mellitus.[3] About one-third of obese PCOS patients have impaired glucose tolerance (IGT), and 7.5–10% have type 2 diabetes mellitus.[4,5] These rates are mildly increased even in non-obese women who have PCOS compared with the general population.

It has also been suggested that PCOS may be a thrombophilic state; in a previous study,[6] 29% of women with PCOS gave a positive family history of thrombosis compared with 8% in the control group. Although this difference was not statistically significant, this may have been because the study was not primarily powered to detect a difference in a family history of thrombosis. In the study, a family history of strokes and myocardial infarction was elicited separately and no difference was found; therefore, family history of thrombosis was assumed to refer to venous thrombosis. Anderson et al.[7] have demonstrated impaired fibrinolysis as shown by elevated circulating levels of plasminogen activator inhibitor.[7]

A number of studies have been conducted that suggest that women with PCOS may also be at increased risk of having a personal history of ovarian and breast cancer,[8,9] especially since these women are hyperandrogenic and infertile, which are risk factors for breast and ovarian cancer, respectively. However, the link is yet to be clearly established.

Clinical Discussion

Clinical phenotypes in PCO families

Legro et al.[10] found hyperandrogenemia with or without oligomenorrhea aggregating in PCOS kindreds and suggested that it can be considered a genetic trait useful in assigning affected status in linkage studies designed to identify PCOS genes. In addition, the fathers tend to be abnormally hairy and female siblings hirsute. Culdoscopy has often shown signs of Stein-Leventhal syndrome, eg. 8 of 12 sisters among the cases showed ovarian changes consistent with that diagnosis.[11] Givens et al.[12] found 41 women (in 2 kindreds) who had hirsutism and/or oligomenorrhea. Ovarian histology, performed in 8 women, showed hyperplasia of theca cells in atretic follicles, a paucity of primordial and developing follicles, and stromal hyperplasia. Elevated levels of androstenedione and/or testosterone and of luteinizing hormone (LH) were found. These levels tended to return to normal after bilateral wedge resection. Some of the men of the families had low plasma testosterone levels and an abnormally high LH-FSH ratio as in the women. The pedigrees were constant with dominant inheritance, probably autosomal, because in one kindred, the disorder was apparently transmitted through a father and son. Mandel et al.[13] excluded linkage to human lymphocyte antigen (HLA). They studied 4 families, each with 2 affected sisters; in 1 family, the mother and a maternal aunt were likewise affected. The diagnosis of polycystic ovaries (PCO) was confirmed by increased serum testosterone, androstenedione, and LH levels compared to those in normal women. Elevated levels of dehydroepiandroandrosterone sulfate (DHEA-S) indicated excess adrenal androgen secretion. Kutten et al.[14] postulated that idiopathic hirsutism, which at times is familial, is sometimes due to increased skin sensitivity to androgen and occurs in the absence of elevated plasma androgens. On the basis of a large family study, Hague et al.[15] arrived at a hypothesis of dominant inheritance with meiotic drive accounting for the anomalous segregation. They found PCO in 96% of daughters of affected families and in 82% of daughters of carrier males. Lunde et al.[16] reported that 19.7% of male first-degree relatives of PCO patients had early baldness or excessive hairiness, as opposed to 6.5% of relatives of controls. For female first-degree relatives, the percentages of PCO-related symptoms were 31.4% and 3.2%, respectively. In a subgroup of 52 families of PCO patients in which one of the parents was reported to have symptoms, 35% of the brothers and 58% of the sisters had symptoms. The findings were considered consistent with autosomal dominant inheritance for a sizeable fraction of families. The possibility of X-linked dominant inheritance was eliminated.

Carey et al.[17,18] described an autosomal dominant syndrome of polycystic ovaries and premature male-pattern baldness. They demonstrated an association with a change in the 5-prime promoter region of the CYP17 gene, which modified the expression of the syndrome in some families but did not appear to be the primary genetic defect.

Govind et al.[19] screened first-degree relatives of women affected with PCO to obtain evidence for the genetic basis of polycystic ovaries and premature male pattern baldness. First-degree female and male relatives of affected individuals had a 61% and 22% chance respectively of being affected. Sisters of PCO probands with polycystic ovarian morphology were more likely to have menstrual irregularity and had larger ovaries and higher serum androstenedione and dehydroepiandrosterone sulfate levels than sisters of non-PCOS women, suggesting a spectrum of clinical phenotypes in PCO families.

Diabetes mellitus and the Polycystic ovary syndrome

Polycystic ovary syndrome is associated with an increased risk of type 2 diabetes mellitus. Several studies have suggested that insulin resistance plays an important role in the pathogenesis of the syndrome. As a consequence of insulin resistance, women affected by PCOS often present abnormalities of glucose metabolism and lipid profile, and have an increased risk of type 2 diabetes and cardiovascular disease over time. Besides insulin resistance, it has been demonstrated that some of these women also have alterations in beta-cell function. Both the disorders (insulin resistance and beta-cell dysfunction) are recognized as major risk factors for the development of type 2 diabetes.[20] Defects in both insulin secretion and insulin action contribute to this predisposition to diabetes. Colilla et al.[21] used the frequently sampled intravenous glucose tolerance test to quantitate insulin secretion,

insulin action, and their product among 33 women with PCOS and 48 nondiabetic first-degree relatives. They then quantitated the heritability of these measures from familial correlations estimated within a genetic model. The sib correlation for insulin secretion was highly significant. In addition, the parameter quantitating insulin secretion in relation to insulin sensitivity was significant among sibs. The authors concluded that there is a heritable component to beta-cell dysfunction in families of women with PCOS, and that heritability of beta-cell dysfunction is likely to be a significant factor in the predisposition to diabetes in PCOS.

Ehrmann et al.[22] examined the effects of race and family history of type 2 diabetes on the risk of impaired glucose tolerance (IGT) and type 2 diabetes in a large cohort of women with PCOS. They found that a family history of type 2 diabetes in a first-degree relative was associated with an increased risk of metabolic abnormality, IGT, and type 2 diabetes in women with PCOS. They also observed higher insulin levels and greater insulin resistance in black women with PCOS than in white women with PCOS; these differences remained statistically significant even after taking the family history of diabetes into account.

A family history of type 2 diabetes is present with a significantly greater frequency among women with PCOS who have IGT or type 2 diabetes when compared with those with normal glucose tolerance. Conversely, a family history of type 2 diabetes in a first-degree relative is associated with a significantly higher risk for IGT or type 2 diabetes in women with PCOS. Even among nondiabetic women with PCOS, a positive family history of type 2 diabetes was strongly associated with metabolic characteristics associated with an increased risk for type 2 diabetes.

In another study conducted in Turkey by Yildiz et al.[23] the authors have not only concluded that a positive correlation exists between PCOS and the finding of glucose intolerance and insulin resistance in first-degree relatives, but they have also recommended screening of first-degree relatives of PCOS patients based on their findings.

They found that PCOS was associated with hyperinsulinemia, insulin resistance, increased risk of glucose intolerance and type 2 diabetes.

Benitez et al.[24] found the prevalence of metabolic disorders such as dyslipidemia, obesity, hypertension and diabetes to be 2.7 fold higher in families of PCOS patients than in control group families. The metabolic disorders were more frequent in parents and grandparents of PCOS patients than in those of normal women.

This finding has, however, not been corroborated by all. Atiomo et al.[25] conducted a study to confirm whether there was a familial association between PCOS and thromboembolic disease, ovarian or breast cancer, diabetes and heart disease. They found no statistically significant difference in the prevalence of a personal or positive family history of diabetes in women with PCOS compared with controls.

PCOS associated neoplasms

A major risk for neoplasms of the reproductive tract, like endometrial, ovarian as well as breast cancer seems to be related to PCOS. While several studies have shown an increased risk for endometrial hyperplasia and cancer in PCOS patients, the variability of the selection criteria for PCOS has been recognized as a potential bias for these data. PCOS women also present clinical characteristics that are related to risk factors for breast cancer and some epidemiological evidences have been described on this issue. However, until now, a clear association between the presence of PCOS and breast carcinoma has not yet been found. High local steroid and growth factor concentrations are considered risk factors for ovarian carcinoma, and are frequently observed in PCOS women. On the other hand, a few studies that have addressed the possibility of a link between PCOS and ovarian cancer, have had results that are conflicting, suggesting that this association is unlikely.[26]

A number of studies provide support to the hypothesis that a family history of breast cancer may be associated with PCOS. Atiomo et al.[25] studied 217 women with and without PCOS under the care of the same consultant gynecologist at a teaching hospital. They found the proportion of women with a positive family history of breast cancer to be significantly greater among women with PCOS compared with controls (20% vs 5% respectively, p < 0.05). They did not find a similar significant difference in the prevalence of a personal or positive family history of ovarian cancer in PCOS women compared with controls. They suggested a genetic basis for this association, as PCOS, breast cancer, and heart disease may be familial. Although it is interesting to speculate on a genetic link between PCOS and breast cancer, it is impossible to be specific at this stage about the mode of inheritance of the risk of breast cancer in women with PCOS without performing detailed genetic studies. An alternative hypothesis to a genetic link between PCOS and breast cancer is that these observations are a secondary event to endocrine risk factors in women with PCOS. These risk factors include elevated testosterone levels, increased levels of insulin, insulin-like growth factor 1, insulin-like growth factor 2, and abdominal obesity, all of which are present in PCOS and have been shown to be tumorigenic.[27]

Association with Cardiovascular Disease

First-degree relatives of PCOS patients carry an increased risk of cardiovascular disease, as do the PCOS patients themselves. These women frequently have dyslipidemia, including borderline or high lipid levels and disproportionately elevated low-density lipoprotein (LDL) cholesterol levels. Sam et al.[28] conducted a study to test the hypothesis that dyslipidemia is a heritable trait in sisters of women with PCOS. Their main outcome measures included lipid and lipoprotein levels and prevalence of the metabolic syndrome. They found that low-density lipoprotein levels were increased in affected sisters of women with PCOS consistent with a heritable trait. The prevalence of the metabolic syndrome was increased in affected sisters. Insulin resistance has been associated with elevated triglyceride levels, increased levels of small, dense LDL cholesterol, and decreased levels of high-density lipoprotein (HDL) cholesterol. The American College of Obstetrics and Gynecology (ACOG) recommends screening for dyslipidemia in all women with PCOS. The finding of an increased prevalence of a family history of heart disease in PCOS women is consistent with studies that demonstrated that several risk factors for heart disease including obesity, insulin resistance, hyperlipidemia, and raised plasminogen activator inhibitor-1 are present in these women.[29] Whether these risk factors are genetic, programmed in utero, or environmental is unclear. Atiomo et al.[25] give support to the hypothesis that these risk factors may be genetic. Yilmaz et al.[30] studied 120 family members consisting of 55 patients with PCOS and 75 unrelated healthy control subjects and found an increased risk of cardiovascular disease in the relatives of PCOS women as compared to the controls.

Conclusion

Polycystic ovary syndrome (PCOS) is a complex and heterogeneous disorder characterized by hyperandrogenemia, hyperinsulinemia, insulin resistance, and chronic anovulation. It is the most common endocrine disorder in women of reproductive age with an enigmatic pathophysiologic and molecular basis. The high prevalence of affected individuals and the wide range of phenotypic expression can be explained by the interaction of a number of key genes with environmental factors. Heritability of PCOS has been inferred from studies of the syndrome in various population groups (ethnic groups, twins, and PCOS families). Although evidence of familial segregation and clustering of the disease in first-degree relatives of women diagnosed with PCOS has been presented, no particular pattern of inheritance has emerged. Some of the problems in genetic studies have been the lack of uniform criteria for diagnosis, heterogeneity of phenotypic features, and the fact that the disorder is only expressed clinically in women during their reproductive years. Even within affected families and among sisters with polycystic ovaries, there is heterogeneity in presentation. However,

regardless of the diagnostic criteria used to identify the propositus and to determine the affected status in the kindred, the genetic studies available suggest a strong familial component.[31] Currently, PCOS is considered a polygenic trait that might result from the interaction of susceptible and protective genomic variants and environmental factors, during either prenatal or postnatal life. A number of studies have shown a positive association between PCOS and a family history of breast cancer and heart attacks. A family history of type 2 diabetes is present with a significantly greater frequency among women with PCOS who have IGT or type 2 diabetes when compared with those with normal glucose tolerance. These associations may be genetic in origin, however, larger studies are required to support this hypothesis. A complex interplay of genetic, intrauterine and environmental factors has also been suggested.

References

1. Stein IF, Leventhal ML. Amenorrhea associated with bilateral polycystic ovaries. *Am J Obstet Gynecol* 1935; 29: 181–191.
2. Zawadski JK, Dunaif A. Diagnostic criteria for polycystic ovary syndrome towards a rational approach. In: Dunaif A, Givens JR, Haseltine FP, et al, eds. *Polycystic ovary syndrome,* Cambridge: Blackwell Science, 1992; 377–384.
3. Kenny SJ, Aubert RE, Geiss LS. Prevalence and incidence of non-insulin-dependent diabetes. In: Harris, et al, editors *Diabetes in America*, 2nd edition Washington DC: US National Institutes of Health, NIH 34, Pub. No. 95: 1468.
4. Ehrmann DA, Barnes RB, Rosenfield RL, et al. Prevalence of impaired glucose tolerance and diabetes in women with polycystic ovary syndrome. *Diabetes Care* 1992; 22: 141–146.
5. Legro RS, Kumselman AR, Dodson WC, et al. Prevalence and predictors of risk for type 2 diabetes mellitus and impaired glucose tolerance in polycystic ovary syndrome: a prospective, controlled study in 254 affected women. *J Clin Endocrinol Metab* 1999; 84: 165–169.
6. Atiomo WU, Condon J, Adekanmi O, Friend J, Wilkin TJ, Prentice AG. Are women with polycystic ovary syndrome resistant to activated protein C? *Fertil Steril* 2000; 74: 1229–1232.

7. Anderson P, Selje Flot I, Abdelnoor M. Increased insulin sensitivity and fibrinolytic capacity after dietary intervention in obese women with polycystic ovary syndrome. *Metabolism* 1995; 44: 611–616.

8. Baron JA, Weiderpass E, Newcomb PA, Stampfer M, Titus-Ernstoff L, Egan KM, et al. Metabolic disorders and breast cancer risk (United States). *Cancer Causes Control* 2001; 12: 875–880.

9. Pierpoint T, McKeigue PM, Issacs AJ, Wild SH, Jacobs HS. Mortality in women with polycystic ovary syndrome at long term follow-up. *J Clin Epidemiol* 1998; 51: 581–586.

10. Legro RS, Driscoll D, Strauss JF, III, Fox J, Dunaif A. Evidence for a genetic basis for hyperandrogenemia in polycystic ovary syndrome. *Proc Nat Acad Sci* 1998; 95: 14956–14960.

11. Cooper HE, Spellacy WN, Prem KA, Cohen WD. Hereditary factors in the Stein-Leventhal syndrome. *Am J Obstet Gynec* 1968; 100: 371–387.

12. Givens JR, Wiser WL, Coleman SA, Wilroy RS, Andersen RN, Fish SA, Watson BS. Familial ovarian hyperthecosis: a study of two families. *Am J Obstest Gynec* 1971; 110: 959–972.

13. Mandel FP, Chang RJ, Dupont B, Pollack MS, Levine LS, New MI, et al. HLA genotyping in family members and patients with polycystic ovarian disease. *J Clin Endocr Metab* 1983; 56: 862–864.

14. Kutten F, Mowszowicz I, Schaison G, Mauvais-Jarvis P. Androgen production and skin metabolism in hirsutism. *J Endocr* 1977; 75: 83–91.

15. Hague W, Adams J, Reeders S, Jacobs H. Non-mendelian segregation ratios in familial polycystic ovaries. (Abstract) *7th Int Cong Hum Genet, Berlin* 1986; 277–278.

16. Lunde O, Magnus P, Sandvik L, Hoglo S. Familial clustering in the polycystic ovarian syndrome. *Gynec Obstet Invest* 1989; 28: 23–30.

17. Carey AH, Chan KL, Short F, White D, Williamson R, Franks S. Evidence for a single gene effect causing polycystic ovaries and male pattern baldness. *Clin Endocr* 1993; 38: 653–658.

18. Carey AH, Waterworth D, Patel K, White D, Little J, Novelli P, Franks S, Williamson R. Polycystic ovaries and premature male pattern baldness are associated with one allele of the steroid metabolism gene CYP17. *Hum Molec Genet* 1994; 3: 1873–1876.

19. Govind A, Obhrai MS, Clayton RN. Polycystic ovaries are inherited as an autosomal dominant trait: analysis of 29 polycystic ovary syndrome and 10 control families. *J Clin Endocr Metab* 1999; 84: 38–43.

20. Pelusi B, Gambineri A, Pasquali R. Type 2 diabetes and the polycystic ovary sydrome. *Minerva Gynecol* 2004; 56: 41–51.

21. Colilla S, Cox NJ, Ehrmann DA. Heritability of insulin secretion and insulin action in women with polycystic ovary syndrome and their first degree relatives. *J Clin Endocr Metab* 2001; 86: 2027–2031.

22. Ehrmann DA, Kasza K, Azziz R, Legro RS, Ghazzi MN, PCOS/Troglitazone Study Group. Effects of race and family history of type 2 diabetes on metabolic status of women with polycystic ovary syndrome. *J Clin Endocr Metab* 2005; 90: 66–71.

23. Yildiz BO, Yarali H, Oguz H, Bayraktar M. Glucose intolerance, insulin resistance, and hyperandrogenemia in first degree relatives of women with polycystic ovary syndrome. *J Clin Endocr Metab* 2003; 88: 2031–2036.

24. Benitez R, Sir Petermann T, Palomino A, Angel B, Maliqueo M, Perez F, Calvillan M. Prevalence of metabolic disorders among family members of patients with polycystic ovary syndrome. *Rev Med Chil* 2001; 129: 707–712.

25. Atiomo WU, El-Mahdi E, Hardiman P. Familial associations in women with polycystic ovary syndrome. *Fertil Steril* 2003; 80: 143–145.

26. Spritzer PM, Morsch DM, Wiltgen D. Polycystic ovary syndrome associated neoplasms. *Arq Bras Endocrinol Metabol* 2005; 49: 805–810.

27. Wong YC, Xie B. The role of androgens in mammary carcinogenesis. *Ital J Anat Embryol* 2001; 106: 111–125.

28. Sam S, Legro RS, Bentley-Lewis R, Dunaif A. Dyslipidemia and metabolic syndrome in the sisters of women with polycystic ovary syndrome. *J Clin Endocrinol Metab* 2005; 90(8): 4797–802.

29. Atiomo WU, Bates SA, Condon J, Shaw S, West JH, Prentice AG. The plasminogen activator system in women with polycystic ovary syndrome. *Fertil Steril* 1998; 69: 236–241.

30. Yilmaz M, Bukan N, Ersoy R, Karakoc A, Yetkin I, Ayvaz G, et al. Glucose intolerance, insulin resistance and cardiovascular risk factors in first degree relatives of women with polycystic ovary syndrome. *Hum Reprod* 2005; 20: 2414–2420.

31. Diamanti-Kandarakis E, Piperi C, Spina J, Argyrakopoulou G, Papanastasiou L, Bergiele A, Panidis D. Polycystic ovary syndrome: the influence of environmental and genetic factors. *Hormones (Athens Greece)* 2006; 5(1): 17–34.

Pathophysiology of PCOS and its Consequences

11

The Pathophysiology of Polycystic Ovary Syndrome

Michel Abou Abdallah, Johnny Awwad

Summary

The Polycystic Ovary Syndrome (PCOS) is by far, the most common and least understood endocrinopathy. Although described some half a century ago, the underlying etiology remains uncertain. Cumulative information and recent advances, however, have shed more light on the pathophysiology of this condition. PCOS is manifested clinically by a combination of ovulatory dysfunction, hyperandrogenic state and abnormal ovarian morphology. Suggested pathogenic mechanisms include disturbances in the hypothalamic gonadotropin-releasing hormone activity, ovarian and adrenal androgen production, and insulin action. Hyperandrogenism and insulin resistance appear to be central to the pathophysiology of the disease, which appears to be multifactorial and polygenic in nature, involving multi-system dysfunctions, namely reproductive, endocrine and metabolic. Although many extra-ovarian factors have been identified to influence the disorder, the ovary remains central to the pathogenic events. The protean manifestations of the disorder amongst women suggest, very likely, a combination of genetic and environmental factors acting together in concert to influence the final expression of the condition.

Introduction

Polycystic Ovary Syndrome (PCOS) remains a loosely defined entity, mostly because it represents a myriad of different clinical and laboratory manifestations, expressed in a spectrum of varying strengths and intensities. This much debated syndrome is one typically defined by consensus, and whose definition varies in relation to our understanding of its underlying pathophysiology. Such pathophysiology appears to be multifactorial and polygenic in nature, involving multi-system dysfunctions, namely reproductive, endocrine and metabolic. Although many extra-ovarian dimensions to the pathophysiology of the syndrome have been identified, the intra-ovarian dysfunction remains the core.

The latest consensus between the American Society for Reproductive Medicine (ASRM) and the European Society for Human Reproduction and Embryology (ESHRE) defined PCOS as the presence of two out of the following three criteria: (i) oligo- and/or anovulation; (ii) hyperandrogenism (clinical and/or biochemical); and (iii) polycystic ovary appearance by ultrasound examination.[1] The typical morphology of a polycystic ovary has been defined as an ovary with 12 or more follicles measuring 2–9 mm in diameter and/or increased ovarian volume

(>10 cm^3).[2] The findings that sonographic criteria of PCOS are also seen in 23% of normal ovulatory women,[3] and that some ovaries from women with PCOS may appear sonographically normal,[4] emphasize the endocrine nature of the disorder, and underlies the fact that ovarian morphology is an expression of a disorder and not the disease itself.

The spectrum of clinical signs and symptoms differs widely amongst women with PCOS and can also vary over time within the same individual woman in the presence of particular precipitating factors, the most significant of which is an alteration in body weight.[5] The association found between PCOS and abnormal insulin metabolism may infer the existence of a complex genetic trait disorder underlying the syndrome.[6] The protean nature of the PCOS phenotype[5] makes it even more difficult to elucidate a genotype. Possibly, different combinations of genetic variants contribute to the differential expression of the different components of the same syndrome.[7]

It is estimated that as many as 6–10% of women of reproductive age group are affected by PCOS. Despite being one of the most common endocrinopathies, a comprehensive and universal approach to its pathophysiology is still lacking. One can summarize our current understanding of the syndrome by four proposed hypotheses: (a) neuroendocrine with exaggerated luteinizing hormone (LH) secretion; (b) ovarian with excessive androgen synthesis (c) adrenal with altered cortisol metabolism, and (d) metabolic with insulin resistance and hyperinsulinemia. Since all advanced hypotheses enjoy wide support, it is likely then that all four concepts are very closely intertwined.

Clinical Discussion

Pathophysiology of PCOS

(a) The Neuroendocrine hypothesis

The gonadotropin releasing hormone (GnRH) 'pulse generator' lies within the arcuate nucleus of the hypothalamus and secretes GnRH in a pulsatile manner, with varying frequencies throughout the normal ovulatory cycle, resulting in variable frequencies and amplitudes of gonadotropin release. Though the underlying mechanisms for this rhythm are poorly understood, peripheral ovarian factors, rather than central elements appear to modulate GnRH action at the pituitary level, and possibly at the hypothalamic too.

Women with PCOS express characteristically elevated tonic LH secretion, manifested both, basally and in response to GnRH administration.[8] This phenomenon was considered as a hall mark of classic PCOS and a cause of androgen excess. This over expression is believed to be partly due to diminished central opioid and dopaminergic tone.[9,10] In normal cycling women, both dopamine receptor antagonist metoclopramide, and opiate receptor antagonist naloxone, yield a rise in serum LH concentration levels, whereas exogenous β-endorphin causes a fall in these levels. In women with PCOS, none of these agents altered LH secretory activity.[10] These findings led some to propose a hypothalamic defect as a possible underlying etiology for the LH hypersecretory state.

Further research demonstrated comparable LH responses to naloxone infusion in women with PCOS and weight-matched controls.[11] Pretreatment with dopa-carbidopa resulted however, in the loss of the naloxone-stimulated LH rise in normal cycling women and an exaggerated LH response in women with PCOS. Such findings suggest that the dopaminergic rather than the opioid tone is altered in PCOS. While evidence of dopamine metabolite abnormalities was found in women with PCOS,[12] other studies nevertheless, failed to demonstrate significant alterations in central dopaminergic activity in these women.[13] The precise role of endogenous opioids and dopamine in the control of LH secretion remains hence, unresolved.

A review of the neuroendocrine control in PCOS identified numerous contradictory findings and hypotheses.[14] Central hypothalamic and pituitary disturbances in PCOS may therefore be influenced by multiple peripheral factors, likely ovarian in origin. An area of further dispute is whether increased tonic LH activity, associated with PCOS, is primarily the result of an increase in GnRH pulse amplitude, pulse frequency, or both. Although most studies have found evidence of increased pulse amplitude, only some have described an increase in pulse frequency,[15,16] which yet others failed to demonstrate.[17–19] An alteration in the circadian rhythm of LH secretion has also been reported with the persistence of high-amplitude LH pulses during the night.[18] Bioactive LH has been further shown to be elevated in many patients with PCOS, in whom immunoactive LH was normal.[20]

In general, it is believed that the frequency and amplitude patterns of the GnRH pulses determine the gonadotropin subunit gene expression and the production of pituitary LH and follicle stimulating hormone (FSH). In normal ovulatory women, an increase in GnRH pulse frequency during the follicular phase favors LH synthesis, while a decrease in GnRH pulse frequency in the luteal phase as a result of progesterone effect favors FSH synthesis. In women with PCOS, GnRH pulse frequency is persistently rapid, favoring LH synthesis and hyperandrogenism. An insensitivity of the GnRH pulse generator to suppression by sex steroid hormones has been suggested.[21] Such insensitivity during pubertal maturation could be a potential mechanism for the perimenarchal abnormalities seen in hyperandrogenic adolescent girls who appear to exhibit early manifestations of PCOS.[22] On the other hand, the pattern of gonadotropin response to GnRH agonist stimulation in women with PCOS appears to be 'masculinized'.[23] Perinatal exposure to excess androgen could program the neuroendocrine system to secrete excessive LH at puberty, resulting in ovarian hyperandrogenism,[23] as also confirmed in primates.[24]

Women with PCOS undergoing laparoscopic ovarian diathermy (LOD) express a significant decrease in LH pulse amplitude[25] and an attenuation of GnRH-stimulated LH secretion.[26] These findings are consistent with an altered ovarian–pituitary feedback via a putative ovarian factor(s) that regulates LH secretion centrally. Although the mechanism of ovulation induction by LOD is uncertain, it appears that minimal damage to the affected ovary, either restores an ovulatory cycle, or improves the ovarian response to stimulation.

(b) The Ovarian hypothesis

The typical morphological features of the enlarged polycystic ovary suggest that the ovary is the primary site of endocrine dysfunction. A dysregulation of the P450c17α enzyme activity, as the main cause of excess ovarian androgen production in PCOS, has been proposed.[27] This has been confirmed by the significant rise in androstenedione and 17-hydroxyprogesterone levels observed in response to a single dose of a gonadotropin-releasing hormone agonist (GnRHa) in hyperandrogenic women with PCOS following dexamethasone adrenal suppression.[28] The same findings were reproduced independent of the ovulatory status of these women, although the 17-hydroxyprogesterone rise was found to be significantly more exaggerated in the presence of anovulation.[29] In contrast, there was no significant increase in both these hormones following adrenocorticotropic hormone (ACTH) stimulation.[29] These findings indicate that the hyperandrogenic state associated with PCOS is predominantly of ovarian origin, and confirm that the primary cause of androgen excess lies within the ovarian theca-interstitial cells independent of LH hypersecretion. This is best exemplified clinically by the observation that some women with PCOS can still express a hyperandrogenic state despite normal LH production, and that those subjected to long-term GnRHa suppression can still display 17-hydroxyprogesterone hyperresponsiveness to human chorionic gonadotropins (hCG).

The finding that increased androgen production is persistently expressed by polycystic ovary theca cells when propagated in long-term culture, strongly supports the hypothesis that the hyperandrogenism associated with PCOS results from an intrinsic steroidogenic abnormality of ovarian theca cells.[30,31] In vitro, P450c17 and 3β-hydroxysteroid dehydrogenase (HSD) enzyme activities were found to be increased by several hundred folds in long-term cultured theca cells from women with PCOS compared to controls; 17β-HSD enzyme activity was unaffected.[31] Since 17β-HSD catalyses the final step in the conversion of androstenedione to testosterone, it can be concluded that the increased synthesis of testosterone precursors may be the primary factor driving the enhanced testosterone secretion in PCOS. C17,20 lyase activity has also been shown to be disproportionately increased in theca cells of women with PCOS.

The presence of numerous follicles with elevated androgen to estrogen ratio was initially considered a manifestation of an active process of follicular atresia. The granulosa cells were later shown to be viable and responsive to FSH stimulation.[32,33] The functional picture of arrested granulosa cells and active theca cells may be consistent with a dysregulation of FSH response, favoring intrafollicular androgen dominance. Since inhibin was found to augment LH-mediated androstenedione production in cultured human theca cells,[34] and inhibit pituitary FSH secretion, increased production of inhibin B by the numerous follicles present in polycystic ovaries could play a significant role in negatively influencing the microenvironment of follicles, contributing to impaired follicular development. The expression of insulin-like growth factors (IGF)s in the follicular fluid of polycystic ovaries was also found to be similar to that in atretic follicles.[35] IGFs are believed to stimulate ovarian cellular mitosis and inhibit apoptosis.

Such ovarian theca cell dysfunction may also be linked to an escape of their normal downregulation of gonadotropins as a result of growth factor dysregulation. This was demonstrated by the decrease in serum LH and androgen levels in women with PCOS following insulin suppression by somatostatin.[36] The generalized overactive steroidogenic state, highly entertained in women with PCOS, is also evidenced by an overproduction of estrone and estradiol in response to a single GnRHa injection.[28] A high serum estradiol level is a common finding in women with PCOS. This is partly due to the availability of excess androgen substrates for aromatase activity and also due to the exaggerated follicular response to FSH stimulation.[37]

(c) The Adrenal hypothesis

In 25% of the women with PCOS, an increase in adrenal androgen production is observed.[38,39] Possible etiologies of the adrenal disorder may lie within a genetic predisposition, ovarian steroidogenic dysfunction,[40] or an alteration in cortisol metabolism. According to this last theory, accelerated peripheral cortisol metabolism could result from increased inactivation of cortisol by excessive 5α-reductase activity[41,42] or even by impaired cortisol conversion due to defective 11β-HSD activity.[43] This situation results in a compensatory increase in ACTH secretion for the purpose of maintaining normal serum cortisol levels at the expense of adrenal androgen overproduction. Evidence for an increase in the total cortisol metabolite excretion in the urine of women with PCOS has been documented indeed, concomitantly with enhanced 5α-reductase activity.[41] This steroidogenic enzyme is responsible for the 5α-reduction of both, testosterone to 5α-dihydrotestosterone in skin and cortisol to 5α-dihydrocortisol in liver. In vitro studies on genital skin fibroblasts suggest that 5α-reductase activity is also unregulated by androgens.[44]

On the other hand, dysregulation of 11β-HSD enzyme activity has also been proposed in women with PCOS,[45] as evidenced by a decreased ratio of 11-hydroxy to 11-oxo cortisol metabolites in these women. Isoenzyme 11β-HSD1, an oxoreductase expressed in human liver and adipose tissue, is responsible for the conversion of inactive cortisone to active cortisol. Impaired activity of this enzyme is expressed through reactive adrenocortical hyperstimulation, and may be influenced by the state of hyperinsulinemia and/or hyperandrogenism.

The actual mechanisms of altered 5α-reductase

and/or 11β-HSD1 activity in women, with PCOS remain nevertheless, uncertain. Obesity, existent in more than half of these women cannot account alone for abnormalities found in these two enzyme activities. Indeed, 5α-reductase activity was found to be significantly more accentuated in women with PCOS compared to weight matched controls,[41] and impaired 11β-HSD1 activity was also confirmed in lean women with PCOS.[45] A putative role for endogenous inhibitors of 11β-HSD1 production[46] and estrone downregulation of its activity in the liver, has been excluded.[47]

(d) The Metabolic hypothesis

The finding of an association between insulin resistance and hyperandrogenism has provided a new approach to the pathogenesis of PCOS.[48] The first recognition of such an association was made by Achard and Thiers in 1921 and was called 'the diabetes of bearded women'.[49] Studies using the euglycemic clamp technique confirm that women with PCOS are more insulin-resistant than age- and weight-matched normal ovulatory women,[50–52] and significantly more so when these women are obese.[53] The observed reduction in insulin sensitivity amongst lean women with PCOS was found to be further decreased in obese normal ovulatory women and even more profoundly decreased in obese women with the syndrome.[54] This indicates that insulin resistance, present in association with PCOS, is independent of obesity and that, the co-existence of obesity is an independent additional contributory factor to the condition. Other studies nevertheless, failed to confirm the existence of insulin resistance in lean women with PCOS. These were based on the use of intravenous glucose tolerance test,[55] continuous glucose infusion model[56] and hyperinsulinemic euglycemic clamp.[57] Reasons for discrepancies could have been caused by the lack of reporting of ethnic variability, central adiposity, and family history of type 2 diabetes.[58] Studies on the molecular mechanisms of insulin resistance in PCOS have shown evidence of a post-binding defect in insulin receptor-mediated signal transduction and a significant decrease in insulin responsiveness.[59] Decreased insulin sensitivity in PCOS appears to be independent of obesity,[51] which may indicate an intrinsic defect, possibly genetically determined in a subset of women with the syndrome.[49] A dysregulation of insulin receptor phosphorylation, resulting in increased insulin-independent serine phosphorylation and decreased insulin-dependent tyrosine phosphorylation, has been suggested to decrease tyrosine kinase activity of the receptor and inhibit normal signaling.[59–60] Only glucose homeostasis is affected as a result with the exclusion of other pleiotropic functions such a cell growth, steroidogenesis and protein synthesis. Increased serine phosphorylation also activates both ovarian and adrenal P450c17 enzymes promoting androgen synthesis.[61] It is therefore possible that a single post-receptor defect, namely serine phosphorylation, can be responsible for both the insulin resistance and androgen excess in PCOS. No structural abnormalities in the insulin receptor per se could be found.[62,63]

A positive correlation between the severity of hyperinsulinemia secondary to insulin resistance and the extent of clinical manifestations of PCOS has been suggested.[64,65] Evidence indicates that hyperinsulinemia is the primary event leading to hyperandrogenism, as the hyperinsulinemic state of women with PCOS remained unchanged following the correction of hyperandrogenemia by bilateral oophorectomy[66] or GnRH-agonist suppression.[67] Hyperinsulinemia increases androgen production directly by acting as a co-gonadotropin, augmenting LH activity within the ovary, and indirectly by enhancing serum LH pulse amplitude. Androgens may in turn contribute at least partially to the insulin resistance state associated with PCOS.[68]

In view of the similarity between the insulin-like growth factor-1 (IGF-1) and insulin receptor, insulin cross-reactivity was suggested as a mechanism for hyperandrogenism.[69] Stimulation of IGF-1 receptors on ovarian theca cells augments LH-mediated androgen production by these cells.[70] Insulin can also modulate steroidogenesis via its own receptors present on both granulosa[71,72] and theca cells.[73,74] Using anti-insulin and anti-IGF-1 receptor antibodies, insulin action was shown to be mediated exclusively via its own receptors.[71] Hyperinsulinemia may stimulate cytochrome P450c17a activity in both the ovaries[75] and adrenals of women with PCOS.[76] Centrally, insulin is thought to enhance LH amplitude in obese women with PCOS.[75,77]

A concordance between the diurnal patterns of LH and insulin has been demonstrated in these women.[78] Insulin receptors have also been identified in pituitary tissues in humans[79] and insulin has been found to stimulate gonadotropin release in rats.[80] More peripherally, by inhibition of hepatic synthesis, insulin reduces serum sex-hormone-binding globulin (SHBG) favoring free circulating androgens, and decreases insulin-like growth factor binding protein-1 (IGFBP-1) allowing more IGF-1 to be available both locally and peripherally.[81]

Although both insulin resistance and hyperinsulinemia have significant pathogenic roles in PCOS, women with hyperinsulinemia are not necessarily all hyperandrogenic. In fact, only 52% of those with type 2 diabetes mellitus (DM) have clinical manifestations of androgen excess.[82] It has been therefore suggested that the effects of type 2 DM and PCOS on insulin-sensitivity are independent, likely involving different mechanisms,[43] possibly reflecting separate genetic defects in which insulin resistance unmasks the PCOS condition in genetically prone women.

Conclusions

Polycystic ovary syndrome is indeed, a diagnosis by consensus owing to the lack of a well-defined homogenous entity. The actual pathophysiologic mechanisms underlying this common endocrinopathy remain unknown and the subject of hectic research. The key features of the disorder include abnormal gonadotropin dynamics, excessive androgen production, and insulin resistance. The ovary represents the main site of dysfunction, but is also influenced by extra-ovarian factors. A familial pattern has been observed, but candidate genes are yet to be identified. The manifestations of PCOS are likely the result of a combination of genetic and environmental factors.

References

1. The Rotterdam ESHRE/ASRM-Sponsored PCOS consensus workshop group. Revised 2003 consensus on diagnostic criteria and long-term health risks related to polycystic ovary syndrome (PCOS). *Hum Reprod* 2004; 19(1): 41–47.
2. Balen AH, Laven JSE, Tan SL, Dewailly D. Ultrasound assessment of the polycystic ovary: international consensus definitions. *Human Reprod Update* 2003; 9: 505–514.
3. Clayton RN, Ogden V, Hodgkinson J, Worswick L, Rodin DA, Dyer S, Meade TW. How common are polycystic ovaries in normal women and what is their significance for the fertility of the population? *Clin Endocrinol* (Oxf) 1992; 37(2): 127–134.
4. Hann LE, Hall DA, McArdle CR, Seibel M. Polycystic ovarian disease: sonographic spectrum. *Radiology* 1984; 150: 531–534.
5. Balen AH, Conway GS, Kaltsas G, Techatrasak K, Manning PJ, West C, Jacobs HS. Polycystic ovary syndrome: the spectrum of the disorder in 1741 patients. *Hum Reprod* 1995; 10(8): 2107–2111.
6. Franks S, Gharani N, McCarthy M. Candidate genes in polycystic ovary syndrome. *Human Reprod Update* 2001; 7: 405–410.
7. Balen AH, Michelmore K. What is polycystic ovary syndrome? Are national views important?. *Human Reprod* 2002; 17: 2219–2227.
8. Yen SS, Vela P, Rankin J. Inappropriate secretion of follicle-stimulating hormone and luteinizing hormone in polycystic ovarian disease. *J Clin Endocrinol Metab* 1970; 30: 435–442.
9. Quigley ME, Rakoff JS, Yen SSC. Increased luteinizing hormone sensitivity to dopamine inhibition in the polycystic ovary syndrome. *J Clin Endocrinol Metab* 1981; 52: 231–234.
10. Cumming DC, Reid RL, Quigley ME, Rebar RW, Yen SS. Evidence for decreased endogenous dopamine and opioid inhibitory influences on LH secretion in polycystic ovary syndrome. *Clin Endocrinol* (Oxf) 1984; 20: 643–648.
11. Barnes R, Lobo R. Central opioid activity in the polycystic ovary syndrome with and without dopaminergic modulation. *J Clin Endocrinol Metab* 1985; 61: 779–782.
12. Yoshino K, Takahashi K, Shirai T, Nishigaki A, Araki Y, Kitao M. Changes in plasma catecholamines and

pulsatile patterns of gonadotropins in subjects with a normal ovulatory cycle and with polycystic ovary syndrome. *Int J Fertil* 1990; 35: 34–39.

13. Barnes RB, Mileikowsky GN, Cha KY, Spencer CA, Lobo RA. Effects of dopamine and metoclopramide in polycystic ovary syndrome. *J Clin Endocrinol Metab* 1986; 63: 506–509.

14. Schoemaker J. Neuroendocrine control in polycystic ovary-like syndrome. *Gynecol Endocrinol* 1991; 5: 277–288.

15. Rebar R, Judd HL, Yen SSC, Rakoff J, Vandenberg G, Naftolin F. Characterization of the inappropriate gonadotropin secretion in polycystic ovary syndrome. *J Clin Invest* 1976; 57: 1320–1329.

16. Burger CW, Korsen T, Van Kessel H, Van Dop PA, Caron FJM, Schoemaker J. Pulsatile luteinizing hormone patterns in the follicular phase of the menstrual cycle, polycystic ovarian disease (PCOD) and non PCOD secondary amenorrhea. *J Clin Endocrinol Metab* 1985; 61: 1126–1132.

17. Kazer RR, Kessel B, Yen SS. Circulating luteinizing hormone pulse frequency in women with polycystic ovary syndrome. *J Clin Endocrinol Metab* 1987; 65: 233–236.

18. Venturoli S, Porcu E, Fabbri R, Magrini O, Gammi L, Paradisi R, et al. Episodic pulsatile secretion of FSH, LH, prolactin, oestradiol, oestrone, and LH circadian variations in polycystic ovary syndrome. *Clin Endocrinol* (Oxf). 1988; 28 (1): 93–107.

19. Murdoch AP, Diggle PJ, White MC, Kendall-Taylor P, Dunlop W. LH in polycystic ovary syndrome: reproducibility and pulsatile secretion. *J Endocrinol* 1989; 121: 185–191.

20. Fauser BC, Pache TD, Hop WC, De Jong FH, Dahl KD. The significance of a single serum LH measurement in women with cycle disturbances: discrepancies between immunoreactive and bioactive hormone estimates. *Clin Endocrinol* (Oxf) 1992; 37: 445–452.

21. Pastor CL, Griffin-Korf ML, Aloi JA, Evans WS, Marshall JC. Polycystic ovary syndrome: evidence for reduced sensitivity of the gonadotropin-releasing hormone pulse generator to inhibition by estradiol and progesterone *J Clin Endocrinol Metab* 1998, 83: 582–590.

22. Marshall JC, Eagleson CA. Neuroendocrine aspects of polycystic ovary syndrome. *Endocrinol Metab Clin North Am* 1999; 28: 295–324.

23. Barnes RB, Rosenfield RL, Ehrmann DA, Cara JF, Cuttler L, Levitsky LL, Rosenthal IM. Ovarian hyperandrogynism as a result of congenital adrenal virilizing disorders: evidence for perinatal masculinization of neuroendocrine function in women. *J Clin Endocrinol Metab* 1994; 79(5): 1328–1333.

24. Dumesic DA, Abbott DH, Eisner JR, Goy RW. Prenatal exposure of female rhesus monkeys to testosterone propionate increases serum luteinizing hormone levels in adulthood. *Fertil Steril* 1997; 67: 155–163.

25. Gadir AA, Khatim MS, Mowafi RS, Alnaser HM, Alzaid HG, Shaw RW. Hormonal changes in patients with polycystic ovarian disease after ovarian electrocautery or pituitary desensitization. *Clin Endocrinol* (Oxf) 1990; 32(6): 749–754.

26. Rossmanith WG, Keckstein J, Spatzier K, Lauritzen C. The impact of ovarian laser surgery on the gonadotrophin secretion in women with PCOD. *Clin Endocrinol* (Oxf) 1991; 34: 223–230.

27. Rosenfield RL, Barnes RB, Cara JF, Lucky AW. Dysregulation of cytochrome P450c17α as the cause of polycystic ovarian syndrome. *Fertil Steril* 1990; 53: 785–791.

28. White DW, Leigh A, Wilson C. Gonadotrophin and gonadal steroid response to a single dose of a long-acting agonist of gonadotrophin-releasing hormone in ovulatory and anovulatory women with polycystic ovary syndrome. *Clin Endocrinol* (Oxf) 1995; 42: 475–481.

29. Franks S, White D, Gilling-Smith C, Carey A, Waterworth D, Williamson R. Hypersecretion of androgens by polycystic ovaries: the role of genetic factors in the regulation of cytochrome P450c17α. *Baillieres Clin Endocrinol Metab* 1996; 10: 193–203.

30. Nelson VL, Legro RS, Strauss JF, McAllister JM. Augmented androgen production is a stable steroidogenic phenotype of propagated theca cells from polycystic ovaries. *Mol Endocrinol* 1999; 13: 946–957.

31. Nelson VL, Qin Kn KN, Rosenfield RL, Wood JR, Penning TM, Legro RS, et al. The biochemical basis for increased testosterone production in theca cells propagated from patients with polycystic ovary syndrome. *J Clin Endocrinol Metab* 2001; 86 (12): 5925–5933.

32. Almahbobi G, Anderiesz C, Hutchinson P, McFarlane JR, Wood C, Trounson AO. Functional integrity of granulosa cells from polycystic ovaries. *Clin Endocrinol* (Oxf) 1996; 44: 571–580.

33. Mason HD, Willis DS, Holly JM, Franks S. Insulin preincubation enhances insulin-like growth factor-II (IGF-II) action on steroidogenesis in human granulosa cells. *J Clin Endocrinol Metab* 1994; 78: 1265–1267.

34. Hsueh AJ, Dahl KD, Vaughan J, Tucker E, Rivier J, Bardin CW, Vale W. Heterodimers and homodimers of inhibin subunits have different paracrine action in the modulation of luteinizing hormone-stimulated androgen biosynthesis. *Proc Natl Acad Sci* USA. 1987; 84(14): 5082–5086.

35. Cataldo NA, Giudice LC. Follicular fluid insulin-like growth factor binding protein profiles in polycystic ovary syndrome. *J Clin Endocrinol Metab* 1992; 74: 695–697.

36. Prelevic GM, Wurzburger MI, Balint-Peric L, Nesic JS. Inhibitory effect of sandostatin on secretion of luteinising hormone and ovarian steroids in polycystic ovary syndrome. *Lancet* 1990; 336(8720): 900–903.

37. Erickson GF, Magoffin DA, Garzo VG, Cheung AP, Chang RJ. Granulosa cells of polycystic ovaries: are they normal or abnormal? *Hum Reprod* 1992; 7(3): 293–299.

38. Ehrmann DA, Rosenfield RL, Barnes RB, Brigell DF, Sheikh Z. Detection of functional ovarian hyperandrogenism in women with androgen excess *N Engl J Med* 1992; 327: 157–162.

39. Turner EI, Watson MJ, Perry LA, White MC. Investigation of adrenal function in women with oligomenorrhea and hirsutism (clinical PCOS) from the north-east of England using an adrenal stimulation test. *Clin Endocrinol* (Oxf) 1992; 36: 389–397.

40. Moran C, Azziz R. The role of the adrenal cortex in polycystic ovary syndrome. *Obstet Gynecol Clin North Am* 2001; 28: 63–75.

41. Stewart PM, Shackleton CH, Beastall GH, Edwards CR. 5α-Reductase activity in polycystic ovary syndrome. *Lancet* 1990; 335: 431–433.

42. Chin D, Shackleton C, Prasad VK, Kohn B, David R, Imperato-McGinley J, et al. Increased 5 alpha-reductase and normal 11beta-hydroxysteroid dehydrogenase metabolism of C19 and C21 steroids in a young population with polycystic ovarian syndrome. *J Pediatr Endocrinol Metab* 2000; 13(3): 253–259.

43. Rodin DA, Bano G, Bland JM, Taylor K, Nussey SS. Polycystic ovaries and associated metabolic abnormalities in Indian subcontinent Asian women. *Clin Endocrinol* (Oxf) 1998; 49: 91–99.

44. Mowszowicz I, Melanitou E, Kirchhoffer MO, Mauvais-Jarvis P. Dihydrotestosterone stimulates 5α-reductase activity in pubic skin fibroblasts. *J Clin Endocrinol Metab* 1983; 56: 320–325.

45. Rodin A, Thakkar H, Taylor N, Clayton R. Hyperandrogenism in polycystic ovary syndrome. Evidence of dysregulation of 11 beta-hydroxysteroid dehydrogenase. *N Engl J Med* 1994; 330: 460–465.

46. Walker BR, Rodin A, Taylor NF, Clayton RN. Endogenous inhibitors of 11β-hydroxysteroid dehydrogenase type I do not explain abnormal cortisol metabolism in polycystic ovary syndrome. *Clin Endocrinol* (Oxf) 200; 52: 77–80.

47. Finken MJ, Andrews RC, Andrew R, Walker BR. Cortisol metabolism in healthy young adults: sexual dimorphism in activities of A-ring reductases, but not 11beta-hydroxysteroid dehydrogenases. *J Clin Endocrinol Metab* 1999; 84: 3316–3321.

48. Balen AH. The pathogenesis of polycystic ovary syndrome: the enigma unravels. *Lancet* 1999; 354: 966–967.

49. Tsilchorozidou T, Overton C, Conway GS. The pathophysiology of polycystic ovary syndrome. *Clin Endocrinol* (Oxf) 2004; 60: 1–17.

50. Chang RJ, Nakamura RM, Judd HL, Kaplan SA. Insulin resistance in nonobese patients with polycystic ovarian disease. *J Clin Endocrinol Metab* 1983; 57: 356–359.

51. Dunaif A, Segal KR, Futterweit W, Dobrjansky A. Profound peripheral insulin resistance, independent of obesity, in polycystic ovary syndrome. *Diabetes* 1989; 38: 1165–1174.

52. Dunaif A, Segal KR, Shelley DR, Green G, Dobrjansky A, Licholai T. Evidence for distinctive and intrinsic defects in insulin action in polycystic ovary syndrome. *Diabetes* 1992; 41: 1257–1266.

53. Dunaif A. Hyperandrogenic anovulation (PCOS): a unique disorder of insulin action associated with an increased risk of non-insulin-dependent diabetes mellitus. *Am J Med* 1995; 98: 33S–39S.

54. Morales AJ, Laughlin GA, Butzow T, Maheshwari H, Baumann G, Yen SS. Insulin, somatotropic, and luteinizing hormone axes in lean and obese women with polycystic ovary syndrome: common and distinct features. *J Clin Endocrinol Metab* 1996; 81: 2854–2864.

55. Herbert CM, Hill GA, Diamond MP. The use of the intravenous glucose tolerance test to evaluate nonobese hyperandrogenemic women. *Fertil Steril* 1990; 53: 647–653.

56. Dale PO, Tanbo T, Vaaler S, Abyholm T. Body weight, hyperinsulinemia, and gonadotropin levels in the polycystic ovarian syndrome: evidence of two distinct populations. *Fertil Steril* 1992; 58: 487–491.

57. Ovesen P, Moller J, Ingerslev HJ, Jorgensen JO, Mengel A, Schmitz O, et al. Normal basal and insulin-stimulated fuel metabolism in lean women with the polycystic ovary syndrome. *J Clin Endocrinol Metab* 1993; 77(6): 1636–1640.

58. Cibula, D. Is insulin resistance an essential

component of PCOS?: The influence of confounding factors. *Hum Reprod* 2004; 19: 757–759.

59. Dunaif A. Insulin resistance and the polycystic ovary syndrome: mechanisms and implication for pathogenesis. *Endocr Rev* 1997; 18: 774–800.

60. Franks S. Polycystic ovary syndrome. *N Engl J Med* 1995; 333: 853–861.

61. Zhang LH, Rodriguez H, Ohno S, Miller WL. Serine phosphorylation of human P450c17 increases 17,20-lyase activitiy: implications for adrenarche and the polycystic ovary syndrome. *Proc Natl Acad Sci* USA. of America 1995; 92: 10619–10623.

62. Conway GS, Avey C, Rumsby G. The tyrosine kinase domain of the insulin receptor gene is normal in women with hyperinsulinaemia and polycystic ovary syndrome. *Hum Reprod* 1994; 9: 1681–1683.

63. Talbot JA, Bicknell EJ, Rajkhowa M, Krook A, O'Rahilly S, Clayton RN. Molecular scanning of the insulin receptor gene in women with polycystic ovarian syndrome. *J Clin Endocrinol Metab* 1996; 81: 1979–1983.

64. Conway GS, Jacobs HS, Holly JM, Wass JA. Effects of luteinizing hormone, insulin, insulin-like growth factor-I and insulin-like growth factor small binding protein 1 in the polycystic ovary syndrome. *Clin Endocrinol* (Oxf) 1990; 33: 593–603.

65. Robinson S, Kiddy D, Gelding SV, Willis D, Niththyananthan R, Bush A, et al. The relationship of insulin insensitivity to menstrual pattern in women with hyperandrogenism and polycystic ovaries. *Clin Endocrinol* (Oxf) 1993; 39 (3): 351–355.

66. Nagamani M, Van Dinh T, Kelver ME. Hyperinsulinemia in hyperthecosis of the ovaries. *Am J Obstet Gynecol* 1986; 154: 384–389.

67. Geffner ME, Kaplan SA, Bersch N, Golde DW, Landaw EM, Chang RJ. Persistence of insulin resistance in polycystic ovarian disease after inhibition of ovarian steroid secretion. *Fertil Steril* 1986; 45: 327–333.

68. Elkind-Hirsch KE, Valdes CT, Malinak LR. Insulin resistance improves in hyperandrogenic women treated with Lupron. *Fertil Steril* 1993; 60: 634–641.

69. Bergh C, Carlsson B, Olsson JH, Selleskog U, Hillensjo T. Regulation of androgen production in cultured human thecal cells by insulin-like growth factor I and insulin. *Fertil Steril* 1993; 59: 323–331.

70. Cara JF, Fan J, Azzarello J, Rosenfield RL. Insulin-like growth factor-I enhances luteinizing hormone binding to rat ovarian theca-interstitial cells. *J Clin Invest* 1990; 86: 560–565.

71. Willis D, Franks S. Insulin action in human granulosa cells from normal and polycystic ovaries is mediated by the insulin receptor and not the type-I insulin-like growth factor receptor. *J Clin Endocrinol Metab* 1995; 80: 3788–3790.

72. Willis D, Mason H, Gilling-Smith C, Franks S. Modulation by insulin of follicle-stimulating hormone and luteinizing hormone actions in human granulosa cells of normal and polycystic ovaries. *J Clin Endocrinol Metab* 1996; 81: 302–309.

73. Barbieri RL, Makris A, Ryan KJ. Insulin stimulates androgen accumulation in incubations of human ovarian stroma and theca. *Obstet Gynecol* 1984; 64: 73S–80S.

74. Nestler JE, Jakubowicz DJ, De Vargas AF, Brik C, Quintero N, Medina F. Insulin stimulates testosterone biosynthesis by human thecal cells from women with polycystic ovary syndrome by activating its own receptor and using inositolglycan mediators as the signal transduction system. *J Clin Endocrinol Metab* 1998; 83: 2001–2005.

75. Nestler JE, Jakubowicz DJ. Decreases in ovarian cytochrome P450c17 alpha activity and serum free testosterone after reduction of insulin secretion in polycystic ovary syndrome. *N Engl J Med* 1996; 335: 617–623.

76. Moghetti P, Castello R, Negri C et al. Insulin infusion amplifies 17α-hydroxycorticosteroid intermediates response to adrenocorticotropin in hyperandrogenic women: apparent relative impairment of 17,20-lyase activity. *J Clin Endocrinol Metab* 1996; 81: 881–886.

77. Nestler JE. Insulin regulation of human ovarian androgens. *Hum Reprod* 1997; 12: 53–62.

78. Yen SS, Laughlin GA, Morales AJ. Interface between extra- and intraovarian factors in polycystic ovarian syndrome. *Ann N Y Acad Sci* 1993; 687: 98–111.

79. Unger JW, Livingston JN, Moss AM. Insulin receptors in the central nervous system: localization, signalling mechanisms and functional aspects. *Prog Neurobiol* 1991; 36(5): 343–362.

80. Adashi EY, Hsueh AJ, Bambino TH, Yen SS. Disparate effect of clomiphene and tamoxifen on pituitary gonadotropin release in vitro. *Am J Physiol* 1981; 240(2): E125–130.

81. Bach LA. The insulin-like growth factor system: basic and clinical aspects. *Aust N Z J Med* 1999; 29(3): 355–361.

82. Conn JJ, Jacobs HS, Conway GS. The prevalence of polycystic ovaries in women with type 2 diabetes mellitus. *Clin Endocrinol* (Oxf) 2000; 52: 81–86.

12

Chronic Complications of Polycystic Ovary Syndrome

Hulusi Bulent Zeyneloglu, Ibrahim Esinler

Summary

Polycystic Ovary Syndrome (PCOS) is the most common reproductive endocrine disorder, affecting approximately 5%–7% of reproductive-aged women. PCOS may be associated with a state of insulin resistance, hyperandrogenism, hyperlipidemia, and hypertension, which are known to be risk factors for the development of cardiovascular disease. PCOS may also be associated with unopposed estrogen which is the main risk factor for endometrial hyperplasia and endometrial cancer.

Therefore, to prevent and reduce the long term complications of PCOS, a physician should not only consider the immediate issues of irregular bleeding, hirsutism, and infertility, but also focus on the long-term goals of preventing diabetes, heart disease, and cancer. Lifestyle modification should be the first-line therapy to reduce the long term effects of PCOS. Calorie restriction and exercise improve insulin sensitivity and decrease central obesity. Insulin sensitizer treatment leads to improvement in glucose tolerance in women with PCOS and decreases circulating androgen and estrogen levels. To minimize the risk of endometrial cancer, women with PCOS and amenorrhea should be encouraged to take exogenous progestogens at least every 3 months, or to take a combined oral contraceptive pill.

Introduction

Polycystic ovary syndrome is the most common reproductive endocrine disorder.[1,2] Approximately 20% of women of reproductive age have polycystic ovarian morphology on ultrasonographic examination,[3] and up to 10% are diagnosed with PCOS.[4]

Polycystic ovary syndrome may be associated with a state of insulin resistance, hyperandrogenism, and hyperlipidemia and with hypertension which are known to be risk factors for the development of diseases such as cardiovascular disease (CVD) and cancers.[5] Therefore, the recognition of its association with long term complications has led to increased recognition of its importance.

Clinical Discussion

The potential long term complications of the PCOS are categorized below:

Cardiovascular disease

Great attention should be exercised to prevent cardiovascular disease (CVD), since it is the leading cause of morbidity and mortality for older women. The American College of Cardiology[6] has determined the following risk factors as being most important for the development of CVD: age, smoking, diabetes, hypertension, obesity, elevated serum low-density lipoprotein cholesterol, and low serum high-density lipoprotein cholesterol. With the exception of age and smoking, which are not related to the presence or absence of PCOS, all of the other factors that increase cardiovascular disease, are probably increased in women with PCOS. Thus, one can assume that women with PCOS have an increased risk for CVD. But we should clearly answer this question: Are the known risk factors for CVD mentioned above really more common in women with PCOS?

Possible predispositions to cardiovascular disease (CVD)

Hypertension (HT)
Recently, Wild[7] summarized the articles related with PCOS and HT in his review paper. Table 12.1 shows these studies. The overall results of these studies revealed that patients with PCOS are more likely to have HT than normal women. However, these studies had several limitations. One of the most important limitations was that factors that affect the risk of HT such as genetics, inactivity, stress, and salt loading were often not controlled in these studies. Thus, the the results should be carefully interpreted. Large prospective data sets are required to determine whether women with PCOS alone are at an increased hypertensive risk. Furthermore, studies in which exercise and diet are controlled, should be undertaken.

Insulin resistance (IR), impaired glucose tolerance (IGT), diabetes mellitus (DM) and gestational diabetes mellitus (GDM):
It is clearly known that women with gestational diabetes mellitus (GDM) have an increased risk of developing type 2 diabetes mellitus (DM) later in life.[17] Furthermore, GDM is thought to present

Table 12.1 Are women with PCOS more prone to hypertension?

Study	Patient population	Findings
Mattsson et al, (1984)[8]	20 PCOS vs 20 normal	Blood pressure higher in PCOS
Zimmermann et al, (1992)[9]	14 PCOS vs 18 normal control	No difference in blood pressure (24-hour ambulatory systolic and diastolic) and left ventricular mass
Conway et al, (1992)[10]	102 lean and obese PCOS	Obese PCOS had higher systolic blood pressure than controls
Sampson et al, (1996)[11]	24 nonobese PCOS with irregular menses; 26 PCOS with regular menses; 10 normal	No difference for 24-hour, daytime, or nighttime ambulatory blood pressure
Holte et al, (1996)[12]	36 PCOS vs 55 control subjects	Higher ambulatory mean arterial blood pressue; higher daytime systolic blood pressure; no difference in diastolic blood pressure
Dahlgren et al, (1992)[13]	33 PCOS; 132 age-matched controls (wedge-resection patients)	Greater prevalence of physician diagnosed hypertension in PCOS group
Loucks et al, (2000)[14]	63 PCOS vs 56 controls	no difference in systolic and diastolic blood pressure
Elting et al, (2001)[15]	346 PCOS patients by telephone vs age-specific Dutch women	Hypertension, 2.5 times higher in PCOS; hypertension, obesity more common in the younger (35–44 y) PCOS group (n = 233)
Vrbikova et al, (2003)[16]	54 PCOS vs 335 controls	Both systolic and diastolic blood pressure higher in PCOS

an early manifestation of the metabolic syndrome (or syndrome X, Table 12.2). Women with PCOS seem to share some of the same metabolic abnormalities as women with GDM. Women with a history of GDM are reported to have an increased frequency of polycystic ovary morphology, hirsutism and irregular cycles, as compared to women with normal pregnancy.[18,19] Some prospective and retrospective data support an increased risk for GDM in PCOS,[20,21] especially if pre-conceptional or early pregnancy hyperinsulinemia exists.[21]

Because of insulin resistance and central obesity, all women with PCOS are considered to be at increased risk for impaired glucose intolerance (IGT) and overt type 2 DM. Dunaif et al.[22] suggested that up to 20% of obese women with PCOS have IGT or DM by their third decade. Women with PCOS have a significantly increased prevalence of IGT and even undiagnosed DM than normal women of the same age, weight and ethnicity.[23,24] It has recently been shown that women with type 2 DM have a higher prevalence of PCOS than that reported in the general population.[25] Recently, Wild[7] summarized the articles related with PCOS and abnormal glucose diabetes mellitus in his review paper. Table 12.3 shows these studies. Ehrmann et al.[26] noted that the prevalence of IGT and non-insulin dependent DM (NIDDM) was considerably higher than expected when compared to age and weight matched women without PCOS. He suggested that the conversion from IGT to diabetes mellitus is accelerated in women with PCOS. Legro et al.[23] similarly noted that women with PCOS are

Table 12.2 Criteria for the metabolic syndrome in women with PCOS

Risk factor	Cut-off
Abdominal obesity (waist circumference)	> 88 cm
Triglycerides	> 150 mg/dl
HDL-C	< 50 mg/dl
Blood pressure	>130/> 85 mmHg
Fasting and 2 h	110 ± 126 mg/dl and/or
glucose from OGTT	2 h glucose 140±199 mg/dl

Note: Three out of five qualify for the syndrome. HDL-C, high density lipoprotein-cholesterol; OGTT, oral glucose tolerance test.

Table 12.3 Are women with PCOS at greater risk for abnormal glucose/diabetes mellitus?

Study	Patient population	Findings
Dahlgren et al, (1992)[13]	33 PCOS; 132 age-matched referents; wedge resection	Greater prevalence of physician diagnosed diabetes mellitus in PCOS
Ehrmann et al, (1999)[26]	122 PCOS	Glucose intolerance 45%; IGT 35%; NIDDM 10%
Legro et al, (1999)[23]	254 PCOS women 14–44 yrs Group 1 = urban, ethnically diverse (n = 110); Group 2 = rural, ethnically homogeneous (n = 144); and 80 control subjects of similar weight, ethnicity, and age	Prevalence of glucose intolerance: IGT 38.6%–31.1%; diabetes mellitus, 7.5%; nonobese PCOS: IGT, 10.3%; diabetes mellitus, 1.5%
Cibula et al, (2000)[27]	28 select patients with ovarian wedge resection compared with 752 control subjects who were selected by age (45–59 yrs) from a random population	PCOS, aged 45–54 yrs (n = 32), prevalence of diabetes mellitus was 4 times higher

at significantly increased risk for IGT and type 2 diabetes mellitus at all weight levels and at a young age. Women with type 1 DM also have been shown to have a high prevalence of hyperandrogenic abnormality (38.8%), including PCOS and hirsutism.[28] Furthermore, Pierpoint et al.[29] noted that the number of deaths in which diabetes was a contributing cause has been demonstrated to be significantly higher among women with PCOS than that expected based on national data (OR, 3.6; 95% CI 1.5 to 8.4).

It can be concluded from the overall results of the studies that, PCOS is frequently associated with central obesity and is associated with varying states of altered glucose metabolism, from minor alterations to overt hyperglycemia with or without diabetes mellitus.

Dyslipidemia

Women with PCOS have higher triglyceride, very low-density lipoprotein (VLDL) cholesterol, and lipoprotein C-III levels and lower high-density lipoprotein (HDL2) cholesterol and apolipoprotein A-I/A-II ratios compared to normal women.[30] Even after correcting for obesity, PCOS is still associated with elevated LDL cholesterol, and there is a synergistic effect of PCOS and obesity in causing hypertriglyceridemia.[31]

Obesity/Metabolic Syndrome

Increased adiposity, particularly visceral adiposity, that is usually measured by an elevated waist circumference (>88 cm) or waist-to-hip ratio, has been associated with hyperandrogenism, insulin resistance, glucose intolerance, and dyslipidemia.[32] Approximately 50–80% women with PCOS are obese, and obesity alone may associated with insulin resistance and hyperinsulinemia.[33] Patients with PCOS usually display central or android pattern obesity (visceral adiposity), which is characterized by an increased waist-hip ratio.[34] This pattern of obesity is an important indicator of the degree of metabolic disturbance and is associated more closely with dyslipidemia and hyperinsulinemia than normal pattern obesity.[35] Despite the fact that obese women have a greater baseline level of

cardiovascular risk, the incremental cardiovascular risk attributable to PCOS may be even greater as the weight increases.

The metabolic syndrome is defined by both lipid and non-lipid criteria that identify individuals at an increased risk for cardiovascular disease and type 2 diabetes (Table 12.2).[36] Ehrmann et al.[37] recently determined the prevalence of metabolic syndrome in 394 PCOS women. Twenty-six (6.6%) subjects had diabetes; among the 368 non diabetics, the prevalence for individual components comprising the metabolic syndrome were: waist circumference > 88 cm in 80%, HDL cholesterol < 50 mg/dl in 66%, triglycerides ≥ 150 mg/dl in 32%, blood pressure ≥ 130/85 mmHg in 21% and fasting glucose concentrations ≥ 110 mg/dl in 5%. Three or more of these individual criteria were present in 123 (33.4%) of the subjects overall. The most important result of the study was that one-third of the non-diabetic women with PCOS developed the metabolic syndrome well before the end of their fourth decade, and usually prior to the end of their third decade of life.[37] This prevalence was markedly higher than the 6.7% prevalence of metabolic syndrome reported in women between the ages of 20 and 30 years and the 15% prevalence reported by the Third National Health and Nutrition Examination Survey in women between the ages 30 and 40.[38] Ehrmann et al.[37] noted that obesity has an independent effect on the risk for the metabolic syndrome. Women with a higher body mass index (BMI) (>27 kg/mg^2) had a nearly 14-fold increased chance of having the metabolic syndrome compared to women with normal BMI.

Recently, Dokras et al.[39] reported that women with PCOS have an 11-fold increase in the prevalence of the metabolic syndrome compared to age-matched controls. The risk of metabolic syndrome is high even at a young age.

Others
C-reactive protein and homocysteine

Serum concentrations of C-reactive protein (CRP) appear to be increased in women with PCOS. As an example, in a retrospective analysis of 116 women with PCOS and 96 BMI matched control women with regular menstrual cycles, serum CRP concentrations were >5 mg/L in 37 percent of PCOS women compared to 10 percent of control subjects.[40] Homocysteine, another marker of cardiovascular disease has also been found to be elevated in women with PCOS.[41]

Obstructive sleep apnea
In a study of 53 women with PCOS compared with 452 premenopausal controls, obstructive sleep apnea and excessive daytime sleepiness were significantly more common in the PCOS group (OR 30.6, p < 0.01; OR 9.0, p < 0.01, respectively).[42] The differences remained significant, even when controlled for BMI. The strongest predictors for sleep apnea were fasting plasma insulin concentrations and glucose-to-insulin ratios. In a another study of 18 obese women with PCOS undergoing overnight polysomnography, subjects were more likely than age and weight-matched controls to have obstructive sleep apnea (44 versus 5.5 percent, p <0.05).[43] The prevalence of obstructive sleep apnea in PCOS is higher than expected and cannot be explained by obesity alone.[44,45] Insulin resistance appears to be a stronger predictor of sleep-disordered breathing than age, BMI, or the circulating testosterone concentration.[34]

Vascular Studies
The combination of dyslipidemia and hyperinsulinemia may predispose women with PCOS to have accelerated vascular disease such as atherosclerosis. Several measures of subclinical atherosclerosis, such as carotid intima-media thickness (IMT) and coronary artery calcium have been studied. Guzick et al.[46] reported increased IMT, which is an indicator of subclinical atherosclerosis, in the carotid artery of PCOS women compared to control women. Similarly, Talbott et al.[47] in a larger study, reported increased IMT in age and BMI matched older women (> 45 years) with PCOS compared to controls. However, in younger women (30–44 years) no significant difference in IMT was found between those with PCOS and controls, although a higher

proportion of those with PCOS had a higher atherosclerotic index (the overall mean of the IMT mean measurements at eight different sites) compared to controls. The authors also reported a higher prevalence of carotid plaque index (sum of plaque grades across right and left carotid arteries) in young women with PCOS compared with age-matched controls.[48]

Lakhani et al.[49] reported increased IMT in the common carotid and femoral arteries in young women with PCOS compared with controls, independent of blood pressure, BMI and lipids. Christian et al.[50] reported increased coronary artery calcification (odds ratio 2.52), assessed using electron beam computed tomography in PCOS women aged 30–45 years who were matched to two control women by age and BMI (odds ratio 5.5).

Reduced vascular compliance[51] and vascular endothelial dysfunction in women with PCOS were also noted in several studies.[51–54] Furthermore, the degree of impairment in vascular reactivity was significantly greater than can be explained by obesity and hyperlipidemia alone[51].

Cardiovascular disease risk and PCOS: Results
The existing data suggest that PCOS may affect or accelerate the development of an adverse cardiovascular risk profile, and even subclinical signs of atherosclerosis, but it does not appear to lower the age of clinical presentation to a premenopausal age group.

Neoplastic risks and PCOS

Endometrial cancer

The risk of developing endometrial cancer has been shown to be adversely influenced by a number of factors including obesity, long-term use of unopposed estrogens, nulliparity and infertility.[55,56] Hypertension and type 2 diabetes mellitus have also long been linked to endometrial cancer, with relative risks of 2.1 and 2.8 respectively;[57] these conditions are now also known to be associated with PCOS. The association between PCOS and endometrial adenocarcinoma has been reported for many years. It appears that PCOS patients have approximately three times the risk of developing endometrial cancer compared to women without PCOS. A cohort study of 1270 women suggested a trebling of the risk of developing endometrial cancer in women with chronic anovulation without hypoestrogenemia (pathological or macroscopic evidence of PCOS, or a clinical diagnosis of chronic anovulation).[58] This study identified the excess risk of endometrial cancer to be 3.1 [95% confidence interval (CI) 1.1±7.3] and proposed that this might be due to abnormal concentrations of unopposed estrogen. Other authors have expanded this theory by suggesting that hyperandrogenism and hyperinsulinemia may further increase the potential for neoplastic change in the endometrium through their effects on concentrations of sex hormone-binding globulin (SHBG), insulin-like growth factor-1 (IGF-1) and circulating estrogens.[59,60]

Endometrial hyperplasia is a precursor of endometrial cancer. In a study of 97 women under the age of 36 years with adenomatous or atypical adenomatous hyperplasia, 25% were found to have typical polycystic ovaries.[61]

Breast cancer

Unopposed estrogen is a risk factor for developing breast cancer. Thus, one can assume that unopposed estrogen stimulation in PCOS patients might therefore be expected to increase the risk of breast cancer in these women. However, no clinical data support this hypothesis. PCOS, by itself, does not appear to be a risk factor for breast cancer.

Ovarian cancer

The Cancer and Steroid Hormone Study[62] and a case-controlled study involving 426 cancer cases and 4081 controls,[63] revealed that the ovarian cancer risk is doubled in PCOS patients. However, studies on the relation between ovarian cancer and PCOS are scarce. Both these studies cited involved patient recall and are therefore, subject to recall bias, but they would be consistent with the gonadotropin theory of incessant stimulation of the ovary leading to the increased risk of development of ovarian cancer. However, no increased risk for ovarian cancer in association with PCOS was noticed in other studies.[29,58,64]

Prevention from risks

To decrease the risks, firsts of all, one should determine the presence or absence of any risk factors associated with PCOS. Thus, early and regular screening for these risk factors in women with PCOS should be carefully performed.

Lifestyle modification should be the first-line therapy to reduce the long term complications of PCOS. Seven percent to 10% weight loss is associated with regular ovulatory cycles in many cases. Exercise improves insulin sensitivity.

Insulin sensitizer treatment leads to improvement in glucose tolerance in women with PCOS[65] and decreases circulating androgen and estrogen levels.[66] Insulin sensitizers also decrease levels of plasminogen activator inhibitor-1 (PAI-1), and improve endothelium-dependent vasodilation.[53]

To minimize the risk of endometrial cancer, women with PCOS and amenorrhea should be encouraged to lose weight first and use exogenous progestogens at least every 3 months, or take a combined oral contraceptive pill.

Recent Advances

To prevent and reduce the long term complications of PCOS, all patients should be screened for insulin resistance (IR) particularly. The euglycemic, hyperinsulinemic glucose clamp test has been accepted as the gold standard to detect IR. However, the use of this test in large-scale clinical practice is time consuming and expensive. Thus, to screen IR in PCOS patients, more accurate and easily performed tests should be used.

The current literature suggests that, the well known risk factors for developing cardiovascular disease are also associated with the PCOS. However, there is paucity of data on the mortality and morbidity due to cardiovascular disease in women with PCOS. There is therefore, an urgent need for studies in this area.

Conclusion

PCOS probably carries an increased long-term risk of developing cardiovascular disease. Modification of the cardiovascular risk profile by treating hypertension, dyslipidemia, hyperinsulinemia and particularly, weight reduction, might help prevent or delay the onset of cardiovascular disease. Lifestyle changes (diet and exercise) should be strongly encouraged to reduce the risk of both type 2 diabetes and cardiovascular disease. A physician should consider the immediate issues of PCOS such as, irregular bleeding, hirsutism, and infertility, but also emphasize on the long-term goals of preventing diabetes, heart disease, and cancer.

References

1. Asuncion M, Calvo RM, San Millan JL, Sancho J, Avila S, Escobar-Morreale HF. A prospective study of the prevalence of the polycystic ovary syndrome in unselected Caucasian women from Spain. *J Clin Endocrinol Metab* 2000; 85: 2434–2448.
2. Knochenhauer ES, Key TJ, Kahsar-Miller M, Waggoner W, Boots LR, Azziz R. Prevalence of the polycystic ovary syndrome in unselected black and white women of the southeastern United States: a prospective study. *J Clin Endocrinol Metab* 1998; 83: 3078–3082.
3. Polson DW, Adams J, Wadsworth J, Franks S. Polycystic ovaries—a common finding in normal women. *Lancet* 1988; 1: 870-872.
4. Futterweit W, Mechanick JI. Polycystic ovarian disease: etiology, diagnosis, and treatment. *Compr Ther* 1988; 14: 12–20.
5. Wild RA. Long-term health consequences of PCOS. *Hum Reprod Update* 2002; 8: 231–241.
6. Grundy SM, Pasternak R, Greenland P, Smith S Jr, Fuster V. Assessment of cardiovascular risk by use of multiple-risk-factor assessment equations: a statement for healthcare professionals from the American Heart Association and the American College of Cardiology. *Circulation* 1999; 100: 1481–1492.
7. Wild RA. Polycystic ovary syndrome: a risk for coronary artery disease? *Am J Obstet Gynecol* 2002; 186: 35–43.
8. Mattsson LA, Cullberg G, Hamberger L, Samsioe G, Silfverstolpe G. Lipid metabolism in women with polycystic ovary syndrome: possible implications for an increased risk of coronary heart disease. *Fertil Steril* 1984; 42: 579–584.
9. Zimmermann S, Phillips RA, Dunaif A, Finegood DT, Wilkenfeld C, Ardeljan M, et al. Polycystic ovary syndrome: lack of hypertension despite profound insulin resistance. *J Clin Endocrinol Metab* 1992; 75: 508–513.
10. Conway GS, Agrawal R, Betteridge DJ, Jacobs HS. Risk factors for coronary artery disease in lean and obese women with the polycystic ovary syndrome. *Clin Endocrinol* (Oxf) 1992; 37: 119–125.
11. Sampson M, Kong C, Patel A, Unwin R, Jacobs HS. Ambulatory blood pressure profiles and plasminogen activator inhibitor (PAI-1) activity in lean women with and without the polycystic ovary syndrome. *Clin Endocrinol* (Oxf) 1996; 45: 623–629.
12. Holte J, Gennarelli G, Berne C, Bergh T, Lithell H. Elevated ambulatory day-time blood pressure in women with polycystic ovary syndrome: a sign of a pre-hypertensive state? *Hum Reprod* 1996; 11: 23–28.
13. Dahlgren E, Johansson S, Lindstedt G, Knutsson F, Oden A, Janson PO, et al. Women with polycystic ovary syndrome wedge resected in 1956 to 1965: a long-term follow-up focusing on natural history and circulating hormones. *Fertil Steril* 1992; 57: 505–513.
14. Loucks TL, Talbott EO, McHugh KP, Keelan M, Berga SL, Guzick DS. Do polycystic-appearing ovaries affect the risk of cardiovascular disease among women with polycystic ovary syndrome? *Fertil Steril* 2000; 74: 547–552.
15. Elting MW, Korsen TJ, Bezemer PD, Schoemaker J. Prevalence of diabetes mellitus, hypertension and cardiac complaints in a follow-up study of a Dutch PCOS population. *Hum Reprod* 2001; 16: 556–560.
16. Vrbikova J, Cifkova R, Jirkovska A, Lanska V, Platilova H, Zamrazil V, Starka L. Cardiovascular risk factors in young Czech females with polycystic ovary syndrome. *Hum Reprod* 2003; 18: 980–984.
17. Damm P, Kuhl C, Bertelsen A, Molsted-Pedersen L. Predictive factors for the development of diabetes in women with previous gestational diabetes mellitus. *Am J Obstet Gynecol* 1992; 167: 607–616.
18. Anttila L, Karjala K, Penttila RA, Ruutiainen K, Ekblad U. Polycystic ovaries in women with

gestational diabetes. *Obstet Gynecol* 1998; 92: 13–16.

19. Kousta E, Cela E, Lawrence N, Penny A, Millauer B, White D, et al. The prevalence of polycystic ovaries in women with a history of gestational diabetes. *Clin Endocrinol* (Oxf) 2000; 53: 501–507.

20. Mikola M, Hiilesmaa V, Halttunen M, Suhonen L, Tiitinen A. Obstetric outcome in women with polycystic ovarian syndrome. *Hum Reprod* 2001; 16: 226–229.

21. Paradisi G, Fulghesu AM, Ferrazzani S, Moretti S, Proto C, Soranna L, et al. Endocrino-metabolic features in women with polycystic ovary syndrome during pregnancy. *Hum Reprod* 1998; 13: 542–546.

22. Dunaif A. Insulin resistance in polycystic ovarian syndrome. *Ann N Y Acad Sci* 1993; 687: 60–64.

23. Legro RS, Kunselman AR, Dodson WC, Dunaif A. Prevalence and predictors of risk for type 2 diabetes mellitus and impaired glucose tolerance in polycystic ovary syndrome: a prospective, controlled study in 254 affected women. *J Clin Endocrinol Metab* 1999; 84: 165–169.

24. Wild S, Pierpoint T, Jacobs H, McKeigue P. Long-term consequences of polycystic ovary syndrome: results of a 31 year follow-up study. *Hum Fertil* (Camb) 2000; 3: 101–105.

25. Conn JJ, Jacobs HS, Conway GS. The prevalence of polycystic ovaries in women with type 2 diabetes mellitus. *Clin Endocrinol* (Oxf) 2000; 52: 81–86.

26. Ehrmann DA, Barnes RB, Rosenfield RL, Cavaghan MK, Imperial J. Prevalence of impaired glucose tolerance and diabetes in women with polycystic ovary syndrome. *Diabetes Care* 1999; 22: 141–146.

27. Cibula D, Cifkova R, Fanta M, Poledne R, Zivny J, Skibova J. Increased risk of non-insulin dependent diabetes mellitus, arterial hypertension and coronary artery disease in perimenopausal women with a history of the polycystic ovary syndrome. *Hum Reprod* 2000; 15: 785–789.

28. Escobar-Morreale HF, Roldan B, Barrio R, Alonso M, Sancho J, de la Calle H, Garcia-Robles R. High prevalence of the polycystic ovary syndrome and hirsutism in women with type 1 diabetes mellitus. *J Clin Endocrinol Metab* 2000; 85: 4182–4187.

29. Pierpoint T, McKeigue PM, Isaacs AJ, Wild SH, Jacobs HS. Mortality of women with polycystic ovary syndrome at long-term follow-up. *J Clin Epidemiol* 1998; 51: 581–586.

30. Wild RA, Bartholomew MJ. The influence of body weight on lipoprotein lipids in patients with polycystic ovary syndrome. *Am J Obstet Gynecol* 1988; 159: 423–427.

31. Legro RS, Kunselman AR, Dunaif A. Prevalence and predictors of dyslipidemia in women with polycystic ovary syndrome. *Am J Med* 2001; 111: 607–613.

32. Sowers JR. Obesity as a cardiovascular risk factor. *Am J Med* 2003; 115 Suppl 8A: 37S–41S.

33. Campbell PJ, Gerich JE. Impact of obesity on insulin action in volunteers with normal glucose tolerance: demonstration of a threshold for the adverse effect of obesity. *J Clin Endocrinol Metab* 1990; 70: 1114–1118.

34. Talbott E, Guzick D, Clerici A, Berga S, Detre K, Weimer K, Kuller L. Coronary heart disease risk factors in women with polycystic ovary syndrome. *Arterioscler Thromb Vasc Biol* 1995; 15: 821–826.

35. Wajchenberg BL. Subcutaneous and visceral adipose tissue: their relation to the metabolic syndrome. *Endocr Rev* 2000; 21: 697–738.

36. Ford ES. The metabolic syndrome and mortality from cardiovascular disease and all-causes: findings from the National Health and Nutrition Examination Survey II Mortality Study. *Atherosclerosis* 2004; 173: 309–314.

37. Ehrmann DA, Liljenquist DR, Kasza K et al. Prevalence and predictors of the metabolic syndrome in women with polycystic ovary syndrome. *J Clin Endocrinol Metab* 2006; 91(1): 48–53.

38. Ford ES, Giles WH, Dietz WH. Prevalence of the metabolic syndrome among US adults: findings from the third National Health and Nutrition Examination Survey. *JAMA* 2002; 287: 356–359.

39. Dokras A, Bochner M, Hollinrake E, Markham S, Vanvoorhis B, Jagasia DH. Screening women with polycystic ovary syndrome for metabolic syndrome. *Obstet Gynecol* 2005; 106: 131–137.

40. Boulman N, Levy Y, Leiba R, Shachar S, Linn R, Zinder O, Blumenfeld Z. Increased C-reactive protein levels in the polycystic ovary syndrome: a marker of cardiovascular disease. *J Clin Endocrinol Metab* 2004; 89: 2160–2165.

41. Schachter M, Raziel A, Friedler S, Strassburger D, Bern O, Ron-El R. Insulin resistance in patients with polycystic ovary syndrome is associated with elevated plasma homocysteine. *Hum Reprod* 2003; 18: 721–727.

42. Ehrmann DA. Polycystic ovary syndrome. *N Engl J Med* 2005; 352: 1223–1236.

43. Fogel RB, Malhotra A, Pillar G et al. Increased prevalence of obstructive sleep apnea syndrome in obese women with polycystic ovary syndrome. *J Clin Endocrinol Metab* 2001; 86: 1175–1180.

44. Vgontzas AN, Legro RS, Bixler EO, Grayev A, Kales

A, Chrousos GP. Polycystic ovary syndrome is associated with obstructive sleep apnea and daytime sleepiness: role of insulin resistance. *J Clin Endocrinol Metab* 2001; 86: 517–520.

45. Gopal M, Duntley S, Uhles M, Attarian H. The role of obesity in the increased prevalence of obstructive sleep apnea syndrome in patients with polycystic ovarian syndrome. *Sleep Med* 2002; 3: 401–404.

46. Guzick DS, Talbott EO, Sutton-Tyrrell K, Herzog HC, Kuller LH, Wolfson SK Jr. Carotid atherosclerosis in women with polycystic ovary syndrome: initial results from a case-control study. *Am J Obstet Gynecol* 1996; 174: 1224–1229.

47. Talbott E, Clerici A, Berga SL, Kuller L, Guzick D, Detre K, Daniels T, Engberg RA. Adverse lipid and coronary heart disease risk profiles in young women with polycystic ovary syndrome: results of a case-control study. *J Clin Epidemiol* 1998; 51: 415–422.

48. Talbott EO, Guzick DS, Sutton-Tyrrell K, McHugh-Pemu KP, Zborowski JV, Remsberg KE, Kuller LH. Evidence for association between polycystic ovary syndrome and premature carotid atherosclerosis in middle-aged women. *Arterioscler Thromb Vasc Biol* 2000; 20: 2414–2421.

49. Lakhani K, Prelevic GM, Seifalian AM, Atiomo WU, Hardiman P. Polycystic ovary syndrome, diabetes and cardiovascular disease: risks and risk factors. *J Obstet Gynaecol* 2004; 24: 613–621.

50. Christian RC, Dumesic DA, Behrenbeck T, Oberg AL, Sheedy PF 2nd, Fitzpatrick LA. Prevalence and predictors of coronary artery calcification in women with polycystic ovary syndrome. *J Clin Endocrinol Metab* 2003; 88: 2562–2568.

51. Kelly CJ, Speirs A, Gould GW, Petrie JR, Lyall H, Connell JM. Altered vascular function in young women with polycystic ovary syndrome. *J Clin Endocrinol Metab* 2002; 87: 742–746.

52. Paradisi G, Steinberg HO, Hempfling A, Cronin J, Hook G, Shepard MK, Baron AD. Polycystic ovary syndrome is associated with endothelial dysfunction. *Circulation* 2001; 103: 1410–1415.

53. Paradisi G, Steinberg HO, Shepard MK, Hook G, Baron AD. Troglitazone therapy improves endothelial function to near normal levels in women with polycystic ovary syndrome. *J Clin Endocrinol Metab* 2003; 88: 576–580.

54. Orio F Jr, Palomba S, Cascella T, De Simone B, Di Biase S, Russo T, et al. Early impairment of endothelial structure and function in young normal-weight women with polycystic ovary syndrome. *J Clin Endocrinol Metab* 2004; 89: 4588–4593.

55. Henderson BE, Casagrande JT, Pike MC, Mack T, Rosario I, Duke A. The epidemiology of endometrial cancer in young women. *Br J Cancer* 1983; 47: 749–756.

56. Dahlgren E, Friberg LG, Johansson S, Lindstrom B, Oden A, Samsioe G, Janson PO. Endometrial carcinoma; ovarian dysfunction—a risk factor in young women. *Eur J Obstet Gynecol Reprod Biol* 1991; 41: 143–150.

57. Elwood JM, Cole P, Rothman KJ, Kaplan SD. Epidemiology of endometrial cancer. *J Natl Cancer Inst* 1977; 59: 1055–1060.

58. Coulam CB, Annegers JF, Kranz JS. Chronic anovulation syndrome and associated neoplasia. *Obstet Gynecol* 1983; 61: 403–407.

59. Gibson M. Reproductive health and polycystic ovary syndrome. *Am J Med* 1995; 98: 67S–75S.

60. Meirow D, Schenker JG. The link between female infertility and cancer: epidemiology and possible aetiologies. *Hum Reprod Update* 1996; 2: 63–75.

61. Chamlian DL, Taylor HB. Endometrial hyperplasia in young women. *Obstet Gynecol* 1970; 36: 659–666.

62. Gammon MD, Thompson WD. Polycystic ovaries and the risk of breast cancer. *Am J Epidemiol* 1991; 134: 818–824.

63. Schildkraut JM, Schwingl PJ, Bastos E, Evanoff A, Hughes C. Epithelial ovarian cancer risk among women with polycystic ovary syndrome. *Obstet Gynecol* 1996; 88: 554–559.

64. Garcea N, Campo S, Panetta V, Venneri M, Siccardi P, Dargenio R, De Tomasi F. Induction of ovulation with purified urinary follicle-stimulating hormone in patients with polycystic ovarian syndrome. *Am J Obstet Gynecol* 1985; 151: 635–640.

65. Ehrmann DA, Schneider DJ, Sobel BE, Cavaghan MK, Imperial J, Rosenfield RL, Polonsky KS. Troglitazone improves defects in insulin action, insulin secretion, ovarian steroidogenesis, and fibrinolysis in women with polycystic ovary syndrome. *J Clin Endocrinol Metab* 1997; 82: 2108–2116.

66. Dunaif A, Scott D, Finegood D, Quintana B, Whitcomb R. The insulin-sensitizing agent troglitazone improves metabolic and reproductive abnormalities in the polycystic ovary syndrome. *J Clin Endocrinol Metab* 1996; 81: 3299–3306.

Frequently Asked Questions

1. What are the long-term complications of the PCOS?

The established complications are cardiovascular diseases, diabetes mellitus and uterine cancer.

2. Are these long-term complications preventible?

Yes

3. What is the most important point to be considered in preventing the development of these complications?

The most important point is, screening the PCOS patients with regard to the risks factors?

4. Is there a screening method available? If so, which is the best screening method?

Several screening methods are recommended by the consensus conferences. However, no one is the best. In large-scale clinical practice, simpler methods such as fasting- and OGTT-based estimates may provide an effective estimate of insulin resistance.

5. What should we do to prevent long-term complications?

Firstly, lifestyle modifications with complimentary diet and exercise should be recommended to women with PCOS. Insulin sensitizers and insulin lowering agents should be prescribed if necessary.

Impaired Glucose Metabolism & Insulin Resistance

13

Glucose Intolerance in the Polycystic Ovary Syndrome: Role of the Pancreatic Beta-Cell

Luís Ruvalcaba, Sandra Cubillos, Alexandra Bermúdez, Silvio Cuneo, Martha García, Julio Chanona

Summary

Nowadays, 5–10% of women of reproductive age have polycystic ovary syndrome (PCOS).[1-4] PCOS is a reproductive disorder with a significant impact on fertility. It is a disorder with a marked increase in risk for diabetes and glucose intolerance. Insulin resistance is not part of the diagnostic criteria for PCOS, but its importance in the pathogenesis of PCOS cannot be denied. Approximately 50–70% of PCOS patients have some degree of insulin resistance, and this hormone insensitivity probably contributes to the hyperandrogenism that is responsible for the signs and symptoms of PCOS. PCOS is associated with insulin resistance independent of total or fat-free body mass. Post-receptor defects in the action of insulin, which are similar to those found in obesity and type 2 diabetes, have been described in PCOS. The discovery that insulin resistance has a key role in the pathophysiology of PCOS has led to a novel and promising form of therapy in the form of insulin-sensitizing drugs. Treatment with insulin sensitizers such as metformin, improve both metabolic and hormonal patterns and also improve ovulation in PCOS. Adequate diagnosis and treatment of glucose intolerance can improve the quality of life of PCOS patients and prevent the development of associated chronic diseases.

Rationale

Insulin resistance is characterized by a post-receptor defect in the action of insulin. The cause of this defect is still under study. Although uncertainty exists, early detection and treatment of insulin resistance present in a large population of PCOS patients, could reduce the incidence or severity of diabetes mellitus, dyslipidemia, hypertension and cardiovascular disease. There are several problems with our current approach to the assessment of insulin sensitivity in PCOS, including the apparent lack of consensus on what defines PCOS and normal insulin sensitivity, ethnic and genetic variability, the presence of other factors such as obesity, stress and aging (Table 13.1) that contribute to insulin resistance, and concern about whether simplified models of insulin sensitivity have the precision to predict treatment needs, responses and future morbidity. The diagnosis of glucose intolerance holds greater prognostic and treatment implications. All obese

Table 13.1 Common disorders associated with insulin resistance

PCOS	Dyslipidemia
Hypertension	Diabetes Mellitus
Pheochromocytoma	Lipodystrophies
Obesity	Cushing's Disease

women with PCOS should be screened for the presence of insulin resistance by looking for other parameters like hypertension, dyslipidemia, central obesity, and glucose intolerance.[5] The present review will address in to the accurate diagnostic and rationale use of insulin sensitizing drugs to treat short term objectives like infertility and long term considerations like prevention and management of the dysmetabolic syndrome with its associate risks of type 2 diabetes and cardiovascular disease.[6]

Introduction

It is estimated that 5–10% of women of reproductive age have polycystic ovary syndrome (PCOS), which is characterized by chronic anovulation and hyperandrogenism in premenopausal women.[1–4] According to the revised guidelines of the PCOS Consensus Workshop Group,[7] to be diagnosed with PCOS, a woman must have 2 of the following 3 manifestations: irregular or absent ovulation, elevated levels of androgenic hormones and/or enlarged ovaries containing at least 12 follicles measuring 2 to 9 mm in diameter and/or have an increased ovarian volume of 10 mL or greater.[1–4] Only one ovary fulfilling these criteria is enough to meet the definition of polycystic ovaries.[1–4] Other hyperandrogenic disorders such as non-classical congenital adrenal hyperplasia and androgen-secreting tumours should be excluded for the diagnosis of PCOS.[3,4]

It should be stressed that polycystic ovaries are not a necessary feature of PCOS and that many women with polycystic ovaries do not have PCOS. Women found to have incidental polycystic ovaries on an ultrasound performed for another indication, should not be considered to have PCOS unless there is corroborating clinical evidence of the syndrome.[1,2]

Around 50% of PCOS women are obese and tend to have an android pattern of obesity. Chronic anovulation may present as irregular menstrual periods or amenorrhea.[1,2] PCOS women are thus in a "chronic estrous state". Constant estrogen exposure leads to proliferation and hyperplasia of the endometrium and this can lead to unpredictable bleeding episodes. Hyperandrogenism is usually suggested by the presence of hirsutism in approximately 80% of the PCOS women and can be documented by measuring androgen levels in the blood. Circulating levels of total testosterone, androstenedione and dehydroepiandrosterone (DHEA) are also elevated.[1–4]

Furthermore, insulin is a negative regulator of the production of sex hormone binding globulin (SHBG) by the liver, and SHBG levels are decreased in hyperinsulinemic conditions, such as metabolic syndrome and visceral obesity. Obese PCOS women do not have elevated luteinizing hormone (LH) levels; therefore, a normal LH level or normal LH/FSH ratio does not rule out PCOS. LH/FSH ratio is now not included in the diagnostic criteria of PCOS.[1–4]

Clinical Discussion

The association between hyperinsulinemia and PCOS was first noted by Burghen et al, in 1980 who found a positive correlation between insulin, androstenedione and testosterone levels among PCOS women. Subsequent studies confirmed insulin resistance as the cause of hyperinsulinemia. It is estimated that 20–40% of PCOS women have impaired glucose tolerance, a number approximately seven-fold higher than the rates in age and weight-matched controls. Prevalence of type 2 diabetes mellitus is also increased in PCOS women (15% versus 2.3% in normal women). Though lean PCOS women have lower rates of carbohydrate intolerance than obese PCOS women, they have higher rates of carbohydrate intolerance than age and weight-matched controls. Thus, PCOS is associated with insulin resistance independent of total or fat-free body mass. Obese PCOS women are more insulin resistant than obese non-PCOS or non-obese PCOS women. Pancreatic beta cell secretory dysfunction has been demonstrated in a subset of PCOS women and this subset probably has the highest risk of developing carbohydrate intolerance and type 2 diabetes. The Rotterdam consensus panel recommends oral glucose tolerance tests for obese PCOS patients.[1,2]

The main function of pancreatic β cells is to synthesize and secrete insulin at appropriate rates to avoid blood glucose fluctuations within a narrow range. Any alteration in β cell function has a profound impact on glucose homeostasis: excessive secretion of insulin causes hypoglycemia and insufficient secretion leads to diabetes. It is therefore, not surprising that insulin secretion is subject to very tight control. This control is primarily ensured by glucose itself but also involves an array of metabolic, neural, hormonal, and sometimes, pharmacological factors. To integrate all these stimulatory and inhibitory influences, β cells rely on a complex stimulus-secretion coupling, between two intracellular pathways that produce triggering and amplifying signals, optimizing adequate insulin secretion to changes in blood glucose concentration, and enable β cells to grade the numerous extracellular messages that they receive. When the extracellular glucose concentration increases, it accelerates the β cell metabolism leading to a decrease in K^+ conductance of the plasma membrane by closure of ATP-sensitive K^+ channels, thus impairing insulin secretion. On the other hand, glucose produces signals that amplify the action of Ca^{2+}, inducing insulin secretion. With the above two mentioned mechanisms, the variation in the glucose concentration allows the typical biphasic and pulsatile insulin secretion. The peculiar biochemical organization of β cells allows intracellular signals to mediate the two pathways that are not redundant but complementary and respect a clear hierarchy. Hormones and neurotransmitters also influence the triggering and amplifying pathways, and this feature enables the use of current therapeutics such as insulin-sensitizing drugs that modify the triggering pathway.[8]

Insulin resistance is characterized by a post-receptor defect in the action of insulin. The cause of this defect is still being elucidated. The first step in the action of insulin action involves binding to the cell-surface receptor. Following insulin binding, the receptor undergoes auto-phosphorylation on specific tyrosine residues (accomplished by the activation of insulin receptor tyrosine kinase). The activated receptor then activates insulin receptor substrates (such as IRS-1,2 and 3), which in turn bind to signalling molecules such as phosphoinositol-3 (PI3) kinase and activate downstream signalling leading to insulin-mediated glucose transport. Abnormalities in both insulin receptor tyrosine kinase (IRTK) activity and in mediators distal to the receptor are present in insulin resistance states. Serine phosphorylation of the insulin receptor decreases IRTK activity.[1,2]

One of the most common prevailing theories regarding the etiology of type 2 diabetes proposes that the primary pathogenetic defect is peripheral insulin resistance resulting in compensatory hyperinsulinemia. Over time, β-cell dysfunction occurs, leading to inadequate secretion of insulin and ultimately, to β-cell exhaustion, insulinopenia, and the development of frank type 2 diabetes mellitus. Substantial literature confirms β-cell dysfunction in PCOS, although as is true in diabetes, there is still considerable debate as to the primacy of the defects and their worsening over time. Basal insulin levels are increased, and insulin secretory response to meals has been shown to be reduced in PCOS women. This dysfunction is independent of obesity.[9]

The hallmark of PCOS is the increased production of testosterone from ovarian theca cells, which can lead to hirsutism and may contribute to anovulation. The use of insulin-sensitizing agents to treat this disorder is based on the theory that insulin can directly stimulate the ovary to augment ovarian androgen production by the stimulation of enzyme P450c17α. Insulin has also been shown to increase luteinizing hormone (LH) stimulated ovarian androgen biosynthesis.[10]

Studies in adipocytes from women with PCOS reveal adipocyte insensitivity to inhibition of lipolysis by insulin as well as a decrease in maximal rates of adipocyte glucose uptake. While these defects are also present in obesity and type 2 diabetes, they can occur in PCOS in the absence of obesity. Dunaif et al.[11] reported decreased insulin receptor autophosphorylation in 50% of fibroblasts removed from PCOS women and this was due to increased receptor serine phosphorylation. Serine phosphorylation, as noted above, has been associated with decreased insulin receptor tyrosine autophosphorylation. In fact, this is the probable mechanism of tumor necrosis factor-alpha (TNF-α) induced insulin resistance. Since serine phosphorylation of P450c17 (the key regulatory enzyme of androgen biosynthesis) increases enzyme activity leading to increased androgen biosynthesis, it is possible that a single defect (serine phosphorylation) can produce both insulin resistance and hyperandrogenism in a subgroup of PCOS women. Lin et al.[12] showed reduced insulin stimulated lactate production in granulosa-lutein cells obtained from women with PCOS, whereas the same cells obtained from normal ovulatory subjects responded with increased lactate production after insulin exposure. *In vitro* human theca cell studies have shown that insulin has direct stimulatory effects on ovarian steroidogenesis. Nestler et al.[13] showed that insulin produced a greater increase in androgen production by theca cells isolated from women with PCOS than in cells obtained from subjects without PCOS, and that this effect is mediated specifically through the insulin receptor rather than through the insulin-like growth factor (IGF) receptor "cross-talk". There is some data to suggest that insulin enhances the effect of LH on preovulatory ovarian follicles, causing premature activation and subsequent follicle arrest. It is possible that hyperinsulinemia (due to insulin resistance) drives the LH effect on ovarian theca cells, which are intrinsically programmed to produce more androgen to cause androgen excess. Excess androgens are known to interfere with the process of follicular maturation, thus inhibiting ovulation and producing more arrested follicles. It has been postulated that the PCOS ovaries are more resistant to the metabolic effects of insulin than to the steroidogenic effects of insulin. Further studies are needed to clarify the "selective insulin resistance" phenomenon.[1,2]

In the last decade, many trials have been held showing the efficacy of insulin sensitizers such as biguanides and thiazolidinediones in improving many aspects of the multifactorial PCOS. Trials have been done with metformin and two thiazolidinediones, troglitazone and rosiglitazone. Metformin is a biguanide, which reduces plasma glucose concentrations in type 2 diabetes patients. Metformin in type 2 diabetes does not lead to weight gain and can induce weight loss in some patients. Metformin predominantly works by reducing hepatic glucose production, inhibiting gluconeogenesis both directly, and indirectly (by decreasing free fatty acid concentrations). There is some data to suggest that it may slightly improve peripheral insulin sensitivity. Various studies on the use of metformin in PCOS patients revealed reductions in androgen levels and improvements in ovulation when metformin was given for a duration of 10-24 weeks. However, only in some of these studies was the effect independent of the weight loss induced by metformin. Metformin has also been found to reduce the high rates of gestational diabetes in PCOS. Thiazolidinediones (TZDs) represent a novel class of drugs that decrease peripheral insulin resistance by enhancing insulin action in the skeletal muscle, liver and adipose tissue. These agents are believed to work by binding and modulating the activity of a family of nuclear transcription factors termed peroxisome proliferator-activated receptors (PPARS). Studies with TZDs in PCOS subjects have shown an improvement in the androgen levels and ovulation rate and enhanced insulin sensitivity without any reduction in the weight of subjects. Troglitazone was the first drug of this class to be studied, however, it was withdrawn from the market in 2000 due to hepatotoxicity. Studies now performed with rosiglitazone have shown a decrease in testosterone, androstenedione and DHEA levels and an increase in SHBG, thereby causing a decrease in free testosterone levels along with an improvement in insulin sensitivity. In a recent study by Ghazeeri et al, rosiglitazone improved both, spontaneous and clomiphene-induced ovulation rates. It is interesting that troglitazone has recently been shown to have independent effects on ovarian steroidogenesis and thus, a direct effect of TZD apart from improvement of insulin resistance cannot be ruled out.[1,2]

Case studies

Practically, hyperinsulinemia (basal or postglucose load) indicates the presence of insulin resistance. Peripheral insulin levels are variable and insulin sensitivity can be more precisely quantified by direct measurement of insulin effects on glucose metabolism in target tissues in vivo and in vitro. Euglycemic glucose clamp studies have demonstrated significant and substantial decreases in insulin-mediated glucose uptake in PCOS. This decrease (35–40%) is of a similar magnitude to that seen in type 2 diabetes, and is independent of obesity, glucose intolerance, increases in waist-hip-girth ratio, and differences in muscle mass. This synergistic negative effect of obesity and PCOS on peripheral glucose uptake, is an important factor in the pathogenesis of glucose intolerance in PCOS.[9]

Insulin resistance has been found in PCOS women of many racial and ethnic groups, however, these results are not universal. Some studies failed to find decreased glucose uptake by the euglycemic glucose clamp in Danish patients. Also, lean and obese women can have normal insulin sensitivity. These differences suggest heterogeneity in PCOS.

It is important to diagnose PCOS patients with impaired glucose tolerance and type 2 diabetes. Unfortunately, fasting glucose test detects only 8% of women with impaired glucose tolerance. For this reason, it is better to use the basal and 2-hour glucose-stimulated levels rather fasting glucose.[9] Although the hyperinsulinemic-euglycemic clamp technique is the gold standard for measuring insulin sensitivity, it is too expensive, time-consuming and labor-intensive to be of practical use in an office setting. Homeostatic measurements (fasting glucose/insulin ratio or homeostatic model assessment [HOMA] value) and minimal model tests (particularly, the oral glucose tolerance test

[OGTT]) represent the easiest office-based assessment of insulin resistance and glucose intolerance in the PCOS patient.[5] (Table 13.2)

PCOS is one of the commonest causes of infertility in females. It is known that anovulation or decreased ovulation is the primary cause of this infertility and as mentioned above, both metformin and TZDs increase the rates of ovulation. Metformin also improves the number of oocytes collected in PCOS women following

Table 13.2 Tests to detect insulin resistance and glucose intolerance

Test	Sensitivity	Difficulty
Hyperinsulinemic-euglycemic clamp	Gold standard	Yes
Insulin tolerance test (ITT)	OK	Yes
Continuous infusion of glucose with model assessment (CIGMA)	OK	Yes
Frequently sampled IV glucose tolerance test (FSIVGTT)	OK	Yes
Oral glucose tolerance test (OGTT)	OK	No
Fasting insulin	OK	No
Fasting glucose/insulin ratio	OK	No
Homeostatic model assessment (HOMA)	OK	No
Quantitative insulin sensitivity check index (QUICKI)	OK	No

FSH stimulation in *in vitro* fertilization. Metformin also improves pregnancy rates. Studies with TZDs on pregnancy rates are currently on.[1,2,14–16]

PCOS women also suffer from early miscarriages. It is possible that PCOS women have a hostile uterine environmental milieu, which causes decreased conception and/or early miscarriages. Plasminogen activator inhibitor-1 (PAI-1) is an endogenous inhibitor of fibrinolysis. Elevated PAI-1 levels have been independently associated with recurrent miscarriages in PCOS women. Hypofibrinolysis due to elevated PAI-1 levels may lead to placental microthrombi and therefore, infertility. Metformin enhances luteal phase uterine vascularity and blood flow and has been shown to reduce the rate of first trimester spontaneous abortions. It is also possible that the reduced rate of pregnancy loss achieved with metformin, may be because of better egg quality.[1,2,14–16]

Recent Advances

Decreased insulin sensitivity is considered to be a regular component of PCOS. Evidence on the presence of insulin resistance in PCOS patients is based on small groups of examined patients, without sufficiently considering significant confounding factors. Several published studies have not confirmed differences in insulin sensitivity when compared with controls, especially in non-obese women.

It is evident that although certain groups of women with PCOS have decreased sensitivity to insulin, other subgroups of women fulfilling the diagnostic criteria for PCOS, have an insulin sensitivity that does not differ from healthy controls. Thus, the finding of insulin resistance in PCOS women is very significant for clinical practice. Their identification is important for the choice of optimal follow-up and for deciding upon the modality of long-term treatment.[17]

Insulin resistance, associated with an increased incidence of cardiovascular disease and atherosclerosis, is now considered to be an inflammatory disorder. Insulin resistance has recently been associated with increased levels of inflammatory mediators in the blood. Studies have therefore been conducted to look for inflammation in PCOS. Gonzelez et al.[18] noted increased levels of tumor necrosis factor alpha, a cytokine that is secreted by the adipose tissue and causes insulin resistance in PCOS women when compared to controls. Interestingly, lean PCOS women had higher TNF-a levels than normal lean women, while the levels were similar in obese PCOS women and obese controls. Kelly

et al.[19] noted increased C-reactive protein (CRP) levels and tissue plasminogen activator (t-PA) levels in PCOS women as compared to healthy weight-matched controls. However, when adjusted for insulin sensitivity, CRP was no longer significantly different between groups but t-PA levels remained significantly different. Women with PCOS also have higher PAI-1 activity and higher fibrinogen levels than controls. However, in another study, when adjusted for body mass index (BMI), PAI-1 levels were not significantly different from controls. Glueck et al.[20] demonstrated that PAI-1 activity was an independent risk factor for miscarriages in PCOS. While the above studies suggest that PCOS is associated with a state of increased inflammation, clinical studies have yet to definitively demonstrate an increased rate of cardiovascular disease in PCOS.

Thiazolidinediones (TZDs) have been shown to decrease inflammation in obese and diabetic subjects. TZDs have also been shown to reduce carotid artery intima media thickness, normalize vascular endothelial function and improve fibrinolytic and coagulation parameters. Rosiglitazone therapy for 26 weeks reduced MMP-9 (a matrix metalloproteinase, implicated in atherosclerotic plaque rupture) and C-RP levels in type 2 diabetics. In studies in PCOS women, troglitazone has been shown to reduce PAI-1 levels and improve endothelial-dependent vasodilation. It is possible that the beneficial effect of TZDs in PCOS may be partly due to the decrease in inflammation. Metformin has also been shown to decrease PAI-1 and C-RP levels in PCOS women.[1,2,14–16]

Several potential markers for insulin resistance (homocysteine, plasminogen activator inhibitor-1, adiponectin, endothelin-1, sex hormone binding globulin, insulin like growth factor binding protein-1) have been evaluated, but their diagnostic credibility for use in routine and clinical applications must await further trials.

Conclusion

Though insulin resistance is not a part of the

diagnostic criteria for PCOS, its importance in the pathogenesis of PCOS cannot be denied. The treatment of PCOS in the past has largely been centered upon anti-androgen therapy for symptomatic control, cyclic hormones for regular menses and ovulation induction for infertility. While weight loss is helpful in PCOS therapy, it may be difficult to achieve. Furthermore, a significant percentage of PCOS women are lean but insulin resistant. Insulin sensitizers are unique in PCOS therapy because they offer both, metabolic and gynecological benefit. Although the use of insulin sensitizers in PCOS has not been approved by the FDA (Food and Drug Administration, USA) yet, it is probable that PCOS will be a recognized indication for TZDs and metformin use in future.[1,2,14-16] Metformin is the first choice drug, however, there is not enough data to support the long term use of metformin. The systematic use of metformin for ovulation induction is not recommended. There is no evidence of improved results following metformin use in women undergoing IVF. The safety of metformin use during pregnancy has been proved.[10]

Women with PCOS and an early diagnosis of insulin resistance, are at a high risk for type 2 diabetes mellitus, therefore, some crucial recommendations for them are: (i) lifestyle measures with weight loss, diet and exercise, (ii) treatment with insulin-sensitizing agents, especially in obese PCOS women.

References

1. Dhindsa G, Bhatia R, Dhindsa M, Bhatia V. Insulin resistance, insulin sensitization and inflammation in polycystic ovarian syndrome. *J Postgrad Med* 2004; 50: 140–144.

2. Bhatia V. Insulin resistance in Polycystic Ovarian Disease. *South Med J* 2005; 98(9): 902–909.

3. Guzick D. Polycystic Ovary Syndrome. *Obstet Gynecol* 2005; 103(1): 181–193.

4. Polycystic Ovary Syndrome. Compendium of selected publications. ACOG Practice Bulletin 2005: 683–696.

5. Legro R, Castaracane V, Kauffman R. Detecting insulin resistance in polycystic ovary syndrome:

purposes and pitfalls. *Obstet Gynecol Surv* 2004; 59(2): 141–154.

6. Baillargeon J, Iuorno M, Nestler E. Insulin sensitizers for Polycystic Ovary Syndrome. *Clin Obstet Gynecol* 2003; 46(2): 325–340.

7. Rotterdam ESHRE/ASRM-Sponsored PCOS Consensus Workshop Group. Revised 2003 consensus on diagnostic criteria and long-term health risks related to polycystic ovary syndrome. *Fertil Steril* 2004; 81: 19–25.

8. Henquin J, Ravier M, Nenquin M, Jonas J, Gilon P. Hierarchy of the β-cell signal controlling insulin secretion. *Europ J Clin invest*. 2003; 33: 742–750.

9. Legro R. Diabetes prevalence and risk factors in polycystic ovary syndrome. Infertility and Reproductive Medicine Clinics of North America. Saunders: Philadelphia 2003; 14(4): 591–602.

10. Iuorno M, Nestler J. Insulin-lowering drugs in polycystic ovary syndrome. Infertility and Reproductive Medicine Clinics of North America. Saunders: Philadelphia 2003; 14(4): 639–652.

11. Dunaif A. Insulin resistance in women with polycystic ovary syndrome. *Fertil Steril* 2006; 86 (1): S13–4.

12. Lin HF, Boden-Albala B, Juo SH, Park N, Rundek T, Sacco RL. Heritabilities of the metabolic syndrome and its components in the Northern Manhattan Family Study. *Diabetologia* 2005; 48 (10): 2006–2012.

13. Nestler JE, Jakubowicz DJ, de Vargas AF, Brik C, Quintero N, Medina F. Insulin stimulates testosterone biosynthesis by human thecal cells from women with polycystic ovary syndrome by activating its own receptor and using inositolglycan mediators as the signal transduction system. *J Clin Endocrinol Metab* 1998; 83(6): 2001–2005.

14. Checa M, Requena A, Salvador C et al. Insulin-sensitizing agents: use in pregnancy an as a therapy for Polycystic Ovary Syndrome. *Hum Reprod* 2005 11(4): 375–390.

15. Barbieri R. Metformin for the treatment of the polycystic ovary syndrome. *Obstet Gynecol* 2003; 101(4): 785–793.

16. McCarthy E, Walker S, McLachlan K, Boyle J, Permezel M. Metformin in obstetric and gynecologic practice: a review. *Obstet Gynecol Surv* 2004; 59(2): 118–127.

17. Cibula D. Is insulin resistance an essential component of PCOS? The influence of confounding factors. *Hum Reprod* 2004; 19(4): 757–759.

18. Gonzalez F, Thusu K, Abdel-Rahman E, Prabhala A, Tomani M, Dandona P. Elevated serum levels of tumor necrosis factor alpha in normal-weight women

with polycystic ovary syndrome. *Metabolism* 1999; 48(4): 437–441.

19. Kelly L, Evans L, Messenger D. Controversies around gestational diabetes: Practical information for family doctors. *Can Fam Physician* 2005; 51(5): 688–695.

20. Glueck CJ, Wang P, Fontaine RN, Sieve-Smith L, Tracy T, Moore SK. Plasminogen activator inhibitor activity: an independent risk factor for the high miscarriage rate during pregnancy in women with polycystic ovary syndrome. *Metabolism* 1999; 48(12): 1589–1595.

14

Risk Factors Related to the Deterioration of Glucose Tolerance in PCOS Women

Jim X Wang, Preeti Dabadghao

Summary

There is a growing concern amongst clinicians and gynecologists in particular, about the long-term health of women being diagnosed to have polycystic ovary syndrome (PCOS). In addition to the usual reproductive problems, it has been established that glucose metabolism is also affected by the presence of PCOS. PCOS women have a higher risk of developing impaired glucose tolerance and non-insulin dependent diabetes mellitus (NIDDM). Follow-up studies have shown that PCOS women have a faster rate of deterioration of glucose tolerance compared with the general population.

To overcome the health problems associated with deteriorating glucose metabolism in PCOS women, clinicians need to be fully aware of the risk factors associated with it. Although it has been known for some time that PCOS is associated with glucose abnormalities, there are few published studies where women with PCOS have been followed up to study changes in their glucose tolerance over time. In addition, there is limited information on all potential risk factors with regard to the changes in glucose tolerance. Here, we discuss the current knowledge on this topic and future research directions. It is clear that more work is needed in order for clinicians to adequately advise patients on how to reduce their individual risk.

Introduction

Polycystic Ovary Syndrome (PCOS) remains one of the most common hormonal disorders in women of reproductive age with an estimated prevalence of 6–10%.[1,2] Variation in prevalence among different populations may reflect the effect of ethnic origin, lifestyle or other demographic or environmental factors on the phenotype. The different diagnostic criteria prior to the recent publication and acceptance of uniform diagnostic criteria,[3] could also contribute to the variation in the reported prevalence. PCOS is well known for its heterogeneous presentation. The most common symptoms are menstrual irregularities, infertility, hirsutism and acne. A large proportion of PCOS women have polycystic ovaries on an ultrasound scan while being generally symptom free.

No single etiological factor fully accounts for the spectrum of abnormalities in PCOS. Excess androgen is one of the most important causes for many symptoms of PCOS. Both, in vivo and in vitro studies have shown that ovarian theca cells in affected women are more efficient at converting androgenic precursors to testosterone than theca cells in normal women.[4] Insulin plays both, direct and indirect roles in the pathogenesis of hyperandrogenemia. Insulin acts synergistically with luteinizing hormone to enhance the androgen production of theca cells. Insulin also inhibits hepatic synthesis of sex hormone-binding globulin (SHBG), the key circulating protein that binds to testosterone and thus increases the proportion of free or bioavailable testosterone.

Seminal studies by Dunaif et al.[5,6] and others indicated that women with PCOS are more insulin resistant than unaffected women matched for body mass index (BMI), fat free body-mass and body-fat distribution.[5–7] Further studies have shown that PCOS women are at a significantly increased risk for impaired glucose tolerance (IGT) and type 2 diabetes mellitus (DM) at all weights and at a young age.[8] A defect in insulin signaling pathway appears to be present in both the adipocytes and skeletal muscle, the primary target tissues of insulin action.[9] Although insulin resistance seemed to be a central pathogenic feature, it is only recently reported that its deterioration is accelerated in women with PCOS. Insulin resistance alone cannot fully account for the predisposition to and development of DM among women with PCOS. In women with normal glucose tolerance, insulin secretion is sufficient for the degree of insulin resistance; when pancreatic beta-cell is no longer able to compensate sufficiently, glucose tolerance begins to deteriorate.[10,11] Like in other populations, most women with PCOS are able to compensate fully

for their insulin resistance at one stage, but a substantial proportion (first-degree relatives with DM) have a disordered and insufficient beta-cell response to meals or glucose challenge. At the same time, women with PCOS are at a substantial risk for the development of metabolic and cardiovascular abnormalities similar to those seen in the metabolic syndrome. PCOS might thus be viewed as a sex specific form of the metabolic syndrome, and the term "syndrome XX" is an apt description for this association.[12]

Cross sectional studies have shown that 30–40% women with PCOS have impaired glucose tolerance (IGT) and as many as 10% have type 2 diabetes (DM). These prevalence rates are among the highest known among women of similar age. It is not clear when PCOS women start having a higher prevalence of impaired glucose metabolism. Table 14.1 is based on several studies which show the prevalence of IGT and DM in the PCOS population.

Metabolic abnormalities associated with PCOS may predispose women to a range of diseases with attendant morbidity and mortality risks. The increased prevalence of several cardiovascular risk factors in PCOS requires our attention. What is important clinically, is to slow the rate of deterioration in glucose tolerance. Understanding the risk factors relating to the rate is therefore, most important.

In the general population, there is progression of IGT to DM (worsening of glucose tolerance) at the rate of 38.2-87.5/1000 person year, depending on the ethnic origins.[15] The

Table 14.1   The prevalence of IGT and DM as reported in several studies

Author and year	Ethnicity	N	Age (range in years)	IGT (%)	DM (%)
Ehrmann et al, (1999)[7]	52% Caucasian 36% African American	122	14–40	35	10
Legro et al, (1999)[8]	57% Caucasian	254	14–44	31	7.5
Weerakiet et al, (2001)[13]	Thai			23	17
Gambineri et al, (2004)[14]	Mediterranean	121	14–37	16	2.5
Dabadghao et al (unpublished)	Caucasian	361	16–42	16	3.5

deterioration rate is associated with some common factors, including advanced age, higher BMI, family history of diabetes and fasting and 2 hours post glucose load blood glucose values.[15]

There are few studies of long-term follow-up of women with PCOS. Our group has reported a follow up study on 69 women; the average duration of follow up was 6.2 years with an overall conversion rate to NIDDM of 2.6% per annum. The conversion rate to NIDDM was particularly high for those women who had IGT at baseline (8.7% per annum). In a small study population (n = 25), Ehrmann et al.[7] have reported the incidence rate for the conversion from normal glucose tolerance (GTT) to IGT or NIDDM as 338 cases/1,000 person years and the conversion of IGT to NIDDM as 372 cases/1,000 person years.[7] On follow up, there was a significant increase in fasting and 2 hours post glucose load plasma glucose values even if they were not in the diagnostic range of IGT or NIDDM,[7] Dabadghao et al. (unpublished data). Cumulative evidence suggests that in PCOS women, the deterioration in glucose tolerance is not only faster, but may also be related to some unique factors. Various scientific organizations, American Diabetes Association (ADA), European Society of Human Reproduction and Embryology (ESHRE) and American Obstetrics and Gynaecology Society, have enlisted PCOS as a risk factor for future development of DM. It is recommended that these women be screened regularly for DM. However, our knowledge on the natural history of glucose tolerance in women with PCOS is scant and more research is needed in this field.

Clinical Discussion

Description of risk or indicating factors for the deterioration of glucose tolerance

In the limited published cross-sectional or longitudinal studies on the change of glucose tolerance status in women with PCOS, the risk factors influencing or associated with the change in glucose concentrations have not been fully assessed. The results have indicated that some risk factors, including obesity, may be the key factors leading to the deterioration. Here, we discuss some known risk factors reported in published or our studies, carried out in the PCOS population.

Age

Insulin resistance increases with advancing age, increasing the incidence of IGT or DM in the older age group. We have followed up 171 women with PCOS for a median period of 6.9 years and the deterioration of GTT was significant in older women.

Body Mass Index/ Waist: Hip Ratio (BMI/WHR)

Obesity, especially abdominal obesity is positively associated with an increased risk of abnormal GTT. In a small group of 25 women, after a mean follow up of 34± 6.6 months, Ehrmann et al.[7] reported that women whose glucose tolerance deteriorated, were more obese than the stable group. Our group has previously shown that the initial extent of obesity (expressed as BMI and waist:hip ratio) had a close association with the change in glucose levels, while the weight gain over the follow-up period was not significantly associated with the increase in glucose concentration. The strong positive relationships of the worsening in GTT with the initial waist:hip ratio and BMI suggested that overweight/obese PCOS women experienced a faster deterioration in their glucose metabolism. This shows that the classification of PCOS based on obesity and metabolic characteristics has long-term implications in predicting the risk of developing NIDDM.[16]

Weight change

Our study showed that the deterioration in glucose tolerance is not linked with the amount of weight gain over a 6-year follow-up period. Since no weight loss occurred in this study population, we cannot assess the effect of weight loss on the possible change in glucose tolerance.

Metabolic Syndrome

Insulin resistance is the main constituent of the metabolic syndrome. Nearly 70% of PCOS women have underlying insulin resistance irrespective of weight and BMI. We have observed that in 171 women with PCOS, the risk of conversion to NIDDM was 2 folds higher in women who had an associated metabolic syndrome.

Many other factors may well be implicated in the deterioration in glucose tolerance in PCOS women, such as ethnic background, severity of clinical symptoms (signifying a severe degree of hyperandrogenism or insulin resistance), infertility and fertility treatment and pregnancy. PCOS women seek medical attention because of clinical hyperandrogenemia or infertility and these factors may be inter-related. Other factors like family history of diabetes, diet and exercise routine, similar to risk factors in general population, could also contribute to the worsening in glucose tolerance. Unfortunately, there seem to be no reported studies on these factors.

Conclusion

Studies on the natural history of glucose tolerance and associated risk factors involved in its deterioration, will help to understand the pathogenesis of NIDDM. In the general population, it has been shown that the implementation of simple lifestyle interventions in high-risk groups (subjects with IGT) delays the development of NIDDM.[17] PCOS provides us with a target population where these and other preventive strategies can be designed and implemented. Further research is needed to elucidate the associated risk factors involved in the deterioration. More information will help us address and rectify them, thus improving the long-term health of these women.

References

1. Asuncion M, Calvo RM, San Millan JL, Sancho J, Avila S, Escobar-Morreale HF. A prospective study of the prevalence of the polycystic ovary syndrome in unselected Caucasian women from Spain. *J Clin Endocrinol Metab* 2000; 85(7): 2434–2438.

2. Diamanti-Kandarakis E, Kouli CR, Bergiele AT, Filandra FA, Tsianateli TC, Spina GG, et al. A survey of the polycystic ovary syndrome in the Greek island of Lesbos: hormonal and metabolic profile. *J Clin Endocrinol Metab* 1999; 84(11): 4006–4011.

3. Anonymous. Revised 2003 consensus on diagnostic criteria and long-term health risks related to polycystic ovary syndrome (PCOS). *Hum Reprod* 2004; 19(1): 41–47.

4. Nelson VL, Qin Kn KN, Rosenfield RL, Wood JR, Penning TM, Legro RS, et al. The biochemical basis for increased testosterone production in theca cells propagated from patients with polycystic ovary syndrome. *J Clin Endocrinol Metab* 2001; 86(12): 5925–5933.

5. Dunaif A, Segal KR, Futterweit W, Dobrjansky A. Profound peripheral insulin resistance, independent of obesity, in polycystic ovary syndrome. *Diabetes* 1989; 38(9): 1165–1174.

6. Dunaif A. Hyperandrogenic anovulation (PCOS): a unique disorder of insulin action associated with an increased risk of non-insulin-dependent diabetes mellitus. *Am J Med* 1995; 98(1A): 33S–39S.

7. Ehrmann DA, Barnes RB, Rosenfield RL, Cavaghan MK, Imperial J. Prevalence of impaired glucose tolerance and diabetes in women with polycystic ovary syndrome. *Diabetes Care* 1999; 22(1): 141–146.

8. Legro RS, Kunselman AR, Dodson WC, Dunaif A. Prevalence and predictors of risk for type 2 diabetes mellitus and impaired glucose tolerance in polycystic ovary syndrome: a prospective, controlled study in 254 affected women [see comments]. *J Clin Endocrinol Metab* 1999; 84(1): 165–169.

9. Dunaif A, Wu X, Lee A, Diamanti-Kandarakis E. Defects in insulin receptor signaling in vivo in the polycystic ovary syndrome (PCOS). *Am J Physiol Endocrinol Metab* 2001; 281(2): E392–399.

10. Kahn SE, Prigeon RL, McCulloch DK, Boyko EJ, Bergman RN, Schwartz MW, et al. Quantification of the relationship between insulin sensitivity and beta-cell function in human subjects. Evidence for a hyperbolic function. *Diabetes* 1993; 42(11): 1663–1672.

11. Polonsky KS, Sturis J, Bell GI. Seminars in Medicine of the Beth Israel Hospital, Boston. Non-insulin–dependent diabetes mellitus - a genetically programmed failure of the beta cell to compensate for insulin resistance. *N Engl J Med* 1996; 334(12): 777–783.

12. Sam S, Dunaif A. Polycystic ovary syndrome: syndrome XX? *Trends Endocrinol Metab* 2003; 14(8): 365–370.

13. Weerakiet S, Srisombut C, Bunnag P, Sangtong S, Chuangsoongnoen N, Rojanasakul A. Prevalence of type 2 diabetes mellitus and impaired glucose tolerance in Asian women with polycystic ovary syndrome. *Int J Gynaecol Obstet* 2001; 75(2): 177–184.

14. Gambineri A, Pelusi C, Manicardi E, Vicennati V, Cacciari M, Morselli-Labate AM, et al. Glucose intolerance in a large cohort of Mediterranean women with polycystic ovary syndrome: phenotype and associated factors. *Diabetes* 2004; 53(9): 2353–2358.

15. Edelstein SL, Knowler WC, Bain RP, Andres R, Barrett-Connor EL, Dowse GK, et al. Predictors of progression from impaired glucose tolerance to NIDDM: an analysis of six prospective studies. *Diabetes* 1997; 46(4): 701–710.

16. Wang JX, Norman RJ. Risk factors for the deterioration of glucose metabolism in polycystic ovary syndrome. *Reprod Biomed Online* 2004; 9(2): 201–204.

17. Tuomilehto J, Lindstrom J, Eriksson JG, Valle TT, Hamalainen H, Ilanne-Parikka P, et al. Prevention of type 2 diabetes mellitus by changes in lifestyle among subjects with impaired glucose tolerance. *N Engl J Med* 2001; 344(18): 1343–1350.

15

Glucose Intolerance in Obese Adolescents with Polycystic Ovary Syndrome

Muralidhar V Pai

Summary

Polycystic Ovary Syndrome (PCOS) is believed to constitute the most frequently encountered endocrinopathy.[1] It is a challenging problem that has far-reaching consequences. Proper understanding of the pathogenesis, pathophysiology and phenotypes is necessary for initiation of appropriate therapy. This chapter addresses the complexities of the syndrome and outlines the mandatory investigations and management options.

Introduction

Women with Polycystic Ovary Syndrome (PCOS), besides having hyperandrogenism and infertility, have profound insulin resistance (IR) and alterations in β-cell function.[2] Moreover, the prevalence of impaired glucose tolerance (IGT) and diabetes is increased in PCOS.[3,4]

Even though PCOS is not as extensively studied in adolescents as it is in older women, it is postulated that the disorder begins at menarche, and its characteristics do not change with age.[5] Adolescents less than 18 years old with PCOS have comparable clinical, neuroendocrine, and ultrasonographic features as adult women with PCOS.[6] Arslanian and co-workers demonstrated that adolescents with PCOS are severely insulin-resistant compared with a control group matched for body composition and abdominal obesity.[7]

Insulin Resistance Syndrome or Metabolic Syndrome is an integral part of PCOS and affects two-thirds of the PCOS women. Decreased insulin-mediated glucose utilization occurs in up to 50% of patients with PCOS.

The Metabolic Syndrome includes any three of the following:

1. Waist circumference >88 cm
2. Triglycerides >150 mg/dl
3. High density lipoprotein (HDL) <50 mg/dl
4. Blood pressure > 130/85 mmHg
5. Fasting blood glucose 110–126 and/or 2-hr glucose 140–199 mg/dl.

Clinical Discussion

Pathology and pathophysiology

Insulin resistance is characterized by decreased sensitivity to insulin in peripheral tissues (muscle and adipose tissue), but not in hepatic tissue.[8] Insulin resistance is considered to be the central player (Fig 15.1), which itself may be due to a genetic predisposition, aging and lifestyle. Insulin resistance leads on to hyperinsulinemia, which in turn, favours altered lipoprotein, cholesterol and steroid hormone metabolisms and increased lipid storage. Thus, body mass index (BMI) is positively correlated to serum insulin and testosterone levels. Both, insulin and insulin-like growth factors, target steps involving thecal P450c17 and potentiate the

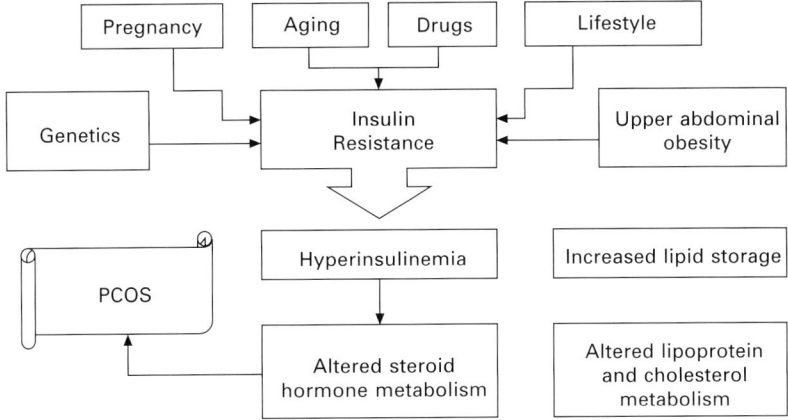

Figure 15.1 The central player-Insulin Resistance

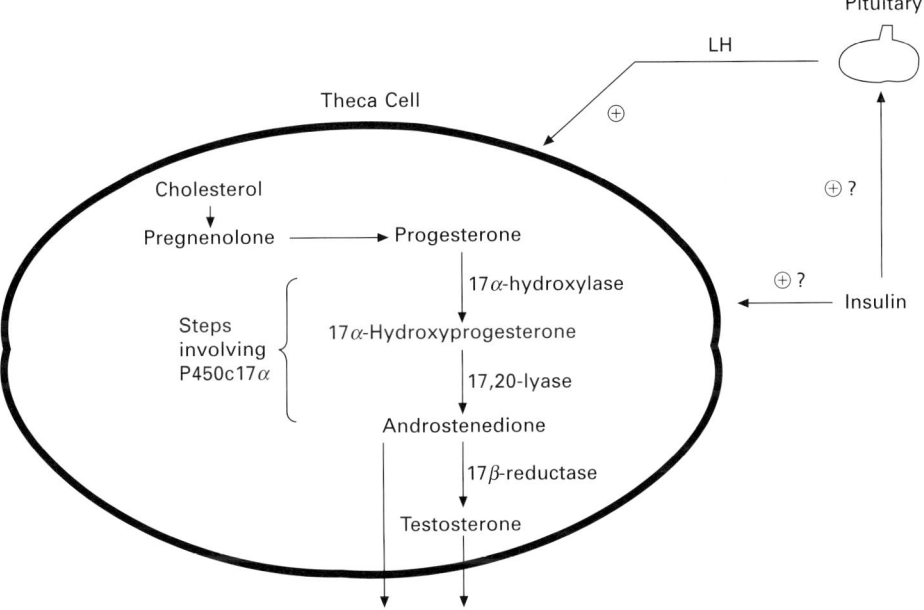

Figure 15.2 The thecal P450c17 as a target for LH and insulin

actions of luteinizing hormone (LH) on theca cell androgen production (Fig 15.2) by favoring and inducing PCOS in predisposed girls. Insulin resistance and hyperinsulinemia decrease hepatic sex hormone–binding globulin (SHBG) and insulin-like growth factor binding globulin -1 (IGFBG –1) levels, which will increase the levels of insulin-like growth factor – 1 (IGF-1). The latter, along with hyperinsulinemia, favors the production of androgens from the ovary and

adrenals. (Fig 15.3). Hyperinsulinemia also favours the production of free fatty acids from adipose tissue.

The other consequences of insulin resistance are increased incidence of type 2 diabetes, hypertension, endothelial dysfunction, acanthosis nigricans, coagulation/ fibrinolytic defects, dyslipidemia, and accelerated atherosclerosis (Fig 15.4), Cushing's syndrome, late-onset congenital adrenal hyperplasia and adrenal tumors.

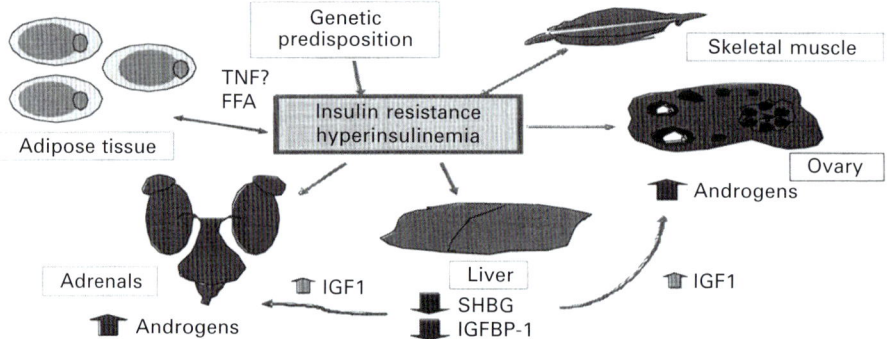

Figure 15.3   Pathogenesis of insulin resistance and role of hyperinsulinemia in the pathophysiology of PCOS

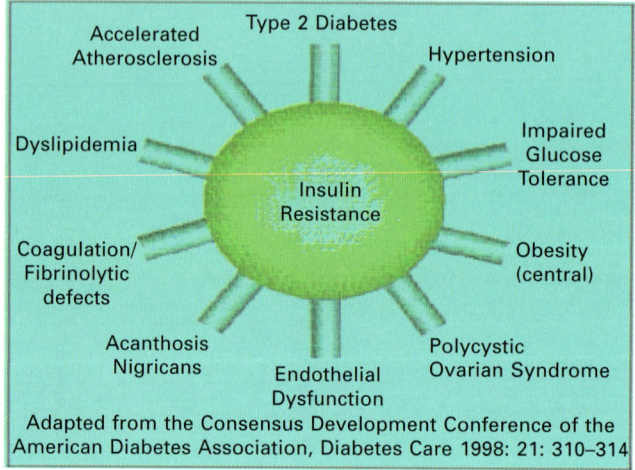

Figure 15.4   Other consequences of Insulin resistance:

Insulin effects related to ovarian function

Insulin directly stimulates ovarian steroidogenesis, potentiates the effect of gonadotropin releasing hormone (GnRH) on pituitary release of luteinizing hormone (LH)/follicle stimulating hormone (FSH), and promotes ovarian growth and cyst formation. It up-regulates LH and type I- IGF receptors in the ovary and acts synergistically with LH/human chorionic gonadotropin (hCG). It stimulates the production of 17-hydroxylase in the ovary and may stimulate or inhibit the production of the enzyme aromatase from the granulosa cells of the ovary, and adipose tissue. It inhibits IGFBP-1 production from the ovary and liver and SHBG production from the ovary.

Hyperandrogenism and PCOS

Hyperandrogenism, present in PCOS, is responsible for the signs/symptoms of androgen excess including anovulation, reduced SHBG, abdominal fat accumulation, lipid abnormalities and perhaps, insulin insensitivity.

The role of hyperinsulinemia and insulin resistance

Hyperinsulinemia and insulin resistance are responsible for the metabolic syndrome and abdominal fat accumulation and serve as co-factors favoring andogen excess, reduced SHBG, and anovulation.

PCOS phenotypes

Based on insulin resistance, there are 2 phenotypes of PCOS, namely

1. PCOS with insulin resistance (IR)
2. PCOS without insulin resistance

PCOS with insulin resistance constitutes about 50–70 % of the cases and are characterized by obesity (may be lean), acanthosis nigricans, hirsutism and resistance to clomiphene citrate. Characteristics of PCOS without IR are lean, euinsulinemic/euglycemic individuals with enhanced ovarian sensitivity to insulin (without hyperinsulinemia).

Symptoms of insulin resistance

Following are the symptoms of insulin resistance in general:

- Early day irritability-late day drowsiness
- Craving for additional sweets after meals
- Eating to over-fullness
- Intense need for food before meals
- Craving for sweets or starchy vegetables
- Poor sleep habits
- Inability to lose weight even on a restricted diet
- Believing that other people eat more than they do.
- Central obesity
- Abnormal hair growth or loss
- Menstrual irregularities
- Hot flushes
- Hyperhydrosis
- Hypertension-mild
- Weight gain
- Depression

Investigations

Insulin resistance is best assessed by an oral glucose tolerance test (OGTT). However, fasting glucose to insulin ratio is a useful measure of insulin sensitivity and is used as a screening test for insulin resistance. A ratio less than 4.5 is considered as abnormal. This screen can be skewed when the patient is fasting, dieting, and exercising, or is slender. Hence, the two-hour post-prandial glucose and insulin level also must be tested. C-peptide and liver enzymes that trigger insulin production may also be estimated.

Management

The management of insulin resistance in general, includes weight reduction, diet management and exercise. The drugs favoring weight loss include sibutramine and orlistat on which studies are absent. Insulin-sensitizing drugs like biguanides (metformin) and thiazolidinediones, D-chiro-inositol, and antiandrogens, have been used to enhance insulin sensitivity. However, the use of antiandrogens in the management of IR is controversial.

Weight reduction

Weight reduction is associated with normalization of hormonal disturbances and the resumption of regular ovulation. It may also help to relieve some of the symptoms of PCOS, such as new hair growth. It also has a beneficial impact on the long-term consequences of PCOS (eg, cardiovascular disease, impaired glucose tolerance, hypertension, dyslipidemia). A weight loss of only 5% of the total body weight is associated with decreased insulin levels, improved menstrual function, reduced hirsutism, acne, and lower testosterone levels.

Diet

A low-calorie diet is recommended for patients with a BMI greater than 25 kg/m, or for patients with truncal obesity. Women with PCOS should decrease their intake of foods high in carbohydrates. Carbohydrates are found in breads, pasta, potatoes, and foods that are sweet. Consultation with a nutritionist may be appropriate, especially in patients who are overweight.

Exercise

No restriction in activity is required, but regular exercise must be encouraged. Aerobic exercise in patients who are overweight is recommended for weight loss. Daily exercise improves the body's use of insulin. Polycystic ovary syndrome may be relieved by daily exercise for at least 30 minutes a day.

Drug Therapy

Drugs that enhance insulin sensitivity, such as insulin-sensitizing drugs, have been most successfully used.

Biguanides

Insulin sensitizers are useful in type 2 diabetes and related insulin resistance. They reduce hepatic glucose output and peripheral resistance to insulin action and lower plasma insulin levels. Among the biguanides, metformin has been extensively used. One may start with a dose of 500 mg per day, twice daily and may go upto a maintenance dose of 850 mg thrice daily, but not to exceed 2550 mg/day.

Potential Advantages of Metformin include:
- Increased glucose tolerance
- Increased insulin sensitivity
- Decreased blood lipid levels
- Increased weight loss or stabilization
- Improved fat distribution
- Decreased blood pressure
- Decreased androgen levels
- Restoration of regular menses
- Postponement of diabetes

The advantages of Metformin continue beyond conception:
- It reduces the miscarriage rate
- Decreases the likelihood of developing gestational diabetes.

Potential Disadvantages of Metformin include:
- Gastrointestinal disturbance in 1/3 of the patients
- Generalized feeling of unwellness
- Decreased absorption of vitamin B-12
- Lactic acid build-up

Contraindications:
Metformin is contraindicated in cases with documented hypersensitivity, renal disease or impairment, ketoacidosis, acute myocardial infarction, septicemia, metabolic acidosis, treatment for congestive heart failure (CHF), concomitant use of parenteral radiographic agents, type 1 diabetes.

Precautions:
Normal renal function must be ensured prior to starting therapy and caution taken in hepatic disease and elderly people. The medication must be discontinued if lactic acidosis, hypoxemia, or sepsis occurs and before performing any surgical procedures

Thiazolidinediones

Thiazolidinediones include rosiglitazone and pioglitazone.

These agents are insulin-sensitizing drugs that increase the disposal of glucose in peripheral tissues and act by activating specific nuclear receptors, the PPAR-gamma (peroxisome proliferator-activated receptor gamma). They have a major effect in the stimulation of glucose uptake in the skeletal muscle and adipose tissue, lowering plasma insulin levels and treating type 2 diabetes associated with insulin resistance. They appear to benefit PCOS patients. A rosiglitazone dosage of 4–8 mg/d per oral qd, or divided bid and a pioglitazone dose of 15–30 mg per oral qd (not to exceed 45 mg/day), may be used

Contraindications
Contraindications to treatment with thiazolidinediones include documented hypersensitivity, active liver disease, ketoacidosis and type 1 diabetes

Precautions
Transaminases must be monitored and therapy discontinued if alanine transaminase (ALT) rises above three times the upper limit of the reference range. Caution must be taken in cases with edema and congestive heart failure (CHF).

Prognosis

PCOS is now recognized as a potentially dangerous syndrome, mostly due to the increased risk (3 – 7 times) of developing type II diabetes mellitus. This risk is increased if the patient has anovulatory vs. ovulatory PCOS. Hence, women with the disorder should have their glucose levels checked regularly to monitor the development of diabetes. However, PCOS has not been definitely linked to an increased risk of cardiovascular disease, endometrial cancer, or death.

Prevention

No known way to prevent PCOS exists, but, if diagnosed and treated early, risks for complications, such as heart disease and diabetes, may be minimized. Weight control through diet and exercise stabilizes hormones and lowers insulin levels.

Conclusion

Gynecologists should categorize any case of PCOS, depending on:

1. Rotterdam definition. The Rotterdam criteria for diagnosis of PCOS include two of the following three manifestations:

   i.   Irregular or absent ovulation
   ii. Hyperandrogenism (clinical or biochemical) and/or
   iii. Polycystic ovaries.

2. Presence or absence of insulin resistance
3. Asymptomatic or symptomatic

Treatment of PCOS should be directed towards causative rather than symptomatic treatment, especially if insulin resistance is proved as the central player.

References

1. Carmina E, Lobo RA. Polycystic ovary syndrome (PCOS): arguably the most common endocrinopathy is associated with significant morbidity in women. *J Clin Endocrinol Metab* 1999; 84: 1897–1899.
2. Dunaif A. Insulin resistance and the polycystic ovary syndrome. mechanism and implications for pathogenesis. *Endocr Rev* 1997; 18: 774–800.
3. Legro RS, Kunselman AR, Dodson WC, Dunaif A. Prevalence and predictors of risk for type 2 diabetes mellitus and impaired glucose tolerance in polycystic ovary syndrome. A prospective, controlled study in 254 affected women. *J Clin Endocrinol Metab* 1999; 84: 165–169.
4. Ehrmann DA, Barnes RB, Rosenfield RL, Cavaghan MK, Imperial J. Prevalence of impaired glucose tolerance and diabetes in women with polycystic ovary syndrome. *Diabetes Care* 1999; 22: 141–146.
5. Yen SSC. The polycystic ovary syndrome. *Clin Endocrinol* (Oxf) 1980; 12: 177–207.
6. Gülekli B, Turhan NÖ, Senöz S, Kükner S, Oral H, Gökmen O. Endocrinological ultrasonographic and clinical findings in adolescent and adult polycystic ovary patients. A comparative study. *Gynecol Endocrinol* 1993; 7: 273–277.
7. Lewy VD, Danadian K, Witchel SF, Arslanian S. Early metabolic abnormalities in adolescent girls with polycystic ovarian syndrome. *J Pediatr* 2001; 138(1): 38–44.
8. Franks S. Polycystic ovary syndrome. *N Engl J Med* 1995; 333(13): 853–861.

16

Type 2 Diabetes Mellitus and The Polycystic Ovary Syndrome

András Szilágyi

Summary

The etiology and pathogenesis of polycystic ovary syndrome (PCOS) is still a matter of controversy, but it is apparent that hyperinsulinemia and insulin resistance (IR) are major determining factors in the development of ovarian hyperandrogenism and chronic anovulation. Follow-up studies have also shown an increase in the incidence of type 2 diabetes mellitus and other elements of the metabolic syndrome in PCOS. Insulin resistance plays a major role in the development of both PCOS and type 2 diabetes mellitus. It is possible that PCOS and type 2 diabetes mellitus are different clinical manifestations of the same IR syndrome, with phenotypic differences due to coincidental genetic defects at different organ levels. It appears that some IR women primarily develop PCOS with hyperinsulinemia and hyperandrogenemia, and to a lesser degree, glucose intolerance. On the other hand, some other IR women will have type 2 DM with or without polycystic ovaries. Thus, reversal of insulin resistance in PCOS, constitutes the fundamental goal in the management of hyperandrogenic anovulatory infertility and in the prevention of long-term consequences. The value of insulin sensitizers such as metformin and/or thiazolidinediones (pioglitazone, rosiglitazone) therapy awaits further evaluation that should be integrated in the spectrum of therapeutic options.

Rationale

Two common disorders that are frequently associated with insulin resistance (IR) are polycystic ovary syndrome (PCOS) and type 2 diabetes mellitus (DM). Insulin resistance plays a major role in the development of both the disorders. The exact nature of the association and differences between PCOS and type 2 DM is unclear, although it appears that some IR women primarily develop PCOS with hyperinsulinemia and hyperandrogenemia, and to a lesser degree, glucose intolerance. On the other hand, type 2 DM may be present in some IR women with or without polycystic ovaries. On the basis of this common origin, the treatment may also have common modalities such as the administration of insulin-sensitizing agents.

The connection and overlapping between the two IR disorders will be discussed in this chapter, as the rationale of the therapy is based on the pathophysiological similarities.

Introduction

Polycystic ovary syndrome (PCOS) is probably the most prevalent endocrinopathy in women and the most common cause of anovulatory infertility.[1] More recent studies, although based on modified criteria of PCOS, report a high prevalence of PCOS ranging from 4% to 9% in the fertile female population.[2,3] Polycystic ovaries (PCO) observed by ultrasound are an even more frequent finding. According to some large studies, the prevalence of PCO in healthy volunteer populations may be upto 33%.[4] 87% of the women presenting with symptoms of oligomenorrhea and hyperandrogenism have polycystic ovaries.[1]

The pathophysiology of the disorder has been thoroughly investigated, but its etiology is still unsettled. There are theories supporting a primary hypothalamic-pituitary defect, a primary ovarian steroidogenic defect, a primary adrenal steroidogenic defect and a primary defect of insulin resistance.[5–8] It has been proven that hyperinsulinemia and insulin resistance play a key role in the pathophysiology of hyperandrogenism and probably, the pathogenesis of PCOS.[5,9] Insulin receptors are present in the ovary[10] and insulin may bind to insulin-like growth factor-1 (IGF-1) receptors and act as a gonadotropic hormone, enhancing induction of ovarian LH receptors and LH binding capacity. Furthermore, the existing literature provides a strong basis for the argument that PCOS clusters in families. However, the mode of inheritance of the disorder is still uncertain. Several loci have been proposed as PCOS genes including CYP11A, the insulin gene, and a region near the insulin receptor.[11] Whatever the pathogenesis of PCOS, the endpoint is an ovary secreting excessive amount of androgens in a hyperinsulinemic, insulin resistant patient. According to the common genetic basis and the characteristic hyperinsulinemia and insulin resistance, PCOS patients are at risk for type 2 diabetes, whereas growing evidence suggests that a significant fraction of the younger patients with type 2 DM, also demonstrate signs of PCOS.[12]

Clinical Discussion

Diagnosis of PCOS and insulin resistance

PCOS has been defined clinically, biochemically, and by ultrasound. The predominantly European diagnosis of PCOS is based on clinical signs of menstrual disturbance and/or hyperandrogenism (hirsutism, acne or alopecia) and established by transvaginal ultrasound examination of the ovaries characterizing the ovarian morphology. Most of the patients with PCO have a clinical or biochemical feature consistent with the ultrasound diagnosis and they are likely to face problems of hyperandrogenism, subfertility and recurrent miscarriage. As for the predominantly North American view, the 1990 National Institute of Health (NIH) conference on PCOS recommended that the diagnostic criteria should include biochemical evidence of hyperandrogenism and ovarian dysfunction without regarding the morphological diagnosis of PCO by ultrasound as an essential part of the diagnosis.[13] A proposal by Homburg[14] attempted to bridge the gap between predominantly American biochemical marker-based diagnosis and the predominantly European reliance on ultrasound as a sine qua non for diagnosis. The final solution was the Rotterdam Consensus on diagnostic criteria for PCOS in 2003.[15] According to these criteria, PCOS can be diagnosed if 2 out of 3 criteria (oligo- or anovulation, clinical and/or biochemical signs of hyperandrogenism, polycystic ovaries) are present, and other etiologies can be excluded. No tests of insulin resistance are necessary to make the diagnosis of PCOS, although they may be considered if additional risk factors for insulin resistance, such as a family history of diabetes, are present. There is currently no clinical test for detecting insulin resistance on a daily basis in the general population. Dynamic invasive tests such as the euglycemic clamp are research procedures because of their intensive use of time and resources. Calculated indices based on fasting levels of insulin and glucose (if <4.5, insulin resistance is indicated) correlate well with dynamic tests of insulin action,[16] although there are multiple flaws that limit their widespread clinical use. However, in a recent study the routine measurement of HOMA-S (homeostasis model assessment) was recommended for identifying insulin resistant PCOS women with a view of targeting them with insulin-sensitizing agents.[17]

According to the Rotterdam Consensus,[15] instead of measuring IR, criteria have been developed for defining a metabolic syndrome in women with PCOS (Table 16.1), that is clinically more relevant and useful.

Table 16.1 Criteria for the metabolic syndrome in women with polycystic ovary syndrome (Three of five qualify for the syndrome)

Risk factor	Cutoff
1. Abdominal obesity (waist circumference)	> 88 cm (>35 inch)
2. Triglycerides	≥150 mg/dl
3. High density lipoprotein cholesterol (HDL-C)	<50 mg/dl
4. Blood pressure	≥130/≥85 mm/Hg
5. Fasting and 2-h glucose from oral glucose tolerance test	110–126 mg/dl and/or 2-h glucose 140–199 mg/dl

2003 Rotterdam consensus[15].

Insulin resistance and metabolic syndrome in PCOS and type 2 diabetes

Insulin resistance (IR), defined as decreased insulin-mediated glucose utilization, is commonly found in the larger population (10–25%).[18] IR can be associated with various features, including low birthweight, short stature, increased upper to lower body ratio, acanthosis nigricans, premature adrenarche, hyperandrogenemia, hirsutism, irregular menstrual cycles, PCOS, central obesity, dyslipidemia (low high-density lipoproteins, high triglycerides), hypertension, microalbuminemia, endothelial dysfunction, glucose intolerance, type 2 diabetes mellitus, early cardiovascular and cerebrovascular disease.[12] As insulin resistance is associated with a cluster of the above mentioned cardiovascular risk factors, the concept of metabolic syndrome (Syndrome X) was first introduced by Reaven.[19] In 1999, the World Health Organization (WHO)[20] proposed a unifying definition for the syndrome and chose to call it the metabolic syndrome, including type 2 diabetes, hypertension, dyslipidemia, central obesity, endothelial dysfunction and the risk of heart disease. The prevalence and etiology of IR in PCOS and type 2 DM is discussed in detail.

Insulin resistance in PCOS

Insulin resistance (IR) and the elements of the metabolic syndrome are present in a great proportion of the PCOS patients. Insulin resistance in women with PCOS, appears to be present in up to 50% of the cases, independent of obesity.[9,21] A 50–70% prevalence of IR has been reported in PCOS.[12] The type of insulin resistance associated with PCOS seems to be unique to this syndrome and is probably characterized by a decrease in insulin sensitivity due to a defect in post-receptor signal transduction between the receptor kinase and the glucose transporter.[22] It seems that lean PCOS patients have a form of insulin resistance that is intrinsic to PCOS,[23] although the exact nature is poorly understood. On the other hand, obese women with PCOS suffer not only from the insulin resistance intrinsic to PCOS, but also that associated with obesity.[23]

Insulin resistance leads to compensatory hyperinsulinemia in PCOS, with the excess insulin causing an exaggerated effect in other responsive tissues as the ovary. Elevated insulin levels appear to directly enhace LH-stimulated androgen secretion from the ovary,[24] and the insulin action contributes to the development of the characteristic hormonal and clinical findings in PCOS patients. The rate limiting enzymes in androgen biosynthesis are 17-hydroxylase and 17/20 lyase that belong to the enzyme complex cytochrome P450c17. Serine phosphorylation of P450c17 selectively increases the 17, 20 lyase activity. Studies in the 1980's demonstrated that serine phosphorylation of the β-chain of the insulin receptor inhibited the receptor's tyrosine phosphorylation and consequent downstream signal transduction. Zhang and co-workers[25] suggested that a gain-of-function mutation in a single cAMP-inducable serine kinase might hyperphosphorylate both P450c17, causing hyperandrogenism, and the β-chain of the insulin receptor, causing insulin resistance, providing a single autosomal dominant mechanism for the two cardinal features of PCOS (serine phosphorylation hypothesis). The genetically increased activity of P450c17 complex may further be increased by several pathways in PCOS.

Among the candidates, LH, insulin-like growth factor-1 (IGF-1) and insulin itself can be listed. In vitro studies have shown that theca-stromal cells respond readily to LH stimulation with androgen production, an increased expression of cytochrome P450c17 activity, with a synergistic effect in the presence of IGF-1 or insulin.[24,26] Furthermore, IGFBP-1, the binding globulin of IGF-1 is suppressed first of all in obese PCOS patients,[26] increasing the potential of IGF-1, which then acts synergistically with LH to stimulate the theca and interstitial cells of the ovary to produce androgens.

Components of the metabolic syndrome can also be found in PCOS patients as a consequence of IR and hyperinsulinemia. The Rotterdam Consensus criteria for the metabolic syndrome in women with PCOS are summarized in Table 16.1.[15] As IR and the metabolic syndrome are characteristic for a subgroup of PCOS women, the term "Syndrome XX" has been proposed.[27]

Insulin resistance in type 2 diabetes mellitus (DM)

Type 2 Diabetes Mellitus (DM) is a heterogeneous metabolic disorder characterized by hyperglycemia resulting from a combination of resistance to insulin action and an insufficient compensatory insulin secretory response. In women of reproductive age, the prevalence of type 2 DM was estimated to be between 1.7% and 6.1%, for the age ranges of 20–39 years and 40 to 49 years, respectively.[28] Insulin resistance is considered to be a fundamental defect in patients with type 2 DM, and by definition, IR would have a prevalence of 100% in these patients. However, there are wide variations in the degree of IR present in diabetic subjects, and therefore, the prevalence of IR in type 2 DM, ranges from 80–100% depending on the definition employed.[12]

As both PCOS and type 2 DM have approximately the same prevalence in women of reproductive age and both the disorders are characterized by different degrees of IR, the risk of type 2 DM in PCOS patients and vice versa

and the percent of reproductive age (or postmenopausal) type 2 diabetic patients affected by PCOS is open to question.

PCOS and the risk of type 2 diabetes

Dunaif and co-workers[29] were the first to report higher ambient glucose levels and a greater than expected frequency of glucose intolerance among PCOS patients compared with normal women. Later, retrospective studies on postmenopausal women with a history of PCOS demonstrated that 15% had type 2 diabetes mellitus compared with a 2.3% prevalence among age-matched controls.[30,31]

Thirty to 40 percent of women with PCOS have impaired glucose tolerance, and as many as 10 percent have type 2 diabetes by their fourth decade.[32] Glucose tolerance also changes over time. Women with PCOS and baseline impaired glucose tolerance (IGT) have a low conversion risk of 6% to type 2 diabetes over approximately 3 years, or 2% per year. The effect of PCOS, given normal glucose tolerance at baseline, is more pronounced with 16% conversion to IGT per year.[33] These findings support that women with PCOS should be periodically rescreened for diabetes due to worsening glucose intolerance over time. A further, indirect evidence for the relationship between PCOS and type 2 DM can be drawn from the Nurses Health Study II, a prospective observational cohort study of health outcomes among 116,671 female nurses, aged 24 to 43 at study inception in 1989. The results indicated that the relative risk for developing type 2 DM among women with long menstrual cycles or highly irregular cycles was 2.08 (95%CI, 1.62–2.66) compared with women with normal cycle length.[34]

Insulin resistance alone cannot fully explain the predisposition to and development of type 2 diabetes among patients with PCOS. Most women with PCOS are able to compensate fully for their insulin resistance, but a substantial proportion (particularly those with first-degree relatives with type 2 diabetes) have a disordered and insufficient beta-cell response to meals or glucose challenge.[32]

A family history of diabetes is present with significantly greater frequency among women with PCOS who had IGT or type 2 DM compared with those with normal glucose tolerance.[35] Furthermore, the fasting glucose concentration is poorly associated with 2-hour glucose concentrations among PCOS women with IGT, suggesting that the fasting glucose concentration is inadequate to predict the presence of IGT in PCOS.[35]

Before the development of frank glucose intolerance, defects in insulin secretion may be latent and revealed only in circumstances that augment insulin resistance, as with the development of gestational diabetes in pregnancy,[36] or glucose intolerance associated with glucocorticoid administration.[32] PCOS with hyperinsulinemia and IR may develop in lean, adolescent girls as well as those who have had premature pubarche, hyperinsulinemia and dyslipidemia before puberty, and a low birth weight even earlier, supporting the hypothesis proposed by Barker[37] that low birth weight or reduced fetal growth is related to the development of type 2 diabetes mellitus, as well as "Syndrome X", in adult life.

In conclusion, patients with PCOS, regardless of ethnicity, appears to have a 5- to 10-fold greater risk for type 2 diabetes mellitus, compared with the case of age and weight-matched women.[12,15] Additionally, a family history of diabetes and the presence of obesity are important predictors for the development of type 2 DM.[12] This finding is consistent with reports noting that many patients with PCOS also demonstrate reduced β-cell function, even in the absence of clinically evident IGT or type 2 DM.

Prevalence of PCOS among patients with DM

If type 2 DM is a frequent finding among PCOS women, and both conditions are characterized by IR, type 2 diabetic patients must have a greater risk of having PCOS than normal women. The common characteristic features of PCOS and type 2 DM are summarized in Table 16.2.

There is growing evidence to support this notion, although there have been few studies addressing this point for the time being. In a group of premenopausal type 2 diabetic women polycystic ovaries were seen by sonography in 82% of the cases, and clinical signs of PCOS were present in 52%.[38] In another study, the prevalence of PCOS among premenopausal type 2 diabetic women was 26.7%,[39] much higher than the 4–9% prevalence in an unselected population of reproductive-aged women.[3,4] Women with previous GDM also show a higher prevalence of polycystic ovaries (41%), hirsutism and irregular menstrual cycles, and a higher body mass index than the controls.[36] According to a small study,

Table 16.2   Common pathophysiological and clinical characteristics of polycystic ovary syndrome (PCOS) and type 2 diabetes mellitus (DM)

PCOS	Type 2 diabetes mellitus
Overlapping in genetic background with type 2 DM[11,25]	Overlapping in genetic background with PCOS
Insulin resistance in 50–70%[9,12,21]	Insulin resistance in 80–100%[12]
Risk of impaired glucose tolerance (IGT): 40%[32]	Risk of having polycystic ovaries: 82%[38]
Risk of type 2 DM: 10%[32] or 5- to 10-fold increased risk[12,15]	Risk of having PCOS: 26–52%[38,39]
Increased risk of metabolic syndrome ("Syndrome XX")[15,27]	Type 2 DM is a component of the metabolic syndrome[20]
Long term management includes: lifestyle modification, insulin sensitizers (metformin)[41–44]	Management includes: lifestyle modification, insulin sensitizers, insulin if needed[45]

women with type 1 diabetes mellitus may also have a higher prevalence of hyperandrogenic disorders, including PCOS (18.8%) and hirsutism.[40] The body mass index was not different among these type 1 diabetic women with or without hyperandrogenic disorders.

With regard to the above mentioned studies, the prevalence of PCOS seems to be significantly higher among reproductive-aged women with type 2 (and probably type 1) DM, resulting in additional reproductive and endocrinologic abnormalities in these women.

Recent Advances and Conclusions

The consequences of the PCOS extend beyond the reproductive axis. Insulin resistance is a prominent feature of PCOS, and women with this disorder are at increased risk for the development of other diaseases that have been linked to insulin resistance, namely type 2 DM and furthermore, metabolic syndrome. On the other hand, type 2 diabetic patients are at a higher risk of having PCOS with its clinical and hormonal consequences. PCOS and type 2 diabetes mellitus are different clinical manifestations of the same IR syndrome. With regard to PCOS, the association between insulin resistance and PCOS must guide the chronic management of the disorder. Interventions that decrease IR are assumed to decrease the metabolic risk and hyperandrogenism, as well as to restore fertility. Accumulating evidence suggests that administration of insulin-sensitizing agents to patients at high risk for type 2 diabetes, decreases the rate of conversion to overt disease. PCOS should be regarded as a general health issue and the use of insulin sensitizing drugs such as metformin should be considered for the prevention of type 2 DM.[41,42] The issue of insulin sensitizer agents is discussed in an other chapter, but as a general conclusion, the highly promising therapeutic profile of metformin deserves further studies and application. According to the accumulating evidence, thiazolidinediones, such as pioglitazone and rosiglitazone should be considered a second line treatment alternative to metformin for the management of women with PCOS who are resistant to insulin, or who are obese.[43] Despite the promising results with short term use of insulin sensitizers, long-term lifetime administration requires further studies.[44] The Diabetes Prevention Program Research Group examined the effects of metformin, lifestyle modification and placebo during a 4-year prospective program on the incidence of type 2 DM among individuals at high risk for diabetes.[45] Subjects treated with metformin had a 31% risk reduction for developing diabetes compared with placebo. However, intensive lifestyle intervention (at least a 7% weight loss and at least 150 min of exercise per week) was associated with a even greater (58%) risk reduction for developing diabetes. It seems logical that the observed efficacy of metformin or lifestyle modification is likely to be applicable to PCOS women as well, and lifestyle modification may be at least as effective as metformin in PCOS patients, too.

Further studies must be carried out in future to evaluate if PCOS and type 2 DM are no more than different clinical manifestations of the same IR syndrome, and the efficacy of insulin senzitizers and/or lifestyle modifications in the lifetime management of IR disorders, including PCOS.

References

1. Adams J, Polson DW, Franks S. Prevalence of polycystic ovaries in women with anovulation and idiopathic hirsutism. *Br Med J* 1986; 293: 355–359.
2. Knochenhauer ES, Key TJ, Kahsar-Miller M, Waggoner W, Boots LR and Azziz R. Prevalence of the polycystic ovary syndrome in unselected black and white women of the Southeastern United States: a prospective study. *J Clin Endocrinol Metab* 1998; 83: 3078–3082.
3. Diamanti–Kandaris E, Kouli CR, Bergiele AT et al. A survey of the polycystic ovary syndrome in the Greek island of Lesbos: hormonal and metabolic profile. *J Clin Endocrinol Metab* 1999; 84: 4006–4011.
4. Michelmore KF, Balen AH, Dunger DB and Vessey MP. Polycystic ovaries and associated clinical and biochemical features in young women, *Clin Endocrinol (Oxf.)* 1999; 51: 779–786.

5. Dunaif A. Insulin resistance in polycystic ovary syndrome. *Ann NY Acad Sci* 1993; 687: 60–64.

6. Ehrmann DA, Barnes RB, Rosenfield RL. Polycystic ovary syndrome as a form of functional ovarian hyperandrogenism due to dysregulation of androgen secretion. *Endocrine Reviews* 1995; 16: 322–353.

7. Homburg R. Polycystic ovary syndrome - from gynaecological curiosity to multisystem endocrinopathy. *Hum Reprod* 1996; 11: 29–39.

8. Szilágyi A, Rossmanith WG. Polyzystisches Ovar-Syndrom: Zentrale oder periphere Regulationsstörung? *Zent bl Gynäkol* 1991; 113: 851–856.

9. Dunaif A. Insulin resistance and polycystic ovary syndrome: mechanism and implications for pathogenesis. *Endocr Rev* 1997; 18: 774–800.

10. Poretsky L, Grigorescu F, Seibel M, Moses AC, Flier S. Distribution and characterization of insulin and insulin -like growth factor-1 receptors in normal human ovary. *J Clin Endocrinol Metab* 1985; 61: 728–734.

11. Legro RS, Strauss JF. Molecular progress in infertility: polycystic ovary syndrome. *Fertil Steril* 2002; 78: 569–576.

12. Ovalle F, Azziz R. Insulin resistance, polycystic ovary syndrome, and type 2 diabetes mellitus. *Fertil Steril* 2002; 77: 1095–1105.

13. Zawadski JK, Dunaif A. Diagnostic criteria for polycystic ovary syndrome: towards a rational approach. In: Dunaif A, Givens JR, Haseltine F. editors. Polycystic Ovary Syndrome, Boston: *Blackwell Scientific* 1992; 377–384.

14. Homburg R. What is polycystic ovarian syndrome? A proposal for a consensus on the definition and diagnosis of polycystic ovarian syndrome. *Hum Reprod* 2002; 17: 2495–2499.

15. The Rotterdam ESHRE/ASRM-Sponsored PCOS Consensus Workshop Group. Revised 2003 consensus on diagnostic criteria and long term health risks related to polycystic ovary syndrome. *Fertil Steril* 2004; 81: 19–25.

16. Legro R, Finegood D, Dunaif A. A fasting glucose to insulin ratio is a useful measure of insulin sensitivity in women with polycystic ovary syndrome. *J Clin Endocrinol Metab* 1998; 83: 2694–2698.

17. Heald AH, Whitehead S, Anderson S et al. Screening for insulin resistance in women with polycystic ovarian syndrome. *Gynecol Endocrinol* 2005; 20: 84–91.

18. Ferrannini E, Natali A, Bell P, Cavallo-Perin P, Lalic N, Mingrone G. Insulin resistance and hypersecretion in obesity. *J Clin Invest* 1997; 30: 1166–1173.

19. Reaven G. Role of insulin resistance in human disease. *Diabetes* 1988; 37: 1595–1607.

20. World Health Organization (WHO). Definition, diagnosis and classification of diabetes mellitus and its complications. Report of a WHO Consultation, part 1: diagnosis and classification of diabetes mellitus. Geneva, Switzerland: WHO, 1999.

21. Dunaif A, Segal KR, Futterweit W, Dobrjansky A. Profound insulin resistance, independent of obesity, in polycystic ovary syndrome. *Diabetes* 1989; 38: 1165–1174.

22. Dunaif A, Segal KR, Green G, Dobjransky A, Licholai T. Evidence for distinctive and intrinsic defects in insulin action in polycystic ovary syndrome. *Diabetes* 1993; 41: 1257–1266.

23. Marsden P, Murdoch A, Taylor R. Tissue insulin sensitivity and body weight in polycystic ovary syndrome. *Clin Endocrinol (Oxf)* 2001; 55: 191–199.

24. Barbieri RL, Makris A, Randall RW, Daniels G, Kistner RW, Ryan KJ. Insulin stimulates androgen accumulation in incubation of ovarian stroma obtained from women with hyperandrogenism. *J Clin Endocrinol Metab* 1986; 62: 904–910.

25. Zhang L, Rodriguez H, Ohno S, Miller WL. Serine phosphorylation of human P450c17 increases 17, 20-lyase activity: Implications for adrenarche and the polycystic ovary syndrome. *Proc Natl Acad Sci USA* 1995; 92: 10619–10623.

26. Homburg R, Pariente C, Lunenfeld B, Jacobs HS. The role of insulin-like growth factor-1 (IGF-1) and IGF binding protein-1 (IGFBP-1) in the pathogenesis of polycystic ovary syndrome *Hum Reprod* 1992; 7: 13791383.

27. Sam S, Dunaif A. Polycystic ovary syndrome: syndrome XX? *Trends Endocrinol Metab* 2003; 14: 365–370.

28. Harris MI, Flegal KM, Cowie CC et al. Prevalence of diabetes, impaired fasting glucose, and impaired glucose tolerance in U.S. adults. The Third National Health and Nutrition Examination Survey, 1988–1994. *Diabetes Care* 1998; 21: 518–524.

29. Dunaif A, Graf M, Mandeli J, Laumas V, Dobrjansky A. Characterization of groups of hyperandrogenic women with acanthosis nigricans, impaired glucose tolerance and/or hyperinsulinemia. *J Clin Endocrinol Metab* 1987; 65: 499–507.

30. Dahlgren E, Johansson S, Lindstedt G et al. Women with polycystic ovary syndrome wedge resected in 1956 to 1965: long term follow-up focusing on natural history and circulating hormones. *Fertil Steril* 1992; 57: 505–513.

31. Szilágyi A, Lubics Gy, Szabó I. Long term follow-up of wedge resected PCOS patients (in Hungarian). *Hungarian J Obstet Gynecol* 1998; 61: 227–231.

32. Ehrmann DA. Medical Progress: Polycystic Ovary Syndrome. *N Eng J Med* 2005; 352: 1223–1236.

33. Legro RS, Gnatuk CL, Kunselman AR, Dunaif A. Changes in glucose tolerance over time in women with polycystic ovary syndrome: a controlled study. *J Clin Endocrinol Metab* 2005; 90: 3236–3242.

34. Solomon CG, Hu FB, Dunaif A et al. Long or highly irregular menstrual cycles as a marker for risk of type 2 diabetes mellitus. JAMA 2001; 286: 2421–2426.

35. Ehrmann DA, Kasza K, Azziz R, Legro RS, Ghazzi MN. Effects of race and family history of type 2 diabetes on metabolic status of women with polycystic ovary syndrome. *J Clin Endocrinol Metab* 2005; 90: 66–71.

36. Holte J, Gennarelli G, Wide L, Lithell H, Berne C. High prevalence of polycystic ovaries and associated clinical, endocrine, and metabolic features in women with previous gestational diabetes mellitus. *J Clin Endocrinol Metab* 1998; 83: 1143–1150.

37. Barker DJP, Hales CN, Fall CHD, Osmond C, Phipp K, Clark PMS. Type 2 (non-insulin-dependent) diabetes mellitus, hypertension and hyperlipidaemia (syndrome X): relation to reduced fetal growth. *Diabetologia* 1993; 36: 62–67.

38. Conn JJ, Jacobs HS, Conway GS. The prevalence of polycystic ovaries in women with type 2 diabetes mellitus. *Clin Endocrinol* 2000; 52: 81–86.

39. Peppard HR, Iuorno MJ, Marfori J, Nestler JE. Prevalence of polycystic ovary syndrome among premenopausal women with type 2 diabetes. *Diabetes Care* 2001; 24: 1050–1052.

40. Escobar-Morreale HF, Roldán B, Barrio R. et al. High prevalence of the polycystic ovary syndrome and hirsutism in women with type 1 diabetes mellitus. *J Clin Endocrinol Metab* 2000; 85: 4182–4187.

41. Nestler JE. Should patients with polycystic ovarian syndrome be treated with metformin?: an enthusiastic endorsement. *Hum Reprod* 2002; 17: 1950–1953.

42. Seli E, Duleba AJ. Should patients with polycystic ovarian syndrome be treated with metformin? *Hum Reprod* 2002; 17: 2230–2236.

43. Stout DL, Fugate SE. Thiazolidinediones for treatment of polycystic ovary syndrome. *Pharmacotherapy* 2005; 25: 244–252.

44. Lam PM, Cheung LP, Haines C. Revisit of metformin treatment in polycystic ovary syndrome. *Gynecol Endocrinol* 2004; 19: 33–39.

45. Knowler W, Barret-Connor E, Fowler S et al. Reduction in the incidence of type 2 diabetes with lifestyle intervention or metformin. *N Eng J Med* 2002; 346: 393–403.

Frequently Asked Questions

1. Does PCOS cluster in families?

Yes, but the mode of inheritance is still uncertain. Several loci have been proposed as PCOS genes including the insulin gene, and the region near the insulin receptor[11] giving basis for the overlapping with the genetic background of type 2 DM.

2. What is the most important pathophysiologic component of PCOS?

Insulin resistance and hyperinsulinemia play a key role in the pathophysiology of hyperandrogenism and probably the pathogenesis of PCOS.[5,9] Fifty to 70% of the PCOS patients are insulin resistant.[9,12,21]

3. Are PCOS patients at risk for diabetes?

Yes, there is a 5- to 10-fold greater risk for type 2 diabetes, compared with age- and weight-matched women.[12,15]

4. Can the development of diabetes be prevented in PCOS patients?

Lifestyle modifications and/or long-term administration of insulin-sensitizer drugs can reduce the risk, but there is not enough data on this issue.[41-45]

17

Hyperinsulinemia and Polycystic Ovary Syndrome

Ibrahim Esinler, Gurkan Bozdag, Hakan Yarali

Summary

Polycystic Ovary Syndrome (PCOS) is a heterogeneous disorder affecting 4–7% of reproductive aged women.[1] It is suggested that the presence of IR and compensatory hyperinsulinemia are responsible for the several adverse effects of PCOS. Insulin resistance and hyperinsulinemia stimulate ovarian androgen production and increase the likelihood of developing diabetes, hypertension and cardiovascular disease (CVD). Thus, great effort should be exercised for the screening and management of IR in patients with PCOS. To detect IR in PCOS, several tests can be used. The euglycemic hyperinsulinemic glucose clamp test is accepted as a gold standard. Whether IR is present or not, lifestyle modification with complementary diet and exercise should be recommended first to patients with PCOS. If IR is detected, to reduce the degree of IR and its long-term adverse effects, insulin-sensitizing agents and insulin-lowering drugs should be prescribed.

Introduction

Polycystic Ovary Syndrome (PCOS) is the most common endocrinopathy in women[2] and characterized by oligomenorrhea and/or chronic anovulation, clinical or biochemical evidence of hyperandrogenism and polycystic ovarian morphology.[3]

There is evidence of insulin resistance (IR) in both lean (30%) and obese (75%) women with PCOS.[4,5] This association was first shown by Burghen et al.[6] in 8 obese PCOS patients in 1980. Later, several studies with larger sample sizes and more accurate tests confirmed this association.[5,7–9] According to John Nestler, PCOS is strongly associated with insulin resistance, which may be exacerbated by the coexistence of obesity, a typical finding among individuals with the syndrome.

Great effort should be exercised for the screening and management of IR in patients with PCOS as IR and hyperinsulinemia stimulate ovarian androgen production and increase the likelihood of developing diabetes, hypertension and cardiovascular disease (CVD) via resulting low high density lipoprotein (HDL) cholesterol, increased triglycerides, and increased plasminogen activator inhibitor 1 (PAI-1), endothelin-1 and C-reactive protein.[10]

Definition of hyperinsulinemia and insulin resistance (IR)

Insulin resistance (IR) basically means that there is an impaired metabolic response to the body's own insulin. The body cells, especially active muscle, liver and fat, do not process glucose as easily as they should. This leads to chronically higher blood insulin levels known as hyperinsulinemia. However, there is no clear reference range for insulin levels to define hyperinsulinemia, but fasting hyperinsulinemia is usually classified as an insulin level greater than 17–20 mU/L.[11] Since hyperinsulinemia in PCOS patients develops as a compensatory mechanism of insulin resistance, the measurement of insulin resistance gives more information than the insulin level measurement alone.[11]

Clinical Discussion

The prevalence of IR in the normal population shows a variation among the ethnic groups, and ranges between 2–16%.[12] However, if the patient has PCOS, the prevalence of IR significantly increases.[10] The prevalence of IR among women with PCOS at the ages <20, 20–29, and 30–39 years is 22%, 45%, and 50% respectively, which is not explained solely by their degree of obesity.[10] However, if the obesity is associated with PCOS, the prevalence may rise up to 75%.[3]

In women with PCOS, basal insulin secretion is increased and hepatic insulin clearance is reduced, resulting in hyperinsulinemia.[13] Despite the hyperinsulinemia, insulin-stimulated glucose utilization is decreased by 35 to 40 percent in women with PCOS.[14]

Hyperinsulinemia stimulates both ovarian and adrenal androgen secretion directly and suppresses sex hormone binding globulin (SHBG) synthesis from the liver, resulting in an increase in free, biologically active androgens. This excess in local ovarian androgen production, augmented by hyperinsulinemia, causes premature follicular atresia and anovulation. Insulin resistance may also be associated with high blood pressure, high blood lipids and type 2 diabetes mellitus (type 2 DM). If all of these symptoms, including excessive weight gain, are clustered together, this is known as Syndrome X, or Metabolic Syndrome. Figure 17.1 illustrates the possible associations, between insulin resistance and hyperinsulinemia and the clinical manifestations of PCOS including both, reproductive and metabolic morbidities.

Mechanisms of insulin resistance and hyperinsulinemia in PCOS

Generally, insulin resistance results from inherited and acquired influences. Hereditary causes include mutations of insulin receptor, glucose transporter, and signaling proteins, although the common forms are largely unidentified. Acquired causes include physical inactivity, diet, medications, hyperglycemia (glucose toxicity), increased free fatty acids, and the ageing process. However, the exact mechanism of development of insulin resistance in PCOS patients cannot be explained yet. Studies in adipocytes have demonstrated no abnormalities in insulin receptor number or affinity in PCOS women, when compared to appropriately weight-matched non-PCOS control women.[15–17] In the adipocytes of PCOS women, maximal rates of glucose transport were significantly decreased, compared to non-PCOS control women.[15–17] This finding suggests the presence of a postbinding defect in insulin receptor-mediated signal transduction in PCOS. Decreased glucose transport in PCOS adipocytes has been shown to be secondary to a significant reduction in the abundance of glucose transporter 4 (GLUT4).[18] Of interest, these defects in PCOS adipocytes are independent of glucose intolerance, obesity, changes in waist-to-hip ratios and circulating levels of sex hormones,[17] suggesting that the abnormalities of insulin action in PCOS adipocytes may reflect intrinsic, rather than acquired defects.

Besides studies in adipocytes, studies on insulin receptor binding in cultured skin fibroblasts from PCOS women have also shown no differences in receptor number and affinity, compared with cultured cells from reproductive aged non-PCOS women.[19] However, in nearly half of the PCOS women, partially purified insulin receptors from cultured fibroblasts had increased basal autophosphorylation and insulin-stimulated autophosphorylation. The insulin receptors in cultured fibroblasts of PCOS women

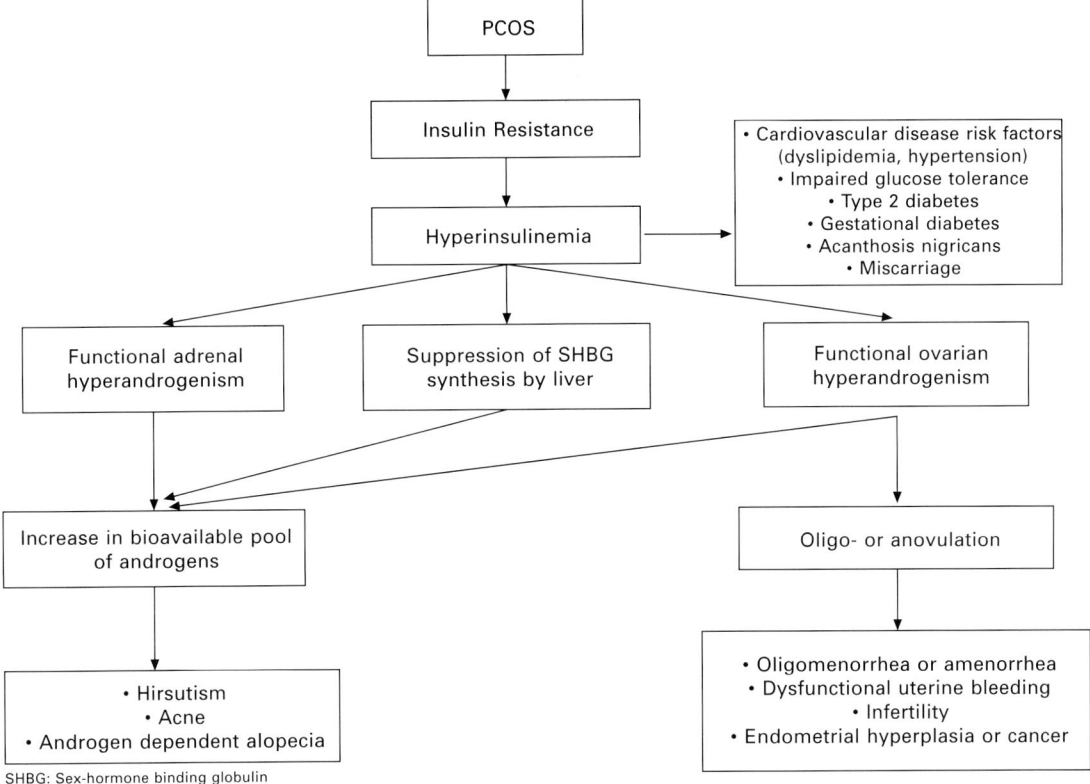

Figure 17.1 The possible associations between insulin resistance, hyperinsulinemia and clinical manifestations of PCOS including both, reproductive and metabolic morbidities.

demonstrated significantly reduced tyrosine kinase activity towards an artificial substrate, compared to partially purified insulin receptors from the fibroblasts of reproductive-age non-PCOS women.[19] Recently, Li et al.[20] noted a 33 percent decrease in insulin-stimulated receptor tyrosine phosphorylation in PCOS fibroblasts, when compared to non-PCOS women. This reduced pattern of phosphorylation has also been detected in insulin receptors of skeletal muscle in PCOS women. Furthermore, it was noted that, these defects in insulin action were independent of obesity and hyperglycemia. All of these studies confirmed the existence of postreceptor abnormalities of insulin signaling in PCOS women. The probable level of postreceptor signaling abnormalities is at the level of insulin receptor substrates 1 (IRS-1) phosphorylation or phosphatidylinositol 3- kinase (PI3-kinase) activation.

Another possible mechanism contributing to the developing insulin resistance in PCOS is free fatty acids (FFAs). Recent studies have reported that the administration of FFAs to healthy subjects can produce insulin resistance and defects in muscle IRS-1-associated PI3-kinase activation.[21] The level of FFAs is increased in obese PCOS women but has not been studied in insulin-resistant, nonobese PCOS women yet.[22,23]

Genetic studies reported no mutations in the coding region of the insulin receptor gene in women with PCOS.[19,24,25]

Case studies

The association between PCOS and

hyperinsulinemia was first shown by Burghen et al.[6] in 8 obese women with PCOS. He reported that obese women with PCOS had significantly elevated basal and post-glucose-load insulin levels, compared to weight-matched control women, suggesting that PCOS women were resistant to insulin.[6] Later, Chang et al.[9] showed higher insulin levels during an oral glucose tolerance test (OGTT) in 10 non-obese PCOS patients compared with 10 height- and weight-matched controls. Dunaif et al.[26] found that obese women with PCOS had significantly increased glucose levels in response to an oral glucose challenge test compared with age- and weight-matched ovulatory control women. They reported that insulin resistance is more pronounced in women with PCOS who are anovulatory than in women who are equally hyperandrogenic but have normal cycles, suggesting that insulin resistance contributes to anovulation.

Legro et al.[27] in his study of 254 women with PCOS, found nearly 40 percent of them to be glucose intolerant, with 31 percent having impaired glucose tolerance and 7.5 percent having type 2 DM. These prevalences were significantly higher than control women matched for age, weight and ethnicity.

In 1996, Dunaif and Finegood[28] examined 28 women with PCOS and 29 age- and weight-matched controls by a modified frequently sampled i.v. glucose tolerance test (IVGTT). They noted significantly increased insulin resistance in women with PCOS and concurrently, an abnormal acute insulin response to glucose. In another study, Diamanti-Kandarkis et al.[29] noticed that the glucose disposal rate values were decreased in both obese and non-obese subgroups of women with PCOS in comparison with controls with similar mean values for weight, body mass index (BMI) and waist -hip ratio (WHR). Another study compared insulin sensitivity in nine women with PCOS, six obese type 2 diabetics and five controls.[30] The insulin sensitivity index (ISI), defined as the ratio of the glucose disposal rate to the insulin concentration at the end of the clamp, was significantly lower in the PCOS group in comparison with the controls. Armstrong et

al.[31] in 2001, documented higher insulin resistance in 11 patients with PCOS in comparison with 13 controls; the controls were, however, not matched by BMI. Toprak et al.[32] focused on 12 non-obese patients with PCOS who they compared with 10 age- and weight-matched controls. Insulin resistance in the PCOS group was significantly higher.

Contrary to the results of these studies mentioned, there is small number of studies with non-confirmatory data on the increased prevalence of insulin resistance in PCOS patients. Ehrmann et al.[33] examined insulin resistance in relation to the presence of a hereditary risk, expressed as a family history of non-insulin-dependent diabetes mellitus (NIDDM). Using IVGTT, they were unable to find any difference in ISI or first phase insulin secretion between women with PCOS and controls. Other studies have also not confirmed increased insulin resistance specifically in lean women with PCOS.[34,35] The potential explanations for the controversy may be several confounding factors such as inter-ethnic variations, variation in the tests used, hereditary risks, and the presence of obesity and life style modifications.

Screening for insulin resistance in women with PCOS

Early detection and treatment of insulin resistance in PCOS can decrease the incidence of short and long-term adverse effects of PCOS. Thus, accurate and reproducible methods of measuring insulin resistance are needed.[36] However, there are presently several obstacles that must be overcome before widespread screening can be recommended. Legro et al.[37] clearly defined these obstacles: (1) the lack of consensus on what defines "normal" insulin resistance, (2) ethnic and genetic variability, (3) the presence of obesity, stress, and ageing (all of which contribute to insulin resistance), (4) the absence of standardized testosterone and insulin assays to assess the presence of PCOS, and (5) concern regarding whether simplified screens for insulin resistance have the precision to predict treatment needs, responses, and future morbidity. Despite these obstacles, we should screen insulin resistance in PCOS patients via the most suitable test for our needs. The tests for insulin resistance are sumarized below.

Methods for clinical assessment of insulin resistance

Several methods have been used for the measurement of insulin resistance (Table 17.1).

Euglycemic hyperinsulinemic glucose clamp (HEGC)

This test is accepted as the gold standard method for the determination of IR. In this technique, IR is measured in the presence of sustained

Table 17.1 The available methods for the assessment of insulin resistance

Euglycemic hyperinsulinemic glucose clamp tests "accepted as gold standard"

Insulin sensitivity test (IST)

Insulin tolerance test (ITT)

Frequently sampled intravenous glucose tolerance test (FSIGT – minimal model)

Fasting-based estimates	
	HOMA-R
	QUICKI

OGTT-based estimates	
	ISIcomp
	MCRest
	OGIS

Fasting insulin

OGTT = oral glucose tolerance test; HOMA = homeostatic model assessment; QUICKI = quantitative insulin sensitivity check index.

hyperinsulinemia. The principle of the test is to keep the glucose concentration constant during increased insulin levels that stimulate glucose disposal, by infusing glucose at a feedback controlled rate. Glucose is frequently measured, and the glucose infusion rate is adjusted to keep glucose close to a target level.[38] In the HEGC, glucose disposal is stimulated by a standardized constant infusion of insulin (40 mU minute/m^2 body surface area), while glucose is kept at a fixed concentration of about 5 mmol/L. After 2–3 hours, insulin concentration and glucose disposal are at a steady state. The glucose and insulin samples are taken in the basal period and in the last 40–60 minutes of the test. The insulin sensitivity (IS) index of the euglycemic clamp is basically the mean glucose infusion rate at steady state. The resulting index, usually termed M (mg/minute or mmol/minute), is then normalized to the lean body mass (LBM) to avoid underestimation of glucose disposal in obese subjects.[39] Thus, the typical units of M are mg/minute/kg LBM. In some cases, M is divided by the steady-state insulin concentration (I) and the so-called M/I index is obtained.

The main difficulty with the clamp tests is its experimental complexity and the expertise required to obtain a stable glucose concentration (and without spills into the hypoglycemic range). Another problem is that 2 hours is often not sufficient to attain a stable steady state.[40]

Insulin sensitivity test (IST)

The insulin sensitivity test involves IV infusion of a defined glucose load and a fixed-rate infusion of insulin over approximately 3 hours. The mean plasma glucose concentration over the last 30 minutes of the test reflects insulin sensitivity. Fewer blood samples and less effort is required for this test as compared with clamp techniques.[40]

Insulin tolerance test (ITT)

The insulin tolerance test (ITT) measures the decline in serum glucose after an IV bolus of regular insulin (0.1–0.5 U/kg) is administered.[40] Several insulin and glucose levels are sampled over the next 15 minutes (depending on the protocol used). Normal ranges for insulin sensitivity in a general population have been published for people with a body mass index below 30 kg/m^2 and for obese subjects (body mass index >30 kg/m^2) at 0.026 to 0.085 mmol/L/min-1 and 0.012 to 0.017 mmol/L/min-1, respectively (7.36). However, no values were determined for PCOS patients.[40]

Frequently sampled intravenous glucose tolerance test (FSIGT – minimal model)

This model requires IV or oral administration of glucose only and is less labor-intensive than clamp techniques.[40] Two main procedures are used: regular and modified FSIGT. In the former, a bolus injection of glucose (0.3 g/kg) is given intravenously in 30–60 seconds and blood samples are collected for 3–4 hours. In the latter, which is a test for subjects with an insufficient insulin response, an insulin injection or short infusion (0.03–0.05 U/kg) is administered at 20 minutes.[41] In both the tests, the number of samples range from 12 to 30.

Fasting-based estimates of insulin sensitivity (IS)

Simple measurements of fasting glucose and insulin concentrations have often been used to derive measures of IS. Fasting insulin concentration has been used as a surrogate for IS, but a more recent approach, the homeostasis model assessment, (HOMA),[40] uses both glucose and insulin concentrations to better account for those conditions in which insulin response is deficient and hyperglycemia is present. One or more consecutive fasting samples are taken and glucose and insulin concentrations are measured. The HOMA index of IS is calculated as: HOMA-R = Glucose (basal) × Insulin (basal)/k. The k is a constant to scale HOMA-R so that it has the value of 1 (or 100%) with mean normal basal glucose and insulin. For glucose in mmol/L and

insulin in mU/mL, the k value is 22.5,[40] but k is sometimes omitted.

QUICKI (quantitative IS check index) is calculated as: QUICKI = Insulin/log Glucose (basal)+ log insulin (basal)

Oral glucose tolerance test (OGTT)-based estimates of insulin sensitivity

The OGTT is a simple test in which both glucose disposal and insulin secretion are stimulated. The OGTT requires ingestion of 75 g glucose and venous blood sampling for 2–3 hours. Glucose and insulin are measured at time zero (preload), 30, 60, 90 and 120 minutes. Also, C-peptide must be measured to calculate insulin secretion.[42] Several methods are used to interpret the results of OGTT such as, ISIcomp, MCRest and OGIS. The most used formulas are given below:

ISI comp = 10.000/square root of [fasting glucose × fasting insulin] × [mean glucose × mean insulin during OGTT]

MCRest = 18.8- 0.271 × BMI- 0.0052 × Insulin (120 min) - 0.27 × Glucose (90 min)

Choosing the most appropriate method for the measurement of insulin sensitivity

Euglycemic hyperinsulinemic glucose clamp (HEGC) is accepted as the gold standard to diagnose the IR. However, it is time-consuming and expensive to perform this test in large-scale clinical practice. Thus, HEGC test should be reserved for intensive physiological studies aiming to measure peripheral insulin resistance on a small number of subjects. In large-scale clinical practice, simpler methods, such as fasting- and OGTT-based estimates may provide an effective estimate of IR. Consensus conferences have recommended screening tests for IR in PCOS in the general and at-risk population. These recommendations are summarized in Table 17.2.

Prevention and treatment of insulin resistance in PCOS

Treatment of PCOS should focus both, on

Table 17.2   The recommended screening tests for IR in PCOS

Group	Screening test	Women requiring screening
American Diabetes Association	Fasting plasma glucose	All
Australian National Health and Medical Research Council	Fasting plasma glucose	Obese (BMI >30 kg/m^2)
Rotterdam Consensus Group	75 g oral glucose tolerance test	Overweight (BMI >28 kg/m^2)

Table 17.3   The recommended conditions for a successful lifestyle modification

Moderate exercise (≥30 min/day or 150 min/week)

Dietary modification (fat ≤30% daily intake, decreased saturated and trans fat and glycemic load, increased fibre and polyunsaturated fat)

Establishing an energy deficit of 500–1000 kcal/day

Reduction of psychosocial stressors

Cessation of smoking

Moderate alcohol consumption

Moderate caffeine consumption

Group interaction/intervention to provide support and assistance in implementing changes

normalizing short-term signs like hyperandrogenism and anovulation, and on reducing the long term metabolic complications. In this manner, lifestyle modifications and/or pharmacological interventions may be useful. As generally expected, pharmacological interventions should be saved for women who failed with simple strategies such as lifestyle modifications.[43] The recent lifestyle modifications have proved as efficacious as pharmacological interventions in reducing the risk of developing IGT and Type 2 DM in subjects with PCOS.[44] The recommended conditions for a successful lifestyle modification are summarized in Table 17.3.[43]

Short-term weight loss (four to eight weeks) has been documented to decrease abdominal fat,[45,46] insulin resistance and serum insulin concentration in recent studies. Norman et al.[43] noted that lifestyle intervention reduced the risk of developing diabetes by 58%. Even in cases with minor weight loss (2–5%), there was invariably an association with decreased insulin resistance and a drop in the blood plasma insulin concentration in PCOS women.[47] Generally, the recommended diet for women with a BMI less than 25 kg/m^2 or higher is 8400 or 6300 J/d (2000 or 1500 kcal/d, respectively), high protein (26% of energy [calories]), low-carbohydrate (44%) diet (42% complex carbohydrates), 30% of the energy (calories) as fat, and a polyunsaturated/saturated fat ratio of 2:1.[48]

Therefore, weight loss is critical in the presence of insulin resistance in patients with PCOS.

In addition to the diet and life-style modifications, several insulin-sensitizing agents and insulin-lowering drugs have been used to treat women with PCOS. Biguanides and thiazolinediones especially, seem to form the basis of medical therapy of PCOS in the near future.[49–52] Metformin is a biguanide and improves insulin sensitivity. The primary effect is a significant reduction in gluconeogenesis, decreasing hepatic glucose production and increasing target tissue sensitivity to insulin. In a study, designed to control the effect of human body weight, the administration of metformin had no effect on IR in extremely overweight women with PCOS. In another study, metformin again had no effect on IR when BMI remained unchanged. In lean, anovulatory women with hyperinsulinemia, metformin treatment reduces hyperandrogenemia although there may be no change in BMI. However, a decrease in the waist to hip ratio is accompanied by a reduction in hyperinsulinemia.[49,51] Therefore, both obese and nonobese patients seem to respond to metformin treatment. Although there is paucity of data, the daily recommended metformin intake is thought to be 1500 mg. The role of metformin in reducing abortion rates and improving in vitro fertilization (IVF) performance is still questionable. When lifestyle modifications fail to achieve spontaneous ovulation and regular cycles, metformin should be prescribed alone or in combination with clomiphene citrate/gonadotropins.

Thiazolidinediones markedly improve insulin sensitivity and insulin secretion mainly via improved peripheral glucose utilization. Troglitazone decreases hyperinsulinemia, androgens, PAI-1, LH, increases SHBG, and improves fibrinolytic capacity. However, liver toxicity is the main reason for the withdrawal of the drug from the markets.[53,54]

Lifestyle modifications with complementary diet and exercise, and insulin sensitizers seem to be well correlated with an improvement in IR in the PCOS population. Both, diet and exercise have been shown to be useful in obtaining regular menstrual cycles, ovulation and improving hyperandrogenemia and hyperinsulinemia. In complex cases, variable combinations should be more effective than single therapy. Of interest, although ovarian drilling is a successful procedure for obtaining regular menses and ovulation for both, short and long-term durations, an improvement in IR is not noted.[55]

Recent Advances

Not all women with PCOS have insulin resistance. However, it has been suggested that IR is often missed by inadequate testing. Today, the gold standard for detecting insulin resistance is the euglycemic hyperinsulinemic glucose clamp (HEGC) test. However, there is no test, including HEGC, that measures the effect of insulin in the ovaries. A woman with very sensitive ovarian function may show adverse insulin related effects even at clinically normal insulin levels. Thus, to evaluate the insulin resistance in PCOS, more tissue based studies with more accurate tests are needed. In addition, more accurate and easily performable tests will enable liberal screening for insulin resistance in all PCOS patients.

Conclusion

The recent literature suggests that insulin resistance and compensatory hyperinsulinemia may be present in both lean and obese women with PCOS. There is no reliable and clinically applicable test for the detection of IR in PCOS to date; hence, PCOS patients should be screened according to the recommendations of consensus conferences. Irrespective of the presence of IR, lifestyle modifications with complementary diet and exercise should be recommended to women with PCOS. If insulin resistance is detected, insulin sensitizers and insulin lowering agents should be prescribed to reduce the degree of IR.

References

1. Knochenhauer ES, Key TJ, Kahsar-Miller M, Waggoner W, Boots LR, Azziz R. Prevalence of the polycystic ovary syndrome in unselected black and white women of the southeastern United States: a prospective study. *J Clin Endocrinol Metab* 1998; 83: 3078–3082.

2. Homburg R. Polycystic ovary syndrome - from gynaecological curiosity to multisystem endocrinopathy. *Hum Reprod* 1996; 11: 29–39.

3. Asuncion M, Calvo RM, San Millan JL, Sancho J, Avila S, Escobar-Morreale HF. A prospective study of the prevalence of the polycystic ovary syndrome in unselected Caucasian women from Spain. *J Clin Endocrinol Metab* 2000; 85: 2434–2438.

4. Conway GS, Jacobs HS, Holly JM, Wass JA. Effects of luteinizing hormone, insulin, insulin-like growth factor-I and insulin-like growth factor small binding protein 1 in the polycystic ovary syndrome. *Clin Endocrinol* (Oxf) 1990; 33: 593–603.

5. Dunaif A, Segal KR, Futterweit W, Dobrjansky A. Profound peripheral insulin resistance, independent of obesity, in polycystic ovary syndrome. *Diabetes* 1989; 38: 1165–1174.

6. Burghen GA, Givens JR, Kitabchi AE. Correlation of hyperandrogenism with hyperinsulinism in polycystic ovarian disease. *J Clin Endocrinol Metab* 1980; 50: 113–116.

7. Shoupe D, Kumar DD, Lobo RA. Insulin resistance in polycystic ovary syndrome. *Am J Obstet Gynecol* 1983; 147: 588–592.

8. Pasquali R, Casimirri F, Venturoli S et al. Insulin resistance in patients with polycystic ovaries: its relationship to body weight and androgen levels. *Acta Endocrinol* (Copenh) 1983; 104: 110–116.

9. Chang RJ, Nakamura RM, Judd HL, Kaplan SA. Insulin resistance in nonobese patients with polycystic ovarian disease. *J Clin Endocrinol Metab* 1983; 57: 356–359.

10. Bloomgarden ZT. Second World Congress on the Insulin Resistance Syndrome: mediators, pediatric insulin resistance, the polycystic ovary syndrome, and malignancy. *Diabetes Care* 2005; 28: 1821–1830.

11. Heald A, Whitehead S, Anderson S et al. Screening for insulin resistance in women with polycystic ovarian syndrome. *Gynecol Endocrinol* 2005; 20: 84–91.

12. Beck-Nielsen H. General characteristics of the insulin resistance syndrome: prevalence and heritability. European Group for the study of Insulin Resistance (EGIR). *Drugs* 1999; 58 (1): 7–10.

13. O'Meara NM, Blackman JD, Ehrmann DA, Barnes RB, Jaspan JB, Rosenfield RL, Polonsky KS. Defects in beta-cell function in functional ovarian hyperandrogenism. *J Clin Endocrinol Metab* 1993; 76: 1241–1247.

14. Dunaif A. Insulin resistance and the polycystic ovary syndrome: mechanism and implications for pathogenesis. *Endocr Rev* 1997; 18: 774–800.

15. Ciaraldi TP, Morales AJ, Hickman MG, Odom-Ford R, Olefsky JM, Yen SS. Cellular insulin resistance in adipocytes from obese polycystic ovary syndrome subjects involves adenosine modulation of insulin sensitivity. *J Clin Endocrinol Metab* 1997; 82: 1421–1425.

16. Ciaraldi TP, el-Roeiy A, Madar Z, Reichart D, Olefsky JM, Yen SS. Cellular mechanisms of insulin resistance in polycystic ovarian syndrome. *J Clin Endocrinol Metab* 1992; 75: 577–583.

17. Dunaif A, Segal KR, Shelley DR, Green G, Dobrjansky A, Licholai T. Evidence for distinctive and intrinsic defects in insulin action in polycystic ovary syndrome. *Diabetes* 1992; 41: 1257–1266.

18. Rosenbaum D, Haber RS, Dunaif A. Insulin resistance in polycystic ovary syndrome: decreased expression of GLUT-4 glucose transporters in adipocytes. *Am J Physiol* 1993; 264: E197–202.

19. Dunaif A, Xia J, Book CB, Schenker E, Tang Z. Excessive insulin receptor serine phosphorylation in cultured fibroblasts and in skeletal muscle. A potential mechanism for insulin resistance in the polycystic ovary syndrome. *J Clin Invest* 1995; 96: 801–810.

20. Li M. Current status of study on polycystic ovary syndrome. *Zhonghua Fu Chan Ke Za Zhi* 2000; 35: 581–582.

21. Dresner A, Laurent D, Marcucci M et al. Effects of free fatty acids on glucose transport and IRS-1-associated phosphatidylinositol 3-kinase activity. *J Clin Invest* 1999; 103: 253–259.

22. Robinson S, Henderson AD, Gelding SV et al. Dyslipidaemia is associated with insulin resistance in women with polycystic ovaries. *Clin Endocrinol (Oxf)* 1996; 44: 277–284.

23. Holte J, Bergh T, Berne C, Lithell H. Serum lipoprotein lipid profile in women with the polycystic ovary syndrome: relation to anthropometric, endocrine and metabolic variables. *Clin Endocrinol (Oxf)* 1994; 41: 463–471.

24. Talbot JA, Bicknell EJ, Rajkhowa M, Krook A, O'Rahilly S, Clayton RN. Molecular scanning of the insulin receptor gene in women with polycystic ovarian syndrome. *J Clin Endocrinol Metab* 1996; 81: 1979–1983.

25. Sorbara LR, Tang Z, Cama A et al. Absence of insulin receptor gene mutations in three insulin-resistant women with the polycystic ovary syndrome. *Metabolism* 1994; 43: 1568–1574.

26. Dunaif A, Graf M, Mandeli J, Laumas V, Dobrjansky A. Characterization of groups of hyperandrogenic women with acanthosis nigricans, impaired glucose tolerance, and/or hyperinsulinemia. *J Clin Endocrinol Metab* 1987; 65: 499–507.

27. Legro RS, Kunselman AR, Dodson WC, Dunaif A. Prevalence and predictors of risk for type 2 diabetes mellitus and impaired glucose tolerance in polycystic ovary syndrome: a prospective, controlled study in 254 affected women. *J Clin Endocrinol Metab* 1999; 84: 165–169.

28. Dunaif A, Finegood DT. Beta-cell dysfunction independent of obesity and glucose intolerance in the polycystic ovary syndrome. *J Clin Endocrinol Metab* 1996; 81: 942–947.

29. Diamanti-Kandarakis E, Mitrakou A, Hennes MM et al. Insulin sensitivity and antiandrogenic therapy in women with polycystic ovary syndrome. *Metabolism* 1995; 44: 525–531.

30. Park KH, Kim JY, Ahn CW, Song YD, Lim SK, Lee HC. Polycystic ovarian syndrome (PCOS) and insulin resistance. *Int J Gynaecol Obstet* 2001; 74: 261–267.

31. Armstrong VL, Wiggam MI, Ennis CN, Sheridan B, Traub AI, Atkinson AB, Bell PM. Insulin action and insulin secretion in polycystic ovary syndrome treated with ethinyl oestradiol/cyproterone acetate. *Qjm* 2001; 94: 31–37.

32. Toprak S, Yonem A, Cakir B, Guler S, Azal O, Ozata M, Corakci A. Insulin resistance in nonobese patients with polycystic ovary syndrome. *Horm Res* 2001; 55: 65–70.

33. Ehrmann DA, Sturis J, Byrne MM, Karrison T, Rosenfield RL, Polonsky KS. Insulin secretory defects in polycystic ovary syndrome. Relationship to insulin sensitivity and family history of non-insulin-dependent diabetes mellitus. *J Clin Invest* 1995; 96: 520–527.

34. Holte J, Bergh T, Berne C, Berglund L, Lithell H. Enhanced early insulin response to glucose in relation to insulin resistance in women with polycystic ovary syndrome and normal glucose tolerance. *J Clin Endocrinol Metab* 1994; 78: 1052–1058.

35. Morin-Papunen LC, Vauhkonen I, Koivunen RM, Ruokonen A, Tapanainen JS. Insulin sensitivity, insulin secretion, and metabolic and hormonal parameters in healthy women and women with polycystic ovarian syndrome. *Hum Reprod* 2000; 15: 1266–1274.

36. Chevenne D, Trivin F, Porquet D. Insulin assays and reference values. *Diabetes Metab* 1999; 25: 459–476.

37. Legro RS. Detection of insulin resistance and its treatment in adolescents with polycystic ovary syndrome. *J Pediatr Endocrinol Metab* 2002; 15 Suppl 5: 1367–1378.

38. DeFronzo RA, Tobin JD, Andres R. Glucose clamp technique: a method for quantifying insulin secretion and resistance. *Am J Physiol* 1979; 237: E214–223.

39. Ferrannini E, Mari A. How to measure insulin sensitivity. *J Hypertens* 1998; 16: 895–906.

40. Pacini G, Mari A. Methods for clinical assessment of insulin sensitivity and beta-cell function. *Best Pract Res Clin Endocrinol Metab* 2003; 17: 305–322.

41. Finegood DT, Hramiak IM, Dupre J. A modified protocol for estimation of insulin sensitivity with the minimal model of glucose kinetics in patients with insulin-dependent diabetes. *J Clin Endocrinol Metab* 1990; 70: 1538–1549.

42. Hovorka R, Jones RH. How to measure insulin secretion. *Diabetes Metab Rev* 1994; 10: 91–117.

43. Norman RJ, Davies MJ, Lord J, Moran LJ. The role of lifestyle modification in polycystic ovary syndrome. *Trends Endocrinol Metab* 2002; 13: 251–257.

44. The Diabetes Prevention Program (DPP): description of lifestyle intervention. *Diabetes Care* 2002; 25: 2165–2171.

45. Andersen P, Seljeflot I, Abdelnoor M, Arnesen H, Dale PO, Lovik A, Birkeland K. Increased insulin sensitivity and fibrinolytic capacity after dietary intervention in obese women with polycystic ovary syndrome. *Metabolism* 1995; 44: 611–616.

46. Holte J, Bergh T, Berne C, Wide L, Lithell H. Restored insulin sensitivity but persistently increased early insulin secretion after weight loss in obese women with polycystic ovary syndrome. *J Clin Endocrinol Metab* 1995; 80: 2586–2593.

47. Buyalos RP, Geffner ME, Bersch N, Judd HL, Watanabe RM, Bergman RN, Golde DW. Insulin and insulin-like growth factor-I responsiveness in polycystic ovarian syndrome. *Fertil Steril* 1992; 57: 796–803.

48. Goldenberg N, Glueck CJ, Loftspring M, Sherman A, Wang P. Metformin-diet benefits in women with polycystic ovary syndrome in the bottom and top quintiles for insulin resistance. *Metabolism* 2005; 54: 113–121.

49. Tasdemir S, Ficicioglu C, Yalti S, Gurbuz B, Basaran T, Yildirim G. The effect of metformin treatment to ovarian response in cases with PCOS. *Arch Gynecol Obstet* 2004; 269: 121–124.

50. De Leo V, La Marca A, Morgante G. Metformin and ovarian steroidogenesis in PCOS women. *Clin Endocrinol* (Oxf) 2000; 52: 243; author reply 4–6.

51. Seli E, Duleba AJ. Treatment of PCOS with metformin and other insulin-sensitizing agents. *Curr Diab Rep* 2004; 4: 69–75.

52. La Marca A, Artensio AC, Stabile G, Volpe A. Metformin treatment of PCOS during adolescence and the reproductive period. *Eur J Obstet Gynecol Reprod Biol* 2005; 121: 3–7.

53. Tarkun I, Cetinarslan B, Turemen E, Sahin T, Canturk Z, Komsuoglu B. Effect of rosiglitazone on insulin resistance, C-reactive protein and endothelial function in non-obese young women with polycystic ovary syndrome. *Eur J Endocrinol* 2005; 153: 115–121.

54. Seto-Young D, Paliou M, Schlosser J et al. Direct thiazolidinedione action in the human ovary: insulin-independent and insulin-sensitizing effects on steroidogenesis and insulin-like growth factor binding protein-1 production. *J Clin Endocrinol Metab* 2005; 90: 6099–6105.

55. Tulandi T, Saleh A, Morris D, Jacobs HS, Payne NN, Tan SL. Effects of laparoscopic ovarian drilling on serum vascular endothelial growth factor and on insulin responses to the oral glucose tolerance test in women with polycystic ovary syndrome. *Fertil Steril* 2000; 74: 585–588.

Frequently Asked Questions

1. Do patients with PCOS have increased risks for developing insulin resistance?

Yes, in the normal population, the rate of IR approximately ranges between 2–16%. However, it is increased to 30% in lean, and 75% in obese women with PCOS.

2. What are the adverse effects of IR in PCOS?

Insulin resistance and hyperinsulinemia stimulate ovarian androgen production with a resultant increase in the likelihood of developing diabetes, hypertension and cardiovascular disease.

3. Is IR acquired in PCOS?

The exact mechanism is not known but the current literature suggests that the cause of IR is postreceptor defects, which are not acquired.

4. Should IR be screened in patients with PCOS

Yes, we should screen patients with PCOS for IR according to recommendations of consensus conferences.

5. What tests should be used to detect IR?

The euglycemic hyperinsulinemic glucose clamp test should be preferred for intensive physiological studies aiming to measure peripheral insulin resistance on a small number of subjects. In large-scale clinical practice, simpler methods, such as fasting- and OGTT-based estimates may provide an effective estimate of insulin resistance.

6. How should we treat IR in PCOS?

If patients have documented IR, first of all, lifestyle modifications with complementary diet and exercise should be recommended. Then, to reduce the degree of IR and to prevent its long term complications, insulin sensitizers and insulin lowering agents should be prescribed.

Obesity

18

Polycystic Ovary Syndrome: What is the Role of Obesity?

Mete Isikoglu, Murat Berkkanoglu, Hasim Cemal,
Kemal Ozgur

Summary

Polycystic Ovary Syndrome (PCOS), which is the most common endocrinopathy in women, also represents the most common cause of anovulatory infertility in young women. In the original description of Stein and Leventhal, obesity was one of the main characteristics of PCOS besides infertility and hirsutism.[1] Since the first description of the syndrome, numerous studies focused on the role of obesity in the pathogenetic process of PCOS. It is known that nearly half of the women with polycystic ovary syndrome (PCOS) are either overweight or obese[2] and when present, obesity worsens the clinical presentation of PCOS.[3] Overweight and obesity contribute to a significant proportion of menstrual disorders in women with PCOS. Mechanisms by which obesity interferes with the pathophysiology and clinical expression of PCOS are complex and not completely understood. There is enough evidence to show that obesity does play a role in the clinical appearance in PCOS women, however, the exact pathogenetic pathways in this process remain to be elucidated. The aim of this chapter is to reveal the facts and theories on the role of obesity in PCOS and to elucidate the probable pathophysiological mechanisms.

Introduction

Polycystic ovary syndrome, is the most common cause of anovulatory infertility in young women. Women with PCOS demonstrate marked clinical heterogeneity. The syndrome is characterized by hyperandrogenism and chronic anovulation and its morbidity may include hyperinsulinemia, insulin resistance, early onset of type 2 diabetes mellitus, dyslipidemia, cardiovascular disease, and infertility.[4–6] Approximately half of all the women with PCOS are overweight or obese. There are endocrine and metabolic differences between lean and obese women with PCOS.

Changes in body weight are a critical factor in regulating menstrual cycles and reproduction. Apparently, there are significant associations between obesity and pubertal development,[7] irregular menstrual cycles, reduced spontaneous and induced fertility. Generally, changes in circulating sex hormones involving androgens, estrogens and those in sex hormone binding globulin (SHBG) levels, appear to underline the obesity-related menstrual and reproductive disorders. Although the exact etiology of PCOS remains unclear, the facts that the history of weight gain frequently precedes the onset of clinical manifestations, obese PCOS women have more severe hyperandrogenism,[8] and the presence of anovulatory cycles, oligomenorrhoea and/or hirsutism are significantly higher in obese than in normal-weight women,[9] suggest a pathogenetic role of obesity in the development of PCOS and related infertility. Obesity in women with PCOS is also associated with adverse effects on the outcome of assisted reproductive technology treatments and an increased risk of miscarriage.[10]

It has been proposed that the pathogenesis of PCOS is different in obese and non-obese women, with insulin resistance and hyperinsulinemia playing a central role in obese women.[11]

Clinical Discussion

Body weight is the major determinant of insulinemia, insulin sensitivity and ovarian hyperandrogenism, independent of PCOS. Although there are several other mechanisms by which obesity contributes to the state of PCOS, it is mainly linked with insulin resistance and hyperinsulinemia. Several studies have shown that obese women with PCOS have more marked hyperinsulinemia, insulin resistance, relative hyperglycemia, and lower levels of SHBG and insulin-like growth factor binding protein-1 (IGFBP-1) compared with lean women with PCOS.[12,13] Some aspects of insulin action in obesity itself resemble those seen in PCOS; e.g. many patients with obesity are insulin resistant and hyperinsulinemic. The pathophysiologic mechanism of obesity-related insulin resistance is not well understood. Dysregulation of the insulin/insulin like growth factor (IGF) system is a key feature in the pathophysiology of PCOS. Hyperinsulinemia (either primary, or secondary to insulin resistance) could interfere with ovulation mechanisms through insulin–insulin-like growth factor (IGF-I) interactions in the ovary,[14] and lead to anovulation, unfavorable estrogen/progesterone balance and further, to the accumulation of abdominal fat.[15]

Obesity is also associated with a more atherogenic lipid profile in women with PCOS.[16] Elevated triglycerides and lower high-density lipoprotein cholesterol (HDL-C) are the most consistently described lipid profile changes in obese compared with lean women with PCOS.[17–19] Metabolic syndrome, which is a constellation of factors including glucose intolerance, dyslipidemia, hypertension and central obesity, is more prevalent in adolescent girls with PCOS. Obesity, hyperandrogenemia and insulin resistance are important risk factors for metabolic syndrome in PCOS.[20]

The degree of insulin resistance correlates with the increase in body mass index.[21] Similar to the insulin resistance seen in normal obesity, a tendency towards higher free fatty acid concentrations and defective suppression of rate of lipid oxidation have been reported during the hyperinsulinemic clamp in obese PCOS subjects, which together with hyperandrogenism, has been associated with abdominal obesity and insulin resistance.[22]

Obesity may induce an insulin-resistant state by several metabolites such as free fatty acids, tumor necrosis factor alpha (TNF-α) and leptin. An impaired rate of both glucose oxidation and non-oxidation contributes to the process. Several molecular mechanisms have also been reported regarding this mechanism.[23] It was proposed that peripheral hyperinsulinemia in obese PCOS women is mainly due to lowered hepatic insulin extraction and to insulin resistance in skeletal muscles.[13] Unlike the target insulin-resistant organs, the ovaries remain responsive to insulin with its own receptors. Hence, increased insulin is capable of stimulating steroidogenesis and excess androgen production in the ovaries of PCOS women, particularly when obesity is present. This may be either by direct stimulation of ovarian androgen synthesis, or via enhancing luteinizing hormone (LH) secretion. In cultures of ovarian stromal tissue obtained from hyperandrogenic women, high concentrations of insulin alone induce androgen accumulation.[24] According to another theory, hyperestrogenism due to obesity, may exert a positive feed-back effect on gonadotropin release resulting in a rise in ovarian androgen production.[25] Increased local ovarian androgen production may lead to premature follicular atresia and consecutively, anovulation.[11] The increase in the delivery of free androgens due to the inhibiting effect of insulin on SHBG synthesis in the hepatic cells, could explain the lower SHBG concentrations observed in obese PCOS women.[26] The relative suppression of IGF binding protein-1 in obese compared with non-obese women with PCOS,[27] can also be accounted for by the more marked hyperinsulinemia demonstrated in the obese group. Thierry van Dessel et al.[28] found a statistically significant inverse correlation between free IGF-I and body mass index (BMI). It was speculated that the relative hyperinsulinemia in obese PCOS subjects compared with the non-obese PCOS subjects suppresses IGFBP-3 proteolysis and thereby lowers the free IGF-I level in this group.[29]

Since obesity worsens the clinical presentation of PCOS by increasing insulin resistance and resulting in a further elevation of ovarian and adrenal androgens and of unbound testosterone, the treatment of obesity is one of the main goals of any therapy for PCOS. That obesity contributes significantly to both insulin resistance and hyperandrogenism in overweight women with and without PCOS, is also evident from the improvement in androgen levels usually seen with weight loss, sometimes to levels observed in weight-matched ovulatory women. Though there is some evidence that androgens may contribute to insulin resistance, however, this finding fails to resolve the question of whether insulin resistance in PCOS is independent of obesity.[30] Obesity has been shown to be an independent predictor of conversion of normoglycemia to impaired glucose tolerance or type 2 DM in women with PCOS.[31] Whether there is a component of insulin resistance in PCOS, independent of the insulin resistance of obesity, will be clarified once the specific molecular mechanisms of insulin resistance in both these conditions are better understood.

Because of hyperandrogenism and insulin resistance, the obesity of PCOS is of the android (central) type, which results in an increased waist-to-hip ratio, and which is highly associated with diabetes mellitus and increased cardiovascular risk. Increased cardovascular risk is worsened by obesity, but appears to be present in all PCOS patients, including those who are not obese. Overweight women with PCOS are predisposed to an increased risk for cardiovascular disease and there is evidence of early cardiovascular disease in these women, potentially related to insulin resistance, when compared to weight-matched controls.[32]

In summary, studies suggest that insulin resistance in PCOS women is, at least partly, related to obesity and fat distribution and not entirely to PCOS itself. Because insulin resistance has not been consistently encountered in populations of lean women with PCOS, the existence of a cause of insulin resistance in PCOS distinct from that associated with obesity remains open to question.

Obesity may also favor hyperandrogenism by genetic or other still undefined factors,[33] or it may act as a secondary factor by amplifying the main factors, such as an increased LH stimulation.[23]

Most studies have shown hypersecretion of adrenal hormones in PCOS subjects compared with healthy women. On the other hand, obesity itself seems to represent a condition of functional hyperandrogenism. There may be various mechanisms by which obesity influences hyperandrogenism in women with PCOS. Although the exact mechanism of this hypersecretion is not well understood, the observed hyperinsulinemia in PCOS subjects, could lead to higher serum concentrations of some adrenal steroids, particularly in obese PCOS subjects.[13] Several studies have reported a higher total and/or free testosterone or free androgen index.[34] The concentration of dihydrotestosterone (DHT) was shown to be higher in the non-obese than in the obese PCOS group, possibly indicating increased peripheral conversion of testosterone. Since obese PCOS patients demonstrate greater suppression of SHBG than the non-obese group, the higher DHT levels can be attributed to the higher SHBG levels in the non-obese group, because DHT has a very high affinity for SHBG.

The history of obesity in the patients's mother during pregnancy,[35] or in utero androgen excess,[36] may be facilitating factors in developing hyperandrogenism and PCOS later in life, suggesting that an ovarian disorder early in life may result in hyperandrogenism later in life. A similar mechanism, suggesting that early onset obesity during peripubertal age may lead to the development of hyperandrogenism via different hormonal pathways including insulin, IGF system, estrogens and cytokines, has been hypothesized.[37]

Several peptides such as leptin and ghrelin have also been claimed to be involved in the pathogenetic process of PCOS.

Leptin is a protein hormone which contributes to the regulation of food intake and energy balance. Serum leptin concentrations correlate positively with total body mass and percentage body fat, and leptin resistance can be involved in the development of obesity.[38] There are indications that hyperinsulinemia[39] and insulin resistance[40] could be associated with increased leptin concentrations. Below a certain BMI, hyperandrogenic women with PCOS have lower leptin levels than controls. Conversely, overweight and obese PCOS subjects appear to produce insufficient leptin for a given fat mass, relative to the degree of hyperinsulinemia, potentially because of the competing effects of adipocyte insulin resistance and androgens on leptin.[41]

Leptin may contribute to the insulin resistance of obesity via several mechanisms; e.g. *ob/ob* mice, which lack functional leptin, develop insulin resistance. Leptin also has a direct interaction with the ovaries. Expression of both leptin and its specific receptors has been found in the human ovary.[42] Leptin may exert a direct inhibitory effect on ovarian steroidogenesis via leptin receptors on the surface of the ovarian cells.[43] It may either antagonize the stimulatory factors,[44] or it may interfere with oocyte maturation.[45] Leptin also regulates the gonadotropin surge initiating pubertal development.[46] Indirect evidence of this issue is that the age of menarche generally occurs at a younger age in obese girls compared with normal weight girls.

The reports are contradictory regarding the leptin levels in PCOS women, and the role of leptin in determining anovulation -if any- in obese PCOS women is elusive so far.

A relatively newly discovered peptide, ghrelin has been showed to enhance appetite and reduce fat utilization.[47] A negative correlation has been shown between ghrelin and androgen levels suggesting that ovaries may be an important target of ghrelin action. Discovery of binding sites for ghrelin in the human ovary, supports this hypothesis. It appears that ghrelin may represent a factor related to gonadal function especially in conditions such as obesity and PCOS.

In conclusion, obese PCOS women have lower ghrelin levels than those expected based on the presence of obesity. Ghrelin negatively correlates with insulin sensitivity only in obese PCOS women. In addition, regardless of the presence of PCOS, a marked negative correlation exists between ghrelin and androstenedione levels, suggestive of an interaction between ghrelin and steroid synthesis or action.[48]

Existing evidence suggests that the opioid system may also be involved in the mechanism of hormonal dysregulation caused by obesity in PCOS patients. Since β-endorphin is able to stimulate insulin secretion, it may also cause hyperandrogenemia via the above mentioned mechanisms. An indirect evidence may be that opioid antagonists may regulate menstrual cycles in obese PCOS women.

It is possible that in some of the obese adolescents, polycystic ovaries may evolve into the full syndrome, with obesity as a risk factor for its development.[29] Obesity in adolescence and in adulthood, and also weight gain after adolescence, particularly in the presence of abdominal obesity, are associated with self-reported PCOS symptoms in adulthood.[49] Thus, obesity-extreme obesity in women, manifest by ages 20–24 years and continuing through 32–41 years, should alert physicians to the likelihood of PCOS.[50]

Conclusion

Taking into account the probable contribution of obesity in the pathogenesis of PCOS, obese patients with PCOS should be encouraged to loose weight. Insulin-sensitizing therapies and a hypocaloric diet have been shown to improve insulin resistance, hyperandrogenism and menstrual disturbances.[51] Indeed, weight loss represents the major factor for improved hyperinsulinemia and insulin resistance in obese PCOS women who are under energy restricted programs. Weight loss also has important beneficial effects on androgen concentrations and related signs and symptoms. Studies revealed an increase in SHBG and a decrease in total and free testosterone following weigth loss. Dietary measures may improve menstrual abnormalities and ovulation as well.[52] Suppression of insulin levels decreases blood androgen concentrations.[16] When metformin, an insulin sensitizing drug, was added to a hypocaloric diet, obese PCOS patients lost weight more significantly than the placebo group.[53] Indeed, metformin treatment also improves ovulation[54] and insulin levels, and decreases LH and testosterone concentrations. Existing data support the use of insulin sensitizers together with dietary measures in obese PCO patients. Nevertheless, dietary measures and weight loss should be the first-line therapy in all obese PCOS women to improve ovulation.

A high fibre diet reduces serum estrogen concentrations and very high lipid intake decreases SHBG levels.[55] Since a high fat and low fibre diet may favour obesity via insulin resistance,[56] the hyperandrogenism cascade may follow this situation.

In conclusion, there is enough evidence to show that obesity does play a role in the clinical appearance in PCOS women, though the exact pathogenetic pathways in this process remain to be elucidated.

References

1. Stein IF, Leventhal ML. Amenorrhea associated with bilateral polycystic ovaries. *Am J Obstet Gynecol* 1934; 29: 181–191.
2. Rogers J, Mitchell GW. The relation of obesity to menstrual disturbances. *N Engl J Med* 1952; 247: 53–56.
3. Ek I, Arner P, Bergqvist A, Carlstrom K, Wahrenberg H. Impaired adipocyte lipolysis in nonobese women with the polycystic ovary syndrome: a possible link to insulin resistance? *J Clin Endocrinol Metab* 1997; 82(4): 1147–1153.
4. Carmina E, Lobo RA Polycystic ovary syndrome (PCOS): arguably the most common endocrinopathy is associated with significant morbidity in women. *J Clin Endocrinol Metab* 1999; 84: 1897–1899.
5. Zawadzki JK, Dunaif A Diagnostic criteria for polycystic ovary syndrome: towards a rational approach. In: Dunaif A, Givens JR, Haseltine FP, Merriam GR, eds. Current issues in endocrinology and metabolism: polycystic ovary syndrome. Boston: Blackwell; 1992; 377–384.
6. Ehrmann DA, Barnes RB, Rosenfield RL, Cavaghan MK, Imperial J Prevalence of impaired glucose tolerance and diabetes in women with polycystic ovary syndrome. *Diabetes Care* 1999; 22: 141–146.
7. Frisch RE. Pubertal adipose tissue: is it necessary for normal sexual maturation? Evidence from the rat and human female. *Fed Proc* 1980; 39: 2395–2400.
8. Pasquali R, Casimirri F. The impact of obesity in hyperandrogenism and polycystic ovary syndrome in premenopausal women. *Clin Endocrinol (Oxford)* 1993; 39: 1–16.
9. Hartz AJ, Barboriak PN, Wong A, Katayama KP, Rimm AA. The association of obesity with infertility and related menstural abnormalities in women. *Int J Obes* 1979; 3 (1): 57–73.
10. Hamilton-Fairley, Kiddy D, Watson H, Paterson C, Franks S. Association of moderate obesity with a poor pregnancy outcome in women with polycystic ovary syndrome treated with low dose gonadotrophin. *Br J Obstet Gynecol* 1992; 99(2): 128–131.
11. Poretsky L, Cataldo NA, Rosenwaks Z, Giudice LC The insulin-related ovarian regulatory system in health and disease. *Endocr Rev* 1999; 20: 535–582.
12. Sengos C, Andreakos C, Iatrakis G Sonographic parameters and hormonal status in lean and obese women with polycystic ovary syndrome. *Clin Exp Obstet Gynecol* 2000; 27: 35–38.
13. Morin-Papunen LC, Vauhkonen I, Koivunen RM, Ruokonen A, Tapanainen JS Insulin sensitivity, insulin secretion, and metabolic and hormonal parameters in healthy women and women with polycystic ovarian syndrome. *Hum Reprod* 2000; 15: 1266–1274.
14. Robinson S, Kiddy D, Gelding SV, et al. The relationship of insulin insensitivity to menstrual pattern in women with hyperandrogenism and polycystic ovaries. *Clin Endocrinol* 1993; 39: 351–355.
15. Rebuffe-Scrive M, Cullberg G, Lundberg P, et al.

Anthropometric variables and metabolism in polycystic ovarian disease. *Horm Metab Res* 1989; 21: 391–397.

16. Gambineri A, Pelusi C, Vicennati V, Pagotto U, Pasquali R. Obesity and the polycystic ovary syndrome. *Int J Obes Relat Metab Disord* 2002l; 26(7): 883–896.

17. Acien P, Qureda F, Matallin P, Villarroya E, Lopez-Fernandez JA, et al Insulin, androgens, and obesity in women with and without polycystic ovary syndrome: a heterogeneous group of disorders. *Fertil Steril* 1999; 72: 32–40.

18. Holte J, Bergh T, Berne C, Lithell H. Serum lipoprotein lipid profile in women with the polycystic ovary syndrome: relation to anthropometric, endocrine and metabolic variables. *Clin Endocrinol (Oxf)* 1994; 41: 463–471.

19. Conway GS, Agrawal R, Betteridge DJ, Jacobs HS. Risk factors for coronary artery disease in lean and obese women with the polycystic ovary syndrome. *Clin Endocrinol (Oxf)* 1992; 37: 119–125.

20. Coviello AD, Legro RS, Dunaif A. Adolescent girls with polycystic ovary syndrome have an increased risk of the metabolic syndrome associated with increasing androgen levels independent of obesity and insulin resistance. *J Clin Endocrinol Metab* 2005 Oct 25; [Epub ahead of print].

21. Rittmaster RS, Deshwal N, Lehman L. The role of adrenal hyperandrogenism, insulin resistance, and obesity in the pathogenesis of polycystic ovarian syndrome. *J Clin Endocrinol Metab* 1993; 76(5): 1295–1300.

22. Holte J, Bergh T, Berne C, Wide L, Lithell H. Restored insulin sensitivity but persistently increased early insulin secretion after weight loss in obese women with polycystic ovary syndrome. *J Clin Endocrinol Metab* 1995; 80 (9): 2586–2593.

23. Pasquali R, Gambineri A. Role of changes in dietary habits in polycystic ovary syndrome. *Reprod Biomed Online* 2004; 8(4): 431–439.

24. Barbieri RL, Makris A, Randall RW, Daniels G, Kistner RW, Ryan KJ. Insulin stimulates androgen accumulation in incubations of ovarian stroma obtainea from women with hyperandrogenism. *J Clin Endocrinol Metab* 1986; 62: 904–910.

25. Yen SSC. The polycystic ovary syndrome. *Clin Endocrinol (Oxf.)* 1980; 12: 177–208.

26. Plymate SR, Matej LA, Jones RE, et al. Inhibition of sex hormone-binding globulin in the hepatoma (Hep G2) cell line by insulin and prolactin. *J Clin Endocrinol Metab* 1988; 67: 460–464.

27. Morales AJ, Laughlin GA, Butzow T, Maheshwari H, Baumann G, Yen SSC. Insulin, somatotropic and luteinizing hormone axes in lean and obese women with polycystic ovary syndrome: common and distinct features. *J Clin Endocrinol Metab* 1996; 81: 2854–2864.

28. Thierry van Dessel HJHM, Lee PDK, Faessen G, Fauser BCJM, Giudice LC. Elevated serum levels of free insulin-like growth factor I in polycystic ovary syndrome. *J Clin Endocrinol Metab* 1999; 84: 3030–3035.

29. Silfen ME, Denburg MR, Manibo AM, Lobo RA, Jaffe R, Ferin M, et al Early endocrine, metabolic, and sonographic characteristics of polycystic ovary syndrome (PCOS): comparison between nonobese and obese adolescents. *J Clin Endocrinol Metab* 2003; 88(10): 4682–4688.

30. Park KH, Kim JY, Ahn CW, Song YD, Lim SK, Lee HC. Polycystic ovarian syndrome (PCOS) and insulin resistance. *Int J Gynaecol Obstet* 2001; 74: 261–267.

31. Norman RJ, Masters L, Milner CR, Wang XJ, Davies MJ. Relative risk of conversion from normoglycemia to impaired glucose tolerance or non-insulin dependent diabetes mellitus in polycystic ovarian syndrome. *Hum Reprod* 2001; 16: 1995–1998.

32. Meyer C, McGrath BP, Teede HJ. Overweight women with polycystic ovary syndrome have evidence of subclinical cardiovascular disease. *J Clin Endocrinol Metab* 2005; 90(10): 5711–5716.

33. Legro RS. The genetics of obesity: lessons for polycystic ovary syndrome. *Annals of the New York Academy of Science* 2000; 900: 193–202.

34. Grulet H, Hecart AC, Delemer B, Gross A, Sulmont V, Leutenegger M, Caron J Roles of LH and insulin resistance in lean and obese polycystic ovary syndrome. *Clin Endocrinol (Oxf)* 1993; 38: 621–626.

35. Creswell JL, Barker DJ, Osmond C, Egger P, Philips DJ, Fraser RB. Fetal growth, length of gestation, and polycystic ovaries in adult life. *Lancet* 1997; 350: 1131–1135.

36. Abbott DH, Dumesic DA, Franks S. Developmental origin of polycystic ovary syndrome- a hypothesis. *J Endocrinol* 2002; 174: 1–5.

37. Pasquali, Pelusi C, Genghini S, Cacciari M, Gambineri A. Obesity and reproductive disorders in women. *Hum Reprod Update* 2003; 9(4): 359–372.

38. Maffei M, Halaas J, Ravussin E, et al. Leptin levels in human and rodent: measurement of plasma leptin and in ob RNA in obese and weight-reduced subjects. *Nat Med* 1995; 1: 1155–1161.

39. Leroy P, Dessolin S, Vilageois P, et al. Expression of ob gene in adipose cells-regulation by insulin. *J Biol Chem* 1996; 271: 2365–2368.

40. Segal KR, Landt M, Klein S. Relationship between insulin sensitivity and plasma leptin concentration in lean and obese men. *Diabetes* 1996; 45: 988–991.

41. Remsberg KE, Talbott EO, Zborowski JV, Evans RW, McHugh-Pemu K. Evidence for competing effects of body mass, hyperinsulinemia, insulin resistance, and androgens on leptin levels among lean, overweight, and obese women with polycystic ovary syndrome. *Fertil Steril* 2002; 78(3): 479–486.

42. Cioffi JA, Van Blerkom J, Antczak M, et al. The expression of leptin and its receptors in pre-ovulatory human follicles. *Mol Hum Reprod* 1997; 3: 467–472.

43. Wiesner G, Vaz M, Collier G, et al. Leptin is released from the human brain: influence of adiposity and gender. *J Clin Endocrinol Metab* 1999; 84: 2270–2274.

44. Spicer LJ, Francisco CC. The adipose obese gene product, leptin: evidence of a direct inhibitory role in ovarian function. 1997; 138: 3374–3379.

45. Duggal PS, Van Der Hoek KH, Milner CR, et al. The in-vivo and in-vitro effects of exogenous leptin on ovulation in rat. *Endocrinology* 2000; 141: 1971–1976.

46. Farooqi IS, Jebb SA, Langmack G, Lawrence E, Cheetham CH, Pentice AM, et al. Effects of recombinant leptin therapy in a child with congenital leptin deficiency. *N Engl J Med* 1999; 341: 879–884.

47. Wren AM, Seal LJ, Cohen MA, et al. Ghrelin enhances appetite and increase food intake in humans. *J Clin Endocrinol Metab* 2001; 86: 5992–5995.

48. Pagotto U, Gambineri A, Vicennati V, Heiman ML, Tschop M, Pasquali R. Plasma ghrelin, obesity and the polycystic ovary syndrome: correlation with insulin resistance and androgen levels. *J Clin Endocrinol Metab* 2002; 87(12): 5625–5629.

49. Laitinen J, Taponen S, Martikainen H, Pouta A, Millwood I, Hartikainen AL, et al. Body size from birth to adulthood as a predictor of self-reported polycystic ovary syndrome symptoms. *Int J Obes Relat Metab Disord* 2003; 27(6): 710–715.

50. Glueck CJ, Dharashivkar S, Wang P, Zhu B, Gartside PS, Tracy T, Sieve L. Obesity and extreme obesity, manifest by ages 20–24 years, continuing through 32–41 years in women, should alert physicians to the diagnostic likelihood of polycystic ovary syndrome as a reversible underlying endocrinopathy. *Eur J Obstet Gynecol Reprod Biol* 2005; 122(2): 206–212.

51. Kowalska I, Kinalski M, Strackowski M, Wolczyski S, Kinalska A. Insulin, leptin, IGF-I and insulin-dependent protein concentrations after insulin-sensitizing therapy in obese women with polycystic ovary syndrome. *Eur J Endocrinol* 2001; 144(5): 509–515.

52. Crosignani PG, Vegetti W, Colombo M, Ragni G. Resumption of fertility with diet in overweight women. *Reprod Biomed Online* 2002; 5: 60–64.

53. Pasquali R, Gambineri A, Biscotti D et al. Effect of long-term treatment with metformin added to hypocaloric diet on body composition, fat distribution, and androgen, and insulin levels in abdominally obese women with and without the polycystic ovary syndrome. *J Clin Endocrinol Metab* 2000; 85: 2767–2774.

54. Batukan C, Baysal B. Metformin improves ovulation and pregnancy rates in patients with polycystic ovary syndrome. *Arch Gynecol Obstet* 2001; 265(3): 124–127.

55. Pasquali R, Gambineri A. Treatment of the polycystic ovary syndrome with lifestyle intervention. *Curr Opin Endocrinol Metab* 2002; 9: 459–468.

56. Abbasi F, McLaughlin T, Lamendola C, et al. High carbohydrate diets, triglyceride-rich lipoproteins, and coronary heart disease risk. *American Journal of Cardiology* 2000; 85: 45–48.

19

The Role of Serum Leptin Elevation in Obese Women with Polycystic Ovary Syndrome

Erbil Dogan, Bulent Gulekli

Summary

Leptin is a hormone secreted mainly from the adipose tissue, and its serum levels reflect the amount of fat stores. Secretion of leptin is affected by various hormones like insulin, androgens and estrogens. Besides regulating the energy metabolism of the body, leptin has important actions on the reproductive system, which makes it an important link between the adipose tissue and hypothalamus – pituitary – gonadal (HPG) axis. Total leptin deficiency, which is very rare in humans, causes profound obesity and reproductive failure in mice, whereas high circulating leptin levels (leptin resistance) may also impair gonadal function.

Most studies indicate that women with polycystic ovary syndrome (PCOS) have similar serum leptin levels compared to age-and weight-matched controls. However, apart from obesity, hyperinsulinism and hyperandrogenemia, common features of these patients, also seem to modulate leptin levels. It seems that, in women with polycystic ovary syndrome, insulin resistance in the adipocytes limits insulin-stimulated leptin secretion. Additionally, higher abdominal fat accumulation in these patients also secretes less leptin, which sends inappropriate satiety signals to the brain resulting in increased body weight and serum leptin levels. The increased circulating leptin levels may impair gonadal function and ovulation in obese patients with PCOS. However, further studies are needed to clarify the role and potential therapeutic application of leptin in PCOS.

Rationale

Leptin is a hormone mainly involved in the regulation of body weight. Its serum levels are influenced by obesity, insulin resistance and the levels of sex steroids. Having direct and indirect effects on the hypothalamus – pituitary – gonadal (HPG) axis, leptin is speculated to have an important role in the pathogenesis of polycystic ovary syndrome (PCOS), which is mainly a state of oligo/amenorrhea, clinical or biochemical signs of hyperandrogenemia, insulin resistance and obesity, leading to metabolic disturbances and infertility.

Introduction

Polycystic ovary syndrome is one of the most common endocrine disorders, affecting 6% to 10% of women of reproductive age.[1] The clinical features of the syndrome include menstrual abnormalities, hirsutism, acne, anovulatory infertility and recurrent miscarriages. Patients with PCOS have elevated androgens, luteinizing hormone (LH), and estrogen levels.[2] There is also a considerable percent of patients with obesity, insulin resistance, lipid abnormalities and increased risk for impaired glucose tolerance and type 2 diabetes mellitus.

The first recognition of an association between glucose intolerance and hyperandrogenism was made in 1921. The association between insulin resistance, which is defined as the reduced response to a given amount of insulin, and PCOS is now well recognized. Studies with the euglycemic clamp technique indicate that insulin resistance is a common feature of the syndrome, and both, obese and nonobese women with the syndrome are more insulin resistant and hyperinsulinemic than the age-and weight-matched women with normal ovaries.[3] Moreover, obese PCOS women are more insulin resistant compared with the nonobese PCOS women. Morales et al.[4] demonstrated that reduced insulin sensitivity was twofold further reduced in obese PCOS patients compared to lean PCOS patients, which suggests that obesity is additive to the insulin resistance related to PCOS. The proposed mechanisms contributing to insulin resistance are peripheral target tissue resistance, decreased hepatic clearance and increased pancreatic sensitivity.

Experimental evidence suggests that the peripheral insulin resistance in these patients is due to serine instead of tyrosine phosphorylation of the insulin receptor, which decreases glucose transport.[5,6] Serine phosphorylation also appears to increase the activity of p450c17, the key regulatory enzyme of androgen biosynthesis, which is present in both, adrenal and ovarian steroidogenic tissue. Therefore, serine phosphorylation partly explains the presence of insulin resistance and hyperandrogenism in a subgroup of PCOS women.

It is already known from rat studies in the 1950s that a hormone from the adipose tissue regulated body weight through an interaction with the hypothalamus. In 1994, *ob* (obesity) gene was identified, which is the gene responsible for obesity in mice.[7] In humans, this gene is known as the Lep gene. Leptin, the name derived from a Greek word "*leptos*" (thin), was discovered by positional cloning of the *ob* gene It is a protein hormone consisting of 167 amino acids, with a molecular weight of 16 kDa. Leptin is exclusively secreted by the adipose tissue, and circulates in the blood, bound to a family of proteins. The main action of leptin is to decrease appetite and increase energy expenditure.[8] Therefore, it was originally thought to be an anti-obesity hormone. Mutations of the *ob* gene (ob/ob) in mice lead to leptin deficiency, which results in hyperphagia, profound obesity, diabetes, insulin resistance and infertility;[9] administration of recombinant leptin to these animals reduces body weight and restores fertility. Another form of obesity and diabetes that occurs in mice is characterized by abnormalities in the leptin receptor (db). These mice are unresponsive to exogenous leptin administration, which indicates leptin resistance.[10] Therefore, ob/ob mouse is obese because it can not produce leptin; on the other hand, db/db mouse is obese because leptin levels are high due to a defective leptin receptor. However, in humans, obesity has not been linked to mutations of the leptin gene, but leptin resistance may be a characteristic of human obesity.

Regulation of leptin secretion

Leptin is predominantly produced by the adipocytes and its serum level is directly related to the fat mass of the body. It has a half life of 30 minutes and is secreted as 3.6 pulses every 24 hours, usually 2-3 hours after meals. There is a diurnal pattern of leptin secretion in humans with a nocturnal rise, which may represent a delayed response to the last meal of the day and may be important for the suppression of appetite during sleep.[11] In both, normal and obese people, food intake does not result in any acute changes in serum leptin levels, but fasting causes a delayed reduction in leptin levels.

It has been shown that serum leptin concentrations correlate significantly with body mass index (BMI) and percentage of body fat. In general, significantly higher leptin concentrations have been found in obese subjects than in lean controls. Loss of weight in obese patients following 8–12 weeks results in a significant reduction in both leptin concentration and expression of *ob* mRNA content in adipocytes. A 10% decrease in body weight can result in approximately 53% reduction in serum leptin concentrations, suggesting that other factors apart from fat tissue, may regulate leptin secretion.[12] This correlation is also significant in patients with eating disorders like anorexia and bulimia nervosa.

In the brain, leptin receptors are located particularly in the arcuate nucleus and ventromedial hypothalamus. These areas are the places where food intake and energy balance are regulated. There are two forms of leptin receptors, long and short forms and these receptors are encoded by the diabetes gene (*db*). Leptin interacts with its receptors within the hypothalamus and inhibits the synthesis and release of neuropeptide Y (NPY), which is a potent stimulator of eating.[13] NPY stimulates food intake, decreases heat and increases insulin and cortisol secretion. Fasting and exercise decrease leptin secretion and increase NPY gene expression in the arcuate nucleus. The increase in NPY levels in the central nervous system (CNS), may have an inhibitory effect on the gonadotropin releasing hormone (GnRH) secretion.[14] It has been also found that leptin accelerates GnRH pulsatility, but not the pulse amplitude, in a dose dependent manner.[13] Insulin stimulates leptin production in humans, both in vitro and in vivo.[15,16] However, only long-term hyperinsulinemia in humans, as is the case in PCOS patients, stimulates leptin secretion from adipose tissue.[17]

Effects of leptin on the reproductive system

Leptin has direct effects on the anterior pituitary and modulates the GnRH pulsatility. Gonadotropic cells express leptin receptors and leptin may directly stimulate LH, and to a lesser extent, follicle stimulating hormone (FSH).[18] These findings suggest that, in addition to conveying information on the energy stores of the body, leptin also has a role in the regulation of the HPG axis. It is speculated that leptin exerts a bimodal action on the HPG axis, depending on its serum levels. Total leptin deficiency, which is very rare in humans, results in HPG dysfunction. At low doses, leptin may have a permissive threshold effect on the CNS that regulates gonadotropin secretion, whereas high serum leptin levels as seen in obese people, may have an inhibitory effect on the gonads.[19]

Human ovarian follicles have leptin receptors; follicular cells express leptin mRNA at the time of dominant follicle selection and granulosa cells have been shown to secrete leptin.[20] This indicates a possible direct paracrine role for leptin in ovarian physiology. Circulating leptin concentrations vary significantly during the menstrual cycle, with a detectable rise in the periovulatory phase and peak concentrations in the midluteal phase of the cycle when progesterone secretion is maximal (Figure 19.1).

Secretion of leptin is affected by various reproductive hormones, growth factors and cytokines. Estrogens increase,[21] whereas androgens[22] suppress leptin production, which causes sexual dimorphism in leptin levels. In fact, there are some other reasons for the increased levels of leptin in women compared to men. First, the pulse amplitude of serum leptin secretion from adipose tissue is two to threefold higher in females than in males. Additionally, fat mass is increased in females and there is differential fat distribution with a higher subcutaneous to visceral fat ratio in women than in men.[23] Leptin mRNA expression is known to be higher in subcutaneous than visceral fat depots. Finally, women have higher total serum leptin levels but lower leptin-binding protein than men indicating higher free leptin levels.[24]

Clinical Discussion

Most of the clinical problems that occur in PCOS patients, are worse in obese patients. Obesity and its metabolic effects are viewed as an important part in the pathophysiology of the syndrome, since 40% of the patients with the syndrome have obesity.[25] The hypersecretion of androgens is also a typical biochemical

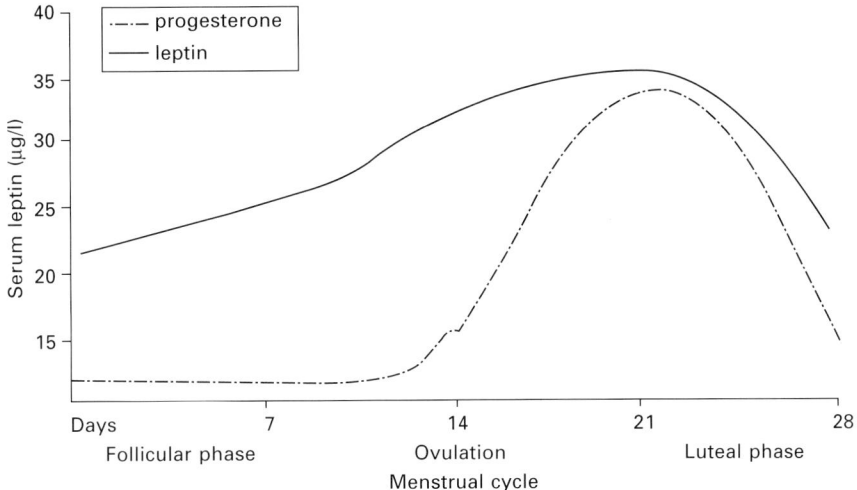

Figure 19.1 Change in the serum leptin level during the menstrual phase.

characteristic of PCOS. Additionally, patients with PCOS often present with hypersecretion of LH and insulin resistance. The combined interaction of obesity, insulin resistance and hyperandrogenism and high basal LH levels in PCOS has led to the suggestion that leptin may play some role in the abnormal ovarian function observed in PCOS.

Initial reports suggested that a substantial proportion of women with PCOS have leptin levels that are higher than expected for their BMI. Brzechffa et al.[26] reported that 29% of women with PCOS had serum leptin values above the 99% prediction interval for their BMI. However, subsequent studies with small groups of patients have not confirmed these data.[27–30] In these studies, serum leptin concentration did not differ significantly between women with PCOS and weight-matched controls. Body mass index seems to be the most important variable responsible for the changes seen in leptin concentrations. Other parameters like hyperandrogenemia, glucose to insulin ratio, fasting insulin and estrogen levels had no effect on leptin levels when controlled for BMI.[31] It has been argued that the distribution of leptin between its bound and free forms, and the pulsatility and circadian rhythm of its secretion and body fat composition (visceral or subcutaneous), has not been incorporated into these studies.[32]

Waist circumference, an index of abdominal fat accumulation and associated insulin resistance in PCOS patients, is found to be strongly and positively correlated with leptin concentration.[33]

As discussed above, the influence of various hormonal parameters on leptin secretion in women with PCOS is not consistent. Majority of the studies did not found significant correlation between leptin and SHBG, androgens and estradiol levels.[27–28] However, significant positive correlations between leptin and the ratios of estradiol/SHBG, estrone/SHBG and testosterone/SHBG were found in PCOS patients.[33] Laughlin et al.[33] reported that independent of body fat, 24 hour mean insulin concentration contributed significantly to leptin levels. Despite this relationship, and the two-fold higher mean insulin concentrations in PCOS patients, the expected increase in serum leptin levels was not observed. These results are explained by the presence of PCOS specific form of insulin resistance in adipocytes, which impairs the stimulatory effect of insulin on leptin secretion.[34] Consistent with this observation, leptin levels were found to be 20% lower in PCOS patients than controls across a wide range of body weights.[35] Similar to these findings, Remsberg et al.[36] demonstrated that, below a certain BMI, hyperandrogenic women with PCOS have lower leptin levels than controls and conversely, obese

PCOS patients appear to produce insufficient leptin for a given fat mass, relative to the degree of hyperinsulinemia. The combined effects of hyperandrogenism, decreased fat mass, and normal insulin levels in PCOS patients, may result in decreased circulating leptin levels. However, in women with PCOS with the highest BMI level, insulin mediated leptin production may be reduced at the level of the adipocyte due to the competing inhibitory effects of both insulin resistance and androgen excess.[36]

Leptin secretion increases with obesity and is stimulated by insulin. In women with PCOS, insulin stimulated leptin secretion is limited by the insulin resistance in adipocytes. An important feature of the obesity in PCOS is the accumulation of visceral fat (increased waist to hip ratio), which secretes less leptin than subcutaneous fat.[24] This may lead to lower than appropriate satiety signals sent to the hypothalamus resulting in progressively severe insulin resistance with eventual decompensation of reproductive function. At the ovarian level, high leptin concentrations may impair ovarian function by reducing the response to gonadotropin stimulation. Beginning from 10ng/mL of serum levels (high physiologic doses), leptin antagonizes the augmenting effect of insulin-like growth factor – 1 (IGF-1) on FSH and LH stimulated steroidogenesis in both granulosa and theca cells.[20,37,38] Thus, high leptin concentration in the ovary may suppress estradiol production and interfere with the development of dominant follicles and oocyte maturation, which may explain the impaired response to gonadotropin stimulation in obese patients with PCOS. Gonadotropin response and leptin levels were studied by Mantzoros et al.[39] in *in vitro* fertilization (IVF) patients and follicular fluid leptin levels were found to be significantly lower in normal women and women with PCOS who succeeded in becoming pregnant within three cycles of IVF compared with those who failed to become pregnant.

Case studies

Improvement in insulin resistance and

hyperinsulinemia by insulin sensitizing agents is expected to alter circulating leptin levels in women with PCOS, but the results are controversial. One study showed a significant reduction in leptin levels after 2 months of treatment with metformin even when the BMI of the patients remained constant.[40] One other study also showed a decrease in leptin levels following metformin use in obese PCOS patients, however, not independent of the decrease in the BMI.[41] A similar reduction was also noted after 10 days of diazoxide treatment.[42] However, troglitazone, the most potent insulin sensitizer, had no effect on serum leptin levels.[43] Unless studies with higher number of subjects are performed, the implementation of these results that use leptin as a marker for response to treatment with insulin sensitizers in clinical studies is limited.

Recent Advances and Conclusion

The contradictory findings regarding the changes in leptin levels in women with PCOS may be related to an incomplete evaluation of the different variables controlling serum leptin levels, mainly insulin and androgens. Since androgens suppress leptin production and long term hyperinsulinemia stimulates it, the net result would be a balance between the effects of BMI, androgens and insulin. Resistance of adipose tissue to the stimulating effect of insulin in PCOS patients, is an issue to be investigated in more detail.

Hence, further studies are required in this area to clarify the complex interaction of adipose tissue and leptin with the HPG axis in PCOS patients before we can use this adipose tissue hormone for therapeutic purposes.

References

1. Tsilchorozidou T, Overton C, Conway GS. The pathophysiology of polycystic ovary syndrome. *Clin Endocrinol* 2004; 60(1): 1–17.
2. Gulekli B, Turhan NO, Senoz S, Kukner S, Oral H, Gokmen O. Endocrinological, ultrasonographic and clinical findings in adolescent and adult polycystic ovary patients: a comparative study. *Gynecol Endocrinol* 1993; 7: 273–7.

3. Dunaif A, Segal KR, Shelley DR, Green G, Dobrjansky A, Licholai T. Evidence for distinctive and intrinsic defects in insulin action in polycystic ovary syndrome. *Diabetes* 1992; 41(10): 1257–1266.

4. Morales AJ, Laughlin GA, Butzow T, Maheshwari H, Baumann G, Yen SS. Insulin, somatotropic, and luteinizing hormone axes in lean and obese women with polycystic ovary syndrome: common and distinct features. *J Clin Endocrinol Metab* 1996; 81(8): 2854–2864.

5. Dunaif A, Xia J, Book CB, Schenker E, Tang Z. Excessive insulin receptor serine phosphorylation in cultured fibroblasts and in skeletal muscle. A potential mechanism for insulin resistance in the polycystic ovary syndrome. *J Clin Invest* 1995; 96(2): 801–810.

6. Dunaif A. Insulin resistance and the polycystic ovary syndrome: mechanism and implications for pathogenesis. *Endocr Rev*, 1997; 18 (6): 774–800.

7. Zhang Y, Proenca R, Maffei M, Barone M, Leopold L, Friedman JM. Positional cloning of the mouse obese gene and its human homologue. *Nature* 1994; 372(6505): 425–432.

8. Caprio M, Fabbrini E, Isidori AM, Aversa A, Fabbri A. Leptin in reproduction. *Trends Endocrinol Metab* 2001; 12(2): 65–72.

9. Halaas JL, Gajiwala KS, Maffei M, Cohen SL, Chait BT, Rabinowitz D, et al. Weight-reducing effects of the plasma protein encoded by the obese gene. *Science* 1995; 269: 543–546.

10. Lee GH, Proenca R, Montez JM, Carroll KM, Darvishzadeh JG, Lee JI, Friedman JM. Abnormal splicing of the leptin receptor in diabetic mice. *Nature* 1996; 379(6566): 632–635.

11. Licinio J, Mantzoros C, Negrao AB, Cizza G, Wong ML, Bongiorno PB, et al. Human leptin levels are pulsatile and inversely related to pituitary-adrenal function. *Nat Med* 1997; 3(5): 575–579.

12. Considine RV, Sinha MK, Heiman ML, Kriauciunas A, Stephens TW, Nyce MR, et al. Serum immunoreactive-leptin concentrations in normal-weight and obese humans. *N Engl J Med* 1996; 334(5): 292–295.

13. Lebrethon MC, Vandersmissen E, Gerard A, Parent AS, Junien JL, Bourguignon JP. In vitro stimulation of the prepubertal rat gonadotropin-releasing hormone pulse generator by leptin and neuropeptide Y through distinct mechanisms. *Endocrinology* 2000; 141(4): 1464–1469.

14. Pierroz DD, Catzeflis C, Aebi AC, Rivier JE, Aubert ML. Chronic administration of neuropeptide Y into the lateral ventricle inhibits both the pituitary-testicular axis and growth hormone and insulin-like growth factor I secretion in intact adult male rats. *Endocrinology* 1996; 137(1): 3–12.

15. Wabitsch M, Jensen PB, Blum WF, Christoffersen CT, Englaro P, Heinze E, et al. Insulin and cortisol promote leptin production in cultured human fat cells. *Diabetes* 1996; 45(10): 1435–1438.

16. Leroy P, Dessolin S, Villageois P, Moon BC, Friedman JM, Ailhaud G, Dani C. Expression of ob gene in adipose cells. Regulation by insulin. *J Biol Chem* 1996; 271(5): 2365–2368.

17. Andersen PH, Kristensen K, Pedersen SB, Hjollund E, Schmitz O, Richelsen B. Effects of long-term total fasting and insulin on ob gene expression in obese patients. *Eur J Endocrinol* 1997; 137(3): 229–233.

18. Iqbal J, Pompolo S, Considine RV, Clarke IJ. Localization of leptin receptor-like immunoreactivity in the corticotropes, somatotropes, and gonadotropes in the ovine anterior pituitary. *Endocrinology* 2000; 141(4): 1515–1520.

19. Moschos S, Chan JL, Mantzoros CS. Leptin and reproduction: a review. *Fertil Steril* 2002; 77(3): 433–444.

20. Agarwal SK, Vogel K, Weitsman SR, Magoffin DA. Leptin antagonizes the insulin-like growth factor-I augmentation of steroidogenesis in granulosa and theca cells of the human ovary. *J Clin Endocrinol Metab* 1999; 84(3): 1072–1076.

21. Shimizu H, Shimomura Y, Nakanishi Y, Futawatari T, Ohtani K, Sato N, Mori M. Estrogen increases in vivo leptin production in rats and human subjects. *J Endocrinol* 1997; 154(2): 285–292.

22. Luukkaa V, Pesonen U, Huhtaniemi I, Lehtonen A, Tilvis R, Tuomilehto J, et al. Inverse correlation between serum testosterone and leptin in men. *J Clin Endocrinol Metab* 1998; 83(9): 3243–3246.

23. Van Harmelen V, Reynisdottir S, Eriksson P, Thorne A, Hoffstedt J, Lonnqvist F, Arner P. Leptin secretion from subcutaneous and visceral adipose tissue in women. *Diabetes* 1998; 47(6): 913–917.

24. McConway MG, Johnson D, Kelly A, Griffin D, Smith J, Wallace AM. Differences in circulating concentrations of total, free and bound leptin relate to gender and body composition in adult humans. *Ann Clin Biochem* 2000; 37: 717–723.

25. Balen AH, Conway GS, Kaltsas G, Techatrasak K, Manning PJ, West C, Jacobs HS. Polycystic ovary syndrome: the spectrum of the disorder in 1741 patients. *Hum Reprod* 1995; 10(8): 2107–2111.

26. Brzechffa PR, Jakimiuk AJ, Agarwal SK, Weitsman SR, Buyalos RP, Magoffin DA. Serum

immunoreactive leptin concentrations in women with polycystic ovary syndrome. *J Clin Endocrinol Metab* 1996; 81(11): 4166–4169.

27. Chapman IM, Wittert GA, Norman RJ. Circulating leptin concentrations in polycystic ovary syndrome: relation to anthropometric and metabolic parameters. *Clin Endocrinol* 1997; 46(2): 175–181

28. Rouru J, Anttila L, Koskinen P, Penttila TA, Irjala K, Huupponen R, Koulu M. Serum leptin concentrations in women with polycystic ovary syndrome. *J Clin Endocrinol Metab* 1997; 82(6): 1697–1700.

29. Mantzoros CS, Dunaif A, Flier JS. Leptin concentrations in the polycystic ovary syndrome. *J Clin Endocrinol Metab* 1997; 82(6): 1687–1691.

30. Telli MH, Yildirim M, Noyan V. Serum leptin levels in patients with polycystic ovary syndrome. *Fertil Steril* 2002; 77(5): 932–935.

31. Pirwany IR, Fleming R, Sattar N, Greer IA, Wallace AM. Circulating leptin concentrations and ovarian function in polycystic ovary syndrome. *Eur J Endocrinol* 2001; 145(3): 289–294.

32. Caro JF. Leptin is normal in PCOS, an editorial about three "negative" papers. *J Clin Endocrinol Metab* 1997; 82(6): 1685–1686.

33. Laughlin GA, Morales AJ, Yen SS. Serum leptin levels in women with polycystic ovary syndrome: the role of insulin resistance/hyperinsulinemia. *J Clin Endocrinol Metab* 1997; 82(6): 1692–1696.

34. Dunaif A, Segal KR, Shelley DR, Green G, Dobrjansky A, Licholai T. Evidence for distinctive and intrinsic defects in insulin action in polycystic ovary syndrome. *Diabetes* 1992; 41: 1257–66.

35. Jacobs HS, Conway GS. Leptin, polycystic ovaries and polycystic ovary syndrome. *Hum Reprod Update* 1999; 5(2): 166–171.

36. Remsberg KE, Talbott EO, Zborowski JV, Evans RW, McHugh-Pemu K. Evidence for competing effects of body mass, hyperinsulinemia, insulin resistance, and androgens on leptin levels among lean, overweight, and obese women with polycystic ovary syndrome. *Fertil Steril* 2002; 78(3): 479–486.

37. Zachow RJ, Magoffin DA. Direct intraovarian effects of leptin: impairment of the synergistic action of insulin-like growth factor-I on follicle-stimulating hormone-dependent estradiol–17 beta production by rat ovarian granulosa cells. *Endocrinology* 1997; 138(2): 847–850.

38. Brannian JD, Zhao Y, McElroy M. Leptin inhibits gonadotrophin-stimulated granulosa cell progesterone production by antagonizing insulin action. *Hum Reprod* 1999; 14(6): 1445–1448.

39. Mantzoros CS, Cramer DW, Liberman RF, Barbieri RL. Predictive value of serum and follicular fluid leptin concentrations during assisted reproductive cycles in normal women and in women with the polycystic ovarian syndrome. *Hum Reprod* 2000; 15(3): 539–544.

40. Morin-Papunen LC, Koivunen RM, Tomas C, Ruokonen A, Martikainen HK. Decreased serum leptin concentrations during metformin therapy in obese women with polycystic ovary syndrome. *J Clin Endocrinol Metab* 1998; 83(7): 2566–2568.

41. Kowalska I, Kinalski M, Straczkowski M, Wolczyski S, Kinalska I. Insulin, leptin, IGF-I and insulin-dependent protein concentrations after insulin-sensitizing therapy in obese women with polycystic ovary syndrome. *Eur J Endocrinol* 2001; 144(5): 509–515.

42. Krassas GE, Kaltsas TT, Pontikides N, Jacobs H, Blum W, Messinis I. Leptin levels in women with polycystic ovary syndrome before and after treatment with diazoxide. *Eur J Endocrinol* 1998; 139(2): 184–189.

43. Nolan JJ, Olefsky JM, Nyce MR, Considine RV, Caro JF. Effect of troglitazone on leptin production. Studies in vitro and in human subjects. *Diabetes* 1996; 45(9): 1276–1278.

Frequently Asked Questions

1. Why do all obese women not develop insulin resistance and why do all insulin resistant women not develop PCOS?

The answer to this question may lie in the genetic susceptibility of the individuals. An example of this susceptibility is the abnormality in serine-threonine phosphorylation involved in the post receptor insulin signal transduction and 17, 20 lyase activity. The presence of such an abnormality may result in both, insulin resistance and abnormal steroid hormone production, leading to the disturbances seen in PCOS.

2. What are the main hormones that change serum leptin levels?

Insulin, thyroid hormones and estrogens increase serum leptin levels, whereas androgens suppress leptin production.

Hyperandrogenemia

20

Hirsutism and Acne in Polycystic Ovary Syndrome

Suresh Nair

Summary

Women, in whom the ovaries exhibit morphological features of multiple small antral follicles with a peripheral distribution (polycystic ovaries), are considered part of a clinical spectrum that is associated with hyperandrogenemia and insulin resistance, particularly when they are obese. This hyperinsulinemia causes, through a lowering of the hepatic production of sex hormone binding globulin (SHBG), an elevation of free unbound testosterone (80% of serum testosterone is bound by SHBG). The resultant hyperandrogenemia in the genetically predisposed, can induce hirsutism and acne. The degree of hirsutism is also influenced by the relative activity of 5α reductase enzyme that converts testosterone to the more active metabolite dihydrotestosterone. As regards the severity of the acne, this is linked largely to the degree of hyperactivity of the sebaceous gland in the pilosebaceous unit. Both these conditions can coexist and are often associated with some degree of disfigurement and hence, substantial loss of self-esteem and resultant psychosocial sequelae. Both these conditions must therefore, be promptly treated, often with similar drug therapies. Hirsutism can initially, and very dramatically, be alleviated by mechanical methods but other general methods, especially in women with polycystic ovaries (PCO), include weight loss, topical treatments, oral contraceptives, anti-testosterone progestational agents such as cyproterone acetate, spironolactone, flutamide, finasteride and insulin sensitizing agents. These agents can also help treat acne but, in addition, appropriate antibiotic therapy and retinoids are essential. Care must be exercised in recognizing whether an individual is pregnant or desirous of pregnancy when administering such treatments, as there are known teratogenic effects that are ubiquitous.

Rationale

Polycystic Ovary Syndrome (PCOS) has been a subject of much debate and controversy, especially with regard to its definition and treatment, ever since the first description of polycystic ovaries by Stein and Leventhal in 1935.[1] It is a heterogeneous condition of unknown etiology characterized by oligo-ovulation and androgen excess. Being the most common endocrinological disorder affecting women in the reproductive age group, it accounts for a prevalence rate of nearly 5 to 10%.[2] Women with PCOS often demonstrate insulin resistance, which results in compensatory hyperinsulinemia. This excess insulin (i) lowers the sex hormone-binding globulin (SHBG) production (hence making available more free unbound circulating testosterone) and also (ii) promotes the secretion of ovarian androgens.[3] The overall impact of the hyperandrogenism is manifested as hirsutism and acne. Whilst these effects are largely cosmetic, they are a cause of significant social embarrassment and emotional distress, such that they warrant an important priority in the overall management of women and adolescents with PCOS.

Introduction

Hirsutism can be defined as hair growth which is excessive involving facial and/or body terminal hair in a male-like distribution.[4] The number of hair follicles usually remains constant, but their size and length increase, as does the pigmentation of hair. Hirsutism is often accompanied paradoxically with androgenic alopecia due to the opposite effect on the scalp follicles. Furthermore, less profound hirsutism found in Eastern Asian women, attests to the ethnic and genetic differences that modify the evaluation of the degree and impact of hirsutism.

There are three hair types, namely,[4]

  (i) lanugo hair – this is lost in early postpartum
 (ii) vellus hair – this is soft, short, non-pigmented hair
(iii) terminal hair – this is pigmented coarse, longer than vellus hair

Vellus hair is transformed into terminal hair in androgen sensitive areas under the influence of testosterone and dihydrotestosterone (DHT). The conversion of vellus hair to terminal hair by testosterone is permanent and occurs over several growth cycles; is of variable distribution e.g. more axillary/pubic hair in puberty, but if there are excessive androgens, this can result in exuberant growth and result in hirsutism on the face, neck and lower abdomen. Hair follicle number, as mentioned before, is fixed, genetically predetermined, forms only during the fetal development and averages around 50 million.[4]

The rate of hair growth varies according to genetic differences in the activity of the 5α-reductase enzyme that converts testosterone to the more potent DHT metabolite.[4] This explains the genetic basis of ethnic variations in hirsutism.

There are three phases in the hair growth cycle:[4]

(a) Anagen phase of active growth (scalp 3 years, face 4 months);
(b) Catagen phase of rest and of variable length of time;
(c) Telogen phase of shedding the hair shaft that has been separating from the dermal papillae at the base during the catagen phase

Furthermore, hyperandrogenism, insulin and insulin-like growth factors all stimulate 5α-reductase activity.[5] There are two isoenzymes of 5α-reductase; type 1 (found in sebaceous glands and pubic skin) and type 2 (found in hair follicles, genital skin, and adult scalp) (Figure 20.1). This explains why there is a variable clinical picture as the hirsutism in some hyperandrogenic women is not commensurate with the severity of the acne.

Acne Vulgaris is a common condition especially in adolescents, caused by hyperactivity of the sebaceous gland in the pilosebaceous unit (PSU) (Figure 20.2). Although acne is a chronic inflammation of the sebaceous glands of the PSU occurring in early adolescence, in most people, it disappears by age 21, but persists in the majority of women with PCOS.[4] The pathogenesis of acne vulgaris begins with overstimulation of the androgen receptors in the PSU resulting in excess sebum production, follicular keratinization, cornification associated with impaired drainage and hence, comedone formation. Abnormal colonization of the PSU with Propionibacterium acnes results in the chronic inflammation.[6]

The main etiological factor in this sequence of events is excess androgen [testosterone, androstenedione, dehydroepiandrosterone (DHEA) and its sulfate (DHEAS)] of ovarian and/or adrenal origin. In addition, testosterone and its 5α reduced metabolite (DHT) are androgens produced in the target tissue itself.

Acne tends to present initially on the face because of increased 5α reductase type 1 activity compared to other skin areas,[6] but 50% of the

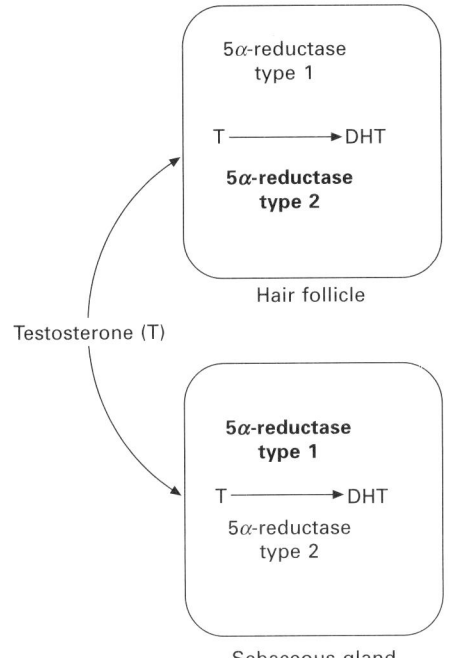

Figure 20.1 Relative enzymatic activities of 5 α-reductase type 1 and type 2 in the hair follicle and sebaceous gland (The predominant enzyme is highlighted in bold).

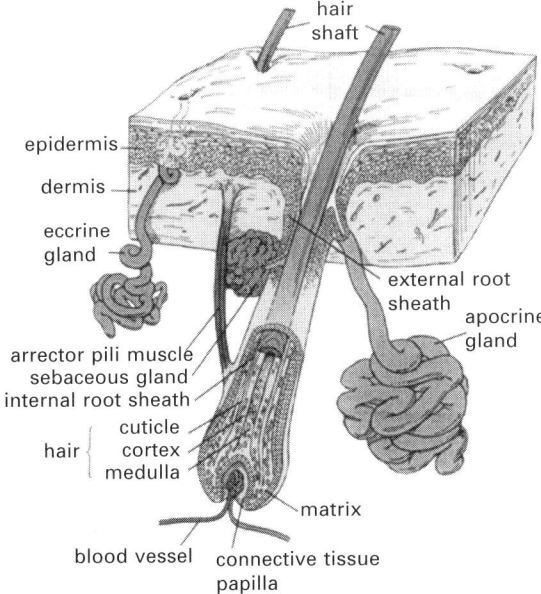

Figure 20.2 The Pilosebaceous Unit (PSU).

women with hyperandrogenism, have acne over the neck, chest and upper back.

A majority of the women presenting with acne will have PCOS. In a study on 82 females presenting with acne vulgaris, 68 (83%) had PCOS compared with 19% in the control group without acne but with polycystic ovaries on ultrasonography. The prevalence of acne in PCOS is less clear with more than 50% of adolescents with PCOS having moderate to severe acne.[7]

Hirsutism and acne, both androgen-driven conditions, manifest their effects through the effect that androgens have on a single morphological entity, the PSU (Figure 20.2). These two clinical scenarios present simultaneously, especially in PCOS, but they do not always appear concomitantly.[7] This is because of the dichotomy in the final pathogenetic pathway where DHT is further reduced to 3α – androstenediol and its glucuroneride only in patients with hirsutism but not with acne. Thus, acne and hirsutism appear to be expressions of the different metabolic fate of DHT.[6]

The PSU comprises of two main structures: the hair follicle and the sebaceous gland, which have different degrees of sensitivity to similar androgenic stimulation. Acne in early adolescence is associated with high circulating DHEAS, whereas hirsutism is linked directly with high concentrations of serum free testosterone hormone in women with ultrasound confirmed polycystic ovaries. Those with acne alone are much less likely to have the biochemical features of PCOS i.e. raised luteinizing hormone (LH) and testosterone, compared with those that have hirsutism.[7]

Evaluation and grading of hirsutism and acne

Hirsutism can be classified as mild, moderate, or severe based on the modified Ferriman-Gallwey (F-G) scoring system,[8] which is a subjective assessment that uses non-midline, non-androgen dependent body hair for diagnosis (Figure 20.3)

Some objective measures of hirsutism include measuring hair shaft diameter, weighed shaved

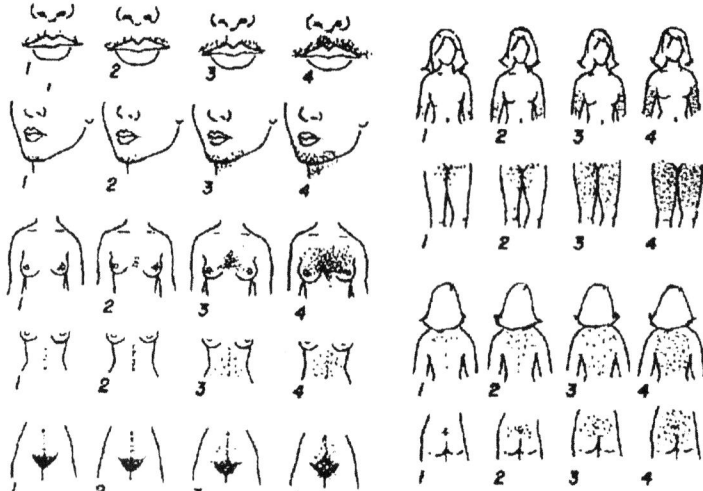

Figure 20.3 Modified Ferriman-Gallwey (F-G) hirsutism scoring system for nine body areas. Each area is rated from 0 (absence of terminal hair) to four (extensive terminal hair growth) and the numbers added. A score of ≥8 indicates hirsutism; only 5% of women qualify by this criteria.[8]

hair from a specific area and computerized assessments of digitalized images of the hirsute areas.[7]

The differential diagnosis of hirsutism is hyperthecosis, non-classical adrenal hyperplasia (NCAH), Cushing's syndrome, thyroid dysfunction, and ovarian or adrenal androgen-secreting tumours.[4]

Should there be rapid hair growth in 3 to 6 months, this suggests an androgen-producing neoplasm. A family history of hirsutism suggests NCAH or PCOS, and a rounded facies, buffalo hump, central obesity and proximal muscle weakness will indicate Cushing's syndrome.[9] In these instances, computerized tomography (CAT) scans of the adrenal gland and pelvic organs is critical to excluding adrenal tumours and detect hyperthecosis (enlarged ovary without follicle formation).

Laboratory analysis must include serum testosterone; DHEAS to exclude a functional adrenal tumour, follicular phase 17-hydroxyprogesterone (17-OHP) picking up NCAH, thyroid stimulating hormone (TSH) to exclude thyroid diseases and a 24 hours urinary free cortisol to screen for Cushing's syndrome. If the total serum testosterone concentration is above 200 ng/dl on 2 separate samplings, then the patient should be evaluated for an androgen-producing tumour – however, a total testosterone concentration of ≥ 250 ng/dl has a positive predictive value of only 9% for an androgen-secreting tumour.

Rapid hirsutism occurring over some months is cause for concern as there might be an androgen secreting tumor. However, hirsutism that is associated with PCOS is more insidious, occuring over a period of several years - hence, a good marker for differential diagnoses.[9]

Acne can be assessed for its clinical severity by evaluating its progress in consecutive phases. A simplified grading system includes:[10]

(i) mild: less than 10 papules on one side of face
(ii) moderate: more than 10 papules and pustules on one side of the face or spread to the shoulders and neck
(iii) severe: above plus deep infiltrates

Clinical Discussion

Treatment of hirsutism

It is important for both, the clinician and the patient to realize that when assessing the outcome of any form of treatment, the growth cycle of hair follicles is 3 months to 6 months – ie. improvements might only be noticeable following treatment continued for at least 3 months.

However, the length of time required to achieve reduced hair growth depends on the number of terminal hair at the different stages (anagen, catagen, telogen). Furthermore, medical treatment has its effect on new terminal hair growth and not on existing follicles that need to be shed first.

Hence, on the face, the anagen phase lasts 16 weeks, catagen, 1 week and telogen, 6 weeks – in this instance, a 6-month treatment interval is required to decrease the F-G scores.[9]

Mechanical hair removal

Mechanical treatments are usually the first line of treatment for hirsutism, or at least a more immediate solution to the problem whilst awaiting the therapeutic effects of medical interventions.

Mechanical hair removing methods include shaving, plucking, waxing, depilatory creams, electrolysis and laser vaporization.

Shaving is the most helpful and most frequently used temporary method. Contrary to popular belief, shaving neither affects the rate or duration of hair growth nor the hair diameter.[9] Hence, shaving should be encouraged as an inexpensive, effective, though temporary method of rapid hair removal that does not thicken or coarsen subsequent hair growth. A dramatic effect to the patient's life is seen particularly after shaving of facial hair.

Plucking of hair is occasionally helpful but results in follicular damage if done repeatedly. The follicle can react either by producing thinner or thicker hair. The skin response is also variable, with some patients developing folliculitis, pigmentary changes, ingrown hair and scarring of skin and follicles that cause resistance to electrolysis treatment.[9,10] Waxing is no different in that it is a "grouped" method of plucking causing the same skin damage.

Chemical depilatories often contain thioglycolates that damage hair follicles. It can

also cause chronic skin irritation as the creams are applied and left for up to 15 minutes after which they are wiped away with the destroyed hair. Chronic skin irritation can worsen the hirsutism and it is poorly tolerated in the armpit and face. The use of waxing, plucking and/or depilatories in androgenized skin should therefore be discouraged.[11]

Electrolysis uses a needle inserted into the hair follicle in the region of the germinative bulb, and destroying it by an electronic current. Whilst it is effective, it is nevertheless expensive, painful and time consuming. In addition, it can result in pit-like scars and pigment changes.[12]

There are three electrolysis techniques:[12]

(i) galvanic electrolysis – a direct current is passed through the needle into the hair follicle.
(ii) thermolysis – a high frequency alternating current is passed through through the needle and produces destructive heat
(iii) blend – combination of (i) and (ii)

Topical lidocaine can minimize pain. Shaving increases the efficacy as it ensures that only anagen hair is targeted; telogen hair is difficult to remove permanently.[9] Electrolysis is unfortunately, tedious, highly operator dependent and impractical for the treatment of large numbers of hair.[11]

Lasers and light-assisted hair removal is based on selective photothermolysis[13] i.e. laser light energy selectively targets the hair follicle preventing lateral damage. The targeted hair must be in the anagen phase. Current lasers are of longer wavelengths so that they can be used on darker skins.

The lasers can be grouped into 3 categories based on the type of laser and light sources.[13]

(i) red light systems (694 mm ruby)
(ii) infrared light systems (755 nm alexandrite, 800 nm semiconductor diode, or 1064 nm neodymium: Yttrium – Aluminium – Garnet (Nd:YAG)
(iii) intensed pulsed light (IPL) source (590 – 120 nm)

After laser treatment, especially repeated episodes,

most patients experience erythema and odema (but not lasting more than 48 hours); blistering and crust formation occur in 10–15% of patients, and temporary pigment changes, such as hyperpigmentation (14–35%) and hypopigmentation (10–17%) develop. Dyspigmentation is less common when lasers such as alexandrite or diode are used at longer wavelengths and pulse durations.[13]

Newer developments in lasers e.g. photoderm and epilight can be used for all skin types (light to dark skinned) and hair colours (black, brown, blonde, mixed). The first treatment removes 20% of hair and an eventual 76% can be removed after 6 treatments. There is minimal sunburn like pain and the treatment is protracted (6 to 12 weeks).[13]

Weight reduction

Lean PCOS women, are generally less hirsute than the obese despite having similar serum total testosterone. Excessive weight gain causes insulin resistance with compensatory hyperinsulinaemia with resultant suppression of sex hormone binding globulin (SHBG) and elevation of free biologically active testosterone – hence the hirsutism. Furthermore, insulin is a growth factor for hair growth. Weight loss reduces serum insulin, increases SHBG, causes a decline in free testosterone levels and improves the hirsutism.

Kiddy et al.[14] reported that in obese PCOS women placed on caloric restriction for 7 months, only those who lost >5% of their initial weight had a significant rise in SHBG, lowered free testosterone, fasting insulin and F-G scores. Nevertheless, the attainment of normal weight is not necessary to observe a fall in serum insulin or hirsutism scores as only one PCOS patient attained a normal body mass index.

Topical treatments

Eflornithine was discovered to be an irreversible inhibitor of ornithine decarboxylase, an enzyme essential for polyamine synthesis, necessary for cell division and differentiation. Introduced in 2001, the eflornithine hydrochloride 13.9% cream-vaniqua, is used as treatment for unwanted hair. It is applied to affected areas twice a day for a minimum of 4 hours each.[15] Balfour et al.[16] used vaniqua in 596 hirsute women for 6 months and showed improvements in facial hair in 58% (34% in the placebo arm) of the women. The side effects were minimal (tingling, burning, erythema, rash) – similar to depilatory agents containing thioglycolates that sever chemical bonds and dissolve the hair shafts. If vaniqua is stopped, hair growth resumes and it is back to pretreatment levels by 8 weeks. Hence, it is an efficacious but transient treatment for hirsutism.

Eflornithine has no known human or animal toxicity or teratogenicity (pregnancy category C). However, by virtue of its anti-mitotic, anti-proliferative and anti-differentiation effect, it should be avoided during pregnancy and appropriate contraception provided in the reproductive age-group.[9]

Pharmacological treatment of hirsutism

Pharmacological therapy for hirsutism can be categorized as:

(A)   androgen suppressive or
(B)   antiandrogen

(A) Androgen suppression

Oral contraception pills (OCPs)- progestins, gonadotropin-releasing hormone analogue (GnRHa) treatment and glucocorticoids can suppress ovarian androgen production. Nevertheless, although high androgen levels can theoretically be reduced in this way, the clinical response of hirsutism treatment may not necessarily correlate with the androgen levels. Furthermore, glucocorticoids are not recommended because they can induce or worsen insulin resistance.

(i) Oral Contraceptive Pills (OCPs)

The estrogen (E_2) and progesterone (P_4) in OCPs act synergistically to suppress ovarian androgen production in PCOS women. They act in the following manner:[9,10]

(1) E_2 and P_4 suppress gonadotropin secretion in the follicular phase and also inhibit the mid cycle gonadotropin surge, which decreases ovarian steroidogenesis.
(2) E_2 acts on the liver, increasing circulating SHBG and hence, reduces free testosterone levels.
(3) P_4 inhibits 5α – reductase activity and also antagonizes the androgen receptor.
(4) P4 increases the metabolic clearance rate of testosterone and DHT.[4]

Hence, OCPs are the only agents that works in a tripartite manner:

• Production (ovary, adrenal glands)
• Bioavailability (SHBG)
• Peripheral metabolism (intracellular 5α – reductase, hepatic transformation)

There are a few studies comparing different types of OCPs but none have been shown to be superior to the other in treating hirsutism in PCOS.[17] For example, OCPs using progestins with lower androgenic activity (e.g. norgestimate, desogestrel, gestodene) have not been shown to be more effective in the treatment of hirsutism compared to those progestins with higher androgenic potential (e.g. levonorgestrel, norgestrel)

With regard to the onset of action, the OCP effect is measured in months and years. An observational study showed that it can take up to 36 to 60 cycles to resolve mild to moderate hirsutism.[5] By 60 cycles, a third of women still had hirsutism but significant resolution was seen in severe cases. Generally, OCP therapy is recommended for 1 to 2 years and there is evidence of continued androgen suppression upto 2 years beyond discontinuation i.e. continued benefit despite cessation of therapy.

The best putative choice of progestins is two unique compounds (i) cyproterone acetate and (ii) drosperinone primarily because the progestins also act as antiandrogens. Cyproterone acetate by itself, or in combination with 35 μg of ethinyl estradiol (Diane-35; Dianette), significantly ameliorates hirsutism in PCOS patients.[17,18] The more recent introduction of Yasmin, a combination of 30 μg of ethinyl estradiol and 5 mg of drosperinone, has shown great promise in significant reduction of facial hair growth, and in some women, complete resolution of their hirsutism.[19] The other beneficial effects that make this drug a popular therapeutic choice is the fact that because drosperinone is derived from 17α – spironolactone, it has an anti androgen activity similar to spironolactone – i.e. blockage of the androgen receptor as well as inhibiting ovarian androgen production and increasing SHBG levels by three to four folds. As an aldosterone antagonist, its diuretic effect decreases premenstrual abdominal bloating and breast tenderness.[19] Furthermore, drosperinone has a pharmacological profile similar to natural progesterone and its antimineralocorticoid effects might favour weight maintenance or extra weight loss.

There are two main concerns in Yasmin therapy; one is thromboembolism and the other is its limited efficacy in the obese PCO patients. However, thromboembolism with Yasmin is possible but rare.[20]

Obese PCOS patients failed to demonstrate an improvement in F-G hirsutism scores even after 6 months of treatment with OCPs compared to a clinically significant change in F-G scores in lean PCOS patients; lean PCOS patients demonstrated a statistically significant decline in serum testosterone ($p < 0.001$) and androstenedione ($p < 0.0001$) levels. The change in serum testosterone levels in the obese PCOS patients was less impressive ($p < 0.05$), while the androstenedione levels remained the same.[21]

In another pilot observational study,[22] in 13 out of 17 patients recruited who completed 6 months of therapy, hirsutism scores did not change significantly in women who were clinically hirsute (i.e. baseline F-G score >10). Nevertheless, acne scores showed significant improvement (ANOVA $p < 0.0001$). Although longer randomized controlled trials are needed to confirm these findings, these preliminary data show that Yasmin provides good cycle control and relief of acne, but cannot provide improvement of hirsutism after 6 months of therapy.[22]

Sadly, there is no data to determine if the addition of an antiandrogen might be more effective than either therapy alone in these obese PCOS. However, there is recent data on combination therapy in idiopathic hirsutism as discussed later.

The *risk factors of OCPs* must always be considered especially in those women who have diabetes, hypertension (especially when uncontrolled), smokers, those who are obese, or have a history of thromboembolism. The risk of myocardial infarction and stroke are increased in the presence of risk factors.[23]

The risk of venous thromboembolism (VTE) and pulmonary thromboembolism (PTE) is slightly increased amongst OCP users. The increased risk of VTE is greatest in the first year of use, and higher in the obese and those with hypertension and diabetes.[23]

OCPs also have a negative effect on carbohydrate metabolism, an important issue in PCOS, where many women are insulin resistant, glucose intolerant or established diabetics. Ethinyl estradiol increases the glucose response by up to 50% in an oral glucose tolerance test (OGTT) and can cause insulin resistance following the intravenous glucose tolerance test (IVGTT).[24] To moderate this effect, lowering the ethinyl estradiol dose from 50 μg to 20 μg lowers the severity of the hyperinsulinemia. The use of progestins as levonorgestrel may have just as great an effect on insulin response with resultant hyperinsulinemia. However, using norethindrone or desogestrel instead, can minimize this effect.[24]

(ii) Progestins alone

When estrogens are contraindicated or not well tolerated, then, progestins alone can be used. Medroxyprogesterone acetate (MPA) as a depot (Depo-Provera 150 mg, intramuscularly every 3 months), or oral MPA (eg. Provera, 10 mg to 30 mg daily), is effective in the treatment of hirsutism.[4] MPA can also inhibit

steroidogenic enzymes i.e. 3 β-hydroxysteroid dehydrogenase. However, the use of MPA has been associated with a decrease in SHBG in PCOS patients.[18]

Cyproterone acetate (CPA) is a progestin that is very effective for the treatment hirsutism and alopecia especially in obese, hyperandrogenic women with alopecia.[25] The dose of CPA given as a progestin is markedly higher (50 mg/day) than in the OCP Diane-35, and usually has a profound suppression on the hypothalamic-pituitary axis. This higher dose of CPA in PCO women is more effective in treating hirsutism than spironolactone alone.[26]

(iii) Gonadotropin-releasing-hormone agonists (GnRHa)

GnRH agonists suppress gonadotropin production, hence reduce ovarian steroidogenesis and androgen levels. The main downside of using GnRHa for the treatment of hirsutism is symptoms of estrogen deprivation and the loss of bone mineral density. Add-back estrogen and progestin therapy as OCPs or supplemental hormone replacement therapy (HRT) can alleviate these side effects to a certain extent.

Lemay et al.[27] used GnRHa (3.6 mg/month) subcutaneously for one year with add-back transdermal estrogen and cyclical MPA from the third month of treatment. In the 8 women studied, F-G scores declined within 90 days, with continued progressive decline for the remainder of the 12-month interval. There was residual benefit even 6 months after discontinuation. A comparative trial of hirsute women treated with only OCPs versus GnRHa + HRT showed a greater improvement in F-G scores and better tolerance of treatment in the GnRHa group. Only the hirsute women in the GnRHa arm of the study showed a statistically significant decrease in F-G scores and hair growth rate but not the OCP treatment arm.[28]

GnRHa with OCPs was less effective than OCPs with antiandrogens like flutamide or CPA.[29] Furthermore, GnRHa is very costly and not a practical initial choice in the treatment of hirsutism.

(B) Antiandrogen therapy

Androgen antagonism prevents the binding of testosterone and other androgens to the receptors and therefore, treats the hyperandrogenism and hirsutism. Other beneficial effects include direct inhibition of steroidogenesis, improvement in insulin sensitivity and circulating lipids.

There is a risk however, of feminization of the external genitalia of a male fetus and because of this teratogenic effect, antiandrogens are often used in combination with OCPs to prevent unexpected pregnancies.

(i) Spironolactone

Spironolactone is an antiandrogen that binds to the androgen receptor with 67% of the affinity of DHT. It is also an aldosterone antagonist and has multiple antiandrogenic effects, namely, inhibition of ovarian and adrenal androgen production, competitive blockade of DHT binding to skin androgen receptors, elevation of SHBG levels, increased testosterone clearance from the body and decreased 5 α-reductase activity.[30]

There was a statistically significant reduction in hair growth and F-G scores in women receiving daily doses of 100 mg and 200 mg spironolactone. Spironolactone (100 mg/day) is more effective than finasteride (5 mg/day) and CPA (12.5 mg/day) in reducing hair growth.[30]

The side effects include polydypsea, polyuria, nausea, headaches, fatigue, gastritis and ovulatory dysfunction causing polymenorrhoea – this effect can be controlled with concomitant OCPs. As it is a diuretic and aldosterone antagonist, it can cause/exacerbate hyperkalemia and must be used judiciously in women with renal impairment.[9]

Spironolactone is less effective in comparison to flutamide (500 mg/day) and takes longer for benefits to be observed i.e. 5 months versus 3 months respectively.

(ii) Flutamide

Flutamide is a non-steroidal antiandrogen. It blocks the androgen receptor, disrupts testosterone and DHT cellular uptake and promotes androgen metabolism to inactive compounds. In contrast to spironolactone, flutamide does not interact with glucocorticoids, progesterone or estrogen receptors when it exerts its blockade of androgen receptors.

Side effects of flutamide include dryness of skin, discoloured urine but more importantly, there have been reports of hepatitis and renal failure.[10]

There have been no reports of fatal hepatotoxicity in doses ≤500 mg/day but mild, transient hepatotoxicity with daily doses between 375 mg to 500 mg, have been reported.[31] However, some authors have reported that long term treatment of PCOS women with flutamide, 500 mg/day for 24 months, was not associated with significant adverse effects. The F-G scores showed significant improvement in 6 months and continued to decline steadily in the remaining 18 months.[32]

Muderris et al.[31,33] showed that flutamide was effective in high (250 mg) and low (125 mg and 62.5 mg/day) doses. There were no reports of hepatotoxicity or other significant side effects at these doses.

Monthly combination therapy i.e. flutamide (250 mg/day) with GnRHa in women with PCO showed a significant reduction in the F-G score, which was maintained even 6 months after the treatment was discontinued.[34]

Another prospective, randomized trial that compared the clinical efficacy of flutamide (250 mg/day) for the first 10 days of the cycle) with spironolactone (100 mg/day) + Diane-35 in the treatment of idiopathic hirsutism, showed that there was a prominent decrease in F-G scores in the flutamide group (from 19.93 ± 4.31 to 15.58 ± 4.28) compared to the spironolactone + Diane-35 group (from 18.77 ± 3.76 to 14.54 ± 3.29), but this difference did not attain statistical significance.[35]

There is a greater risk of teratogenicity with flutamide and women should be counseled about its effects on the male fetus and must use contraception.[9]

(iii) Finasteride

The enzyme 5 α-reductase that converts testosterone to DHT (see Figure 20.1) exists in two isoforms, type 1, found predominantly in the skin, and type 2, found predominantly in the prostate and reproductive tissues. Finasteride, first introduced in 1992 to treat prostatic disorders, is a potent inhibitor of both these isoenzymes.[36] As finasteride blocks the conversion of testosterone to DHT, serum testosterone levels tend to rise. Furthermore, inhibition of 5 α-reductase can cause feminization of a male fetus – hence, effective contraception must be used. Other side effects are mild gastrointestinal disturbances, headaches, dry skin and decreased libido.[37] Finasteride is better tolerated than other anti androgens with minimal hepatic and renal toxicity. It is available as a 5 mg tablet for the treatment of prostate cancer and a 1 mg tablet for the treatment of male alopecia.[10]

Wong et al.[36] showed that both, finasteride (5 mg/day) and spironolactone (100 mg/day) were equally efficacious in reducing F-G scores and hair shaft diameters in 14 hirsute women after only 3 months of treatment. Continuous therapy for a further 3 months produced continued improvement of both the hair growth parameters.

In another study, half the standard dose (2.5 mg/day) of finasteride was just as efficacious in the treatment of hirsutism as the higher dose.[37] Hence, both the 2.5 mg and 5 mg doses accomplish an equivalent reduction in hirsutism scores at 6 months and 12 months post-treatment. As expected, the side effects and medication cost was decreased in the group on the lower dose.

Insulin sensitizing agents

Women with PCOS tend to exhibit insulin resistance and compensatory hyperinsulinemia, which in turn increases serum total and free testosterone by stimulating ovarian androgen synthesis and lowering circulating SHBG levels. Insulin is also a growth factor for hair. Hence, therapies that improve insulin sensitivity, might decrease hyperandrogenemia and hence, improve hirsutism. Metformin, pioglitazone and acarbose are examples of some of the insulin sensitizing agents used for treatment.

The most commonly used agent in this class

of drugs is metformin. It belongs to the biguanide class of antihyperglycemics and acts by inhibiting hepatic gluconeogenesis. Minor complaints following the initiation of metformin, generally include gastrointestinal symptoms (i.e. nausea, diarrhoea, abdominal bloating). Major complications such as lactic acidosis, albeit rare, can be serious. Precautions include preliminary serum creatinine estimation and liver function tests, which should be repeated 6 and 12 months into treatment.[38]

The trials involving metformin use for the treatment of hirsutism have generally been small, some showing no significant change in the hirsutism scores,[39,40] and others detecting only slight improvements in hirsutism scores.[41,42] In the Cochrane review of trials for the efficacy of metformin, only one study was appropriately designed to evaluate hirsutism; this showed no treatment effect.[38] In this review, there were no studies available for the assessment of the impact of metformin on androgenic alopecia. However, in one trial, where metformin was administered 1000 mg/day for 3 months and 2000 mg/day for the subsequent 3 months, there was no change in F-G scores, but there was a significant improvement in hyperinsulinemia and free androgen levels in women with PCO.[40]

Kelly et al.[43] used metformin at 1500 mg/day in PCOS women whose hirsutism was unresponsive to OCPs. In this cohort of patients, there was a statistically significant, albeit minor (10%) decline in F-G scores with an associated decrease in hair growth velocity after 6 months therapy. A comparative trial[44] in PCOS women using OCPs versus metformin (1500 mg/day), showed a significant reduction in F-G scores and mean hair diameter in both the treatment arms. Metformin was better tolerated, as the dropout rate was 3 and 7 for metformin and OCPs respectively.

Another group of compounds, the thiazolidinediones, e.g. pioglitazone and rosiglitazone improve insulin sensitivity with a post-insulin receptor mechanism. Pioglitazone and rosiglitazone are selective ligands for the peroxisome proliferator – activated receptor γ (a nuclear hormone receptor expressed predominantly in adipose tissue), and play a central role in controlling the adipocyte gene expression and differentiation.[45]

Furthermore, this group of drugs markedly improves muscle insulin sensitivity, resulting in increased glucose disposal in muscles.

Pioglitazone is very effective in increasing insulin action in PCOS women and is not associated with hepatotoxicity as is the case with troglitazone. Romualdi et al.[45] showed that when pioglitazone, 45 mg/day was used in obese PCOS women, there was a significant improvement in F-G scores within just 2 months of therapy, irrespective of whether the patients were normo- or hyperinsulinemic and hirsutism scores continued to fall throughout the treatment phase of 6 months. This drug is well tolerated and can be successfully used for hirsutism in PCOS patients with no evidence hyperinsulinemia.

Acarbose is an α – glucosidase inhibitor that decreases the absorption of carbohydrates from the intestinal tract, negating the post-prandial rise in glucose and insulin. Acarbose, 300 mg/day in PCOS women was found to normalize the insulin response during an OGTT.[46] This was associated with a significant decline in serum testosterone and androstenedione levels but Ciotta et al.[46] could not demonstrate an improvement in F-G scores at the end of 3 months. The likely explanation for the lack of response proposed by the authors[47] was that, 3 months treatment is insufficient time to notice a change in F-G scores.

Treatment of acne

As mentioned earlier, acne is a disease of the PSU. The PSU is influenced by not only androgen pro-hormones (dehydroepiandrosterone, androstenedione) and androgens (testosterone, dihydrotestosterone), but also estrogens, insulin, insulin-like growth factor, growth hormones, glucorticoids and prolactin. The majority of women with acne have androgenic circulating hormones in the high upper limit range. Upto 50% of women with hyperandrogenism will have acne lesions on the neck, chest and upper back,

excessive sebum production being the precipitating factor for acne lesion formation.

Drugs that are able to decrease circulating levels of pro-androgens and androgens can be used to treat acne, e.g. OCPs. Similarly, drugs such as cyproterone acetate, and pure anti-androgens like flutamide, acting directly at the skin level to decrease DHT action on the PSU, are even better candidates for treatment.[47]

Acne vulgaris and OCPs

Virtually, all OCPs combining an estrogen and a progestin, can ultimately improve the acne as they all increase the hepatic synthesis of SHBG, hence decrease free serum testosterone, and also inhibit FSH and LH production, which in turn decreases ovarian androgen synthesis.[47]

OCPs should be the first-line therapy in young women with acne and who desire contraception. Although the efficacy of OCPs in the treatment of acne has been available since 1980s, it was only in 1997 when the first randomized placebo-controlled trial was published.[48] When norgestimate was compared against a placebo, both treatments worked in reducing the lesion counts. It is likely that the placebo effect was a result of proper skin-care practice. Nevertheless, the OCP group had a statistically significant improvement over the placebo group, i.e. 46% reduction in lesion count. Some studies suggest that there is an added advantage with formulations that contain a low androgenic progestin.[49]

Rosen et al.[49] have also shown that OCPs containing levonorgestrel or desogestrel produce a 50% reduction in acne lesions after nine cycles of therapy. The improvements are brought about largely from reduction in sebum production and probably, by alterations in follicular cell desquamation, the impact being greater in the upper chest and forehand, where there are more and larger sebaceous glands.

In nearly all the currently available OCPs, the estrogen component is ethinyl estradiol, present in low dosages ranging from 20 μg to 35 μg. These low doses of estrogen only have a subtle effect on inhibition of sebum secretion, which is mediated by the estrogenic stimulation of the hepatic synthesis of SHBG, resulting in lowered circulating levels of testosterone.

The progestin components in OCPs are derivatives of testosterone or progesterone. The androgenic effect of these testosterone derivatives ranges from almost none (e.g. norgestimate, desogestrel) to mild and moderate ones. The only progesterone derivative contained in an OCP is cyproterone acetate – CPA (Diane-35) whose effect is such that it is categorized as an anti-androgen. Cyproterone acetate alone, is a potent progesterone that decreases LH secretion and testosterone production, blocks androgen receptor binding and inhibits 5α reductase activity. CPA at high daily doses of 50 mg to 100 mg for 10 days each month is associated with a 75% improvement.[50] Androcur is a CPA, which is used in doses ranging from 10 mg to 50 mg owing to its anti androgenic action upon acne. Most of the commonly used OCPs can be used for contraceptive purposes as well as for the treatment of moderate acne. The best choice of an OCP for acne treatment should be one containing a non-androgenic progestin or better, an anti androgenic one. Here, Diane-35, the only hormone for which the sole indication is acne, is regarded as the gold standard for acne treatment.[50] As Diane-35 also inhibits ovulation, it carries a concomitant contraceptive benefit. Diane 35 is indicated for the treatment of severe acne not responding to oral antibiotics. Furthermore, in conditions such as polycystic ovarian disease (PCOD), or in patients in whom there is significant acne, seborrhoea and hirsutism, Diane-35 is the ideal choice of treatment.

Acne and other agents

Spironolactone, an antiandrogen and aldosterone antagonist, decreases sebum production and improves acne.[50] Although some women experience positive benefits with just 25 mg daily, the therapeutic dose for acne can vary between 50 mg to 100 mg a day. Addition of spironolactone to OCPs for resistant cases can increase the efficacy of OCPs in alleviating acne. Further, because spironolactone is teratogenic, combining it with OCPs provides contraception as well. One such combination is the new OCP (Yasmin) containing drosperinone, which is a progestin derived from 17α – spironolactone with anti androgenic activity similar to spironolactone.[9]

Flutamide, a non-steroidal antiandrogen, is associated with hepatotoxicity and hence, best used at lower doses than those for hirsutism. Daily doses of 62.5 mg or 125 mg have been shown to be effective for mild to moderate acne.[50] Combination therapy with an OCP makes flutamide more effective in the treatment of acne than if used alone. Furthermore, its potential effects on the normal development of a male fetus, warrants concomitant OCPs use.

Finasteride inhibits 5-α reductase through its affinity for the type 1 isoenzyme that is involved in the formation of acne. The dosages need to be high to block this enzyme, as its receptor affinity is low. A comparative study of 5 mg of finasteride with 250 mg of flutamide showed a 36% decrease in acne scores compared to the 60% decrease with flutamide.[51] In this study, the significant placebo effect apparent in acne clinical trials had prompted the authors to conclude that 5 mg of finasteride is no more efficacious than the placebo in acne score improvement and hence, this drug is not recommended for acne.[51]

Insulin sensitizing agents like metformin, 1500 mg daily for 12 months, have produced improvements in acne scores without much change in the sebum excretion rate.[44]

Poulin[47] summarized the practical treatment of acne in female patients as follows. Be it "mild" or "moderate to severe" acne, benzoyl peroxide is used in conjunction with an antibiotic whose effect can be topical for mild acne but systemic for moderate to severe acne. Topical retinoids (tretinoin, adapalene, tazarotene) are good for mild and moderate to severe acne, but in the more severe form of disease, the clinician must consider a course of oral isotretinoin, in which case, two reliable forms of contraception must be used.

In moderate to severe acne, hormonal treatment

in the form of Diane-35 or other OCPs is combined with systemic antibiotics.

The following table (table 20.1) summarizes the step-wise approach to acne management.

Table 20.1 The step-wise approach to acne management

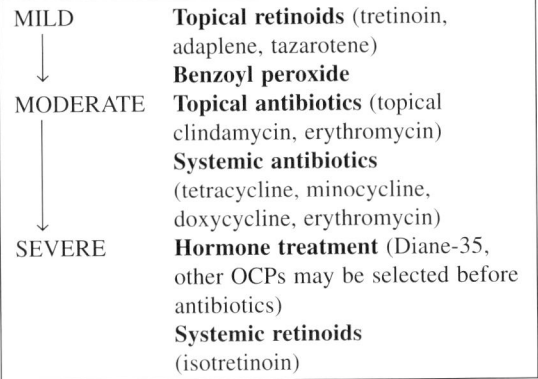

MILD	**Topical retinoids** (tretinoin, adaplene, tazarotene)
↓	**Benzoyl peroxide**
MODERATE	**Topical antibiotics** (topical clindamycin, erythromycin)
↓	**Systemic antibiotics** (tetracycline, minocycline, doxycycline, erythromycin)
SEVERE	**Hormone treatment** (Diane-35, other OCPs may be selected before antibiotics)
	Systemic retinoids (isotretinoin)

Hirsutism and acne in menopause

There is a tendency for the development of hirsutism in the menopausal period due to high LH levels inducing ovarian androgen production. However, a sudden onset of hirsutism should be investigated to exclude an androgen-secreting tumor. In post menopausal women who have PCOS, cyproterone acetate in a sequential regimen with hormone replacement dosages of estrogen can be used.[52]

Some women with PCOS have ovarian hyperthecosis with the ovaries packed with luteinized theca cells, which under the influence of high LH from ovarian failure increase androgen synthesis. Here, medication is inefficacious and oophorectomy must be seriously considered.[52]

Conclusion

Women with PCOS not only have to grapple with obesity and its attendant metabolic problems, but sometimes, also have to go through fertility treatments. For overweight PCOS women, even a 5% weight reduction can result in improvement in the metabolic parameters and F-G scores.

Hirsutism and acne, a frequent accompanying problem, exert tremendous psychosocial effects in addition to all the other metabolic disturbances.

The ultimate goal of medical therapy is to reduce the time spent in mechanically removing unwanted hair – an endeavour that must not be discouraged. The simple measure of shaving provides immediate visual improvement of hirsutism, does not lead to its worsening and provides at least a quick short-term option for facial (especially chin) hirsutism.

The first line pharmacological treatment should be OCPs, particularly those containing cyproterone acetate, with the inclusion of anti-androgens (spironolactone, flutamide, finasteride) at the lowest effective dose to enhance clinical efficacy. Antiandrogens overall, are more effective than androgen suppression therapy for hirsutism and acne. Metformin is a useful second-line therapy in hyperinsulinemic PCOS women.

Patients must be counseled that medical treatment takes time to exert its full effects and that hirsutism, and sometimes acne, is likely to recur if treatment is stopped. Maintenance therapy such as OCPs with or without low dose CPA is indicated. Treatment to stem worsening hirsutism is likely to be more successful than reversing an already established and prolific hirsutism. It is therefore, more prudent to start medical therapy early in young mildly hirsute adolescents, particularly when they have a family history of moderate to severe hirsutism.

With regard to acne, the gold standard of treatment is CPA with ethinyl estradiol. OCPs have been proven to provide safe and effective long-term control of acne. Combination therapy with other systemic and topical agents as prescribed in the algorithm is the clinical approach of choice.

References

1. Stein IF, Leventhal ML. Amernorrhoea associated with bilateral polycystic ovaries. *Am J Obstet Gynecol* 1935; 29: 181–191.
2. The Rotterdam ESHRE/ASRM-sponsored PCOS consensus workshop group: Fauser B, Tarlatzis B, Chang J, Azziz R et al. Revised 2003 consensus on diagnostic criteria and long-term health risks related to polycystic ovary syndrome (PCOS). *Hum Reprod* 2004; 19: 41–47.

3. Dunaif A. Insulin resistance and the polycystic syndrome: mechanism and implications for pathogenesis. *Endocr Rev* 1997; 18: 774–800.

4. Azziz R. The evaluation and management of hirsutism. *Obstet Gynecol* 2003; 101: 995–1007.

5. Falsetti L, Gambera A, Andrico S, Sartoni E. Acne and hirsutism in polycystic ovary syndrome: clinical, endocrine-metabolic and ultrasonographic differences. *Gynecol Endocrin* 2002; 16: 275–284.

6. Toscano V, Balducci R, Bianchi P et al. Two different pathogenic mechanisms may play a role in acne and hirsutism. *Clin Endocrinol* 1993; 39: 551–556.

7. Bunker CB, Newton J, Kilborn J et al. Most women with acne have polycystic ovaries. *Br J Dermatol* 1989; 121: 675–680.

8. Ferriman D, Gallwey JD. Clinical assessment of body hair growth in women. *J Clin Endocrinol Metab* 1961; 21: 1440–447.

9. Archer JS, Chang RJ. Hirsutism and acne in polycystic ovary syndrome. *Best Pract and Research Clin Obstet Gynecol* 2004; 18(5): 737–754.

10. Balen AH, Conway GS, Homburg R, Legro R S (eds). Polycystic ovary syndrome. A guide to clinical management: Disorders of the Pilosebaceous unit: hirsutism and androgenic alopecia, Thomson Publishers (UK), 2005; 143–158.

11. Richards RN, Uy M, Meharg G. Temporary hair removal in patients with hirsutism: a clinical study. *Cutis* 1990; 45(3): 199–202.

12. Richards RN. Electrolysis for the treatment of hypertrichosis and hirsutism. *Skin Therapy Lett* 1999; 4 (6): 3–4.

13. Schroeter CA, Raulin C, Thurlimann W, Reineke T, De Potter C, Neumann HA. Hair removal in 40 hirsute women with an intense laser-like light source. *Eur J Dermatol* 1999; 9(5): 374–379.

14. Kiddy DS, Hamilton-Fairley D, Bush A, Short F, Anyaoku V, Reed MJ, Franks S. Improvement in endocrine and ovarian function during dietary treatment of obese women with polycystic ovary syndrome. *Clin Endocrinol* (Oxf). 1992; 36(1): 105–111.

15. Shapiro J, Lui H. Vaniqa—eflornithine 13.9% cream. *Skin Therapy Lett* 2001 Apr; 6(7): 1–3, 5. Erratum in: *Skin Therapy Lett* 2001; 6(8): 5.

16. Balfour JA, McClellan K. Topical eflornithine. *Am J Clin Dermatol* 2001; 2(3): 197–201.

17. Sobbrio GA, Granata A, D'Arrigo F, Arena D, Panacea A, Trimarchi F, Granese D, Pulle C. Treatment of hirsutism related to micropolycystic ovary syndrome (MPCO) with two low-dose oestrogen oral contraceptives: a comparative randomized evaluation. *Acta Eur Fertil* 1990; 21(3): 139–141.

18. Dahlgren E, Landin K, Krotkiewski M, Holm G, Janson PO. Effects of two antiandrogen treatments on hirsutism and insulin sensitivity in women with polycystic ovary syndrome. *Hum Reprod* 1998; 13(1O): 2706–2711.

19. vanVioten WA, van Haselen CW, van Zuuren EJ et al. The effect of 2 combined oral contraceptives containing either drosperinone or cyproterone acetate on acne and seborrhea *Cutis* 2002; 69: 2–15.

20. van Grootheest K, Vrieling T. Thromboemoblism associated with the new contraceptive Yasmin. *Br Med J* 2003; 326–35.

21. Cibula D, Hill M, Fanta M, Sindelka G, Zivny J. Does obesity diminish the positive effect of oral contraceptive treatment on hyperandrogenism in women with polycystic ovarian syndrome? *Hum Reprod* 2001; 16(5): 940–944.

22. Palep-Singh M, Barth JH, Mook K, Balen H. An observational study of Yasmin in the management of polycystic ovarian syndrome. *J Fam Plann Reprod Health Care* 2004; 30: 163–165.

23. Petitti DB. Combination estrogen-progestin oral contraceptives. *New Engl J Med* 2003; 349: 1443–1450.

24. Cook D and Godsland I. Safety evaluation of modern oral contraceptives. *Contraception* 1998; 57: 189–201.

25. Vexian P, Chaspoux C, Boudou P, Fiet J et al. Effects of minoxidil 2% vs cryproterone acetate treatment on female androgenetic alopecia: a controlled, 12-month randomized trial. *Br J Dermatol* 2002; 146: 992–999.

26. Spritzer PM, Lisboako, Mattiello S, Lhullier F. Spironolactone as a single agent for long term therapy of hirsute patients. *Clin Endocrinol (oxf)* 2000; 52: 587–594.

27. Lemay A and Faure N. Segmental oestrogen-progestin addition to gonadotrophin-releasing hormone agonist suppression for the chronic treatment of ovarian hyperandrogenism: a pilot study. *J Clin Endocrinol Metab* 1994; 79: 1716–1722.

28. Azziz R, Ochoa TM, Bradley EL Jr, Potter HD, Boots LR. Leuprolide and estrogen versus oral contraceptive pills for the treatment of hirsutism: a prospective randomized study. *J Clin Endocrinol Metab* 1995; 80(12): 3406–3411.

29. Pazos F, Escobar-Morreale HF, Balsa J. A prospective randomized controlled trial comparing the long acting GnRH agonist triptorelin, flutamide and CPA used in combination with OCPs in the treatment of hirsutism. *Fertil Steril* 1999; 71: 122.

30. Farquhar C, Lee O, Toomath R, Jepson R. Spironolactone versus placebo or in combination with steroids for hirsutism and/or acne. *Cochrane Database Syst Rev*. 2003; (4): CD000194.

31. Muderris II B, Ayram F and Guven M. A prospective randomized trial comparing flutamide (250 mg/d) and finasteride (5 mg/d) in the treatment of hirsutism. *Fertil Steril* 2000; 73: 984–987.

32. Pucci E, Genazzani AD, Monzani F, Lippi F, Angelini F, Gargani M, Barletta D, Luisi M, Genazzani AR. Prolonged treatment of hirsutism with flutamide alone in patients affected by polycystic ovary syndrome. *Gynecol Endocrinol* 1995; 9(3): 221–228.

33. Muderris II B, Ayram F. Clinical efficacy of lower dose flutamide 125 mg/day in the treatment of hirsutism. *J Endocrin Invest* 1999; 22: 165–168.

34. De Leo V, Fulghesu AM, la Marca A, Morgante G, Pasqui L, Talluri B, Torricelli M, Caruso A. Hormonal and clinical effects of GnRH agonist alone, or in combination with a combined oral contraceptive or flutamide in women with severe hirsutism. *Gynecol Endocrinol* 2000; 14(6): 411–416.

35. Inal MM, Yildirim Y and Taner EC. Comparison of the clinical efficacy of flutamide and spironolactone plus Diane-35 in the treatment of idiopathic hirsutism: a randomized controlled study. *Fertil Steril* 2005; 84: 1693–1697.

36. Wong IL, Morris RS, Chang L, Spahn MA, Stanczyk FZ, Lobo RA. A prospective randomized trial comparing finasteride to spironolactone in the treatment of hirsute women. *J Clin Endocrinol Metab* 1995; 80(1): 233–238.

37. Muderris II BF, Guven M, Kelestimur F. Comparison of high-dose finasteride (5 mg/day) versus low-dose finasteride (2.5 mg/day) in the treatment of hirsutism. *European Journal of Endocrinology* 2002; 147: 467–471.

38. Lord JM, Flight IH, Norman RJ. Metformin in polycystic ovary syndrome: systematic review and meta-analysis. *BMJ* 2003 25; 327(7421): 951–953.

39. Morin-Papunen LC, Koivunen RM, Ruokonen A, Martikainen HK. Metformin therapy improves the menstrual pattern with minimal endocrine and metabolic effects in women with polycystic ovary syndrome. *Fertil Steril* 1998; 69: 691–696.

40. Morin-Papumen LC, Vauhkonen I, Koivunen RM, Ruckonen A et al. Endocrine and metaboliic effects of metformin versus ethinyl estradiol – cyproterone acetate in obese women with polycystic ovary syndrome: a randomized study. *Journal of Clinical Endocrinology Metabolism* 2000; 85: 3161–3168.

41. Ibanez L, Vallas C, Potau N, Marcos MV, de Zegher F. Sensitization to insulin in adolescent girls to normalize hirsutism, hyperandrogenaemia, oliogemenorrhoea, dyslipidemia, and hyperinsulinism after precocious pubarche. *J Clin Endocrinol Metab* 2000; 85: 3256–3530.

42. Kolodziejczk B, Duleba AJ, Spaczynski RZ, Pawelczyk L. Metformin therapy decreases hyperandrogenism and hyperinsulinemia in women with polycystic ovary syndrome. *Fertil Steril* 2000; 73: 1149–1154.

43. Kelly CJ, Gordon D. The effect of metformin on hirsutism in polycystic ovary syndrome. *Eur J Endocrinol* 2002; 147(2): 217–221.

44. Harborne L, Fleming R, Lyall H, Sattar N, Norman J. Metformin or antiandrogen in the treatment of hirsutism in polycystic ovary syndrome. *J Clin Endocrinol Metab* 2003; 88(9): 4116–4123.

45. Romualdi D, Guido M, Ciampelli M, Giuliani M, Leoni F, Perri C, Lanzone A. Selective effects of pioglitazone on insulin and androgen abnormalities in normo- and hyperinsulinaemic obese patients with polycystic ovary syndrome. *Hum Reprod* 2003; 18(6): 1210–1218.

46. Ciotta L, Calogero AE, Farina M, De Leo V, La Marca A, Cianci A. Clinical, endocrine and metabolic effects of acarbose, an alpha-glucosidase inhibitor, in PCOS patients with increased insulin response and normal glucose tolerance. *Hum Reprod* 2001; 16(10): 2066–2072.

47. Poulin Y. Practical approach to the hormonal treatment of acne. *J Cutan Med Surg* 2004; 8 Suppl 4: 16–21.

48. Redmond GP, Olson WH, Lippman JS, Kafrissen ME, Jones TM, Jorizzo JL. Norgestimate and ethinyl estradiol in the treatment of acne vulgaris: a randomized, placebo-controlled trial. *Obstet Gynecol* 1997; 89(4): 615–622.

49. Rosen MP, Breitkopf DM, Nagamani M. A randomized controlled trial of second- versus third-generation oral contraceptives in the treatment of acne vulgaris. *Am J Obstet Gynecol* 2003; 188(5): 1158–1160.

50. Thiboutot D, Chen W. Update and future of hormonal therapy in acne. *Dermatology* 2003; 206(1): 57–67.

51. Carmina E, Lobo RA. A comparison of the relative efficacy of antiandrogens for the treatment of acne in hyperandrogenic women. *Clin Endocrinol* (Oxf). 2002; 57(2): 231–234.

52. Nikolaou D, Gilling-Smith C. Hirsutism. Current Obstet and Gynecol 2005; 15: 174–182.

Dyslipidemia

21

Predictors of Dyslipidemia in Women with Polycystic Ovary Syndrome

Hashim Jamal, Kemal Ozgur

Summary

There is a growing body of epidemiological evidence supporting the link between dyslipidemia and polycystic ovary syndrome (PCOS). Dyslipidemia seems to be a feature of PCOS, but its pathogenesis remains controversial.

There has been little hypothesis-generating research exploring the interplay between lipid dysfunction and PCOS. Many mechanisms have been speculated. Insulin resistance and hyperandrogenism seem to play a key role in the pathophysiology of PCOS and its related endocrine and metabolic abnormalities including dyslipidemia.

In previous studies and clinical trials, investigators have confounded hyperlipidemia in PCOS women. However, further studies are needed to elucidate the physiopathogenesis of dyslipidemia and its prevention and determine the appropriate medical therapies and drug combinations to reduce the risk of dyslipidemia and cardiovascular disease in these women.

Rationale

The purpose of this chapter is to evaluate the literature pertinent to dyslipidemia in women with PCOS. Medline, Current Contents, and Pub-Med were searched.

This chapter focuses on:
- the epidemiological evidence linking dyslipidemia with PCOS and the identification of issues relevant to dyslipidemia.
- the underlying mechanisms of dyslipidemia in PCOS women.
- the current and future trends in the use of combination and adjunctive therapies.

Introduction

Polycystic ovary syndrome, defined as the combination of oligo/anovulation and hyperandrogenism, affects more than 5% of women of reproductive age.[1] The syndrome is a heterogeneous disorder with widespread systemic manifestations. Although originally considered a gynecological disorder, it is associated with a wide range of endocrine and metabolic abnormalities, including coronary heart disease (CHD), diabetes mellitus, dyslipidemia, visceral obesity, and hypertension.[2]

Dyslipidemia is a disorder of lipoprotein metabolism, including lipoprotein overproduction or deficiency. These changes may be manifested by the elevation of serum total cholesterol, low-density lipoprotein (LDL) cholesterol and triglycerides (TG) concentration, and a decrease in the high density lipoprotein (HDL) cholesterol concentration.[3]

Although abnormalities in lipid and lipoprotein levels have been widely reported in women with PCOS, several studies have reported conflicting views with regard to the features of dyslipidemia.[4,5] Some studies have described elevated total cholesterol concentrations, while other previous investigators have been fairly consistent in their reports of hypertriglyceridemia.[6–8] Other researchers have demonstrated significantly lower levels of HDL cholesterol in women with PCOS compared with weight-matched controls.[6,9] Nevertheless, in several studies, investigators have failed to find differences in circulating lipid levels in women with PCOS as compared with weight-matched control women.[7,9,10]

These conflicting studies are reviewed in this article for a better understanding of dyslipidemia and medication that may be used alone or in conjunction to decrease the risk of dyslipidemia in women with PCOS.

Clinical Discussion

Women with polycystic ovary syndrome are at an increased risk for atherosclerosis and should be targeted for primary prevention of CHD.[11] Dyslipidemia was found to be a major prognostic risk factor for cardiovascular disease (CVD). Hypertension, dyslipidemia and diabetes must be treated in PCOS women and these women must be followed carefully all through their life.

Women with PCOS are at an increased risk for metabolic syndrome.[12] Additionally, the prevalence of metabolic syndrome is increased in sisters with PCOS.[13] Metabolic Syndrome, also called Syndrome X or Insulin Resistance Syndrome, is a combination of insulin resistance diabetes mellitus, dyslipidemia, hypertension, and central obesity. Insulin resistance (71%) is the most common metabolic abnormality in PCOS patients followed by obesity (52%) and dyslipidemia (46.3%), with an incidence of (31.5%) for the metabolic syndrome.[1] The lipid profile of patients with the metabolic syndrome is often characterized by the appearance of hypertrygliceridemia and small, dense LDL,

together with low HDL. Patients with these abnormalities are at an increased risk for premature CHD.[14] As compared to women without PCOS, 85% of PCOS women have dyslipidemia characteristic of the metabolic syndrome.[15]

Although most studies suggest an association between dyslipidemia and PCOS, their results are somewhat conflicting. Most studies suggest that PCOS patients are hyperlipidemic with higher total cholesterol, LDL and TG concentrations and lower HDL levels than controls.[16,17] On the other hand, Bickerton et al.[18] have demonstrated that there are no significant differences in lipid, or lipoprotein concentrations between patients with PCOS and weight-matched controls.

To what extent are PCOS, obesity and dyslipidemia related?

Obesity has an important influence on the lipid profile. Dyslipidemia of obesity is characterized by low levels of HDL, increased TG, increased subfractions of small, dense LDL, and increased levels of apolipoprotein B-100 (ApoB-100).[19,20]

Approximately 50% of patients with PCOS are overweight or obese with abdominal fat accumulation.[21] In several studies, investigators demonstrated that lipid and lipoprotein concentrations did not differ in obese, overweight and non obese PCOS women compared to the normal groups, while HDL was decreased in obese PCOS and obese control women.[9,22,23]

Robinson et al.[7] evaluated lipids and lipoproteins in women with PCOS, compared the results with weight-matched controls, and related the findings to indices of insulin secretion and action, and menstrual history. In this study, total serum cholesterol levels were similar in obese and non obese PCOS women, while total HDL was decreased significantly only in the obese PCOS group. The authors concluded that PCOS is associated with biochemical risk factors for premature vascular disease, which cannot be explained by obesity alone.

In a large study of non-Hispanic White women, elevations in LDL levels were the predominant lipid abnormality in women with PCOS, independent of obesity.[24] In addition, a significant finding was the decrease in ApoA1/ApoB ratio among women with PCOS compared to women with obesity, but with normal ovarian morphology and regular menstrual cycles.[25]

In non-obese patients with PCOS, serum TG levels correlated with visceral fat and preperitoneal fat thickness. The mean HDL levels correlated negatively with visceral fat and preperitoneal fat thickness. In a multiple regression analysis, visceral fat thickness contributed significantly to high serum TG. The authors concluded that intra-abdominal, preperitoneal, and visceral fat accumulation may contribute to the development of lipid metabolism disorders in nonobese patients with PCOS.[26].

Previous reports of lipid abnormalities in PCOS patients have produced conflicting results, which may, in part, be related to the lack of appropriate controls. We conclude that dyslipidemia is found more frequently in women with PCOS, independent of the excess weight that is often found in this patient group, and cannot be explained by obesity alone.

Are first-degree relatives of PCOS women at increased risk for dyslipidemia?

There is a strong familial component of PCOS, but the mode of inheritance is still uncertain.[1] Hahn and colleagues presented a characterization of PCOS from North Rhine-Westphalia in Germany. Clinical features, family history as well as endocrine and metabolic parameters were prospectively recorded from 200 successive patients. PCOS patients showed significantly higher body mass index (BMI), body fat mass and androgen levels, as well as impaired glucose and insulin metabolism.

Sam et al.[13] enrolled a study to test the hypothesis that dyslipidemia is a heritable trait in sisters of women with PCOS. They found that low-density lipoprotein levels are increased in affected sisters of women with PCOS consistent with a heritable trait. The prevalence of the metabolic syndrome is also increased in affected sisters. The probability of finding a metabolic disorder in the families of PCOS patients, is 2.7 fold higher than in the control group families. Metabolic disorders are more frequent in parents and grandparents of PCOS patients than in those of normal women.[27] The brothers of women with PCOS also have insulin resistance, which is associated with abnormalities in serum lipid concentrations.[28]

Dyslipidemia in postmenopausal PCOS women

Polycystic ovary syndrome is common in post-menopausal women attending outpatient clinics, and is a marker for a metabolic profile that is associated with a high-risk for CVD. Dyslipidemia in ageing women with PCOS is not related to the menstrual cycle pattern but rather, to obesity. A significant association of obesity, rather than raised testosterone, with dyslipidemia was also confirmed.[29]

Is hyperinsulinemia or hyperandrogenism responsible for dyslipidemia in PCOS women?

Meirow et al.[16] reported that obesity with marked hyperandrogenism was the predominant feature in patients with insulin resistance (IR). Non insulin resistance (NIR) patients were not obese and had a significantly lesser degree of hyperandrogenism. Insulin was positively correlated with total cholesterol, LDL and TG, and negatively correlated with HDL in IR patients. In NIR subjects, insulin was not correlated with any of the lipids.[16]

Graf et al.[9] clarified the independent effects of hyperandrogenemia, hyperinsulinaemia, and obesity on lipid and lipoprotein levels in women with PCOS. They demonstrated that non-obese PCOS women had significant positive correlations between testosterone and LDL levels, and insulin and TG levels.[9]

In many studies, hyperinsulinemia due to IR has been associated with lipid and lipoprotein abnormalities in women with PCOS.[5,7,30] Insulin related lipid changes in PCOS women account to no more than about 25%.[24] Robinson et al.[7] found that insulin sensitivity accounted for 22% of the lipid variance, while BMI accounted for 54%.[7] Therefore, a relationship between insulin and lipid abnormalities was reported, but the significance of this finding still not clear.

Markers of insulin resistance were found to be higher in classic anovulatory polycystic ovary syndrome(C-PCOS) than ovulatory polycystic ovary syndrome (OV-PCOS) patients. Lipid abnormalities were high in both C-PCOS and OV-PCOS women.[31] Among hyperandrogenic women, the prevalence of abnormal metabolic parameters was higher in C-PCOS than OV-PCOS,[31] and the severity of lipid abnormalities was expected to be much more in women with C-PCOS.

Hyperandrogenemia, in terms of significantly raised total testosterone levels, was found in 30% of the PCOS women. Altered lipid profiles in women with PCOS may result from the independent effects of androgen excess and insulin resistance, which may be a possible explanation for the occurrence of dyslipidemia in PCOS women.[32] Data from other studies have concluded that circulating androgen levels affect lipid and lipoprotein levels in women with PCOS.[4,9,23] Moreover, other researchers suggest that dyslipidemia is secondary to excess androgen action,[33] while still others others have demonstrated no direct correlation of this increase with changes in the lipid-lipoprotein profile.[25]

On the other hand, Rojkowa et al.[23] speculate that altered activity of hepatic lipase or lipid transfer protein can explain the pathophysiogenesis of dyslipidemia in women with the PCOS.

Several theories have been proposed to explain the pathophysiogenesis of dyslipidemia in PCOS women. However, all of these hypotheses are still speculative. The most widely accepted one seems to be that attributing hyperinsulinemia and hyperandrogenemia to dyslipidemia.

Should we use homocysteine (Hcy) or C-reactive protein (CRP) as a risk factor indicator for dyslipidemia in PCOS women?

There is an increase in Hcy levels and CRP levels in PCOS patients. Positive correlations among serum Hcy, insulin and androgen levels have been found in PCOS patients.[34] According to Bayraktar et al.[34], the reason for hyperhomocysteinemia seems to be related to insulin resistance, but not to high androgen levels. However, in another sudy enrolled by a Czech group, Vrbikova et al.[35] pointed that hyperhomocysteinemia is linked to androgen levels.

Other Turkish investigators have determined that patients with PCOS have elevated insulin resistance, plasma Hcy levels, and changes in serum lipid profile, which play an important role in the development of cardiovascular disease, but they observed no correlation between plasma Hcy, BMI, and lipid and lipoprotein levels.[36]

Three recent studies evaluated the association between CRP levels and PCOS. CRP is a marker of inflammation that has been demonstrated in multiple, prospective, epidemiological studies to predict the incident myocardial infarction, stroke, peripheral arterial disease, and sudden death.[37] In a German PCOS cohort study, CRP was frequently elevated in young PCOS patients.[1] Studies have reported that PCOS patients have significantly higher serum CRP levels than healthy women.[38,39] High CRP levels in the PCOS group suggest that women with PCOS may indeed be at risk for early-onset CVD. These results suggest that CRP may be a precursor for dyslipidemia but Boulman et al.[40] did not find any significant relationship between CRP levels and lipid profile in a large group of PCOS patients. Both CRP and Hcy have been shown as independent risk factors for CVD, but the investigation did not conclude a relation with dyslipidemia.

Prevention and treatment of dyslipidemia in PCOS

Short-term trials of metformin have shown promising effects in lowering insulin secretion, improving insulin sensitivity, restoring normal menstrual cycles, and correcting lipid abnormalities.[41] Other studies have shown that metformin reduces circulating levels of free fatty acid (FFA)[42] and decreases fatty acid oxidation.[43,44] Triglyceride levels are also reduced by metformin; hepatic triglyceride synthesis is reduced and clearance of very low-density lipoproteins (VLDL) is increased.[45]

According to Santana and colleagues,[46] metformin use in PCOS patients decreased serum total cholesterol and LDL and increased HDL. Aruna et al.[47] reported an increase in HDL levels and a decrease in total cholesterol following six months of metformin use.

In a prospective, randomized study, aimed to investigate the effects of metformin and ethinyl estradiol-cyproterone acetate on lipid levels in obese and non-obese women with PCOS, thirty-five women with PCOS(18 obese and 17 non-obese) were randomized to six-month treatments with metformin or ethinyl estradiol-cyproterone acetate oral contraceptive pills. Authors demonstrated that metformin treatment has beneficial effects on the lipid profile and therefore, it can be used in the prevention of cardiovascular complications in PCOS women.[48]

Several antiandrogens have been used for the treatment of hirsutism in PCOS treatment. The oral pure androgen receptor blocker, flutamide, inhibits peripheral action of androgens by binding and blocking the androgen receptor. The apparent protective effect of flutamide against dyslipidemia can be explained by the possibility that dyslipidemia is secondary to excess androgen action.[33] Perhaps, the most compelling direct evidence that flutamide may reduce the risk for dyslipidemia comes from two studies. Low dose flutamide [Pubertas praecox (PP)] treatment was found to be an effective and safe approach to reduce hirsutism and circulating androgen, LDL, and TG levels in 18 nonobese adolescent girls

with functional ovarian hyperandrogenism.[49] In another prospective study, seventeen women with PCOS (10 obese and 7 lean) received a 12-week course of flutamide. It was found that flutamide treatment was also associated with an increase in HDL, decrease in the LDL/HDL ratio, decrease in total cholesterol, LDL, and TG. The effects of flutamide on the lipid profile were found regardless of obesity, and were not associated with a change in weight.[50]

The association between flutamide use and dyslipidemia was also evaluated in 12 other obese PCOS women in another study. There was no significant change in total cholesterol, HDL, LDL and TG following 2 months of treatment with a daily dose of 250 mg flutamide. In this study, flutamide did not appear protective against dyslipidemia.[51]

In teenage girls with ovarian hyperandrogenism, low-dose combined flutamide-metformin therapy attenuated a spectrum of abnormalities, including insulin resistance and hyperlipidemia. Furthermore, after nine months of flutamide-metformin therapy, body fat decreased and ovulation rate increased.[52] Lv et al.[53] determined that after six months of treatment with cyproterone acetate(CPA) combined with metformin, BMI and WHR (waist hip ratio) were significantly decreased.

In a study population of 24 women, non-obese, young women with PCOS were randomized to receive a combination of flutamide-metformin and a low-dose oral contraceptive(OC). A total of 12 women elected to receive the OC, and this subgroup (OC+) was matched to a subgroup continuing on flutamide-metformin alone (OC-). In (OC+) women, the beneficial effects of flutamide-metformin on hyperandrogenemia, hyperinsulinemia and dyslipidaemia were maintained, with an additional increase in sex hormone-binding globulin (SHBG) and thus, a further drop in the free androgen index.[54] In a more recent clinical trial, ethinylestradiol (EE) combined with the antiandrogenic progestin cyproterone acetate (CPA), showed a decrease in LDL and total cholesterol/ HDL index, and increases in HDL and TG in PCOS patients.[55]

There now exists a compelling body of evidence of therapy for the prevention of dyslipidemia in PCOS patients. The administration of troglitazone (TGZ), an insulin-sensitizing agent of the thiazolidinedione class, improves dyslipidemia associated with insulin resistance in PCOS.[56] Atherosclerotic lipid levels were also normalized after troglitazone administration.[57] Yilmaz and colleagues[58] demonstrated that these agents are effective in PCOS patients with 'high' baseline lipid measurements.

There is a paucity of studies that have reported long-term changes in lipid profile after weight loss in PCOS women. Following a hypocaloric diet and exercise, the addition of metformin, flutamide or the combined metformin + flutamide treatment, appears to have a more favorable outcome on body fat distribution, androgens, lipids, hirsutism and menses in PCOS women.[59,60] Brown et al.[61] reported a case of biopsy-documented nonalcoholic steatohepatitis (NASH) that improved appreciably through moderate exercise and weight loss in a young woman with PCOS. This case report suggests that fatty liver and NASH may be another important disease to identify in PCOS women, and it also demonstrates the improvement in this condition with moderate exercise and weight loss.[61]

The point, of course, is that metformin and other insulin-sensitizing agents in combination with antiandrogens and low-dose oral contraceptives, may lower the risk of dyslipidemia through unknown mechanisms. These drugs may be recommended for use in, either the prevention, or the treatment of dyslipidemia in PCOS patients. However, more prospective studies are required to establish the link between the use of metformin and other drugs, and the consequent reduction in dyslipidemia.

Conclusion

PCOS is much more than just menstrual irregularity or infertility. PCOS encompasses many long-term health problems such as, the development of dyslipidemia, type 2 diabetes mellitus, and cardiovascular disease.

We argue that, at present, dyslipidemia should be included as a part of the work-up in patients with PCOS. Undoubtedly, all the data available up to the present, suggest that hyperandrogenism and hyperinsulinism possess the intrinsic conditions that lead to an increased incidence of dyslipidemia in PCOS.

Treatment regimens directed toward lowering hyperlipidemia should probably be more aggressive in the future. Of course, in the prevention and treatment of PCOS-related dyslipidemia, the applicability and efficiency of insulin sensitizing agents, antiandrogens and other treatment regimens await the results of long-term clinical studies.

References

1. Hahn S, Tan S, Elsenbruch S, Quadbeck B, Herrmann BL, Mann K, Janssen OE. Clinical and biochemical characterization of women with polycystic ovary syndrome in North Rhine-Westphalia. *Horm Metab Res* 2005; 37(7): 438–444.
2. Lefebvre P, Raingeard I, Renard E, Bringer J. Long-term risks of polycystic ovaries syndrome. *Gynecol Obstet Fertil* 2004; 32(3): 193–198.
3. Jialal I. A practical approach to the laboratory diagnosis of dyslipidemia. *Am J Clin Pathol* 1996; 106(1): 128–138.
4. Wild RA, Painter PC, Coulson PB, Carruth KB, Ranney GB. Lipoprotein lipid concentrations and cardiovascular risk in women with polycystic ovary syndrome. *J Clin Endocrinol Metab* 1985; 61(5): 946–951.
5. Talbott E, Guzick D, Clerici A, Berga S, Detre K, Weimer K, Kuller L. Coronary heart disease risk factors in women with polycystic ovary syndrome. *Arterioscler Thromb Vasc Biol* 1995; 15(7): 821–826
6. Conway GS, Agrawal R, Betteridge DJ, Jacobs HS. Risk factors for coronary artery disease in lean and obese women with the polycystic ovary syndrome. *Clin Endocrinol (Oxf)* 1992; 37(2): 119–125.
7. Robinson S, Henderson AD, Gelding SV et al. Dyslipidaemia is associated with insulin resistance in women with polycystic ovaries. *Clin Endocrinol (Oxf)* 1996; 44(3): 277–284.
8. Pirwany IR, Fleming R, Greer IA, Packard CJ, Sattar N. Lipids and lipoprotein subfractions in women with PCOS: relationship to metabolic and endocrine

parameters. *Clin Endocrinol (Oxf)* 2001; 54(4): 447–453.

9. Graf MJ, Richards CJ, Brown V, Meissner L, Dunaif A. The independent effects of hyperandrogenaemia, hyperinsulinaemia, and obesity on lipid and lipoprotein profiles in women. *Clin Endocrinol (Oxf)* 1990; 33(1): 119–131.

10. Holte J, Bergh T, Berne C, Lithell H. Serum lipoprotein lipid profile in women with the polycystic ovary syndrome: relation to anthropometric, endocrine and metabolic variables. *Clin Endocrinol (Oxf)* 1994; 41(4): 463–471.

11. Christian RC, Dumesic DA, Behrenbeck T, Oberg AL, Sheedy PF, Fitzpatrick LA. Prevalence and predictors of coronary artery calcification in women with polycystic ovary syndrome. *J Clin Endocrinol Metab* 2003; 88(6): 2562–2568.

12. Dokras A, Bochner M, Hollinrake E, Markham S, Vanvoorhis B, Jagasia DH. Screening women with polycystic ovary syndrome for metabolic syndrome. *Obstet Gynecol* 2005; 106(1): 131–137.

13. Sam S, Legro RS, Bentley-Lewis R, Dunaif A. Dyslipidemia and metabolic syndrome in the sisters of women with polycystic ovary syndrome. *J Clin Endocrinol Metab* 2005; 90(8): 4797–4802.

14. Erbas T. Metabolic syndrome. *Acta Diabetol* 2003; 40 Suppl 2: S401–404.

15. Margolin E, Zhornitzki T, Kopernik G, Kogan S, Schattner A, Knobler H. Polycystic ovary syndrome in post-menopausal women—marker of the metabolic syndrome. *Maturitas* 2005; 50(4): 331–336.

16. Meirow D, Raz I, Yossepowitch O, Brzezinski A, Rosler A, Schenker JG, Berry EM. Dyslipidaemia in polycystic ovarian syndrome: different groups, different aetiologies? *Hum Reprod* 1996; 11(9): 1848–1853.

17. Orio F Jr, Palomba S, Spinelli L et al. The cardiovascular risk of young women with polycystic ovary syndrome: an observational, analytical, prospective case-control study. *J Clin Endocrinol Metab* 2004; 89(8): 3696–3701.

18. Bickerton AS, Clark N, Meeking D et al. Cardiovascular risk in women with polycystic ovarian syndrome (PCOS). *J Clin Pathol* 2005; 58(2): 151–154.

19. Miller WM, Nori-Janosz KE, Lillystone M, Yanez J, McCullough PA. Obesity and lipids. *Curr Cardiol Rep* 2005; 7(6): 465–470.

20. Howard BV, Ruotolo G, Robbins DC. Obesity and dyslipidemia. *Endocrinol Metab Clin North Am* 2003; 32(4): 855–867.

21. Faloia E, Canibus P, Gatti C, Frezza F, Santangelo M, Garrapa GG, Boscaro M. Body composition, fat distribution and metabolic characteristics in lean and obese women with polycystic ovary syndrome. *J Endocrinol Invest* 2004; 27(5): 424–429.

22. Esposito V, Federico P, Lo Iudice G, Rispoli C, Sabatino P, D'Alessandro B. Correlation between hormonal and metabolic profiles in women with polycystic ovary syndrome. *Minerva Endocrinol* 1992; 17(1): 21–29.

23. Rajkhowa M, Neary RH, Kumpatla P, Game FL, Jones PW, Obhrai MS, Clayton RN. Altered composition of high density lipoproteins in women with the polycystic ovary syndrome. *J Clin Endocrinol Metab* 1997; 82(10): 3389–3394.

24. Legro RS, Kunselman AR, Dunaif A Prevalence and predictors of dyslipidemia in women with polycystic ovary syndrome. *Am J Med* 2001; 111(8): 607–613.

25. Maitra A, Pingle RR, Menon PS, Naik V, Gokral JS, Meherji PK. Dyslipidemia with particular regard to apolipoprotein profile in association with polycystic ovary syndrome: a study among Indian women. *Int J Fertil Womens Med* 2001; 46(5): 271–277.

26. Yildirim B, Sabir N, Kaleli B. Relation of intra-abdominal fat distribution to metabolic disorders in nonobese patients with polycystic ovary syndrome. *Fertil Steril* 2003; 79(6): 1358–1364.

27. Benitez R, Sir-Petermann T, Palomino A, Angel B, Maliqueo M, Perez F, Calvillan M. Prevalence of metabolic disorders among family members of patients with polycystic ovary syndrome. *Rev Med Chil* 2001; 129(7): 707–712.

28. Kaushal R, Parchure N, Bano G, Kaski JC, Nussey SS. Insulin resistance and endothelial dysfunction in the brothers of Indian subcontinent Asian women with polycystic ovaries. *Clin Endocrinol (Oxf)* 2004; 60(3): 322–328.

29. Elting MW, Korsen TJ, Schoemaker J. Obesity, rather than menstrual cycle pattern or follicle cohort size, determines hyperinsulinaemia, dyslipidaemia and hypertension in ageing women with polycystic ovary syndrome. *Clin Endocrinol (Oxf)* 2001; 55(6): 767–776.

30. Legro RS, Blanche P, Krauss RM, Lobo RA. Alterations in low-density lipoprotein and high-density lipoprotein subclasses among Hispanic women with polycystic ovary syndrome: influence of insulin and genetic factors. *Fertil Steril* 1999; 72(6): 990–995.

31. Carmina E, Chu MC, Longo RA, Rini GB, Lobo

RA. Phenotypic variation in hyperandrogenic women influences the findings of abnormal metabolic and cardiovascular risk parameters. *J Clin Endocrinol Metab* 2005; 90(5): 2545–2549.

32. Wu X, Zhang Z, Su Y. Lipoprotein lipids in polycystic ovarian syndrome: independent associations with androgen excess and insulin resistance. *Zhonghua Fu Chan Ke Za Zhi* 1998; 33(1): 25–27.

33. Ibanez L, Valls C, Ferrer A, Ong K, Dunger DB, De Zegher F. Additive effects of insulin-sensitizing and anti-androgen treatment in young, nonobese women with hyperinsulinism, hyperandrogenism, dyslipidemia, and anovulation. *J Clin Endocrinol Metab* 2002; 87(6): 2870–2874.

34. Bayraktar F, Dereli D, Ozgen AG, Yilmaz C. Plasma homocysteine levels in polycystic ovary syndrome and congenital adrenal hyperplasia. *Endocr J* 2004; 51(6): 601–608.

35. Vrbikova J, Tallova J, Bicikova M, Dvorakova K, Hill M, Starka L. Plasma thiols and androgen levels in polycystic ovary syndrome. *Clin Chem Lab Med* 2003; 41(2): 216–221.

36. Yilmaz M, Biri A, Bukan N, Karakoc A, Sancak B, Toruner F, Pasaoglu H. Levels of lipoprotein and homocysteine in non-obese and obese patients with polycystic ovary syndrome. *Gynecol Endocrinol* 2005; 20(5): 258–263.

37. Ridker PM. Clinical application of C-reactive protein for cardiovascular disease: detection and prevention. *Circulation* 2003; 107: 363–369.

38. Bahceci M, Tuzcu A, Canoruc N, Tuzun Y, Kidir V, Aslan C. Serum C-reactive protein (CRP) levels and insulin resistance in non-obese women with polycystic ovarian syndrome, and effect of bicalutamide on hirsutism, CRP levels and insulin resistance. *Horm Res* 2004; 62(6): 283–287.

39. Fenkci V, Fenkci S, Yilmazer M, Serteser M. Decreased total antioxidant status and increased oxidative stress in women with polycystic ovary syndrome may contribute to the risk of cardiovascular disease. *Fertil Steril* 2003; 80(1): 123–127.

40. Boulman N, Levy Y, Leiba R, Shachar S, Linn R, Zinder O, Blumenfeld Z. Increased C-reactive protein levels in the polycystic ovary syndrome: a marker of cardiovascular disease. *J Clin Endocrinol Metab* 2004; 89(5): 2160–2165.

41. Kent SC, Legro RS. Polycystic ovary syndrome in adolescents. *Adolesc Med* 2002; 13(1): 73–88, vi.

42. Bailey CJ, Turner RC. Drug therapy: metformin. *N Engl J Med* 1996; 334: 574–579.

43. Perriello G, Misericordia P, Volpi E et al. Acute antihyperglycemic mechanisms of metformin in NIDDM. Evidence for suppression of lipid oxidation and hepatic glucose production. *Diabetes* 1994; 43(7): 920–928.

44. Reaven GM, Johnston P, Hollenbeck CB, Skowronski R, Zhang JC, Goldfine ID, Chen YD. Combined metformin-sulfonylurea treatment of patients with noninsulin-dependent diabetes in fair to poor glycemic control. *J Clin Endocrinol Metab* 1992; 74(5): 1020–1026.

45. Wiernsperger NF, Bailey CJ. The antihyperglycemic effect of metformin: therapeutic and cellular mechanisms. *Drugs* 1999; 58 (suppl 1): 31–39.

46. Santana LF, de Sa MF, Ferriani RA, de Moura MD, Foss MC, dos Reis RM. Effect of metformin on the clinical and metabolic assessment of women with polycystic ovary syndrome. *Gynecol Endocrinol* 2004; 19(2): 88–96.

47. Aruna J, Mittal S, Kumar S, Misra R, Dadhwal V, Vimala N. Metformin therapy in women with polycystic ovary 1syndrome. *Int J Gynaecol Obstet* 2004; 87(3): 237–241.

48 Rautio K, Tapanainen JS, Ruokonen A, Morin-Papunen LC. Effects of metformin and ethinyl estradiol-cyproterone acetate on lipid levels in obese and non-obese women with polycystic ovary syndrome. *Eur J Endocrinol* 2005; 152(2): 269–275.

49. Ibanez L, Potau N, Marcos MV, de Zegher F. Treatment of hirsutism, hyperandrogenism, oligomenorrhea, dyslipidemia, and hyperinsulinism in nonobese, adolescent girls: effect of flutamide. *J Clin Endocrinol Metab* 2000; 85(9): 3251–3255.

50. Diamanti-Kandarakis E, Mitrakou A, Raptis S, Tolis G, Duleba AJ. The effect of a pure antiandrogen receptor blocker, flutamide, on the lipid profile in the polycystic ovary syndrome. *J Clin Endocrinol Metab* 1998; 83(8): 2699–2705.

51. Vrbíková J, Hill M, Dvoráková K, Stanická S, Vondra K, Stárka L. Flutamide suppresses adrenal steroidogenesis but has no effect on insulin resistance and secretion and lipid levels in overweight women with polycystic ovary syndrome. *Gynecol Obstet Invest* 2004; 58: 36–41.

52. Ibanez L, Ong K, Ferrer A, Amin R, Dunger D, de Zegher F. Low-dose flutamide-metformin therapy reverses insulin resistance and reduces fat mass in nonobese adolescents with ovarian hyperandrogenism. *J Clin Endocrinol Metab* 2003; 88(6): 2600–2606.

53. Lv L, Liu Y, Sun Y, Tan K. Effects of metformin combined with cyproterone acetate on clinical features, endocrine and metabolism of non-obese

women with polycystic ovarian syndrome. *J Huazhong Univ Sci Technolog Med Sci* 2005; 25(2): 194–197.

54. Ibanez L, de Zegher F. Low-dose combination of flutamide, metformin and an oral contraceptive for non-obese, young women with polycystic ovary syndrome. *Hum Reprod* 2003; 18(1): 57–60.

55. Villaseca P, Hormaza P, Cardenas I, Oestreicher E, Arteaga E. Ethinylestradiol/cyproterone acetate in polycystic ovary syndrome: lipid and carbohydrate changes. *Eur J Contracept Reprod Health Care* 2004; 9(3): 155–165.

56. Legro RS, Azziz R, Ehrmann D, Fereshetian AG, O'Keefe M, Ghazzi MN. Minimal response of circulating lipids in women with polycystic ovary syndrome to improvement in insulin sensitivity with troglitazone. *J Clin Endocrinol Metab* 2003; 88(11): 5137–5144.

57. Hasegawa I, Murakawa H, Suzuki M, Yamamoto Y, Kurabayashi T, Tanaka K. Effect of troglitazone on endocrine and ovulatory performance in women with insulin resistance-related polycystic ovary syndrome. *Fertil Steril* 1999; 71(2): 323–327.

58. Yilmaz M, Bukan N, Ayvaz G, Karakoc A, Toruner F, Cakir N, Arslan M. The effects of rosiglitazone and metformin on oxidative stress and homocysteine levels in lean patients with polycystic ovary syndrome. *Hum Reprod* 2005; 20(12): 3333–3340.

59. Gambineri A, Pelusi C, Genghini S, Morselli-Labate AM, Cacciari M, Pagotto U, Pasquali R. Effect of flutamide and metformin administered alone or in combination in dieting obese women with polycystic ovary syndrome. *Clin Endocrinol* (Oxf) 2004; 60(2): 241–249.

60. Legro RS. Polycystic ovary syndrome: current and future treatment paradigms. *Am J Obstet Gynecol* 1998; 179(6 Pt 2): S101–S108.

61. Brown AJ, Tendler DA, McMurray RG, Setji TL. Polycystic ovary syndrome and severe nonalcoholic steatohepatitis: beneficial effect of modest weight loss and exercise on liver biopsy findings. *Endocr Pract* 2005; 11(5): 319–324.

Risk of Cardiovascular Disease

22

Coronary Heart Disease – Risk Factors in Women with Polycystic Ovary Syndrome

Dov Feldberg

Summary

Major features of Polycystic ovary syndrome (PCOS) as obesity, hyperinsulinism and diabetes mellitus, have a grave prognosis on women's health. Nevertheless, a large number of publications concerning the metabolic status in PCOS women, failed to present a consensus on the impact and correlation between these biochemical changes and coronary or carotid artery morbidity.

Future longitudinal trials including genetic factors are needed to explore the natural history of PCOS with its sequelae on women's well being around the globe.

Introduction

During recent years, the correlation between PCOS and coronary heart disease (CHD) has become more and more obvious nevertheless, there exists controversy in the literature.[1] Risk factors as diabetes, insulin resistance, hypertension and hyperlipidemia have a tremendous impact on coronary artery function and the pathophysiology of CHD. The basic research on the connection between PCOS and CHD usually included small cohorts of patients without statistical power. The major problem is that women with PCOS are treated for infertility in their reproductive years, but are "neglected", in terms of research in their elderly phase of life when the clinical expression of CHD comes into reality.

One recent large study, dealing with heart disease and women's health, is the "Nurse Study".[2] This study, despite the size, ignored in terms of database, the clinical symptoms of PCOS as hyperandrogenism and menstrual irregularity or sonographic ovarian imaging. For these reasons, extrapolation of PCOS patients from the general cohort became impossible.

The contrary approach is well expressed in the literature and risk factors as obesity, hyperinsulinism, diabetes mellitus, hypertension and hyperlipidemia have a grave prognosis for the future health of women. However, in this context, there is no possibility of figuring out the importance of PCOS diagnosis and CHD performance and complications.

A survey of the literature concerning PCOS and the etiology of CHD in these patients provokes three major questions that demand adequate answers:

1. Are known risk factors for CHD in women more common in PCOS patients?
2. Do women with PCOS diagnosis have an increased risk for CHD?
3. Can we control the CHD events by correcting risk factors in PCOS patients?

Clinical Discussion

In order to find the appropriate answers to these thorough questions, a full survey of the relevant literature was performed on the connection between PCOS and CHD using the Medline and Internet facilities. Using the database in the literature, 4 correlations of pathophysiological performance in women with PCOS diagnosed by world accepted criteria[3] were examined: hypertension, glucose intolerance/diabetes mellitus, dyslipidemia and coronary or carotid plaques.

Analyzing the results of the list of studies addressing the correlation between PCOS and hypertension, it was observed that the results were conflicting and non-persistent. Some studies[4,5,7–10] (Table 22.1), were based on a small number of patients and even in the large studies,[6,11] (Table 22.1), an accurate diagnosis of PCOS could not be made on the basis of the histological data from ovarian wedge resections or the telephone interview questionnaires, which had a problem of selection bias. Large prospective studies are needed to definitely answer the possible correlation between PCOS and hypertension.

The correlation between glucose intolerance or diabetes mellitus in PCOS, concluded by the various studies,[10,12–15] is presented in Table 22.2. Based on the data from the literature, we can conclude that from the standpoint of pathophysiology, obesity with an ovarian structure suggestive of PCOS, increases the risk for glucose intolerance and diabetes. But, from the data that was drawn, it was impossible to conclude that women with diabetes mellitus, obesity and PCOS have increased risk of death from CHD compared to obese diabetic women without PCOS. From the UK prospective diabetes study,[2] it seems clear that hyperglycemic control and prevention of hypertension, reduces the chances for CHD in obese women with or without PCOS diagnosis.

The correlation between PCOS and dyslipidemia as concluded by the various studies,[16–21] is presented in Table 22.3 Most of the dyslipidemia and PCOS studies are on a top level of confidence although again, most of the cohorts are not big enough. The confidence power

Table 22.1 Correlation between PCOS and hypertension

No.	Study	Patient Population	Findings
1.	Mattsson et al, (1984)[4]	20 PCOS vs 20 normal	Blood pressure higher in PCOS
2.	Zimmermann et al, (1992)[5]	14 PCOS vs 18 normal control (similar age, race, BMI)	No difference in blood pressure, left ventricular hypertrophy
3.	Conway et al, (1992)[6]	102 Lean and obese PCOS; 19 Lean PCOS	Lean PCOS with higher insulin than normal; obese PCOS had higher blood pressure
4.	Sampson et al, (1996)[7]	24 Nonobese PCOS with irregular menses; 26 PCOS by ultrasound scan, regular menses; 10 normal	No difference for 24-hr ambulatory blood pressure; PCOS with menstrual disturbance had higher fasting insulin and plasminogen activator inhibitor levels
5.	Holte et al, (1996)[8]	36 PCOS vs 55 control subjects, matched for BMI	Higher ambulatory mean arterial blood pressure; higher daytime systolic blood pressure; no difference in diastolic blood pressure
6.	Fridstrom et al, (1999)[9]	33 PCOS vs 66 normal	Higher blood pressure, third trimester of pregnancy in PCOS retrospective
7.	Dahlgren et al, (1992)[10]	33 PCOS; 132 age-matched referents; wedge resection	Greater prevalence of physician diagnosed hypertension, PCOS
8.	Elting et al, (2001)[11]	346 PCOS patients by telephone; age-specific; rates of Dutch women	Hypertension, 2.5 times higher in PCOS; hypertension, obesity more in the younger (35-44 y) PCOS group (n = 233)

Table 22.2 Correlation between glucose intolerance or diabetes mellitus in PCOS

No.	Study	Patient Population	Findings
1.	Dahlgren et al, (1992)[10]	33 PCOS; 132 age-matched referents; wedge resection	Greater prevalence of physician-diagnosed diabetes mellitus in PCOS
2.	Ehrmann et al, (1999)[12]	122 PCOS	Glucose intolerance, 45%; IGT, 35%; NIDDM, 10%
3.	Legro et al, (1999)[13]	254 PCOS 14–44 y; prospectively, 1 urban ethnically diverse (n = 110); 1 rural ethnically homogenous (n = 144); rural PCOS and 80 control subjects of similar weight, ethnicity and age	Prevalence of glucose intolerance: IGT, 38.6%–31.1%; diabetes mellitus, 7.5%; nonobese PCOS: IGT, 10.3%; diabetes mellitus, 1.5%
4.	Cibula et al, (2000)[14]	28 Select patients with ovarian wedge resection compared with 752 control subjects who were selected by age (45–59 y) from random population	Prevalence of diabetes mellitus 4 times higher in PCOS women aged 45–54 y (n = 32).
5.	Legro, (2002)[15]	46 PCOS compared with 80 controls	High prevalence of glucose intolerance. Not treated enough

Table 22.3 Correlation between PCOS and dyslipidemia

No.	Study	Patient Population	Findings
1.	Wild et al, (1985)[16]	29 PCOS vs 30 control subjects	Higher triglyceride, lower HDL cholesterol levels in PCOS
2.	Wild et al, (1988)[17]	13 PCOS; 13 control subjects, matched for BMI	Higher triglyceride and VLDL cholesterol levels, lower HDL, cholesterol levels in PCOS
3.	Slowinska-Srzednicka et al, (1991)[18]	49 Glucose tolerant women, lean and obese, PCOS vs normal	Lower HDL_2 and higher apolipoprotein B levels in obese and nonobese PCOS; obese PCOS had higher triglyceride and VLDL cholesterol, lower HDL cholesterol levels
4.	Wild et al, (1992)[19]	47 Hirsute vs 15 control subjects	Higher triglyceride, VLDL cholesterol, apolipoprotein C-III, AI/AII levels, and lower HDL cholesterol levels
5.	Talbott et al, (1995)[20]	206 PCOS and control subjects, voter registration tapes and directories of households; subjects matched by age, race and neighbourhood	Increased triglyceride, decreased total HDL and HDL_2 cholesterol, increased total cholesterol and LDL levels
6.	Velazquez et al, (2000)[21]	18 Hispanic PCOS vs 9 control subjects	Lean and obese PCOS subjects had increased triglyceride levels after fat load

Table 22.4   Correlation between PCOS and coronary or carotid plaques

No.	Study	Patient Population	Findings
1.	Wild et al, (1990)[22]	102 Consecutive patients underwent angiography	PCOS more likely positive; hirsutism, acne, waist/hip; CAD
4.	Talbott et al, (1995)[20]	46 PCOS vs 59 control subjects by carotid scanning	Carotid artery index worse in PCOS; correlated with age, BMI, diastolic blood pressure and LDL cholesterol level
2.	Birdsall et al, (1997)[23]	143 Consecutive patients underwent angiography; pelvic ultrasound scan, <60; none with oophorectomy	PCOS in 42%, associated with hirsutism; previous hysterectomy; higher free testosterone triglyceride, and C-peptide levels; lower HDL cholesterol levels; PCOS more CAD
5.	Christian et al, (2000)[24]	EBCT (30–45 y), PCOS and normal; historic community control subjects that were age and BMI matched; women, 175; men, 154; previous EBCT	Coronary calcification more prevalent in PCOS (odds ratio, 2.52) vs community dwelling women (odds ratio, 5.5); similar age; equivalent to men
6.	Talbott et al, (2004)[25]	61 PCOS patients and 85 controls; metabolic and ultrasound studies	Increase in metabolic syndrome and coronary calcification in PCOS patients
7.	Vryonidou, (2005)[26]	130 PCOS patients compared with 55 controls; Metabolic studies with carotid artery ultrasound scan	PCOS women had a significant increase in cardiovascular risk and increase in intima-media thickness

comes from the possibility of performing precise metabolic studies on groups of women with or without PCOS. As we can conclude from the studies, dyslipidemia is present in cohorts of PCOS patients all over the world, but CHD with cardiac event complications occurs in women with extreme values of hyperlipidaemia. One of the prominent symptoms of PCOS is obesity that includes 50% of the patients. The frequency of metabolic syndrome[5] in obese women of reproductive age is about 20%. High free testosterone concentrations were recorded in the majority of PCOS women with metabolic syndrome. The combination of all the risk factors mentioned, increases without any doubt, the incidence of CHD in the PCOS population of obese women. Table 22.4 presents the results of various studies,[20,22–26] on the correlation between PCOS and coronary of carotid plaques.

From the data that was accumulated, PCOS is associated with an increased prevalence of calcium deposits in the coronary vessels that comes to expression in a relatively early age,

before menopause.[27] The same observation is true for the carotid artery deposition of calcium plaques in the PCOS cohort of patients.

Figure 22.1 depicts the various factors that contribute to insulin resistance, its effects and their correlation with CHD. Taking all the risk factors into consideration, the death from CHD is positively associated with obesity, glucose intolerance, elevated triglyceride levels and PCOS diagnosis by ovarian ultrasonography.[28]

In order to summarize the results of this extensive survey of literature, we have to focus on the answers to the three basic questions that were asked at the beginning of this chapter:

1. Are the known risk factors for CHD in women more common in PCOS patients?
    Until recent years, all the information that was accumulated in the literature indicated that, despite the increased prevalence of diabetes and other cardiovascular risk factors, the risk for premature coronary heart disease in women with PCOS is not as high as

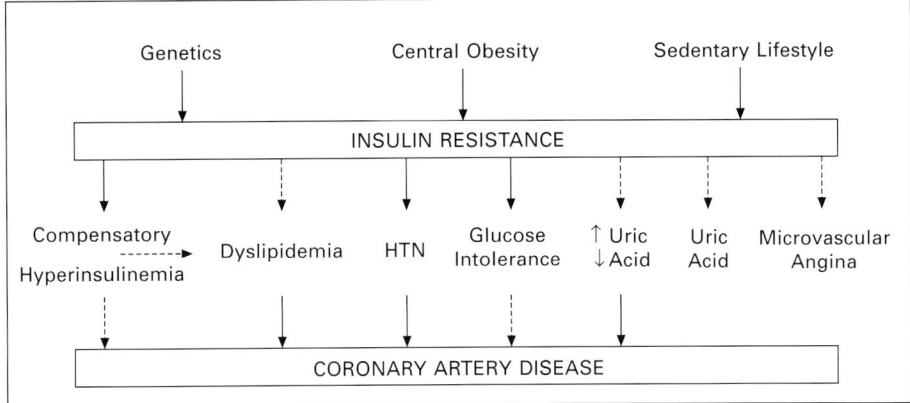

Figure 22.1 Components of insulin resistance syndrome. ⟶ indicates probable or established causal relationship. − − →indicates association present, but causal relationship not determined.
Dyslipidemia includes: increased triglyceride levels, decreased HDL cholesterol levels, small dose LDL particles, and large postprandial triglyceride-rich lipoprotein particles.
HTN = hypertension; PAI-1 = plasminogen activator inhibitor, type 1; tPA = tissue plasminogen activator.
Source: Davidson et al [28].

previously predicted. Furthermore, there is no data that suggests that heart disease mortality is higher in women with PCOS, unless they also have severe diabetes and metabolic disorders.

2. Do women with a diagnosis of PCOS have an increased risk for CHD?
    Data collected from contemporary literature shows that the unfavorable distribution of cardiovascular risk factors in women with PCOS, compared with age-matched controls, persists into middle-age. These findings are consistent in all studies on middle-aged women with a history of PCOS. Possible explanations for the discrepancy between the prevalence of cardiovascular risk factors and the expected prevalence of CHD could include inaccuracy of predictive models for CHD in women. We comprehend the presence of protective factors against CHD in women with PCOS, such as prolonged exposure to unopposed estrogen, or elevated levels of vascular endothelial growth factor.[29]

3. Can we control the CHD events by correction of risk factors in PCOS patients?
    This thorough question is the major aspect of this chapter and literature survey. Until today, no study has had the appropriate statistical power to analyze the net effect of preventive therapy on CHD morbidity or mortality in the PCOS cohort of patients. Therapeutic agents that lower lipid levels are common practice in the primary and secondary prevention of heart diseases in men and women since the mid-nineties. The predicted life-years saved by lowering the lipid levels and hypertension are most important. Primary prevention should include assessment of CHD risk rather than individual risk factors.

Conclusion

The metabolic status of PCOS women is reflected by presence of insulin resistance, central obesity and hyperlipidemia.[30,31] These risk factors seem to elevate the prevalence of diabetes and CHD. After a careful analysis of the literature, one can conclude that retrospective long-term follow-up studies have confirmed the higher incidence of diabetes, but have not shown a higher risk of mortality from CHD.

Cross sectional studies have presented only some association between PCOS and CHD.

Prospective long-term randomized double blind control studies, established by evidence-based approach, are still awaited.[32]

There is no doubt that we have enough evidence regarding the association of the long-term risks of CHD with diabetes mellitus, which should be taken into consideration when counseling women with PCOS. Pharmacological interventions as metformin (glucophage) or other insulin sensitizing drugs, together with lipid lowering agents, appear to present potentially effective measures in ameliorating insulin resistance with an improvement in the clinical and hormonal parameters, and a possible decline in the incidence of cardiovascular pathology.[33] Nevertheless, in this global approach, additional research and investigation is needed. Weight loss is a universal first line preventive therapeutic intervention in this cohort of PCOS women. Future longitudinal trials, including genetic factors, need to be performed to explore the natural history of PCOS with its sequelae on women's health around the globe.

References

1. Balen A, Rajkowha M. Polycystic ovary syndrome—a systemic disorder? *Best Pract Res Clin Obstet Gynaecol* 2003; 17(2): 263–274.

2. Wild S, Pierpoint T, McKeigue P, Jacobs H. Cardiovascular disease in women with polycystic ovary syndrome at long-term follow-up: a retrospective cohort study. *Clin Endocrinol* (Oxf). 2000; 52(5): 595–600.

3. Speroff L, Fritz MA, editors. Clinical Gynecologic Endocrinology and Infertility. 7th ed. Philadelphia: Lippincott Williams and Wilkins, 2005.

4. Mattsson LA, Cullberg G, Hamberger L, Samsioe G, Silfverstolpe G. Lipid metabolism in women with polycystic ovary syndrome: possible implications for an increased risk of coronary heart disease. *Fertil Steril* 1984; 42(4): 579–584.

5. Zimmermann S, Phillips RA, Dunaif A, Finegood DT, Wilkenfeld C, Ardeljan M, et al. Polycystic ovary syndrome: lack of hypertension despite profound insulin resistance. *J Clin Endocrinol Metab* 1992; 75(2): 508–513.

6. Conway GS, Agrawal R, Betteridge DJ, Jacobs HS. Risk factors for coronary artery disease in lean and obese women with the polycystic ovary syndrome. *Clin Endocrinol* (Oxf). 1992; 37(2): 119–125.

7. Sampson M, Kong C, Patel A, Unwin R, Jacobs HS. Ambulatory blood pressure profiles and plasminogen activator inhibitor (PAI-1) activity in lean women with and without the polycystic ovary syndrome. *Clin Endocrinol* (Oxf). 1996; 45(5): 623–629.

8. Holte J, Gennarelli G, Berne C, Bergh T, Lithell H. Elevated ambulatory day-time blood pressure in women with polycystic ovary syndrome: a sign of a pre-hypertensive state? *Hum Reprod* 1996; 11(1): 23–28.

9. Fridstrom M, Nisell H, Sjoblom P, Hillensjo T. Are women with polycystic ovary syndrome at an increased risk of pregnancy-induced hypertension and/or preeclampsia? *Hypertens Pregnancy* 1999; 18(1): 73–80.

10. Dahlgren E, Johansson S, Lindstedt G, Knutsson F, Oden A, Janson PO, et al. Women with polycystic ovary syndrome wedge resected in 1956 to 1965: a long-term follow-up focusing on natural history and circulating hormones. *Fertil Steril* 1992; 57(3): 505–513.

11. Elting MW, Korsen TJ, Bezemer PD, Schoemaker J. Prevalence of diabetes mellitus, hypertension and cardiac complaints in a follow-up study of a Dutch PCOS population. *Hum Reprod* 2001; 16(3): 556–560.

12. Ehrmann DA, Barnes RB, Rosenfield RL, Cavaghan MK, Imperial J. Prevalence of impaired glucose tolerance and diabetes in women with polycystic ovary syndrome. *Diabetes Care* 1999; 22(1): 141–146.

13. Legro RS, Kunselman AR, Dodson WC, Dunaif A. Prevalence and predictors of risk for type 2 diabetes mellitus and impaired glucose tolerance in polycystic ovary syndrome: a prospective, controlled study in 254 affected women. *J Clin Endocrinol Metab* 1999; 84(1): 165–169.

14. Cibula D, Cifkova R, Fanta M, Poledne R, Zivny J, Skibova J. Increased risk of non-insulin dependent diabetes mellitus, arterial hypertension and coronary artery disease in perimenopausal women with a history of the polycystic ovary syndrome. *Hum Reprod* 2000 Apr; 15(4): 785–789.

15. Legro RS, Urbanek M, Kunselman AR, Leiby BE, Dunaif A. Self-selected women with polycystic ovary syndrome are reproductively and metabolically abnormal and undertreated. *Fertil Steril* 2002; 78(1): 51–57.

16. Wild RA, Painter PC, Coulson PB, Carruth KB,

Ranney GB. Lipoprotein lipid concentrations and cardiovascular risk in women with polycystic ovary syndrome. *J Clin Endocrinol Metab* 1985; 61(5): 946–951.

17. Wild RA, Bartholomew MJ. The influence of body weight on lipoprotein lipids in patients with polycystic ovary syndrome. *Am J Obstet Gynecol* 1988; 159(2): 423–427.

18. Slowinska-Srzednicka J, Zgliczynski S, Wierzbicki M, Srzednicki M, Stopinska-Gluszak U, Zgliczynski W, et al. The role of hyperinsulinemia in the development of lipid disturbances in nonobese and obese women with the polycystic ovary syndrome. *J Endocrinol Invest* 1991; 14(7): 569–575.

19. Wild RA, Alaupovic P, Parker IJ. Lipid and apolipoprotein abnormalities in hirsute women. I. The association with insulin resistance. *Am J Obstet Gynecol* 1992; 166(4): 1191–1196.

20. Talbott E, Guzick D, Clerici A, Berga S, Detre K, Weimer K, Kuller L. Coronary heart disease risk factors in women with polycystic ovary syndrome. *Arterioscler Thromb Vasc Biol* 1995; 15(7): 821–826.

21. Velazquez ME, Bellabarba GA, Mendoza S, Sanchez L. Postprandial triglyceride response in patients with polycystic ovary syndrome: relationship with waist-to-hip ratio and insulin. *Fertil Steril* 2000; 74(6): 1159–1163.

22. Wild RA, Grubb B, Hartz A, Van Nort JJ, Bachman W, Bartholomew M. Clinical signs of androgen excess as risk factors for coronary artery disease. *Fertil Steril* 1990; 54(2): 255–259.

23. Birdsall MA, Farquhar CM, White HD. Association between polycystic ovaries and extent of coronary artery disease in women having cardiac catheterization. *Ann Intern Med* 1997; 126(1): 32–35.

24. Christian RC et al. Clinical hyperandrogenism and body mass index predict coronary calcification in premenopausal women with polycystic ovary syndrome (PCOS) [abstract]. *Endocr Soc Abstracts* 2000: 400.

25. Talbott EO, Zborowski JV, Rager JR, Boudreaux MY, Edmundowicz DA, Guzick DS. Evidence for an association between metabolic cardiovascular syndrome and coronary and aortic calcification among women with polycystic ovary syndrome. *J Clin Endocrinol Metab* 2004; 89(11): 5454–5461.

26. Vryonidou A, Papatheodorou A, Tavridou A, Terzi T, Loi V, Vatalas IA, et al. Association of hyperandrogenemic and metabolic phenotype with carotid intima-media thickness in young women with polycystic ovary syndrome. *J Clin Endocrinol Metab* 2005; 90(5): 2740–2746.

27. Wild RA. Polycystic ovary syndrome: a risk for coronary artery disease? *Am J Obstet Gynecol* 2002; 186(1): 35–43.

28. Davidson MB. Clinical implications of insulin resistance syndromes. *Am J Med* 1995; 99(4): 420–426.

29. Paradisi G, Steinberg HO, Hempfling A, Cronin J, Hook G, Shepard MK, Baron AD. Polycystic ovary syndrome is associated with endothelial dysfunction. *Circulation* 2001; 103(10): 1410–1415.

30. Korhonen S, Hippelainen M, Niskanen L, Vanhala M, Saarikoski S. Relationship of the metabolic syndrome and obesity to polycystic ovary syndrome: a controlled, population-based study. *Am J Obstet Gynecol* 2001; 184(3): 289–296.

31. Jahanfar S, Eden JA, Nguyen T, Wang XL, Wilcken DE. A twin study of polycystic ovary syndrome and lipids. *Gynecol Endocrinol* 1997; 11(2): 111–117.

32. Wild S, Pierpoint T, McKeigue P, Jacobs H. Cardiovascular disease in women with polycystic ovary syndrome at long-term follow-up: a retrospective cohort study. *Clin Endocrinol* (Oxf). 2000; 52(5): 595–600.

33. Talbott EO, Guzick DS, Sutton-Tyrrell K, McHugh-Pemu KP, Zborowski JV, Remsberg KE, Kuller LH. Evidence for association between polycystic ovary syndrome and premature carotid atherosclerosis in middle-aged women. *Arterioscler Thromb Vasc Biol* 2000; 20(11): 2414–2421.

23

Polycystic Ovary Syndrome and Carotid Artery Stenosis

Jairam K Aithal, AV Ganesh Kumar

Summary

Polycystic Ovary Syndrome (PCOS), a common endocrinopathy affecting 5–10% of women of reproductive age, is also characterized by a clustering of risk factors associated with an adverse lipid profile and blood pressure. It is also found to be associated with selective insulin resistance, obesity, type 2 diabetes mellitus, increased levels of serum markers of premature atherosclerosis, as well as endothelial dysfunction. These associated factors are responsible for the development of premature atherosclerosis in the carotid/coronary vasculature causing cardiovascular disease (CVD). Significant carotid artery disease mainly affects older women with PCOS, though at a younger age, metabolic derangements lead to a measurable increase in carotid intima-media thickness. Along with modifications in lifestyle, including weight loss, diet and exercise, treatment of antecedent conditions like insulin resistance, hypercholesterolemia and hypertension is of paramount importance in keeping carotid artery stenosis at bay.

Introduction

Polycystic Ovary Syndrome (PCOS) is characterized by chronic anovulation, androgen excess, polycystic ovaries and infertility.[1] Moreover, it is often associated with selective insulin resistance leading to metabolic alterations.[2] Obesity, type 2 diabetes mellitus (T2DM), dyslipidemia, increased levels of serum markers of premature atherosclerosis, hypertension, as well as endothelial dysfunction, are all responsible for the development of premature atherosclerosis in the carotid/coronary vasculature causing cardiovascular disease (CVD).[3–12] This unique model of disease with androgen excess, insulin resistance and dyslipidemia is termed *female metabolic syndrome* or *syndrome XX*.[13] It presents early in adolescents and can be the cause of premature CVD in the same.

Pathogenesis

Diabetes mellitus, hypertension, tobacco in any form, dyslipidemia, age, a family history, stress, certain metabolic derangements and endothelial dysfunction, are known risk factors for the development of premature atherosclerosis in humans. Of these, a number of metabolic derangements are present in women with PCOS. These are as follows:

PCOS and Insulin Resistance Syndrome (IRS)

The IRS is defined as a cluster of abnormalities and clinical syndromes that are more likely to occur in patients with insulin resistance than in others.[14] It identifies patients with an increased risk of T2DM and CVD. On the basis of the American College of Endocrinology (ACE) position statement in 2003, the identifying features of this syndrome are as follows[14,15]:

1. reduction of serum HDL cholesterol level to < 50 mg/dl
2. increase of serum triglyceride level to > 150 mg/dl
3. hypertension, defined as a blood pressure >130/85 mmHg
4. insulin resistance and increased tendency to have T2DM
5. fasting blood glucose of 110–125 mg/dl
6. glucose levels of 140–199 mg/dl, 120 minutes after a 75 g glucose challenge.

The incidence of IRS and compensatory hyperinsulinemia is high in people with PCOS. Most reports indicate that at least 75% of women with PCOS fulfill the criteria for IRS.[16] Both, obesity and physical inactivity are major factors that work synergistically with the inherent post-receptor defect and lead to insulin resistance in women with PCOS.[17] While obesity increases the chances of occurrence of insulin resistance, most non-obese women with PCOS also have insulin resistance.[18] It is interesting to note that the converse is not true. Not all women with IRS have PCOS.[19] This may be due to genetic differences in susceptibility of the ovaries and the pancreas. The incidence of IRS in the PCOS population may be underestimated as it may be difficult to assess the same in the absence of hyperinsulinemic-euglycemic clamp studies and this is found only in a few advanced centers.[20]

Type 2 Diabetes Mellitus (T2DM) and PCOS

Impaired glucose tolerance (IGT) and frank DM occur when the pancreatic beta cell is unable to compensate for insulin resistance.[21] There is a high prevalence (30–40%) of IGT and T2DM in women with PCOS, including young teens as well as post-menopausal women.[22–24] The incidence is particularly higher in women with a family history of T2DM or obesity. Oligomenorrhea, a surrogate marker for PCOS (almost 80% of patients with oligomenorrhea have PCOS), may predict a 2 to 2.5 fold increase in risk for T2DM, particularly in the presence of a family history of T2DM.[25] Obesity synergistically adds to this risk.[26] The presence of T2DM in concurrence with IRS, abolishes the gender gap and precludes development of CVD in this subset of patients.[27,28]

Dyslipidemia and PCOS

Women with PCOS are frequently found to have atherogenic lipid abnormalities that may reflect underlying IRS as well as effects of ethnicity, genetics, obesity and lifestyle factors. These are characterized by high triglycerides[6,29] and low HDL levels.[30] This reciprocal relationship between triglycerides and HDL is strongly associated with IRS and is one factor that contributes to accelerated atherogenesis in PCOS. Obesity exacerbates high triglyceride levels. A ratio of triglycerides to HDL of greater than 3 appears to predict IRS effectively.[31] Other lipid abnormalities include predisposition toward higher amounts of circulating smaller, denser LDL cholesterol.[32] This is particularly seen in women below 45 years of age. This early and prolonged exposure to dyslipidemia, is a significant risk factor in the development of CVD in PCOS.

Endothelial dysfunction and PCOS

Insulin-dependent vascular relaxation occurs due to insulin-regulating endothelial nitric oxide synthesis.[33] Due to IRS, this metabolic dysregulation leads to decreased vascular compliance of large vessels as well as reduced vasodilation. Increased endothelin 1 (ET 1), a marker of vasculopathy in patients with IRS,[34] has been noted in patients with PCOS. In obese patients, it is increased by almost 5-fold. Decreased vascular compliance is known to correlate with early CVD.

Hypertension and PCOS

Women with PCOS are known to have a higher incidence of systolic blood pressure.[35] Reduced vasodilation as a result of endothelial dysfunction and obesity is seen in women with PCOS, though the correlation is not strong.

Pro-inflammatory and atherogenic markers and PCOS

Low grade inflammation, increased oxidative stress[36] [raised levels of adipokines like tumor necrosis factor (TNF) alpha, interleukin (IL)-6, adiponectin],[37] altered inflammatory markers [elevated serum C-reactive protein (CRP) levels],[38] raised homocysteine, altered circulating divalent cations, altered hemostasis and fibrinolysis and increased tissue plasminogen activator – 1,[22,39] can all contribute to the process of accelerated atherosclerosis.

HDL cholesterol, Dehydroepiandrosterone sulfate (DHEAS) and delta 4 androstenedione (delta 4A)

It has been observed that high levels of these moieties have shown reduced intima-media thickness (IMT) in women with PCOS.[40,41] It has been postulated that these precursors of testosterone and estradiol have a lipid lowering potential. These precursors also improve endothelial function as they have the characteristics of a peroxisome proliferator with antiproliferative and chemoprotective effects.[41] They also have a favorable effect on obesity and diabetes.

Incidence

Women with PCOS have a seven-fold increase in T2 DM (15% vs 2%),[42] a three-fold increase in hypertension, a significantly higher waist-hip ratio and a four fold increase in CVD (21% vs 5%).[43]

Studies have shown that the incidence of CVD with an IMT of 1 mm compared to 0.6 mm showed a hazard ratio of 7.4, and that the risk of stroke increased with an IMT of > 0.75 mm.[44–46]

Increased carotid IMT is seen in women with PCOS above the age of 45, except in those women whose CRP levels were elevated where it was seen prematurely, as also in cases where women had an increased waist-hip ratio. Women with IRS and an increased IMT have a higher incidence of stroke.

Clinical Discussion

Natural history of carotid stenosis

Amongst asymptomatic patients with >60% carotid stenosis, the annual rate of ipsilateral stroke is 2%.[47] Amongst symptomatic patients, the annual rate of ipsilateral stroke in patients with >50% carotid stenosis is around 18% in spite of medical therapy, increased stenosis severity being associated with an increased risk of stroke.[48] Also, this incidence was observed to be higher in patients with increased inflammatory markers or heterogenous appearance of the plaque on ultrasound or magnetic resonance (MR) angiography.

Clinical presentation

Most patients will be asymptomatic and a clinical finding of carotid bruit points to the diagnosis. Symptomatic patients present with a history of transient ischemic attacks or frank strokes.[48]

Diagnosis

Diagnosis of carotid artery stenosis is most commonly made clinically when a person presents with a transient ischemic attack or stroke and auscultation shows a carotid bruit. The easiest modality of non-invasive estimation of carotid artery stenosis is the carotid Doppler ultrasound.[48] This measures carotid intima-media thickness (IMT) as well as delineates the extent (percentage) of stenosis.[46] With new tools such as power Doppler ultrasound, magnetic resonance imaging and CT angiography being available, this diagnosis has become more precise and treatment friendly.[48] The gold standard remains carotid angiography, which helps delineate the extent of plaque, its morphology and presence of concomitant plaques. It also helps delineate the status of the aortic arch and other arch vessels.[46]

Medical management

Aggressive management of risk factors with medications is recommended in all patients of PCOS to delay/retard progression of atherosclerosis. Statins are recommended in all these patients with low density lipoprotein (LDL) cholesterol levels of 130 mg/dL or above.[49] Apart from cholesterol reduction, statins also have a pleiotropic effect on plaques rendering them less volatile and dangerous. Mono-antiplatelet therapy with aspirin is useful in primary prevention of atherosclerosis of the carotid artery. In patients with proven plaques, dual antiplatelet therapy with aspirin and clopidogrel is the preferred line of management.[49] Anticoagulants are not shown to be more effective than dual antiplatelet therapy. In fact, there seems to be an increased incidence

of bleeding with anticoagulants. Adequate level of control over hypertension and diabetes is of paramount importance in preventing the development of atherosclerosis in the carotids.[47]

Surgical management

Carotid end-arterectomy (CEA) was for long the preferred form of treatment of severe symptomatic carotid artery stenosis and asymptomatic stenosis of > 60%.[48]

Endovascular revascularization

Carotid stenting has come into vogue only in the last decade. Initially, due to problems of dissection of the artery, stent recoil and restenosis, and distal embolisation and stroke, the procedure was not the preferred form of treatment. With the advent of nitinol and elgiloy self expanding stents, and distal protection devices, and a rise in technical success to almost 100%, today a lot of centers prefer this form of therapy to CEA.[48] These stents exert a radial force on the carotids and prevent

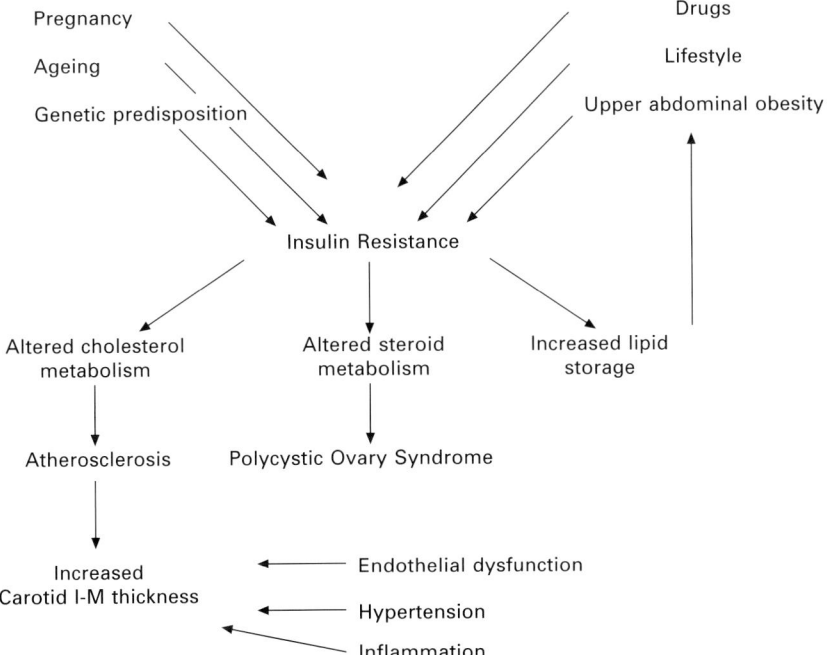

Figure 23.1   Risk factors and cardiovascular complications associated with Polycystic Ovary Syndrome

recoil. Distal protection devices prevent downstream flow of embolic material during the stenting procedure, trapping these particles in filters which can be removed post-procedure.

Major trials have also demonstrated that when distal embolisation protection devices are used, carotid stenting is superior to CEA.

According to current recommendations, all symptomatic carotid artery stenosis more than 50% should undergo revascularisation in the form of stenting or CEA. It is also recommended in patients with asymptomatic carotid stenosis with a blockage of more than 60%. In patients with concurrent coronary artery disease, a coronary artery bypass along with CEA is the recommended treatment. In all other patients, the treatment of choice today is carotid artery stenting with a distal embolisation protection device. In all these patients, lifelong anti-platelets and statins are recommended.

Conclusion

PCOS is a disorder characterized by a clustering of risk factors that is associated with an adverse lipid profile and blood pressure (Figure 23.1). Carotid artery wall thickness has been shown to be strongly associated with obesity, increased waist-to-hip ratio and increased lipids. It is further increased by deranged inflammatory markers and other mediators. Significant carotid artery disease mainly affects older women with PCOS, though at a younger age, metabolic derangements lead to measurable increases in carotid intima-media thickness.

Along with modifications in lifestyle, including weight loss, diet and exercise, treatment of antecedent conditions like insulin resistance, hypercholesterolemia and hypertension is of paramount importance in keeping carotid stenosis at bay.

References

1. Carmina E, Lobo RA. Polycystic ovary syndrome (PCOS). *J Clin Endocrinol Metab* 1999; 84: 1897–1899.

2. Book CB, Dunaif A. Selective insulin resistance in the polycystic ovary syndrome. *J Clin Endocrinol Metab* 1999; 87: 3110–3116.

3. Dunaif A, Thomas A. Current concepts in the polycystic ovary syndrome. *Annu Rev Med* 2001; 52: 401–419.

4. Dunaif A. Insulin resistance and the polycystic ovary syndrome mechanism and implications for pathogenesis. *Endocr* 1997; Rev 18: 774–800.

5. Ehrmann DA, Barnes RB, Rosenfield RL. Prevalence of impaired glucose tolerance and diabetes in women with polycystic ovary syndrome. *Diabetes Care* 1999; 22: 141–146.

6. Talbott E, Clerici A, Berga, et al. Adverse lipid and coronary heart disease risk profiles in young women with polycystic ovary syndrome: results of a case – control study. *J Clin Epidemiol* 1998; 51: 415–422.

7. Conway GS, Agrawal R, Betteridge DJ. Risk factors for coronary heart disease in lean and obese women with the polycystic ovary syndrome. *Clin Endocrinol (Oxf)* 1992; 37: 119–125.

8. Kelly CC, Lyall H, Petrie JR. Low grade inflammation in women with polycystic ovarian syndrome. *J Clin Endocrinol Metab* 2001; 86: 2453–2455.

9. Escobar-Morreale HF, Botella-Carretero J, Villuendas G. Serum interleukin. *J Clin Endocrinol Metab* 2004; 89: 806–811.

10. Schachter M, Raziel A, Friedler S, Strassburger D. Insulin resistance in patients with polycystic ovary syndrome is associated with elevated plasma homocysteine. *Hum Repord* 2003; 18: 721–727.

11. Paradisi G, Steinberg HO, Hempfling A, et al. Polycystic ovary syndrome is associated with endothelial dysfunction. *Circulation* 2001; 103: 1410–1415.

12. Orio F, Palomba S, Cascella T, et al. Early impairment of endothelial structure and function in young normal weight women with polycystic ovary syndrome. *J Clin Endocrinol Metab* 2004; 89: 4588–4593.

13. Sam S, Dunaif A. Polycystic ovary syndrome: syndrome XX? *Trends Endocrinol Metab* 2003; 14: 365–370.

14. Insulin Resistance Syndrome Task Force: American College of Endocrinology position statement on Insulin Resistance Syndrome. *Endocrinol Pract* 2003; 9: 236–252.

15. Expert Panel on Detection, Evaluation and Treatment of High Blood Cholesterol in Adults. Executive summary of the Third Report of the National cholesterol Education Program (NCEP). JAMA 2001; 285: 2486–2497.

16. Glueck CJ, Papanna R, Wang P. Incidence and treatment of the metabolic syndrome in newly referred women with confirmed polycystic ovarian syndrome. *Metabolism* 2003; 52: 908–915.

17. McLaughlin T, Abbasi F, Kim HS. Relationship between insulin resistance, Weight loss, and coronary heart disease risk in healthy, obese women. *Metabolism* 2001; 50: 795–800.

18. Dunaif A, Segal KR, Futterweit W. Profound peripheral insulin resistance, independent of obesity, in polycystic ovary syndrome. *Diabetes* 1989; 38: 1165–1174.

19. Ovalle F, Azziz R. Insulin resistance, polycystic ovary syndrome, and type 2 diabetes mellitus. *Fertil Steril* 2002; 77: 1095–1105.

20. Diamanti – Kandarakis E, Kouli C. Failure of mathematical indices to accurately assess insulin resistance in lean, overweight, or obese women with polycystic ovary syndrome. *J Clin Endocrinot Metab* 2004; 89: 1273–1276.

21. Dunaif A, Finegood DT. Beta-cell dysfunction independent of obesity and glucose intolerance in the polycystic ovary syndrome. *J Clin Endocrinol Metab* 1996; 81: 942–947.

22. Ehrmann DA, Barnes RB, Rosenfield RL. Prevalence of impaired glucose tolerance and diabetes in women with polycystic ovary Syndrome. *Diabetes Care* 1999; 22: 141–146.

23. Legro RS, Kunselman AR, Dodson WC. Prevalence and predictors of risk for type 2 diabetes mellitus and impaired glucose tolerance in polycystic ovary syndrome. *J Clin Endocrinol Metab* 1999; 84: 165–169.

24. Palmert MR, Gordon CM, Kartashov AI. Screening for abnormal glucose tolerance in adolescents with polycystic ovary syndrome. *J Clin Endocrinol Metab* 2002; 87: 1017–1023.

25. Solomon CG, Hu FB, Dunaif A, et al. Long or highly irregular menstrual cycles as a marker for risk of type 2 diabetes mellitus. JAMA 2001; 286: 2421–2426.

26. Talbott EO, Zborowski JV, Boudreaux MY. Do women with polycystic ovary syndrome have an increased risk of cardiovascular disease? *Minerva Ginecol* 2004; 56: 27–39.

27. Mak KH, Haffner SM. Diabetes abolishes the gender gap in coronary heart disease. *Eur Heart J* 2003; 24: 1385–1386.

28. Alexander CM, Landsman PB, Teutsch SM. NCEP – defined metabolic syndrome, diabetes, and prevalence of coronary heart disease among NHANES III participants age 50 years and older. *Diabetes* 2003; 52: 1210–1214.

29. Mather KJ, Kwan F, Corenblum B. Hyperinsulinemia in polycystic ovary syndrome correlates with increased cardiovascular risk independent of obesity. *Fertil Steril* 2000; 73: 150–156.

30. Wild RA, Painter PC, Coulson PB. Lipoprotein lipid concentration and cardiovascular risk in women with polycystic ovary syndrome. *J Clin Endocrinol Metab* 1985; 61: 946–951.

31. McLaughlin T, Abbasi F, Cheal K. Use of metabolic markers to identify over-weight individuals who are insulin resistant. *Ann Intern Med* 2003; 139: 802–809.

32. Dejager S, Pichard C, Giral P, et al. Smaller LDL particle size in women with polycystic ovary syndrome compared to controls. *Clin Endocrinol* 2001; 54: 455–462.

33. Paradisi G, Steinberg HO, Hempfling A, et al. Polycystic ovary syndrome is associated with endothelial dysfunction. *Circulation* 2001; 103: 1410–1415.

34. Diamanti – Kandarakis E, Spina G. Increased endothelin – 1 levels in women with polycystic ovary syndrome and the beneficial effect of metformin therapy. *J Clin Endocrinol Metab* 2001; 86: 4666–4673.

35. Holte J, Gennarelli G, Berne C. Elevated ambulatory day time blood pressure in women with polycystic ovary syndrome; a sign of a pre-hypertensive state? *Hum Reprod* 1996; 11: 23–28.

36. Kelly CC, Lyall H, Petrie JR. Low grade chronic inflammation in women with polycystic ovarian syndrome. *J Clin Endocrinol Metab* 2001; 86: 2453–2455.

37. Ridker PM. Clinical application of C – reactive protein for cardiovascular disease detection and prevention. *Circulation* 2003; 107: 363–369.

38. Boulman N, Levy Y, Leiba R, et al. Increased C-reactive protein levels in the polycystic ovary syndrome : a marker of cardiovascular disease. *J Clin Endocrinol Metab* 2004; 89: 2160–2165.

39. Ehrmann DA, Schneider DJ, Sobel BE, et al. Troglitazone improved defects in insulin action, insulin secretion, ovarian steroidogenesis, and fibrinolysis in women with polycystic ovary syndrome. *J. Clin Endocrinol Metab* 1997; 82: 2108–2116.

40. Talbott EO, Guzick DS, Sutton – Tyrrell K, et al. Evidence for association between polycystic ovary syndrome and premature carotid atherosclerotic in middle aged women. *Arterioscler Thromb Vasc Biol* 2000; 20: 2414–2421.

41. Vryonidou A, Papatheodorou A, Tavridou A, et al.

Association of hyperandrogenemic and metabolic phenotype with carotid intima. *J Clin Endocirnol Metab* 2005; 90: 2740–2746.

42. Dahlgren E, Johansson S, Lindstedt G, et al. Women with polycystic ovary syndrome wedge resected in 1956 to 1965. *Fertil Steril* 1992; 57: 505–513.

43. Cibula D, Cifkova R, Fanta M. Increased risk of non insulin dependent diabetes mellitus. *Hum Reprod* 2000; 15: 785–789.

44. Chambless LE, Heiss G, Fulson AR. Association of coronary heart disease incidence and arterial wall thickness and major risk factors. *Am J Epidemiol* 1997; 146: 583–494.

45. Aminbakhsh A, Mancini GB. Carotid intima-media thickness. *Clin Invest Med* 1999; 22: 149–157.

46. O'Leary DH, Polak JK, Kronmal RA. Carotid artery intima and media thickness as a risk factor for myocardial infarction and stroke in older adults. Cardiovascular Health Study Collaborative Research Group. *N Engl J Med* 1999; 340: 14–22.

47. Bonora E, Kiechl S, Willeit J, et al. Carotid atherosclerosis and coronary heart disease in the metabolic syndrome. *Diabetes Care* 2003; 26: 1251–1257.

48. Colledge J, Grehalgh RM, Davies AH. The symptomatic carotid plaque. *Stroke* 2000; 31: 774–781.

49. Hess DC, Demchuk AM, Brass LM. HMG CoA inhibitors: a promising approach to stroke prevention. *Neurology* 2000; 54: 790–796.

Infertility

24

The Pathogenesis of Infertility and Early Pregnancy Loss in Polycystic Ovary Syndrome

Andrea Borini, Luca Dal Prato

Summary

Polycystic Ovary Syndrome (PCOS) is probably the most common cause of anovulatory infertility and is associated with an increased risk of miscarriage after either spontaneous or assisted conception. PCOS ovaries contain a significantly higher number of follicles, but the growth of these follicles is arrested when they reach a diameter of 5–8 mm. The factors involved in the process have not been fully elucidated. Hypersecretion of luteinizing hormone (LH), secondary to dysregulation of gonadotropin releasing hormone (GnRH) pulse generator has been initially blamed, but more recently, increasing evidence of a primary ovarian defect disturbing both folliculogenesis and steroidogenesis has emerged.

A series of intra and extra-ovarian factors seems to act together in a process that triggers anovulation or early pregnancy loss through the impairment of folliculogenesis, oocyte maturation, steroidogenesis, and endometrial receptivity.

Excessive androgen production seems to be the key determinant in the evolution of this disorder, but hyperinsulinemia (often associated with obesity) also plays an important role in its interaction with LH. Intraovarian growth factors, such insulin-like growth factors (IGF), anti Mullerian hormone (AMH), growth differentiation factor 9 (GDF-9), or inhibin may participate in the process by acting through paracrine mechanisms, but whether these abnormalities are the direct cause of anovulation and pregnancy loss, or the consequence of deranged steroidogenesis, is still to be determined.

Rationale

Infertility is one of the main features of polycystic ovary syndrome (PCOS). Failure to achieve pregnancy in women with this disorder is chiefly associated with anovulation, though an increased incidence of spontaneous pregnancy loss, the mechanism of which is unknown, has also been found in PCOS women. The present chapter aims to shed light on the multiple factors involved in the development of infertility and the difficulty in child-bearing in women suffering from PCOS.

Introduction

Polycystic ovary syndrome (PCOS) is a very common endocrine disorder of women in reproductive years and probably, the most common cause of anovulatory infertility and hyperandrogenism. Polycystic ovaries have been associated with about 75% of the cases of anovulatory infertility.[1] The prevalence of the syndrome in the general population is about 4–10%.[2,3] The phenotypic expression of the disorder varies considerably. The main clinical manifestations are hyperandrogenism and menstrual irregularity though metabolic dysfunctions, including insulin resistance and obesity, are often associated. Polycystic ovaries have also been found in about 25% of normal ovulatory women with no history of hyperandrogenism.[4]

Anovulation would seem to be the main cause of failed pregnancy in this disorder.[5] There is evidence however, that in addition to a problem in conceiving, women with PCOS are at increasing risk of miscarriage after either spontaneous or assisted conception. The cause of miscarriage in PCOS has not been fully understood though the potential link between insulin resistance and recurrent pregnancy loss has been suggested in studies that showed a significant reduction of first trimester miscarriage in women treated with metformin.[6]

Clinical Discussion

Pathogenesis of infertility in PCOS

The polycystic ovary has been defined by ultrasound examinations. Women with PCOS have enlarged ovaries with multiple peripheral small follicles, 2–10 mm in diameter around an enlarged central stroma.[7] Endocrine abnormalities of the reproductive axis include accelerated GnRH pulsatile activity, hypersecretion of luteinizing hormone (LH), theca-stromal cell hyperactivity and hypofunction of the FSH-granulosa cell axis. These abnormalities result in higher androgen secretion with hirsutism, follicular arrest and ovarian acyclicity.

Obesity is common but is not a prerequisite for the development of PCOS, since 50% of PCOS women are not obese.[8] Its association with insulin resistance/hyperinsulinemia and impaired growth hormone (GH) secretion is well established. A clear explanation for the pathogenesis of PCOS remains elusive, though there is evidence that genetic factors have an important role.[8] Its effective treatment by both, anti-estrogens and exogenous follicle stimulating hormone (FSH) suggests that a primary disorder of FSH regulation may be central. It has been postulated that altered inputs to the GnRH neural system by a series of factors such as insulin, insulin-like growth factor (IGF) and estrogens during the critical development phase of adrenarche and puberty may induce dysregulation of the GnRH pulse generator. This peripubertal hyperactivity of the GnRH/LH axis may be an important determining factor in the pathogenesis of PCOS, a view compatible with the *exaggerated adrenarche theory* by which adrenal androgens provide substrates for peripheral conversion to estrogens prompting inappropriate feedback to the hypothalamic-pituitary unit.[8]

There is however, evidence that the PCOS mechanism involves a primary ovarian defect.[9] Other extraovarian factors such as GH, IGF-1 and insulin seem to be co-gonadotropins and act in synergy with LH on theca cells to stimulate excessive androgen secretion. The existence of a vicious circle in the pathophysiology of PCOS has thus been recognized.

While the key determinant in the evolution of this disorder is excessive androgen production, closely tied to disordered folliculogenesis prompting chronic anovulation, the factors involved in the process and how they act in the ovary have not been fully understood.

Histology provides us with 2 findings (Table 24.1):

1. PCOS ovaries contain a significantly higher number of primary and secondary follicles.[9,10]
2. The growth of these follicles is arrested when they reach a diameter of 5–8 mm.

Table 24.1　Characteristics of ovarian follicles in PCOS

• Primordial follicles	Normal number
• Primary and secondary follicles	Significantly increased
• Follicle growth	Arrested
• Follicular atresia	Decreased

Contrary to the findings in previous studies in rats, that pointed to an atretogenic action of high intraovarian androgen levels on growing follicles, more recent studies in monkeys have shown that testosterone increases follicular FSH receptors, suggesting that androgens indirectly promote follicular growth and estrogen biosynthesis by enhancing the action of FSH[11] and stimulating the expression of insulin-like growth factor (IGF) and its intrafollicular receptors.[12] Follicles in PCOS are in fact, vital and are able to produce steroids in response to gonadotropins.

Causes of excessive follicular growth

Polycystic ovaries are characterized by an excessive number of growing follicles upto a size of 2–5 mm, and are typically visualized as multifollicular ovaries at ultrasonography. The actual number has been reported as 2-3 fold[10] or even 6-fold[9] that of normal ovaries and is correlated with the high serum levels of testosterone and androstendione.[13] The pool of primordial follicles on the other hand, seems to be normal. Webber[9] found a significant increase

in the percentage of early growing (primary) follicles in both ovulatory and anovulatory women with polycystic ovaries compared with normal ovaries suggesting that the initiation of follicle growth could be excessively stimulated in these patients. This finding indicates that there are fundamental differences between polycystic and normal ovaries in early follicular development, suggesting an intrinsic ovarian abnormality. The increased recruitment of follicles in polycystic ovaries does not, however, accelerate menopause, since the increased density of small preantral follicles might be the result of a larger number of germ cells in the fetal ovary or a lower rate of oocyte loss during late gestation, childhood, and puberty.

There is growing evidence that intra-ovarian hyperandrogenism plays the most important role in excessive follicular growth in PCOS,[13] but paracrine factors may also be involved (Table 24.2). Alterations in steroidogenesis in

Table 24.2   Factors involved in the pathogenesis of chronic anovulation in PCOS

Factor	Defect	Site of action	Effect
FSH	Insufficiency	Granulosa cells	Follicular arrest
LH	Hypersecretion	Granulosa cells Theca cells	Premature response: follicular arrest Hyperandrogenism
Androgens	Hypersecretion	Granulosa cells Pituitary	Follicular arrest Abnormal gonadotropin secretion
Estrogens	Hypersecretion	Pituitary	Increased LH secretion Suppressed FSH secretion
Insulin	Hypersecretion	Granulosa cells Theca cells	Premature maturation: follicular arrest Hyperandrogenism
IGFBP	Higher levels	Granulosa cells	Inhibitory effect on IGF and FSH actions: follicular arrest
Inhibin	Hypersecretion	Pituitary Theca cells	Suppressed FSH secretion Hyperandrogenism?
Anti-Mullerian Hormone	Higher levels	Theca cells Granulosa cells	Hyperandrogenism Inhibition of aromatase, inhibition of E2 synthesis: follicular arrest

FSH   : Follicle stimulating hormone
LH   : Luteinizing hormone
IGFBP : Insulin-like growth factor binding protein
IGF   : Insulin-like growth factor
E2   : Estradiol

PCOS involve both theca and granulosa cells and may be prompted by intra or extra-ovarian factors.

Extra-ovarian factors

Earlier reports pointed to increased LH pulse frequency and amplitude as the cause of excessive androgen biosynthesis in theca cells. Recent data, however, suggest that hypersecretion of LH, which is not present in all cases of anovulatory PCOS, is not the primary cause, but rather a consequence of impaired feedback due to abnormal ovarian function.[14] Hyperinsulinemia (and insulin resistance) is another extra-ovarian factor that may induce hyperandrogenism by amplifying the effects of LH on theca cell steroid production. Confirmation of this comes from the finding that improvement in insulin sensitivity through the administration of insulin-lowering agents or weight loss decreases serum androgen levels with no effect on LH levels.[15]

Intra-ovarian factors

The finding that cultures of theca cells from PCOS ovaries (excluded from in vivo hormonal stimulation) produce more androgens and progesterone than theca cells isolated from normal ovaries, suggests that dysregulation of androgen biosynthesis is an intrinsic property of theca cells from PCOS[5]. Hyperandrogenism may therefore be genetically determined.[16]

Moreover, granulosa cells produce inhibin, which is thought to modulate follicular steroidogenesis directly. Inhibin might prompt excess intra-ovarian androgens in PCOS by enhancing basal and LH-induced androgen production by theca cells through a paracrine effect from granulosa cells.[13]

Finally, Anti-Mullerian hormones (AMH), produced by granulosa cells, may be involved in the production of excess androgens in PCOS. Recent studies reported an excessive production of AMH in PCOS[17,18] with a positive and significant relationship between AMH and serum testosterone and androstenedione levels

in PCOS patients versus controls, suggesting a positive paracrine effect of AMH on theca cells.

A partial protection from atresia by unknown factors has been hypothesized.[19] The hyperexpression of some growth factors, such as epidermal growth factor (EGF) and transforming growth factor alpha (TGFα), in PCOS, thought to be survival or antiapoptotic factors, led to the belief that they were involved in the blocking of apoptosis and atresia, leading to an accumulation of multiple small antral follicles.

It has also been suggested that oocytes may play a role in regulating follicular activity. Growth differentiation factor 9 (GDF-9) is selectively expressed in developing oocytes and stimulates both basal and LH-stimulated androgen biosynthesis in rat theca cells. It has been reported that GDF-9 expression is reduced and delayed in polycystic ovaries and that GDF-9 deficiency can arrest folliculogenesis before granulosa cells gain competence to initiate apoptosis.[20]

Follicular arrest

Follicular growth arrest is the second folliculogenesis defect reported in PCOS and may account for anovulation by impairing the selection of a single dominant follicle, though no clear explanation has to date been found for it (Table 24.2).

Relative FSH insufficiency

There is evidence that the functional integrity of granulosa cells in PCOS is fully intact when assessed in vitro.[8] The follicles are probably arrested by inadequate FSH secretion and by the inhibition of IGF and FSH actions by intrafollicular insulin-like growth factor-binding proteins (IGFBPs).[8]

The disproportionately low and constant FSH levels in PCOS may be the critical abnormality leading to follicular arrest. The lack of any inter-cycle FSH rise has been described in these women,[8] though this might be due to increased inhibin production or the result of hypothalamic–pituitary feedback from increased ovarian steroid concentrations.

Inhibin selectively inhibits FSH secretion, but its role in the pathogenesis of anovulation in PCOS remains ambiguous. Both, raised and normal inhibin-B concentrations have been reported in the serum or follicular fluid of women with PCOS. It has been shown that inhibin-B is secreted in a pulsatile manner in normal ovulating women. In women with ovulatory dysfunction due to PCOS, no such pattern of regular pulsatility was seen, though it did recover after laparoscopic ovarian diathermy. Lockwood's study concluded that the abnormal pattern of inhibin-B secretion, together with high basal levels due to multiple small follicles, may enhance the process of abnormal folliculogenesis.[21]

Action of growth factors

Recent reports have highlighted the role of local inhibitory factors of FSH activity.[22] Epidermal growth factor (EGF) and transforming growth factor (TGFα and β) are produced in the ovary and correlate inversely with follicular size. They have inhibitory effects on estrogen production from in vitro granulosa cells while TGFα also inhibits LH-stimulated androgen production from theca cells. Cytokines such as tumour necrosis factor-α (TNF-α) seem to modulate theca cell steroidogenesis. Increased levels of TNF-α have been found in serum and follicular fluid of PCOS women and they are inversely correlated with estradiol levels. All these factors may play a role in follicular arrest in PCOS, though this role is still unknown.

Greater importance has recently been attached to AMH, a product of granulosa cells in growing follicles involved in follicle growth. AMH expression is marked in preantral and early antral follicles, reduced in larger antral and preovulatory follicles and absent in primordial or atretic follicles. Women with PCOS have significantly higher serum and follicular fluid AMH levels than normal women, and an inverse AMH-E2 levels relationship.[17] This finding suggests that AMH may modulate ovarian E2 synthesis and may play a role in the typically disordered folliculogenesis of PCOS by exerting a paracrine inhibitory effect on nearby follicles.

A recent study put forward a new explanation for follicular arrest in PCOS.[18] AMH concentration correlated positively with 2 to 5 mm follicles both, in PCOS subjects and controls, but not with 6 to 9 mm follicles, and was *negatively correlated* to serum FSH levels. AMH was also positively correlated with the serum testosterone and androstenedione levels in PCOS only.

The authors postulate that excessive AMH is involved in the inhibition of FSH-induced aromatase activity, thus reducing estradiol synthesis in granulosa cells. The ratio of AMH/number of follicles was not increased, suggesting that each follicle produces a normal amount of AMH while excessive AMH production arises from the greater number of 2–5 mm follicles. Therefore, the inhibitory effect of AMH might not result from an intra-follicular excess of this hormone but rather, from an excessive AMH tone within the microenvironment of the selected follicles.[13]

Premature action of LH

High LH levels are often, but not always, observed in women with PCOS, and are not therefore, indispensable for anovulation. There is evidence of increased theca cell responsiveness to LH stimulation versus normal theca tissue, indicating a primary defect in these cells.[5] The precise nature of the defect is not clear, but an increase in P450 activity induced by genetic factors may be involved. Besides theca cells, granulosa cell behaviour is also abnormal in PCOS. Some reports suggest that anovulatory PCOS patients acquire LH receptors in granulosa cells prematurely and that the number of such receptors is higher than in normal women. This premature response of small antral follicles to LH may indicate that they are in a prematurely advanced stage of development, triggering premature luteinization and arrest of cell proliferation and follicle growth.

Insulin

There is evidence that insulin plays an important role in the arrest of follicular growth. Insulin and IGFs appear to act as co-gonadotropins in the ovary. In theca cells, they act synergistically with LH in stimulating androgen production. The result is an increased androgen substrate in the granulosa cells. Improvement in insulin sensitivity through the administration of insulin-lowering drugs has led to a reduction of serum androgens with no effect on LH levels.

In the granulosa cells, insulin has been found to increase FSH-induced estradiol secretion, both in vitro and in vivo. Hyperinsulinemia, acting in synergy with LH, may induce premature maturation of granulosa cells in vivo in anovulatory women with PCOS and may be a cause of follicular arrest.[22]

In PCOS follicles, IGF is in the physiologic range. In the presence of androstendione, aromatase activity and estradiol secretion by granulosa cells are very low. However, in vitro, these cells respond normally to IGF and FSH. These findings indicate that the functional integrity of granulosa cells in PCOS is fully preserved and that inhibitors of FSH or IGF are present in vivo in the follicles. Intrafollicular IGFBPs have been found to exert an inhibitory effect on IGF and FSH actions. In PCOS follicles, high IGFBP and low IGF levels have been found, as in the androgen-dominated follicles of ovulating woman, whereas the opposite is found in estrogen-dominated follicles. High levels of IGFBP would segregate IGF, thus reducing its facilitatory effect on FSH action and contributing to follicular arrest.[8]

Whether or not insulin resistance is the main etiologic factor in anovulation in PCOS is unclear, because not all PCOS patients have been found to present abnormal insulin secretion. Conversely, hyperinsulinemia and insulin resistance have been found in some ovulatory patients.

Obesity

Insulin resistance in PCOS is frequently associated with obesity. Anovulatory subjects have greater central obesity than women with regular ovulation, higher glucose increment after glucose challenge, lower insulin sensitivity index, higher plasma LH, and lower plasma sex hormone-binding globulin (SHBG). Weight reduction and exercise have been shown to improve menstrual disturbance and infertility in obese women with polycystic ovary syndrome. Lifestyle modification without rapid weight loss leads to a reduction of central fat and improved insulin sensitivity, which restores ovulation in overweight infertile women with PCOS. Lifestyle modification is therefore, the best initial management for obese women seeking to improve their reproductive function.[23]

Pathogenesis of early pregnancy loss in PCOS

Early pregnancy loss, defined as the failure to confirm the presence of an embryonic sac by ultrasound scan at 6–7 weeks gestation, occurs in 18–22% of all positive pregnancy tests.[24] Early pregnancy loss, defined as miscarriage during the first trimester, has been reported to occur in 10–15% of all clinically recognized pregnancies in normal women.[25]

Recurrent pregnancy loss, usually defined as 3 or more consecutive pregnancy losses, occurs in 1% of the pregnant women. Several potential etiologies for recurrent pregnancy loss have been put forward, including chromosomal abnormalities, uterine malformations or cervical incompetence, diabetes mellitus, hypothyroidism, antiphospholipid antibody syndrome or thrombophilia. Women with polycystic ovaries or PCOS have a higher incidence of first trimester spontaneous abortions ranging from 25 to 73%.[26] Polycystic ovaries have been detected in 82% of women suffering from recurrent pregnancy loss.[27]

The precise role of PCOS in the pathogenesis of miscarriage is still uncertain. Some studies have shown a relationship with high LH levels, but several intra or extra-ovarian interconnected factors may also play a role (Table 24.3).

High LH levels

It has been reported that women with either higher

Table 24.3 Factors involved in the pathogenesis of early pregnancy loss in PCOS

Factor	Effect
LH hypersecretion	Premature oocyte maturation Increased endometrial advancement
Androgens hypersecretion	Premature oocyte maturation Inhibition of endometrial cell growth and secretory activity
Insulin hypersecretion	Potentiation of LH and androgens effects
Obesity	Increased androgen free fraction Insulin resistance
PAI hyperactivity	Impaired trophoblastic development, thrombotic placental insufficiency

LH : Luteinizing hormone
PAI : Plasminogen Activator Inhibitor

LH levels or hyperandrogenism are at increased risk of miscarriage following either spontaneous or assisted conception. More recent studies, however, have failed to confirm these reports. In a group of women with recurrent miscarriage,[25] PCOS was diagnosed by ultrasound in 21% of the patients, while 80% of them showed no significant alteration in LH and FSH levels.

As LH is secreted in a pulsatile manner, a single measurement may not detect increased serum LH levels. For this reason, Watson[28] evaluated LH urinary excretion during the cycle and mean follicular phase serum testosterone on a daily basis, and found them to be significantly higher in cases of early pregnancy loss versus control group, the difference in LH being greatest in the early luteal phase. Abnormalities in LH secretion were found in 81% of women with recurrent fetal loss.

Pre-pregnancy pituitary suppression of high endogenous LH by GnRH agonist has been suggested as a way of reducing pregnancy loss after ovulation induction or in vitro fertilization (IVF), but the results are not clear-cut. Homburg[29] reported a reduction in miscarriage rates from 39.1% to 17.6% and an improvement in live birth rates after co-treatment with GnRH agonist and human menopausal gonadotropin (hMG) compared with treatment with gonadotropins alone.

Clifford,[30] however, found no improvement in pregnancy rates using pre-pregnancy suppression of high LH concentrations in ovulatory women with recurrent miscarriage and hypersecretion of LH.

Inappropriately raised LH levels may have an adverse effect on the developing oocyte or endometrium, either directly, or indirectly by triggering an increase in testosterone and estrogen levels. Inhibition of oocyte maturation inhibitor may cause premature oocyte maturation, while hyperandrogenemia may impair folliculogenesis and granulosa cell function.

Alternatively, hypersecretion of LH might exert a negative effect on the endometrium, since LH receptors have been found on the endometrium. This possibility has recently received confirmation from a report analysing the effect of late administration of GnRH antagonist in IVF cycles and indicating that, the higher exposure of the genital tract to LH and E_2 in the mid-follicular phase, might adversely affect implantation rates by altering endometrial receptivity. The different endocrine environment present in these cycles might prompt earlier initiation of progesterone action on the endometrium, enhancing endometrial advancement, which in turn, may significantly compromise the chances of ongoing pregnancy.[31]

The role of high LH levels and PCOS has been recently reconsidered in a study showing similar live birth rates in women with PCOS (60.9%) compared to women with normal ovarian morphology (58.5%). Neither elevated serum LH concentration nor elevated serum testosterone concentration was associated with increased miscarriage rates. The conclusion of the study was that polycystic ovarian morphology is not predictive of pregnancy loss in ovulatory women with recurrent miscarriage.[32]

Hyperandrogenism

Hyperandrogenism is a common feature of PCOS.

The actual mechanism linking hyperandrogenism to increased risk of miscarriage is not known, but for some time, it was thought to be the result of a direct action on the oocyte, possibly a reflection of premature oocyte maturation.[33] However, more recent studies have focused on endometrial receptivity. Androgen levels are higher in women who have recurrent miscarriages, both with and without PCOS, than they are in normal fertile controls, suggesting that this may be a feature of women at risk for recurrent miscarriage, and not simply with PCOS. These high levels of androgens may have a detrimental effect on endometrial function,[34] as has been confirmed by an in vitro study suggesting that, androstenedione can inhibit human endometrial cell growth and secretory activity.[35]

Hyperinsulinemia and obesity

Insulin resistance with compensatory hyperinsulinemia is a key feature of PCOS. It is frequently, but not always, linked with obesity, and has been reported to be an independent risk factor for recurrent pregnancy loss.[26] The potential link between insulin resistance and recurrent pregnancy loss in PCOS has been suggested in studies showing a significant reduction in first trimester miscarriage in women treated with metformin.[6,36]

Hyperinsulinemia boosts the effect of LH and of hyperandrogenemia and has been reported to adversely affect endometrial function.[6]

It is very difficult to distinguish the effects of obesity alone from those of hyperandrogenism and hyperinsulinism. Obesity, is in fact, often present in PCOS and induces a reduction in sex hormone binding globulin (SHBG), increasing the free fraction of circulating androgens. Obesity itself has been described as increasing the risk of miscarriage either after spontaneous or assisted conception.[37] A recent study[38] evaluated the independent effect of PCOS on the risk of miscarriage after adjustment for body mass and other possible confounding factors using multivariate logistic regression analysis in 1018 women; it concluded that the higher risk of miscarriage observed in women with PCOS is probably due to the high prevalence of obesity and high levels of estradiol obtained through ovarian stimulation. Since weight reduction and exercise have been shown to improve insulin sensitivity, it would be advisable for obese patients to reduce weight before planning conception.

Other factors

High levels of plasminogen activator inhibitor (PAI), a significant inhibitor of fibrinolysis, have been reported in women with early recurrent unexplained miscarriage. Recent studies have detected high levels of PAI activity in women with PCOS, and a positive association between PAI activity and miscarriages/adverse pregnancy outcome has been found in PCOS patients.[39]

High levels of PAI may therefore, play a direct role in the pathophysiology of spontaneous miscarriages by provoking thrombotic placental insufficiency. Such an abnormality, occurring in early pregnancy, may also lead to impaired trophoblastic development and poor placentation.[36]

Hyperinsulinemia influences PAI activity. Metformin therapy in patients with PCOS, reduces the levels of PAI activity, fasting serum insulin levels and insulin resistance.[36,39] Moreover, a decrease in the incidence of first trimester spontaneous miscarriages has been reported.[36]

Recent Advances

The role of AMH in the pathogenesis of anovulation in PCOS has recently been examined. One study indicates that insulin might be the key factor in PCO development and that AMH is only a marker of ovarian follicular activity. Administration of metformin induces a rapid decrease in androgen secretion and increases the ovulation rate within four months, reducing circulating AMH only after four months of treatment. From these findings, the authors postulated that the critical ovarian process that is influenced by protracted metformin administration is initial follicular recruitment. The decrease in AMH levels after four months of metformin treatment seems to reflect the replacement of the original cohort (recruited under conditions of insulin resistance and high androgen concentrations) with a new smaller cohort recruited under the normalised insulin regime.[40] However, another very recent study observed AMH in follicles from the primordial stage onward and not in the early antral stage. A relative deficiency of AMH was found in primordial and transitional follicles in ovaries from anovulatory women with polycystic ovaries compared with ovulatory women. This deficiency may contribute to disordered early follicle development in PCOS.[41]

Conclusion

PCOS has been intensively studied for several decades and there have been a lot of new insights in recent years with regard to its pathogenesis. The intimate mechanisms by which it reduces the chances of child-bearing however, have not yet been fully elucidated.

The presence of increased LH pulsatility and FSH deficiency pointed to a possible key role of the GnRH pulse generator dysregulation, but more recently, increasing evidence of a primary ovarian defect has emerged. Both, folliculogenesis and steroidogenesis are disturbed in PCOS.

Hyperandrogenism seems to be the key to both anovulation and pregnancy loss, but hyperinsulinemia also plays an important role in its interaction with LH. Involvement of local intraovarian paracrine factors has recently been detected.

It might be plausible that a series of factors act together in a process that triggers anovulation or early pregnancy loss through the impairment of folliculogenesis, oocyte maturation, steroidogenesis, and endometrial receptivity in a sort of "vicious cycle" where just what actually activates the pathological process still remains to be clarified.

References

1. Hull MG. Epidemiology of infertility and polycystic ovarian disease: endocrinological and demographic studies. *Gynecol Endocrinol* 1987; 1(3): 235–245.
2. Knochenhauer ES, Key TJ, Kahsar-Miller M, Waggoner W, Boots LR, Azziz R. Prevalence of the polycystic ovary syndrome in unselected black and white women of the southeastern United States: a prospective study. *J Clin Endocrinol Metab* 1998; 83(9): 3078–3082.
3. Diamanti-Kandarakis E, Kouli CR, Bergiele AT, et al. A survey of the polycystic ovary syndrome in the Greek island of Lesbos: hormonal and metabolic profile. *J Clin Endocrinol Metab* 1999; 84(11): 4006–4011.
4. Polson DW, Adams J, Wadsworth J, Franks S. Polycystic ovaries–a common finding in normal women. *Lancet* 1988; 1(8590): 870–872.
5. Chang RJ. Polycystic Ovary Syndrome and Hyperandrogenic States. In: Strauss JF, Barbieri RL, editors. Yen and Jaffe's Reproductive Endocrinology, 5th Edition. Philadelphia: *Elsevier Saunders* 2004; p. 597–632.
6. Jakubowicz DJ, Iuorno MJ, Jakubowicz S, Roberts KA, Nestler JE. Effects of metformin on early pregnancy loss in the polycystic ovary syndrome. *J Clin Endocrinol Metab* 2002; 87(2): 524–529.
7. Balen AH, Laven JS, Tan SL, Dewailly D. Ultrasound assessment of the polycystic ovary: international consensus definitions. *Hum Reprod Update* 2003; 9(6): 505–514.
8. Yen SSC. Polycystic Ovary Syndrome. In: Yen SSC, Jaffe RB, Barbieri RL, editors. Reproductive Endocrinology, 4th Edition. Philadelphia: *Saunders* 1999; p. 436–478.
9. Webber LJ, Stubbs S, Stark J, et al. Formation and early development of follicles in the polycystic ovary. *Lancet* 2003; 362(9389): 1017–1021.
10. Hughesdon PE. Morphology and morphogenesis of the Stein-Leventhal ovary and of so-called "hyperthecosis". *Obstet Gynecol Surv* 1982; 37(2): 59–77.
11. Weil S, Vendola K, Zhou J, Bondy CA. Androgen and follicle-stimulating hormone interactions in primate ovarian follicle development. *J Clin Endocrinol Metab* 1999; 84(8): 2951–2956.
12. Vendola K, Zhou J, Wang J, Bondy CA. Androgens promote insulin-like growth factor-I and insulin-like growth factor-I receptor gene expression in the primate ovary. *Hum Reprod* 1999; 14(9): 2328–2332.
13. Jonard S, Dewailly D. The follicular excess in

polycystic ovaries, due to intra-ovarian hyperandrogenism, may be the main culprit for the follicular arrest. *Hum Reprod Update* 2004; 10(2): 107–117.

14. Eagleson CA, Gingrich MB, Pastor CL, et al. Polycystic ovarian syndrome: evidence that flutamide restores sensitivity of the gonadotropin-releasing hormone pulse generator to inhibition by estradiol and progesterone. *J Clin Endocrinol Metab* 2000; 85(11): 4047–4052.

15. Moghetti P, Castello R, Negri C, et al. Metformin effects on clinical features, endocrine and metabolic profiles, and insulin sensitivity in polycystic ovary syndrome: a randomized, double-blind, placebo-controlled 6-month trial, followed by open, long-term clinical evaluation. *J Clin Endocrinol Metab* 2000; 85(1): 139–146.

16. Legro RS, Spielman R, Urbanek M, Driscoll D, Strauss JF, 3rd, Dunaif A. Phenotype and genotype in polycystic ovary syndrome. *Recent Prog Horm Res* 1998; 53: 217–256.

17. Cook CL, Siow Y, Brenner AG, Fallat ME. Relationship between serum Mullerian-inhibiting substance and other reproductive hormones in untreated women with polycystic ovary syndrome and normal women. *Fertil Steril* 2002; 77(1): 141–146.

18. Pigny P, Merlen E, Robert Y, et al. Elevated serum level of anti-Mullerian hormone in patients with polycystic ovary syndrome: relationship to the ovarian follicle excess and to the follicular arrest. *J Clin Endocrinol Metab* 2003; 88(12): 5957–5962.

19. Homburg R, Amsterdam A. Polysystic ovary syndrome–loss of the apoptotic mechanism in the ovarian follicles? *J Endocrinol Invest* 1998; 21(9): 552–557.

20. Teixeira Filho FL, Baracat EC, Lee TH, et al. Aberrant expression of growth differentiation factor-9 in oocytes of women with polycystic ovary syndrome. *J Clin Endocrinol Metab* 2002; 87(3): 1337–1344.

21. Lockwood GM, Muttukrishna S, Groome NP, Matthews DR, Ledger WL. Mid-follicular phase pulses of inhibin B are absent in polycystic ovarian syndrome and are initiated by successful laparoscopic ovarian diathermy: a possible mechanism regulating emergence of the dominant follicle. *J Clin Endocrinol Metab* 1998; 83(5): 1730–1735.

22. van der Spuy ZM, Dyer SJ. The pathogenesis of infertility and early pregnancy loss in polycystic ovary syndrome. Best Pract *Res Clin Obstet Gynaecol* 2004; 18(5): 755–771.

23. Huber-Buchholz MM, Carey DG, Norman RJ. Restoration of reproductive potential by lifestyle modification in obese polycystic ovary syndrome: role of insulin sensitivity and luteinizing hormone. *J Clin Endocrinol Metab* 1999; 84(4): 1470–1474.

24. Winter E, Wang J, Davies MJ, Norman R. Early pregnancy loss following assisted reproductive technology treatment. *Hum Reprod* 2002; 17(12): 3220–3223.

25. Diejomaoh MF, Al-Azemi M, Jirous J, et al. The aetiology and pattern of recurrent pregnancy loss. *J Obstet Gynaecol* 2002; 22(1): 62–67.

26. Glueck CJ, Wang P, Goldenberg N, Sieve-Smith L. Pregnancy outcomes among women with polycystic ovary syndrome treated with metformin. *Hum Reprod* 2002; 17(11): 2858–2864.

27. Sagle M, Bishop K, Ridley N, et al. Recurrent early miscarriage and polycystic ovaries. *BMJ* 1988; 297(6655): 1027–1028.

28. Watson H, Kiddy DS, Hamilton-Fairley D, et al. Hypersecretion of luteinizing hormone and ovarian steroids in women with recurrent early miscarriage. *Hum Reprod* 1993; 8(6): 829–833.

29. Homburg R, Levy T, Berkovitz D, et al. Gonadotropin-releasing hormone agonist reduces the miscarriage rate for pregnancies achieved in women with polycystic ovarian syndrome. *Fertil Steril* 1993; 59(3): 527–531.

30. Clifford K, Rai R, Watson H, Franks S, Regan L. Does suppressing luteinising hormone secretion reduce the miscarriage rate? Results of a randomised controlled trial. *BMJ* 1996; 312(7045): 1508–1511.

31. Kolibianakis EM, Albano C, Kahn J, et al. Exposure to high levels of luteinizing hormone and estradiol in the early follicular phase of gonadotropin-releasing hormone antagonist cycles is associated with a reduced chance of pregnancy. *Fertil Steril* 2003; 79(4): 873–880.

32. Rai R, Backos M, Rushworth F, Regan L. Polycystic ovaries and recurrent miscarriage—a reappraisal. *Hum Reprod* 2000; 15(3): 612–615.

33. Stanger JD, Yovich JL. Reduced in-vitro fertilization of human oocytes from patients with raised basal luteinizing hormone levels during the follicular phase. *Br J Obstet Gynaecol* 1985; 92(4): 385–393.

34. Okon MA, Laird SM, Tuckerman EM, Li TC. Serum androgen levels in women who have recurrent miscarriages and their correlation with markers of endometrial function. *Fertil Steril* 1998; 69(4): 682–690.

35. Tuckerman EM, Okon MA, Li T, Laird SM. Do androgens have a direct effect on endometrial

function? An in vitro study. *Fertil Steril* 2000; 74(4): 771–779.

36. Glueck CJ, Phillips H, Cameron D, Sieve-Smith L, Wang P. Continuing metformin throughout pregnancy in women with polycystic ovary syndrome appears to safely reduce first-trimester spontaneous abortion: a pilot study. *Fertil Steril* 2001; 75(1): 46–52.

37. Fedorcsak P, Storeng R, Dale PO, Tanbo T, Abyholm T. Obesity is a risk factor for early pregnancy loss after IVF or ICSI. *Acta Obstet Gynecol Scand* 2000; 79(1): 43–48.

38. Wang JX, Davies MJ, Norman RJ. Polycystic ovarian syndrome and the risk of spontaneous abortion following assisted reproductive technology treatment. *Hum Reprod* 2001; 16(12): 2606–2609.

39. Glueck CJ, Wang P, Fontaine RN, Sieve-Smith L, Tracy T, Moore SK. Plasminogen activator inhibitor activity: an independent risk factor for the high miscarriage rate during pregnancy in women with polycystic ovary syndrome. *Metabolism* 1999; 48(12): 1589–1595.

40. Fleming R, Harborne L, MacLaughlin DT, et al. Metformin reduces serum Mullerian-inhibiting substance levels in women with polycystic ovary syndrome after protracted treatment. *Fertil Steril* 2005; 83(1): 130–136.

41. Stubbs SA, Hardy K, Da Silva-Buttkus P, et al. Anti-Mullerian hormone protein expression is reduced during the initial stages of follicle development in human polycystic ovaries. *J Clin Endocrinol Metab* 2005; 90(10): 5536–5543.

42. Adams JM, Taylor AE, Crowley WF, Jr., Hall JE. Polycystic ovarian morphology with regular ovulatory cycles: insights into the pathophysiology of polycystic ovarian syndrome. *J Clin Endocrinol Metab* 2004; 89(9): 4343–4350.

Frequently Asked Questions

1. Do all the women with PCO suffer from anovulation?

Polycystic ovaries have been found in about 25% of normal ovulatory women without hyperandrogenism. Moreover, some patients with PCOS ovulate regularly and have normal fertility, despite the presence of clinical and/or biochemical hyperandrogenism. A recent study demonstrated that a polycystic aspect of the ovaries is associated with normal E2, P4, and gonadotropin dynamics, but higher androgen and insulin levels and lower SHBG levels in non-hirsute women with documented ovulatory cycles. These findings suggest that polycystic ovaries with ovulatory cycles exist as a discrete entity, represent the mildest form of ovarian hyperandrogenism, and are associated with greater insulin resistance than in women with normal ovarian morphology.[42]

2. Is anovulation constant in PCOS?

PCOS is more often a cause of oligo-ovulation, rather than of anovulation. Sometimes, for unknown reasons, a dominant follicle is able to elude the inhibitory intra-ovarian influence and proceeds towards ovulation and development of a corpus luteum.

3. Should metformin be suggested as the first line treatment to increase the chances of child-bearing in obese PCOS women?

No, it would be better to suggest weight loss as the first line treatment.

Therapy

25

Treatment of Polycystic Ovary Syndrome in Adolescence

Roy Homburg

Summary

Polycystic Ovary Syndrome (PCOS) in the adolescent is a frequent cause of menstrual irregularity (mostly persistent oligomenorrhea), acne, hirsutism, and even premature pubarche. Typical ultrasound findings in the ovary can complete the clinical diagnosis. The obese especially, should be examined for impairment of insulin sensitivity and glucose tolerance as these, if untreated, may compromise long-term health. The androgen excess of PCOS acts on the pilosebaceous unit to cause acne and hirsutism, which often have a disturbing psychosocial effect on the teenager. Early detection of the syndrome and its treatment with antiandrogens can save much anguish and for the overweight, loss of weight is an integral part of correct management. The long-term use of metformin for adolescents is still hotly debated, but preliminary data suggest that it may have a role in symptomatic, and perhaps, preventative treatment.

Rationale

Polycystic Ovary Syndrome (PCOS) is a very prevalent syndrome, which often presents around the time of the menarche. The pathogenesis of this heterogeneous syndrome is still incompletely determined, and although the symptomatic management in adult women is now fairly well determined, the management of PCOS in adolescents leaves many questions unanswered.

Introduction

As some of the accepted symptoms of PCOS (menstrual irregularities, acne) have been associated with a "normal" adolescence, definitive diagnostic criteria have been blurred. Biochemical features such as increased androgen and insulin secretion, typical of PCOS, are also often, a feature of a normal adolescence. Even when the diagnosis of PCOS has been well established, should the condition be managed symptomatically, prophylactically or not at all, at such a young age? Following a short discourse on the symptomatology, diagnostic criteria, prevalence and pathophysiology of PCOS, these are the questions which will be tackled here.

Clinical Discussion

Symptoms and signs of PCOS in adolescence

Menstrual irregularities and/or symptoms of hyperandrogenism are the commonest form of presentation of PCOS in adolescence.

The menstrual irregularities usually consist of oligomenorrhea (>35 days between menstruation) or amenorrhea (>6 months without bleeding). These symptoms reflect ovulatory dysfunction. Oligomenorrhea in adolescents has widely been regarded as a stage in the physiological maturation of the hypothalamic pituitary-ovarian axis. However, today, following close investigation of oligomenorrheic adolescents, it seems that a very large proportion of these have biochemical markers typical of PCOS and eventually develop the further clinical features of the syndrome. For example, 57% of 52 oligomenorrheic, 15 year olds, had luteinzing hormone (LH) and testosterone levels above the 95th percentile of girls with regular menstrual cycles.[1] Similarly, 32% of adolescents with oligomenorrhea were found to have clinically obvious hirsutism[2] and 21% had acne.[3] If the oligomenorrhea of adolescence does "correct itself", it is most likely to do so in the first two post-menarchal years. After this time, oligomenorrhea may be regarded as a possible early clinical sign of PCOS and is worth investigating.

The commonest forms of clinical expression of hyperandrogenism, the fundamental problem in PCOS, are mainly expressed at the level of the skin in the form of hirsutism and acne.

Hirsutism is an excess of pigmented, thick terminal hair that appears in a male distribution pattern in androgen sensitive areas. These areas include face, chest, abdomen and thighs. Before puberty, body hair is primarily composed of fine, short, unpigmented vellus hair, which during pubarche, is stimulated by androgens to become coarse, pigmented, thickened terminal hair. An excess of androgens will produce such hair growth in a male distribution pattern.

Acne vulgaris is a very common condition, particularly in adolescents. It is basically caused by increased activity in sebaceous glands, which is a manifestation of cutaneous androgenization. It often appears in the teenage years, induced by the burst of pubertal androgenic activity, but if persistent, particularly severe, or of late onset it is commonly associated with PCOS.

Overweight [body mass index (BMI) 26–30 kg/m^2], and frank obesity (BMI > 30 kg/m^2) are associated features in about 40% of adults, but are less common and less pronounced in adolescents.

The typical, ultrasonically-diagnosed, morphological features of the polycystic ovary are the single most prevalent diagnostic sign of this syndrome, whose presentation may have many facets and combinations of signs and symptoms. Biochemical features include raised serum testosterone, androstendione or free androgen index, raised serum LH concentrations and hyperinsulinemia. Again, in a similar fashion to the presentation of the symptoms, the biochemical features are inconsistently present, especially when a single blood sample is analyzed.

Adolescents with PCOS manifest clinical, metabolic and endocrine features similar to those of the adult women and differences between non-obese and obese women with PCOS may be detected in adolescence.[4]

The earliest recognized sign of PCOS is a premature pubarche. Girls who present in mid-childhood with premature growth of pubic hair, elevated dehydroepiandrosterone (DHEA) levels and hyperinsulinemia, are at high risk for developing the full PCOS phenotype, including ovarian hyperandrogenism and chronic anovulation.[5–7]

Diagnosis

The heterogeneity of the signs and symptoms has made the uniform use of diagnostic criteria for PCOS difficult. However, a meeting in Rotterdam in 2003 has created a consensus proposal, in which any 2 of the following features will make the diagnosis of PCOS:

1. Oligo- or anovulation.
2. Hyperandrogenism – clinical and/or biochemical.
3. Polycystic ovaries.

Other disorders with a similar presentation, congenital adrenal hyperplasia, Cushing's syndrome and androgen secreting tumours, should be excluded.

Investigations

Thorough history taking and physical examination are essential. Persistent oligo-or amenorrhea accompanied by symptoms of hyperandrogenism such as hirsutism and acne, virtually make the diagnosis. Hirsutism may be quantified using the Ferriman-Gallwey score and acne should be persistent. The typical ultrasound features of the polycystic ovary, 12 or more follicles of 2–8 mm diameter and/or an ovarian volume of >10cc,[8] are best seen using the vaginal ultrasound but can be amply viewed trans-abdominally in adolescents.

Biochemical features of PCOS may include increased serum concentrations of testosterone, androstendione and LH and low sex hormone binding globulin (SHBG) <35 nmol/L, as well as evidence of insulin resistance. These biochemical features are very heterogeneous and inconsistent and therefore, I do not regard them as essential to make the diagnosis. An estimation of serum testosterone is helpful if an androgen producing tumour is suspected; 17-hydroxy-progesterone concentrations can rule out congenital adrenal hyperplasia to a large extent and Cushing's syndrome, if suspected, can be confirmed in the usual fashion. While insulin resistance and impaired glucose intolerance are not essential features of the diagnosis, their unveiling may be important at an early stage for the prevention of future health hazards, especially in the obese. Screening can be performed relatively easily, by employing a fasting glucose:insulin ratio of <7 as a useful index of insulin resistance in adolescents.[9] If present, regular checks with a 2-hour oral glucose challenge test and fasting lipid profiles should be contemplated.

Prevalence

In adults, PCOS is very prevalent and it has been estimated to be present in some 5–10% of women in the fertile age group.[10] Although data on the prevalence of PCOS in adolescence is very limited, there is no reason to suspect that this is any different at this time to that in adult life, as the symptoms are mostly obvious during this early period in life. In the fertile age group, 92% of women presenting with hirsutism had polycystic ovaries diagnosed by ultrasound scanning as had 87% of those presenting with oligomenorrhea and 26% of those with amenorrhea.[11]

The prevalence of acne in women with PCOS has been less clearly documented, probably due to the fact that it is usually accompanied by more dominant hyperandrogenic symptoms such as hirsutism. However, more than 50% of adolescents who had PCOS, were found to have moderate to severe acne.[12]

The majority of women who have acne will have polycystic ovaries. The most informative large study[13] examined the ultrasound appearance of the ovaries in 82 females with acne vulgaris as the presenting symptom, who were referred to a dermatology clinic. Of these 82 women, 68 (83%) had polycystic ovaries. This staggering figure compares with 19% of women in a control group with no acne who had polycystic ovaries on ultrasound examination. Smaller studies[14–15] have found a prevalence of ultrasound diagnosed polycystic ovaries in 52–80% of women with persistent, moderate to severe acne. To my mind, these types of study have revolutionized much of the treatment of acne, by informing and emphasizing for dermatologists and gynaecologists alike, the role of PCOS in its etiology and applying anti-androgenic therapeutic principles accordingly.

Because of different definitions that have been used, it is difficult to estimate the prevalence of menstrual disturbances in PCOS. However, in the largest series published, using ultrasonically diagnosed polycystic ovaries as the marker[16] 29.7% of such women had normal cycles, 47% had oligomenorrhea, 19.2% had amenorrhea, 2.7% had polymenorrhea and 1.4% had menorrhagia. These figures are remarkably consistent with those of a smaller study that examined the prevalence of menstrual disturbance in women who had both, ultrasound features of polycystic ovaries and clinical and/or biochemical evidence of hyperandrogenism, i.e. PCOS.[17] In this study, 73.6% of the women had oligo/amenorrhea and 26.4% had regular menses.

Clearly, in adolescents, menstrual disturbance is a very prevalent presenting feature of PCOS and polycystic ovaries are found in the vast majority of adolescents with persistent oligomenorrhea.

Pathophysiology

At the heart of PCOS is an overproduction of ovarian androgens. The source of this basic dysfunction is unknown, but some progress has been made in elucidating the consequent pathophysiology.

Ovarian androgen production is basically dictated by the level of activity of the enzyme cytochrome p450c17α, working through the enzymes 17-hydroxylase and 17,20 lyase. The activity of p450c17α is, in turn, influenced by LH, and particularly in PCOS, by the combination of insulin and LH, which hyperactivate the enzyme. The amount of free (bioavailable) testosterone in the circulation is regulated by SHBG whose levels are decreased by both high insulin and high androgen concentrations.

Hirsutism and acne

Paradoxically, hirsutism may be seen in the presence of total testosterone levels in the normal range. It is the amount of biologically active free testosterone (normally about 1% of total testosterone) that dictates the severity of the clinical symptoms, and even small changes in the concentration of SHBG can make a significant difference. Alternatively, hyperandrogenism may be expressed as a result, not of elevated androgen levels, but rather, of increased sensitivity of the pilo sebaceous unit to androgen. This is the probable explanation of the ethnic and genetic differences in the incidence of hirsutism in PCOS which, for example, is much lower in Asian women. High androgen concentrations have a deleterious effect on the development, growth and activity of the sebaceous glands and hair follicles. Testosterone is a strong androgen, which binds to intracellular androgen receptors in the skin and is converted by 5α reductase to dihydrotestosterone (DHT), which has even more potent androgen effects on the hair follicle and sebaceous gland. Two iso-enzymes of 5α reductase are found in the skin cells, type I mostly in sebaceous glands, and type II mostly in the hair follicles themselves.[18]

Increased sebaceous gland function is of major importance in the etiology of acne. Fueled by overstimulation of the androgen receptors, an excess of sebum is produced.

The etiology of acne in early adolescence has been associated with increasing serum levels of dehydroepiandrosterone sulfate (DHEAS), whereas hirsutism has been more directly linked with high concentrations of free testosterone. The two structures comprising the pilosebaceous unit may have different degrees of sensitivity to similar androgenic stimulation.[19]

The hormonal profile of women who have acne and ultrasonically demonstrated polycystic ovaries compared with women who have acne but morphologically normal ovaries differs.[14] Those with polycystic ovaries had raised concentrations of androstendione, DHEA, DHEAS, and LH:FSH ratio compared to those with normal ovaries. Those with polycystic ovaries and acne without other clinical characteristics of PCOS may be a distinct sub-population of women with PCOS.[20]

Menstrual disturbances

The presence and severity of menstrual disturbances have variously been associated with a number of factors. These include obesity, insulin resistance, androgen and LH concentrations and the size of the follicle cohort.

The intimate association of obesity and its exacerbating effect on insulin resistance in women with PCOS has prompted a number of studies to investigate whether insulin insensitivity influences menstrual regularity. Insulin sensitivity was significantly decreased in women with PCOS with oligomenorrhea compared with women with PCOS but regular cycles and compared with controls with normal ovaries.[17] The combination of insulin insensitivity and polycystic ovaries is thus associated with anovulation and irregular cycles. Menstrual irregularity may be related to the magnitude of insulin sensitivity or insulin secretion.[21]

High LH concentrations have also been associated with menstrual irregularity. In a series of 1741 women with ultrasonically detected polycystic ovaries, those with LH concentrations >10IU/l had a very significantly increased incidence of cycle disturbance compared with those who had an LH concentration <10IU/l.[16] In adolescents, hypersecretion of LH is the most common abnormality in those with oligomenorrhea with or without hyperandrogenism.

Management

There is little that can be more devastating to a young woman than the stigmata of hyperandrogenemia. Hirsutism, acne and obesity are there for all to see and may have an often disturbing effect on the social life and psychological make up of a teenager. In addition, hyperandrogenism will often upset the menstrual rhythm, hinder ovulation and consequently, cause infertility. Long term sequelae of hyperandrogenism, often accompanied by hyperinsulinemia, are now coming to light and a failure to relate to the symptoms and signs at an early stage may threaten general health over the age of 40. The management options in adolescent PCOS are numerous, usually symptomatic and, possibly, preventative. Weight loss for the obese and treatment with antiandrogens are well established, whereas the use of insulin sensitizers for adolescents with PCOS is still a debatable topic.

Weight loss

Some 80% of obese women with PCOS have insulin resistance and consequently hyperinsulinemia. They almost inevitably have the stigmata of hyperandrogenism and irregular menstruation. Insulin stimulates LH and ovarian androgen secretion and decreases SHBG.[22] In addition, high levels of insulin lower insulin-like growth factor binding protein I (IGFBP-I) concentrations, releasing more free IGF-1, which in turn promotes the action of LH. Central obesity and BMI are major determinants of insulin resistance, hyperinsulinemia and hyperandrogenemia. As obesity therefore expresses and exaggerates the signs and symptoms of insulin resistance, loss of weight can reverse this process by improving ovarian function and the associated hormonal abnormalities. This is good strategy in order to achieve short and long-term goals such as, reduction in hirsutism and acne, return of ovulation and consequent conception, and almost certainly, a decreased prevalence of cardiovascular disease, hypertension and diabetes mellitus in later life. Curiously, in obese women with PCOS, a loss of 5–10% of body weight is enough to restore reproductive function in 55–100% of the women[23–24] and greatly improve hirsutism in 40–55% within 6 months of weight reduction.[24] This weight loss can be successfully achieved with a low calorie diet, exercise and a change in lifestyle, pioneered in a program with impressive results.[25] Weight loss has the undoubted advantages of being effective and cheap with no side effects.

Insulin sensitizing agents

Metformin is an oral biguanide used for the treatment of diabetes as it is an antihyperglycemic, which inhibits hepatic glucose production and increases the number of insulin receptors. Insulin concentrations are therefore decreased as a secondary phenomenon with a resulting decrease in androgen and LH concentrations and increase in sex hormone binding globulin. Metformin may also have a direct action on theca cells, reducing androgen production. There are now many reports of clinical improvement with metformin in, mostly obese, adult women with PCOS.[26–27] In doses of 1500–2550 mg/day, gastrointestinal side effects have proved troublesome and common, but serious side effects have not been reported in an adolescent population.[28]

While adolescents with PCOS will inevitably be disturbed by the obvious and blatant stigmata, acne and hirsutism, and be worried by menstrual irregularity or absence of menstruation, the long-term sequelae of the syndrome are of less immediate concern to them. A debate has now evolved regarding the use of insulin sensitizing agents, notably metformin, in this age group.[29] Theoretically, this treatment, as evidenced in adults, will reduce hyperandrogenism and therefore, will improve hirsutism, acne and ovulatory dysfunction in the short-to medium-term. In the long-term, it would hypothetically help to prevent the onset of type-2 diabetes, beta cell exhaustion and maybe, cardiovascular disease after the age of 40, by eliminating persistent hyperinsulinemia. While traditional treatments with oral contraceptives and antiandrogens correct menstrual irregularity and hyperandrogenemia and consequently, acne and hirsutism, they do not positively affect hyperinsulinemia and its consequences.

The decision whether to employ metformin as part of the therapeutic armamentarium in adolescent PCOS, is a difficult one based on today's knowledge. There are no large, randomized, controlled trials in adolescents. A handful of short-term studies, and with small numbers, have shown a distinct improvement in obese and non-obese adolescents with PCOS in restoring menstrual regularity and improving androgen concentrations. Glueck et al.[30] gave metformin for a mean of 10 months to 11 oligo- or amenorrheic adolescents with PCOS. Ten responded by resuming regular, ovulatory cycles. Although this sounds encouraging, the results are confounded by a concomitant diet-induced weight reduction. Ibanez et al.[31] gave metformin for 6 months to 18 non-obese girls with anovulatory, hyperinsulinemic hyperandrogenism with success in that, 14 started ovulating regularly and no serious side effects were noted. A recent study by the same team[32] examined the effects of a low-dose combination of flutamide and metformin on 30 teeenagers who had hyperinsulinemic hyperandrogenism. Hirsutism, serum androgens, insulin sensitivity, lipid profile, abdominal fat and ovulation rate, all showed marked improvement following this treatment.

However, several questions still remain unanswered. Will metformin be effective in preventing the long-term sequelae of the syndrome? Will it prove as completely safe as present data suggest? What will be the effect of committing a teenager to maybe 20 years of medication? Time and well controlled, randomized, long-term trials are needed to answer these questions. A further question relates to the fact that a correct diet and lifestyle have already proven to be of value in the prevention of diabetes, hypertension and cardio vascular disease in adults. If this education could be impressed upon adolescent girls with PCOS and continued into the reproductive years, there is much to be gained.

Antiandrogens

As the acne associated with PCOS undoubtedly arises from over stimulation of the pilosebaceous unit by androgens, then antiandrogens are the most effective long-term treatment option.

Figure 25.1 indicates the possibilities and sites of action of a number of antiandrogen medications that block the synthesis or action of androgens: cyproterone acetate (CPA), spironolactone, flutamide, finasteride and ketoconazole.

Excluding North America, a combination of CPA (an orally active progestogen), is probably, the most widely used antiandrogen used in combination with ethinyl estradiol (EE). CPA has an anti androgen action at several sites[33]: 1. in combination with EE, it suppresses LH release by the anterior pituitary, 2. competes for the androgen receptor which it blocks, 3. suppresses the action of 5α reductase as a progestogen, and 4. with EE, it increases SHBG concentrations. The combination of CPA (2 mg/day) and EE (35 μg/day) given cyclically, has proved very effective in the treatment of hirsutism and acne in addition to serving as an excellent contraceptive.[34] A reduction of more than 50% in the hirsutism score has been demonstrated after 9 months of treatment,[35] and acne has been successfully treated in almost 100% of the cases using this minimal

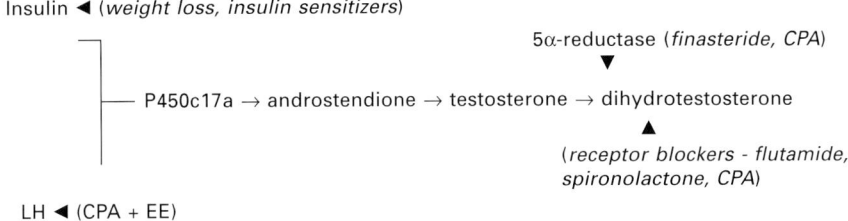

Insulin ◄ (*weight loss, insulin sensitizers*)

5α-reductase (*finasteride, CPA*)
▼
P450c17a → androstendione → testosterone → dihydrotestosterone
▲
(*receptor blockers - flutamide, spironolactone, CPA*)

LH ◄ (CPA + EE)

Figure 25.1   Sites of action of anti-androgen agents. Possible treatments are in parentheses and italics. (CPA = cyproterone acetate, EE = ethinyl estradiol).

dose.[36] The addition of CPA in a dose of 10–100 mg/day on the first 10 days of the combined medication has proved effective in more severe cases. Success rates in reversing or severely diminishing symptoms and maintaining improvement are high with minimal side effects, but patients need to be informed that this treatment is not "instant", and that, at least 4–9 months are needed to see an improvement in hirsutism and 3–5 months for acne. Acne will be cleared in 60% of the patients in six months and after 12 months, 95% should be free of acne.

Side effects of CPA in combination with ethinyl estradiol are similar to those of oral contraceptives, are usually mild and transient and include mastodinia, increased appetite and headaches. The effects on the lipid profile are usually slight and probably clinically irrelevant, and include an increase in triglycerides and a small increase in cholesterol, mainly due to an increase in the high density lipoprotein (HDL) fraction. No significant hepatotoxicity has been reported in a woman using CPA cyclically.

Spironolactone is an aldosterone antagonist but its antiandrogen action is exerted by competitive inhibition of testosterone and DHT binding to the androgen receptor. In the usual dose of 100 mg/day, spironolactone does not seem to suppress either androgen or LH levels.[37] Spironolactone has been widely used for the treatment of hirsutism. A recent, randomised, double-blind, placebo controlled trial reported a 41% reduction in the hirsutism score after 6 months of treatment with spironolactone. These improvements following spironolactone treatment were very similar to those obtained with flutamide and finasteride.[38]

Flutamide is a non steroidal anti androgen, which has primarily been used in advanced prostatic carcinoma in that, it inhibits DHT binding to the androgen receptors. It has also proved effective in the treatment of hirsutism and acne in women.[39] Similar improvements in hirsutism have been reported whether doses of 250 mg or 500 mg/day were used. The efficacy, non-interference with ovulation and generally good tolerance of flutamide, have been tempered by rare reports of hepatotoxicity,[40] which may be severe, and the incidence of which seems to increase with higher doses.[39] Careful monitoring of liver function is therefore advised if flutamide is to be used for the treatment of hisutism or acne.

Finasteride has quite a different site of action. It acts by inhibiting the activity of 5α reductase, the enzyme responsible for the conversion of testosterone to DHT, which is particularly potent at the hair follicle level. This treatment is taken orally in a dose of 1–5 mg/day and is effective without any appreciable side effects although it may need more prolonged treatment to achieve the goal. Finasteride is effective in the treatment of hirsutism as 5α reductase has a vital role in the androgen regulation of hair growth, and its inhibition is thus, potentially effective.

In PCOS patients, a higher efficacy has been reported with CPA and flutamide compared with finasteride.[40] Others have reported no therapeutic differences between finasteride and flutamide,[41] nor between CPA and spironolactone.[42] The lower the dose of any of these drugs, the lower the prevalence of side effects.

However effective these antiandrogen medicines may be, they ameliorate symptoms while they are being taken, but fail to "cure" the cause. After the withdrawal of treatment with spironolactone, flutamide or CPA, hirsutism relapses to 60–80% of the original score, regardless of which antiandrogen therapy is used.[43] What is now becoming clear is that the longer the duration of treatment (at least with CPA/EE) the lesser the chance of relapse within a given time. Using long-term treatment with CPA (25–50 mg/day) and EE (0.01–0.02 mg/day) in a reverse sequential regimen, hirsutism was absent for 6 months in all patients.[44] After 12 months without treatment, hirsutism had worsened in 28% of the patients and after 24 months, 44% were still showing an improvement on the original hirsutism score. A further study, using standard treatment with CPA/EE (2 mg/35 μg), followed-up 34 patients after cessation of treatment.[45] Six patients had had no relapse within the follow up period of 19 months. The only significant difference was in the duration of treatment between those who relapsed (mean 26 months) and those who did not (40 months).

An essential element in the successful compliance of the patient on anti androgen treatment is the accuracy and fullness of information given to her by the physician. First and foremost, the fact that a good clinical response to treatment takes time, is essential. Secondly, the need for long term maintenance treatment of 3-4 years, even when obvious clinical improvement has been achieved. Thirdly, the possibility of relapse, some time after treatment is terminated.

Restoring menstrual regularity

The aim of treatment for the menstrual disturbances associated with PCOS, is to provide a regular menstrual cycle. This can be achieved using measures, which will also relieve symptoms associated with hyperandrogenism, particularly hirsutism and acne, will prevent endometrial hyperplasia, and may help prevent long-term health consequences.

As with the treatment of all other symptoms associated with PCOS in obese patients, weight loss should be the first line of treatment. This alone has an excellent chance of restoring normal menstrual regularity in patients who succeed in losing >5% of their body weight.[23] This improvement is associated with a reduction in circulating insulin and androgen levels, which can also be achieved using insulin sensitizing drugs. Although evidence is still flimsy, metformin does appear to improve cyclicity in about 50% of patients with oligo/amenorrhea (see above). In a compilation of data from controlled trials, Harborne et al.[46] found that women on metformin had 41 cycles per 100 patient months compared with 21 cycles per 100 patient months in those receiving placebo. They concluded that these improvements were variable and modest. It seems therefore, that insulin sensitizers cannot as yet be recommended for treatment when menstrual irregularity is the primary complaint.

For those who have symptoms of hyperandrogenism associated with their menstrual irregularity, the cyclical administration of the combination of ethinyl estradiol (EE) and the anti-androgen cyproterone acetate (CPA) would seem to be the optimal treatment. This has been described in length above. As untreated PCOS may be regarded as a progressive syndrome, at least up to the age of 40, it is reasonable to assume that treatment with this combination of EE and CPA, which markedly reduces androgen concentrations and their untoward effects, will put the syndrome "on hold" so improving the prospects of success of fertility treatment when it is discontinued. All other cyclically administered contraceptive pills will of course, regularize the cycle.

Mainly due to the lack of availability of CPA in the United States, other antiandrogenic drugs have been employed for the treatment of PCOS. These include spironolactone, flutamide and finasteride, but again, these are not usually utilized as first line treatment when menstrual irregularity is the primary complaint, especially for adolescents.

Conclusions

Persistent oligomenorrhea is a common symptom

of PCOS in adolescence and PCOS also underlies many a case of moderate to severe acne. Awareness of the early symptoms of PCOS is essential for diagnosis and correct symptomatic management.

The combination of cyproterone acetate and ethinyl estradiol is very effective for the treatment of acne, hirsutism and cycle disturbances. Treatment with insulin sensitizers for the adolescent is a possibility, but not yet scientifically established; for the obese adolescent, loss of weight is equally as effective.

References

1. Van Hooff MHA, Voorhoorst FJ, Kaptein MBH, Hirasing RA, Koppenaal C, Schoemaker J. Endocrine features of polycystic ovary syndrome in a random population sample 14-16 year-old adolescents. *Hum Reprod* 1999; 14: 2223–2229.
2. Siegberg R, Nilsson CG, Stenman UH, Widhold O. Endocrinologic features of oligomenorrheic adolescent girls. *Fertil Steril* 1986; 46: 852–857.
3. Apter D, Vihko R. endocrine determinants of fertility: serum androgen concentrations during follow-up of adolescents into the third decade of life. *J clin Endocrinol Metab* 1990; 71: 970–974.
4. Silfen ME, Denburg MR, Manibo AM, et al. Early endocrine, metabolic, and sonographic characteristics of polycystic ovary syndrome: comparison between nonobese and obese adolescents. *J Clin Endocrinol Metab* 2003; 88: 4682–4688.
5. Legro RS. Detection of insulin resistance and its treatment in adolescents with polycystic ovary syndrome. *J Pediatr Endocrinol Metab* 2002; 15 Suppl 5: 1367–1378.
6. Rosenfield RL, Ghai K, Ehrmann DA, Barnes RB. Diagnosis of the polycystic ovary syndrome in adolescence: comparison of adolescent and adult hyperandrogenism. *J Pediatr Endocrinol Metab* 2000; 13 Suppl 5: 1285–1289.
7. Ibanez L, Ong KK, Mongan N, et al. Androgen receptor gene CAG repeat polymorphism in the development of ovarian hyperandrogenism. *J Clin Endocrinol Metab* 2003; 88: 3337–3338.
8. Jonard S, Robert Y, Cortet C, Decanter C, Dewailly D. Ultrasound examination of polycystic ovaries: Is it worth counting the follicles? *Hum Reprod* 2003; 18: 598–603.
9. Kent SC, Legro RS. Polycystic ovary syndrome in adolescents. *Adolesc Med* 2002; 13: 73–88.
10. Erkokola R, Ruutiainen K. Hirsutism: definitions and etiology. *Ann Med* 1990; 22: 99–103.
11. Adams J, Polson DW, Franks S. Prevalence of polycystic ovaries in women with anovulation and idiopathic hirsutism. *Brit Med J* 1986; 293: 355–359.
12. Dramusic V, Rajan U, Chan P, Ratnam SS, Wong YC. Adolescent polycystic ovary syndrome. *Ann NY Acad Sci* 1997; 816: 194–208.
13. Bunker CB, Newton J, Kilborn J, et al. Most women with acne have polycystic ovaries. *Brit J Dermatol* 1989; 121: 675–680.
14. Betti R, Bencini PL, Lodi A, Urbani CE, Chiarelli G, Crosti C. Incidence of polycystic ovaries in patients with late-onset or persistent acne: hormonal reports. *Dermatologica* 1990; 181: 109–111.
15. Jebraili R, Kaur S, Kanwar AJ, Kataria S, Dash RJ. Hormone profile & polycystic ovaries in acne vulgaris. *Indian J Med Res* 1994; 100: 73–76.
16. Balen AH, Conway GS, Kaltsas G, Techatrasak K, Manning PJ, West C, Jacobs HS. Polycystic ovary syndrome: the spectrum of the disorder in 1741 patients. *Hum Reprod* 1995; 10: 2705–2711.
17. Robinson S, Kiddy D, Gelding SV, et al. The relationship of insulin insensitivity to menstrual pattern in women with hyperandrogenism and polycystic ovaries. *Clin Endocrinol* 1993; 39: 351–355.
18. Paus R, Cotsarelis G. The biology of hair follicles. *N Engl J Med* 1999; 341: 491–497.
19. Toscano V, Balducci R, Bianchi P, Guglielmi R, Mangiantini A, Rossi FG, Colonna LM, Sciarra F. Two different pathogenetic mechanisms may play a role in acne and in hirsutism. *Clin Endocrinol* (Oxf). 1993 Nov; 39(5): 551–556.
20. Bunker CB, Newton JA, Conway GS, Jacobs HS, Greaves MW, Dowd PM. The hormonal profile of women with acne and polycystic ovaries. *Clin Exp Dermatol* 1991; 16: 420–423.
21. Legro RS, Bentley-Lewis R, Driscoll D, Wang SC, Dunaif A. Insulin resistance in the sisters of women with polycystic ovary syndrome: Association with hyperandrogenemia rather than menstrual irregularity. *J Clin Endocrinol Metab* 2002; 87: 2128–2133.
22. Poretsky L, Cataldo NA, Rosenwaks Z, Giudice LC. The insulin related ovarian regulatory system in health and disease. *Endoc Revs* 1999; 20: 535–582.
23. Kiddy DS, Hamilton-Fairley D, Bush A et al. Improvement in endocrine and ovarian function during dietary treatment of obese women with

polycystic ovary syndrome. *Clin Endocrinology* 1992; 36: 105–111.

24. Pasquali R, Antenucci D, Casmirri F, et al. Clinical and hormonal characteristics of obese amenorrheic hyperandrogenic women before and after weight loss. *J Clin Endocrinol Metab* 1989; 68: 173–179.

25. Clark AM, Thornley B, Tomlinson L, Galletley C, Norman RJ. Weight loss in obese infertile women results in improvement in reproductive outcome for all forms of fertility treatment. *Hum Reprod* 1998; 13: 1502–1505.

26. Pasquali R, Gambineri A, Biscotti D, et al. Effect of long term treatment with metformin added to hypocaloric diet on body composition, fat distribution and androgen and insulin levels in abdominally obese women with and without polycystic ovary syndrome. *J Clin Endocrinol Metab* 2000; 85: 2767–2774.

27. Moghetti P, Castello R, Negri C, et al. Metformin effects on clinical features, endocrine and metabolic profiles and insulin sensitivity in polycystic ovary syndrome: a randomized, double blind, placebo-controlled 6-month trial, followed by open, long term clinical evaluation. *J Clin Endocrinol Metab* 2000; 85: 139–146.

28. Legro RS. Polycystic ovary syndrome: current and future treatment paradigms. *Am J Obstet Gynecol* 1998; 1795: S101.

29. Jamieson MA. The use of metformin in adolescents with polycystic ovary syndrome. *J Pediatr Adolesc Gynecol* 2002; 15: 109–114.

30. Glueck CJ, Wang P, Fontaine R, Tracy T, Sieve-Smith L. Metformin to restore normal menses in oligo-amenorrheic teenage girls with polycystic ovary syndrome. *J Adolesc Health* 2001; 29: 160–169.

31. Ibanez L, Valls C, Ferrer A, Marcos M V, Rodriguez-Hiero F, de Zegher F. Sensitization to insulin induces ovulation in nonobese adolescents with anovulatory hyperandrogenism. *J Clin Endocrinol Metab* 2001; 86: 3595–3598.

32. Ibanez L, Ong K, Ferrer A, Amin R, Dunger D, de Zegher F. Low dose flutamide-metformin therapy reverses insulin resistance and reduces fat mass in nonobese adolescents with ovarian hyperandrogenism. *J Clin Endocrinol Metab* 2003; 88: 2600–2606.

33. Diamanti-Kandarakis E, Tolis G, Duleba A. Androgens and therapeutic aspects of anti-androgens in women. 1995; 2: 577–592.

34. Golland IM, Elstein ME. Results of an open one-year study with diane-35 in women with polycystic ovarian syndrome, 1993; 687: 263–8.

35. Sarih Y, Diber S, Kelestimur F. comparison of Diane 35 and Diane 35 plus finasteride in the treatment of hirsutism. *Fertil Steril* 2001; 75: 496–500.

36. Van Waygen RG, van den Ende A. Experience in the long term treatment of hisutism and/or acne with cyproterone acetate-containing preparations. Efficacy, metabolic and endocrine effects. *Expl Clin Endocrinol Diabetes* 1995; 103: 241–251.

37. Spritzer PM, Opperman-Lisboa K, Mattiello S, Lhulier F. Spironolactone as a single agent for long term therapy of hirsute patients. *Clin Endocrinol* 2000; 52: 587–594.

38. Moghetti P, Tosi F, Tosti A, et al. Comparison of spironolactone, flutamide and finasteride efficacy in the treatment of hirsutism: a randomized, double-blind, placebo controlled trial. *J Clin Endocrinol Metab* 2000; 85: 89–94.

39. Moghetti P, Castello R, Negri C, et al. Flutamide in the treatment hirsutism: long term clinical effects, endocrine changes and androgen receptor behaviour. *Fertil Steril* 1995; 64: 511–517.

40. Venturoli S, Marescalchi O, Colombo FM, et al. A prospective randomized trial comparing low dose flutamide, finasteride, ketoconazole and cyproterone acetate-estrogen regimens in the treatment of hirsutism. *J clin Endocrinol Metab* 1999; 84: 1304–1310.

41. Falsetti L, De Fusco D, Eleftheriou G, et al. Treatment of hirsutism by finasteride and flutamide in women with polycystic ovary syndrome. *Gynecol Endocrinol* 1997; 11: 251–257.

42. Erenus M, Yucelten D, Gurbuz O, et al. Comparison of spironolactone-oral contraceptive versus cyproterone acetate-estrogen regimens in the treat-ment of hirsutism. *Fertil Steril* 1996; 66: 216–219.

43. Yucelten D, Erenus M, Gurbuz O, Durmusoglu F. Recurrence rate of hirsutism after 3 different antiandrogen therapies. *J Am Acad Dermatol* 1999; 41: 64–68.

44. Flagmini C, Venturoli S, Fabbri R. Long term management of hirsute patients with cyproterone acetate. In: Spona J, Aydinlik S eds. Hirsutism and endocrine dermatological problems. Parthenon Press, Carnforth, *Lancs* 1988; pp 29–37.

45. Kokaly W, McKenna TJ. Relapse of hirsutism following long-term successful treatment with oestrogen-progesterone combination. *Clin Endocrinol* 2000; 52: 379–382.

46. Harborne L, Fleming R, Lyall H, Norman J, Sattar N. Descriptive review of the evidence for the use of metformin in polycystic ovary syndrome. *Lancet* 2003; 361: 1894–1900.

Frequently Asked Questions

1. How can PCOS be distinguished from 'normal' adolescent stigmata?

The presence of persistent oligomenorrhea, more than 2 years after the menarche and/or acne, which is particularly severe, persistent or of late onset, are very suggestive of PCOS.

2. Should testing for insulin resistance be performed in all cases of adolescent PCOS?

This is not mandatory except for girls who are overweight or frankly obese.

3. Does every adolescent who has a diagnosis of PCOS need treatment?

The treatment of PCOS at this stage of life is symptomatic. If the patient is disturbed by the symptoms, it is worthwhile treating. Prophylactic treatment with a combination of CPA+E2, or life-style change if overweight or frankly obese, are obvious options. Long-term treatment with insulin sensitizers has not yet been established.

4. What is the earliest age that treatment should be started?

I, personally, do not treat before the age of 15 years.

26

Pharmacologic Treatment of Polycystic Ovary Syndrome in the Reproductive Years

Cem S Atabekoglu, Aydin Arici

Summary

In clinical practice, patients with polycystic ovary syndrome (PCOS) frequently require medical therapy for menstrual irregularity, infertility, obesity, excess hair growth, hair loss and acne. The selection of therapy for PCOS generally depends on the physical symptoms and patient's desire for childbearing. In addition, patients with PCOS have noteworthy long-term risks such as diabetes, coronary artery disease, endometrial or breast cancer. Long-term follow-up of women with PCOS has revealed that approximately 40% of patients develop impaired glucose tolerance (IGT) or frank non-insulin dependent diabetes mellitus (NIDDM) by the time they arrive at the age of 40.[1] For this reason, PCOS is represented as a major health issue that affects young women. The medical treatment of PCOS has long centered upon only symptoms and on producing a hypoandrogenic environment. Recently, however, the approach has changed. We now have a much greater depth of understanding of the pathogenesis of PCOS. Developments in molecular biology have greatly expanded our understanding of this syndrome. The relationship between insulin resistance and PCOS has been known since 1980. Nowadays, insulin-sensitizing drugs have gained popularity because they both, ameliorate symptoms of PCOS and correct probable main

pathogenetic factors. Several unresolved controversies persist regarding the treatment of women with PCOS. This article addresses a review of the pharmacologic treatment of PCOS in accordance with current knowledge.

Introduction

Treatment of oligomenorrhea and amenorrhea

Menstrual irregularity is the most common gynecological presentation of PCOS. Dysfunctional bleeding and amenorrhea have been noted in 29% and 51% of patients with PCOS respectively.[2] It should be kept in mind that chronic anovulation may increase the risk of endometrial hyperplasia and carcinoma. Although endometrial cancers occur in 5% or fewer women under the age of 40 years, PCOS is common in these patients.[3] Hence, endometrial evaluation should be considered if patients with PCOS do not have regular menstrual bleeding for a year or longer. Ultrasonography may help to establish the risk and need for biopsy. These anovulatory women are required to take medication in order to reduce their endometrial carcinoma risk. Classically, administering either cyclic progestin or oral contraceptives with a combination of estrogen and progestin can inhibit endometrial proliferation. If progestin only treatment is chosen, it should be given at least for 12 to 14 days every month. Combined oral contraceptives have traditionally been used for menstrual disorders, in cases where fertility is not desired. Combined oral contraceptive use both, achieves inhibition of endometrial proliferation and reduces ovarian androgen production, which ameliorates the symptoms relevant to hyperandrogenism. Although combined oral contraceptives are efficacious in cycle control and protect against endometrial hyperplasia, there may be some drawbacks of long-term use due to the undesired effects of the pill on insulin resistance and obesity. It is increasingly recommended that the use of combined oral contraceptives be reviewed for long-term treatment and if possible, alternative methods be taken into consideration in the patient with PCOS.

Obesity is observed 4-times more frequently in women with menstrual disturbances compared to women with normal cycles. Women with PCOS are often overweight and obesity is present in at least 30% and, some series have reported percentages up to 75%. Both, PCOS and obesity are independent risk factors for insulin resistance. The presence of obesity may worsen the effect of PCOS on menstrual functions. It has been shown that if women with PCOS have a body mass index (BMI) higher than 30 kg/m^2, 70% of these patients have menstrual disturbances and only 22% have normal menstrual function.[4] It has also been shown that if these obese women with PCOS lose weight, they are more likely to resume regular menstruation. Studies related to weight loss through lifestyle modification have indicated an improvement in menstrual regularity. If patients have been classified as overweight or obese at the time of therapy, weight management with dietary intervention and increased physical activity should be offered as a first line treatment option. Large changes in weight may not be needed to restore reproductive function. A relatively small or modest (2 to 7%) weight loss can improve insulin resistance, hyperandrogenism, menstrual function and fertility.[5,6] Moreover, weight loss is also important to reduce long-term risks; therefore,

weight loss must be a rational and available goal for obese PCOS patients.

There is a correlation between menstrual irregularity and infertility with increased serum androgens and luteinizing hormone (LH) in obese patients with PCOS. Another endocrinological disturbance in obese PCOS patients is insulin resistance. Insulin resistance is strongly influenced by obesity in non-PCOS subjects.

Lately, insulin resistance and compensatory hyperinsulinemia have been well documented in lean and obese women with PCOS in comparison to weight-matched controls. Owing to both, poor long-term compliance with the weight reduction program, and the fact that 10 to 30% of women with PCOS are non-obese, weight loss is not a treatment option for all PCOS patients. Besides, insulin resistance of PCOS appears to impart an increased risk of glucose intolerance, diabetes, and lipid abnormalities, and may enhance the development of macrovascular disease. Given the strong evidence that hyperinsulinemia plays a crucial pathogenic role in the development of PCOS, it is reasonable to assume that interventions that reduce circulating insulin levels in women with PCOS may restore normal reproductive functions and decrease long-term complications of PCOS.

Insulin sensitizers have been utilized for many years to prevent the long-term complications of diabetes and consequent cardiovascular disease and are now becoming popular in PCOS. However, there has not yet been any consensus about the efficacy of insulin sensitizers on long-term cardiovascular risks associated with PCOS. The most commonly used insulin sensitizer in PCOS is metformin. Metformin is an oral biguanide, which is well established for the treatment of hyperglycemia and does not cause hypoglycemia in normoglycemic patients. The majority of studies related to metformin have demonstrated a significant improvement in insulin sensitivity, serum insulin and androgen levels, accompanied by decreased LH and increased sex hormone binding globulin (SHBG) concentrations. On the contrary, some studies did not find any significant change in fasting insulin or insulin response to glucose challenge and testosterone levels, except for weight loss. Authors speculated that the amelioration of clinical features in response to metformin might take place independent of insulin sensitivity or circulating insulin concentrations.

The restoration of regular menstrual cycles by metformin has been reported in approximately 60% of the patients and the restoration of ovulation occurred in 78–96% of the patients in the published series. Recently, Kriplani et al.[7] has shown that a six-month metformin therapy improves menstrual cyclicity by 85% in oligomenorrheic, hypomenorrheic, amenorrheic and infertile women with PCOS. Moreover, 62% of responders achieved regular periods. Glueck et al.[8,9] showed that metformin treatment allowed resumption of normal menses in most teenagers (91%) with PCOS, who were previously amenorrheic and in 74% of who had fasting hyperinsulinemia. The same researchers described their clinical experience with metformin combined with a high protein–low carbohydrate diet in a similar population. After at least 6 months follow-up, all treated patients had normal fasting blood glucose and glycohemoglobin levels, and 91% resumed regular normal menses.[8,9] Recently, Kayshap et al.[10] evaluated this topic in their meta-analysis and showed that metformin treatment has beneficial effects on cycle regulation in patients with PCOS, who did not have complaints of infertility as compared with placebo (RR 1.45; 95% CI 1.11-1.90).

Two recent large studies have shown that decreasing insulin resistance through diet, exercise, or metformin, can decrease the development of diabetes in individuals at high risk.[11,12] Knowler et al.[12] showed that the use of metformin decreased the risk of developing frank diabetes by 31%. It has also been shown by the UK Prospective Diabetes Study (UKPDS) Group that diabetics treated with metformin have significantly fewer cardiovascular events.[13] According to these limited data, although long-term use of metformin treatment seems to be beneficial in women with PCOS and glucose intolerance, further studies are needed to show additional health benefits and safety of the drug for long-term use.

Clinical Discussion

Treatment of infertility

PCOS is known to be the most common cause of anovulatory infertility. Similar to the management of menstrual irregularity of any origin, lifestyle modification with caloric restriction and exercise is extremely important in the first stage of intervention. This should be considered as active medical therapy and not as an alternative to other medical interventions. Regardless of the indication and type of treatment, this was clearly shown in the study by Clark et al.[14] which was performed on patients with a body mass index (BMI) >30 kg/m^2 who were infertile for more than 2 years. However, approximately three-fourths of the patients had PCOS. These patients were considered for a six months lifestyle modification program before the conventional medical treatment for infertility. Of the 67 patients who completely obeyed the program, 60 ovulated and 52 (77.6%) became pregnant, compared with none in the dropout group.[14] Unfortunately, many women with PCOS find lifestyle intervention difficult to institute and maintain. Besides, quite a few patients are in the normal weight range and may not benefit from weight loss.

There are number of medical or surgical therapies to induce ovulation and accomplish pregnancy in women with PCOS. All gynecologists are interested in the most effective therapy for anovulatory patients with PCOS who wish to become pregnant.

Ovulation induction

There are two reasons for conducting ovulation induction (OI) in a patient with PCOS. One is to restore normal ovulation, with the purpose of maintaining a single follicle for timed intercourse. The other is to obtain multiple follicles through controlled ovarian hyperstimulation (COH), for in vitro fertilization (IVF)/intracytoplasmic sperm injection (ICSI). Obviously, you should not start with the same approach in these two groups.

Clomiphene citrate

Clomiphene citrate (CC) has been used for induction of ovulation since 1962. Because of the cheap, safe and incomplex management, CC is still used as a first line treatment for infertile anovulatory PCOS patients. CC significantly increases ovulation by interfering with the feedback mechanisms in the hypothalamic pituitary ovarian axis. The success rate of CC treatment in anovulatory PCOS women is very high. It has been shown that approximately 60%–85% of the patients ovulate, but only 30%–40% of them conceive following CC therapy. Women, who fail to ovulate on low doses of CC, are given higher doses of the drug. If patients still do not ovulate, they are described as CC resistant. Rates of CC resistance are approximately 15 to 40% in women with PCOS.

In these CC-resistant women, other treatment modalities such as laparoscopic electrocautery or ovulation induction with gonadotropins have been proposed as alternative therapies for women with PCOS. Laparoscopic ovarian drilling has potential side effects, including serious surgical complications and anesthetic risks. Injection of gonadotropins has been employed as a very effective treatment over the years, but especially in PCOS, this treatment requires a high degree of skill, extensive hormone and ultrasound monitoring, since follicular response tends to be initially slow, but explosive in the later stages of stimulation, which may be associated with multiple pregnancies and ovarian hyperstimulation syndrome (OHSS).

Gonadotropins

The first choice of treatment in patients with CC resistant PCOS is still controversial. According to review of Farquhar et al.[15] six cycles of gonadotropin treatment give higher ongoing cumulative pregnancy rates than laparoscopic treatment for a short-term follow-up period of six months (OR 0.48, 95% CI 0.28–0.81). However, three or six cycles of gonadotropin use have not been found to be better than ovarian cautery at the longest length of follow up of

either 6 or 12 months (OR 1.27, 95% CI 0.77–2.09). Very recently, Bayram et al.[16] compared the effectiveness of an electrocautery strategy with ovulation induction using recombinant follicle stimulating hormone (r-FSH) in patients with CC resistant PCOS in a randomized controlled clinical trial. If anovulation persisted eight weeks after the operation, CC was used at first for six cycles. If the patient remained anovulatory, r-FSH treatment was started. The cumulative rate of ongoing pregnancy was found to be 67% at 12 months in both groups. Nevertheless, the ongoing pregnancy rate after six months was lower with electrocautery than r-FSH, and approximately more than half the patients had to receive CC and r-FSH. Because of the fact that all multiple-pregnancies were found in patients who received r-FSH, the authors proposed that multiple pregnancies could largely be avoided by electrocautery and CC before this treatment.[16] In addition, it has been proposed that the use of gonadotropin as a second line therapy for anovulatory CC-resistant PCOS is more expensive than laparoscopic ovarian diathermy. Farquhar et al.[17] suggested that the cost per pregnancy for laparoscopic ovarian diathermy is approximately one-third less than that for ovulation induction with gonadotropins.[17] However, laparoscopic treatment has some risk with regard to the surgery and anesthesia involved. Therefore, some patients and physicians prefer gonadotropin treatment. Injection of gonadotropins has been employed as a very effective treatment over the years. However, due to the exaggerated response of gonadotropins in later stages of stimulation in PCOS patients and the risk of multiple pregnancies and ovarian hyperstimulation syndrome (OHSS), this treatment requires a high degree of skill, extensive hormone and ultrasound monitoring. The most important aim is to achieve a singleton live birth and not to cause OHSS at the end of the gonadotropin treatment. At this point, it may be extremely difficult to set a gonadotropin threshold. To reduce these risks, low-dose protocols have been recommended. This issue will be discussed more extensively under the title of '*Controlled ovarian stimulation with gonadotropins in PCOS*'.

Metformin

Studies establishing the relationship between PCOS and insulin resistance and the association between high insulin concentrations and anovulatory infertility, have led to the use of insulin-sensitizing medications for ovulation induction. Between 50 to 80% of women with PCOS have been found to have insulin resistance, and a large majority of these women are obese. The synergistic interaction between luteinizing hormone (LH) and insulin in promoting androgen secretion from theca lutein cells in patients with and without PCOS has also been shown. We know that CC resistance is more common in women who are obese, have higher androgen concentrations, excess LH, and insulin resistance. Because of these relationships, numerous studies were performed related to metformin use in the treatment of infertility in patients with PCOS. Initially, metformin was used chiefly for CC-resistant women with PCOS, and majority of these studies showed that the addition of metformin was more effective than CC alone treatment. The relationship between weight loss and metformin treatment has been shown in the vast majority of the studies. It is possible that weight loss may account for some of the beneficial effects observed in many metformin studies. In several studies, the ovulation rate increased with no change in weight, which suggests that the effect is independent of weight loss. Recently, Attia et al.[18] showed that metformin directly inhibits androgen production in human thecal cells. Nestler et al.[19] performed a controlled study with the administration of metformin 500 mg three times daily or placebo for 35 days. Women who failed to ovulate spontaneously were given 50 mg of CC daily for 5 days, concomitant with metformin or placebo. This regimen was successful in 19 of 21 women (90%) in the metformin group and 2 of 25 (8%) in the placebo group. Overall, 31 of the 35 women (89%) treated with metformin ovulated spontaneously, or in response to CC, as compared with 3 of the 26 women (12%) treated with placebo.[19] Furthermore, this improvement was associated with decreased insulin secretion in the metformin group.

Lord et al.[20] compared CC plus metformin treatment with clomiphene alone in a systematic review and found a significant effect of combination treatment on both, ovulation and pregnancy rates. Ovulation occurred in 76% of the patients in the combination group, but only 42% of those receiving CC alone group (OR 4.41, 95% CI 2.37–8.22, p < 0.0001). Similarly, pregnancy rates were found to be four times higher in combination treatment compared to CC alone group (OR 4.40, 95% CI 1.96–9.85, p = 0.0003). However, the authors also clarified that when these studies were re-evaluated in respect of whether patients were resistant to CC, these rates increased in studies related to resistant patients (OR 9.34, 95% CI 3.97–21.97, p < 0.00001). On the contrary, in another trial in the meta-analysis, in which participants were not selected on the basis of being CC resistant, the ovulation rate in the placebo and CC arm was high (64%) and did not show any evidence of benefit following addition of metformin compared with CC (OR 1.90, 95% CI 0.77 to 4.70). The number needed to treat (NNT) was 3.0, with a range of 1.6 in the trial with the lowest rate of ovulation with CC alone (the participants were selected as having been previously resistant to CC) to 8.6 in a trial in which the participants' previous sensitivity to clomiphene was unknown.[20] After this review, Kayshap et al.[10] published their meta-analysis and showed that metformin plus CC treatment was 3-4-fold superior to CC alone for ovulation induction (RR 3.04; 95% CI 1.77–5.24) and pregnancy (RR 3.65; 95% CI 1.11–11.99) in women with PCOS.[10]

Although Şahin et al.[21] could not demonstrate the effectiveness of metformin plus CC treatment over treatment with CC alone on ovulation [(38 of 51 cycles (74.4%) versus 34 of 55 cycles (61.8%) respectively] and pregnancy rates [5 of 11 women (45.5%) versus 3 of 10 women (30%) respectively] in their small study, they showed that all the patients in the metformin plus CC group who conceived had insulin resistance but three women in the CC group who conceived were non-insulin-resistant. They concluded that metformin therapy could be recommended in PCOS patients with insulin resistance.[21]

Since patients using metformin achieve spontaneous ovulation without superovulation, it has been proposed that metformin does not confer the same risks of ovarian hyperstimulation and multiple pregnancies as does CC treatment. Moreover, metformin does not have the same negative effects on the cervical mucus and endometrium as CC. Therefore, CC-resistant PCOS patients may benefit more from treatment with metformin. Besides, metformin appears to be as effective as laparoscopic drilling in inducing ovulation and may increase the number of pregnancies and reduce the prevalence of miscarriage, resulting in a higher live birth rate. It may be stated that metformin should be the first line of therapy for a CC-resistant patient. If ovulation does not occur after several months, laparoscopic ovarian drilling or gonadotropins may be considered to be an effective option. IVF should be considered as a last option for women with PCOS who are unable to ovulate effectively. Pasquali et al.[22] have shown that the addition of metformin is more effective than placebo alone when dietary intervention is attempted in women with PCOS. More weight loss, greater reduction in waist circumference, a higher decrease in visceral fat mass, and lower levels of testosterone were found in women who took metformin rather than placebo.[22] Ovulation was achieved in 46% of those who received metformin alone compared with 24% who received placebo. The numbers needed to treat for ovulation was 4.4. Ovulation rate increased in the metformin group (OR 3.88, 95% CI 2.25–6.69, p < 0.0001), but there was no difference in the clinical pregnancy rate in the metformin group compared to the placebo group (OR 2.76, 95% CI 0.85–8.98, p = 0.09). There was an improvement in serum insulin levels and a reduction in free testosterone in response to metformin in the meta-analysis of Lord et al.[20] In another meta-analysis,[10] it has been shown

that metformin is 50% better than placebo for ovulation induction in infertile PCOS patients [RR 1.50; 95% CI 1.13–1.99], but this beneficial effect of metformin versus placebo was not proved with regard to the achievement of pregnancies (RR 1.07; 95% CI 0.20–5.74). Nevertheless, the data so far, do not demonstrate a benefit of metformin on placebo when the outcome considered is related to pregnancy. The follow-up time to pregnancy was short, and in the quantitatively summarized studies, pregnancy was not the primary outcome, nor were these studies powered to assess pregnancy as an outcome.[10]

Despite widespread acceptance and zealous use of such medications, metformin had not been compared to CC in a direct, randomized controlled trial. Very recently, Polamba et al.[23] published their prospective, randomized, double-blind, double-dummy, controlled clinical trial comparing CC and metformin as the first-line treatment for ovulation induction in non-obese anovulatory women with PCOS. In that study, one hundred non-obese primary infertile anovulatory women with PCOS were included and all participants took metformin cloridrate (850 mg twice daily) plus placebo or placebo plus CC (150 mg for five days from the 3rd day of a progesterone withdrawal bleed) for six months. Although the ovulation rate was not statistically different between the treatment groups (62.9% versus 67% respectively, p = 0.38), metformin treatment was shown to be effective in increasing the cumulative pregnancy rate when compared to CC (68.9% versus 34.0% respectively, p < 0.001) and the abortion rate was found to be significantly lower in the metformin group compared to that in the CC group.[23]

There are few studies on the subject of whether metformin treatment may improve reproductive outcome when used together with FSH. Dale et al.[24] examined the possible correlation between insulin resistance and the outcome of gonadotropin stimulation in infertile CC-resistant women with PCOS. In that study, the insulin-resistant PCOS women required more gonadotropin and a longer time to achieve follicular maturation than non- insulin-resistant

PCOS women. Although ovulation rates in completed cycles were similar between the insulin-resistant and non-insulin-resistant PCOS women, the conception rates were significantly higher in the non-insulin-resistant PCOS women.[24] In accordance with this data, De Leo et al.[25] have shown in their randomized prospective trial that pre-treatment with metformin improves FSH-induced ovulation in women with CC-resistant PCOS. The number of dominant follicles, cycle cancellation rate and peak estradiol level were significantly lower in cycles treated with FSH and metformin than in those treated with FSH alone. That study also showed that metformin leads to an orderly FSH-induced ovulation in patients with PCOS.[25] On the contrary, Yarali et al.[26] suggested that metformin did not improve insulin resistance, ovulation and pregnancy rate during a low-dose step-up protocol using r-FSH. Yarali et al.[26] treated infertile CC-resistant women with PCOS with r-FSH using the low-dose step-up protocol. They gave placebo or metformin for only a six weeks period before a single r-FSH treatment cycle. They found that the overall ovulation rates were 75% and 94% in the placebo and metformin groups respectively, with pregnancy rates of 6.3% and 31.3% respectively. However, this improvement was not statistically significant. Thus, the authors concluded that in CC-resistant PCOS patients with normal glucose tolerance, metformin may restore ovulation with no improvement in insulin resistance, but it has no the significant effect on the ovarian response during r-FSH treatment.[26]

Controlled ovarian stimulation with gonadotropins

The most important aim is to achieve a singleton live birth without causing OHSS at the end of the gonadotropin treatment. At this point, it may be extremely difficult to establish the gonadotropin threshold. Conventional protocols commence with 75–150 IU/day gonadotropin and dose is increased by 75 IU every 5–7 days. This protocol has a potentially unacceptable multiple pregnancy rate and is associated with life threatening OHSS that reaches a peak level of 12%. Hence, chronic low-dose protocols have been proposed to minimize the risk of multiple follicular developments. There are two chronic low-dose protocols in clinical practice:

Chronic low-dose step up protocol

In this protocol, the starting gonadotropin dose is 75 IU/day that is commenced on the third day of a spontaneous or progesterone induced withdrawal bleeding. The initial dose is maintained for the first 14 days unless follicular maturity warrants human chorionic gonadotropin (hCG) administration. If there is no evidence of an ovarian response on ultrasound, the daily dose is increased by 37.5 IU after 14 days of therapy. Further dose adjustments are made if necessary after a period of 5–7 days to a maximum of 225 IU/day. This stepwise increase continues until ovarian activity is seen on ultrasound; then, the same dose (i.e. the threshold dose) is continued until the follicular diameter is >17 mm. Human chorionic gonadotropin (hCG), 10,000 IU i.m. is given to induce ovulation. The hCG injection is withheld, when there are more than three follicles >15 mm in diameter because of the risk of multiple pregnancy and/or OHSS, or if there is no response after 35 days of treatment. As some women respond excessively to treatment, the starting dose may be decreased to 37.5 IU and increments lesser than usual (18.75 IU) are made. Though the conventional starting dose of gonadotropin is 75 IU/day, several authors proposed a lower starting dose (37.5–52.5 IU), since these give similar outcomes in effect with regard to ovulation, pregnancy and miscarriage rates. This approach is associated with privileged monovulatory cycles.

Chronic low-dose step down protocol

In this protocol, a higher initial dose of gonadotropins (150IU) than that employed in the step-up protocol is used after spontaneous or progesterone-induced withdrawal bleeding and this dose is maintained until a dominant follicle, measuring ≥ 10 mm diameter on transvaginal ultrasound, is identified. The gonadotropin dose is then gradually decreased by 37.5IU and the same dose decrement is made every 3 days until hCG administration.

The low dose step-up protocol using urinary follicular stimulating hormone (u-FSH), has the advantage of more controlled stimulation, resulting in the development of fewer multiple follicles and therefore, a decreased risk of OHSS and multiple pregnancies. Recently, the step-up protocol has been found to be approximately twice more effective than the low dose step-down protocol in obtaining monofollicular development (68% versus 32% respectively) with a lower cancellation rate (15% versus 38% respectively). Besides, the low-dose step-up protocol yielded a higher ovulation rate than step-down protocol (70% versus 62% respectively) in this multicentric study. Ovarian hyperstimulation syndrome developed only in 2% of patients treated with the low-dose step-up protocol. On the contrary, OHSS was observed in 11% of patients treated with the low-dose step-down protocol.[27]

Nonetheless, when we deduce the consequence of these results, we ought to bear in mind that these studies include patients who have different PCOS characteristics. Imani et al.[28] showed that in patients who may have more serious ovarian abnormality and fail to ovulate with CC, a higher threshold dose of exogenous follicular stimulating hormone (FSH) is necessary. On the contrary, if the patients ovulate but do not conceive after CC treatment, a lower dose of exogenous FSH will be sufficient. According to Imani et al,[28] BMI, response to the preceding CC cycle, insulin like growth factor (IGF)-1 level and basal FSH concentrations are important parameters to predict the FSH response.[28] It has been suggested that, the first cycle should be performed with a low-dose step-up regime to evaluate the FSH threshold level. After the threshold is determined, the step down cycle may be commenced with 37.5 IU above this level. If the commenced dose is sufficient and an incremental dose is not required for ovulation in the first cycle, this dose regime is fixed in following cycle.

Sequential step-up and step-down protocol
FSH dependence gradually decreases in the dominant follicle during follicle growth. Hugues et al.[29] tried to mimic this physiological change and developed a sequential step-up and step-down protocol. In the primary stage, they applied the step-up regime to obtain the threshold dose. After the dominant follicle reached 14 mm diameter, they reduced FSH dose by 37.5 IU in order to mimic this physiological feature. When they compared low dose step up protocol with this sequential step-up and step-down protocol, they found a significantly lower estradiol level and decreased number of medium-sized follicles at the time of hCG administration in the sequential protocol. The authors suggested that this type of regime might increase the chances of monofollicular development.[29]

Choice of gonadotropin

Exogenous gonadotropins are essential for standard ovulation induction. Human menopausal gonadotropin (hMG), u-FSH and recombinant FSH (r-FSH) preparations have been used successfully for controlled ovarian hyperstimulation. hMG, u-FSH, and r-FSH appear to be equally effective in achieving pregnancy. hMG contains 75 IU FSH and 75 IU luteinizing hormone (LH), but the majority (90%) of the protein content of this preparation consists of gonadotropin-unrelated urinary proteins. It may be thought that these non-relevant proteins can give rise to unwanted side effects, including allergic or other hypersensitivity reactions during an ovarian stimulation cycle. According to the two-cell, two gonadotropin theory, both FSH and LH are necessary for normal follicular development and steroidogenesis. Indeed, administration of FSH with LH is a rule in hypogonadotropic women. On the contrary, in normogonadotropic women, it has been suggested that very low amounts of LH are sufficient for normal follicular development. Furthermore, elevations in serum LH during the follicular phase of the menstrual cycle have been associated with lower fertility rates and an increase in the probability of spontaneous abortion. With regard to whether LH is necessary for patients induced with gonadotropin-releasing hormone agonist (GnRH-a) and FSH, although circulating LH concentrations are much lower than in the normal menstrual cycle, recent trials have revealed that pure FSH is effective in these suppressed cycles. It has been suggested that endogenous LH levels are sufficient for folliculogenesis in these women. Since women with PCOS have elevated LH concentrations, gonadotropin preparations devoid of LH may in theory be more physiological. Nevertheless, it has been suggested that an appreciable proportion of normogonadotropic women acquire slight endogenous LH levels for follicle development following GnRH-a down-regulation. Laml et al.[30] succeeded in carrying out oocyte retrieval and embryo transfer by the additional administration of recombinant LH to r-FSH in six women who had previously failed to respond to r-FSH hyperstimulation.[30] According to the previous Cochrane review, u-FSH preparations do not improve pregnancy rates when compared with traditional and less expensive hMG preparations. However, the use of u-FSH has a reduced risk of OHSS.[31] There is no evidence to show that r-FSH is better than hMG in achieving ongoing pregnancy/live birth rates. The clinical pregnancy rate was shown to be of borderline significance in favor of hMG (summary OR 1.28; 95% CI 1.00–1.64) in the latest Cochrane review related to this issue.[32] M van Wely et al.[33] has also suggested that there is yet, insufficient evidence to conclude that r-FSH is more effective than u-FSH in women with CC-resistant PCOS.[33] Recently, Gerli et al.[34] compared u-FSH with r-FSH in order to determine which preparation is more cost-effective in ovarian stimulation for intrauterine insemination (IUI) in patients with PCOS. They found that although a greater amount of gonadotropins had been used, the urinary preparation was more cost- effective than r-FSH. Authors have also shown that there were no differences between u-FSH and r-FSH in the number of follicles >17 mm, stimulation days, number of ampoules per cycle, clinical pregnancy rate, multiple pregnancy rate, spontaneous abortions and canceled cycles in PCOS patients.[34]

GnRH-agonist treatment
Although PCOS patients respond substantially well to low-dose gonadotropin therapy for ovulation induction, multiple gestation and spontaneous abortion rates are quite high, and range from 20 to 35%. Down-regulating the pituitary-ovarian axis with gonadotropin releasing hormone agonist (GnRH-a) prior to the initiation of gonadotropin therapy may decrease the likelihood of spontaneous abortions. GnRH-a administration in controlled ovarian stimulation (COS) protocols, suppress elevated LH and androgen levels and prevent the premature LH surge. Balen et al.[35] showed that spontaneous abortion rates following IVF are significantly higher in patients with PCO compared to those of women with normal ovaries. Long buserelin protocol plus gonadotropin treatment results in lower miscarriage rates compared to patients with PCOS who are treated with CC.[35] Similarly, Homburg et al.[36] found that pregnant women who received only hMG for superovulation had higher miscarriage rates than patients who received GnRH-a in addition to hMG (39.1% versus 17.6% respectively).[36] Furthermore, patients with PCO who do not receive GnRH-a therapy may have higher cancellation and lower fertilization rates than that normal patients. Therefore, GnRH-a treatment is required in patients with PCOS, who will receive gonadotropins for ovarian stimulation in IVF cycles.

Gonadotropin releasing hormone antagonists
Gonadotropin releasing hormone antagonists have several theoretical advantages over the agonists because they act by the mechanism of competitive binding and this allow a modulation of the degree of hormonal suppression by dose adjustment. Further, antagonists suppress gonadotropin release within a few hours, have no flare-up effect, and gonadal functions resume without a delay following their discontinuation. All patients opt for a simple protocol to achieve good clinical results and GnRH antagonists provide an opportunity for a much shorter treatment cycle with lower doses of gonadotropin injections. It

has been shown in the Cochrane meta-analysis that there was a statistically significant reduction in incidence of severe OHSS (RR 0.36, 95% CI 0.16–0.80) using antagonist regimens as compared to the long GnRH-a protocol.[37] It is also proposed that GnRH-antagonists can be used to prevent a premature LH surge, to trigger ovulation and reduce the risk of OHSS. Albeit, there is no real prospective study that shows the superiority of GnRH antagonist to GnRH agonist treatment yet. On the contrary, it has been shown that there were significantly fewer clinical pregnancies in patients treated with GnRH-antagonists (OR 0.78, 95% CI 0.62–0.97).[37]

There are only a few reports regarding GnRH antagonist use during IVF cycles in PCOS patients. GnRH antagonists have been administered in the late follicular phase to prevent or interrupt the LH surge successfully during COS. If a similar application was performed in PCOS patients undergoing IVF treatment, early follicular phase high tonic LH secretion would probably, still be present. Recently, Hwang et al.[38] compared a combination of Diane-35 and GnRH antagonist with the GnRH-a long protocol. They used three consecutive cycles of Diane-35 pre-treatment in an attempt to decrease serum LH and androgens. Afterwards, in order to both augment the suppressive effect of Diane-35 and prevent progressive tonic LH elevation in the early follicular phase and a premature LH surge in the late follicular phase, they administered cetrorelix acetate concomitantly with exogenous gonadotropins. According to the authors, Diane-35/cetrorelix protocol had a similar pregnancy outcome compared to the GnRH-a long protocol in women with PCOS undergoing IVF treatment. However, significantly fewer days of injection, lower amounts of gonadotropin usage and lower estradiol levels on the day of hCG injection, following the Diane/cetrorelix protocol, were the advantages of that protocol, while the major drawback may be the long-term administration of Diane-35.[38]

In vitro fertilization (IVF)

IVF is an effective treatment after repeated failure of ovulation induction by CC and gonadotropin. It should be kept in mind that weight reduction should decrease the gonadotropin requirements and difficulties associated with oocyte retrieval, although this opinion has not been supported by a randomized controlled study in patients with PCOS.

Measures regarding problems related to ovulation induction in IVF

Several problems may be encountered during the superovulation of patients with PCOS undergoing IVF treatment. It has been supposed that the quality of eggs and embryos is reduced in these patients. We know that local high androgen concentrations have a detrimental effect on follicle growth and oocyte quality. Studies conducted in mice have shown that atretic follicles have higher androgen/estrogen levels than the other foolicles. A recent mouse follicle culture study has demonstrated that local androgen increase affects the fertilization of in vitro cultured oocytes under the stable gonadotropin tonus.[39] Additionally, human studies revealed that the follicular steroid environment is correlated with oocyte quality. Another problem in PCOS patients is tonic hypersecretion of LH that is proposed as one of the major factors responsible for a high miscarriage rate, poor oocyte quality, and a low fertilization and cleavage rate. Increased number of follicles may develop during superovulation cycles and result in very high estradiol levels. This untimely high estradiol level may trigger an LH surge, which is inappropriate for the stage and size of the follicle. A significant reduction in the fertilization rate of mature oocytes has been observed in patients whose basal LH was greater than one standard deviation above the mean. Therefore, suppression of endogenous LH is important in patients with PCOS who are candidates for IVF.

Because of the different selection criteria of PCOS patients, there is no consensus about whether oocyte quality is affected in PCOS patients. Some researchers suggest that the number of follicles is higher, while the fertilization rate is low in PCOS patients. In contrast, several investigators have not found a negative effect of PCOS on the fertilization, cleavage and pregnancy rates. When studies regarding the experience with oocyte donation are addressed, no differences in the chances of fertilization and implantation among oocytes produced by patients with PCOS, polycystic ovaries and normal ovaries are observed. Under the light of these observations, although several studies have found decreased fertilization rates, we cannot say that oocytes and embryos from patients with PCOS are reduced in quality.

A vast majority of studies agree that PCOS is a major risk factor for the development of OHSS, which may lead to a hazardous life-threatening situation against which precautions must be taken. Each patient, who undergoes ovarian stimulation with gonadotropins for IVF, gives a different response to therapy. The crucial point is individualization of treatment and careful review of the history of stimulation, in order to estimate the patient's propensity for an exaggerated response. Today, the most preferred regime is the low-dose gonadotropin stimulation accompanied by GnRH-a long-protocol. Besides, one group has proposed the use of the combination of oral contraceptive and GnRH-a with initial oral contraceptive treatment of the patient, followed by an overlap of the oral contraceptive with the GnRH-a for approximately 1 week and finally, followed by the continuation of the agonist in the absence of the oral contraceptive. Gonadotropin stimulation with FSH is initiated at any time following withdrawal bleed of the patient. The results with this protocol have suggested not only an improvement in the stimulation of the ovaries, which leads to better egg quality, embryo development and pregnancy rates, but also a decrease in the incidence of OHSS.[40] However, in spite of these approaches, some patients still exhibit an exaggerated response to gonadotropin therapy. If this happens, measures should be taken to prevent the development of the hyperstimulation syndrome. If the response is aggravated and takes place too early with multiple small follicles on ultrasonography and estradiol levels greater than 1000 pg/mL, cycle cancellation without the administration of hCG may be an advisable option. The exaggerated response might be observed at a later stage of stimulation with multiple follicles larger than 15 mm in average diameter and extremely elevated serum estradiol concentration. At this point, different strategies such as reduction in the hCG dose from 10,000 IU to 5,000 or 3,000 IU may be used according to patient characteristics. Unfortunately, this approach may decrease the incidence of OHSS merely due to the hCG injection and it does not prevent the problem if the patient gets pregnant. Nowadays, recombinant LH is commercially available for clinical use. Thus, the induction of final maturation of the follicles and oocytes may be triggered with recombinant LH after the administration of GnRH-a. The other alternative is retrieval of all the oocytes and cryopreservation of all the embryos thus produced. This approach may be an opportunity to deal with the hyperstimulated patient without the undesirable effect of the syndrome on pregnancy. It has been postulated that the continuation of GnRH-a after hCG administration, for approximately 2 weeks until menses ensue, gives added protection against the development of OHSS. Sometimes, patients are at a risk of OHSS, but the risk is not too high to cancel embryo transfer. In these patients, a single embryo transfer may be a rational step to prevent multiple gestations. Moreover, it has been postulated that this transfer should be performed at the blastocyst stage on day 5 or 6. Coasting may be considered as an alternative method in these patients. It involves withdrawing exogenous gonadotropins and postponing hCG administration until the patient's serum estradiol level decreases to a 'safer' level, which is 3000 to 4000 pg/mL. However, it should be kept in mind that it has been suggested that prolonged coasting (more than 4 days) is associated with poor results. Finally, numerous studies have been published related to the retrieval and in vitro maturation and fertilization of immature oocytes recovered from unstimulated PCO patients to treat high responding women with PCO. The use of glucocorticoids for the prevention of hyperstimulation syndrome immediately after retrieval does not appear promising. This treatment did not yield any significant difference in the rate of OHSS.

Stadtmauer et al.[41] hypothesized that metformin may improve the quality of oocytes retrieved from patients with PCOS by reducing hyperinsulinism, and by modulating the local insulin and IGF levels. They retrospectively analyzed 46 women with CC-resistant PCOS, who underwent 60 cycles of IVF-embryo transfer with intracytoplasmic sperm injection. In half of the cycles, patients received metformin 1000–1500 mg daily, starting with the cycle prior to the gonadotropin treatment cycle. The authors found that the metformin cycles were associated with a decrease in the total number of follicles on the day of hCG administration, with no change in the mean follicular diameter. Metformin treatment did not affect the mean number of oocytes retrieved, although, the mean number of mature oocytes and embryos cleaved was higher. Fertilization rates (64% versus 43% respectively) and clinical pregnancy rates (70% versus 30% respectively) were also increased following metformin use. Metformin led to the modulation of preovulatory follicular fluid IGF levels, with increases in IGF-I and decreases in IGF-binding protein 1 (IGFBP-1).[41] Contrary to these findings, Fedorcsak et al.[42] reported that in women with PCOS who received long-term down regulation and stimulation with r-FSH, insulin resistance was not related to either hormone levels or IVF outcome. Obesity was independently associated with relative gonadotropin resistance.[42]

Treatment of hirsutism

Hirsutism in women is defined as excessive facial and/or body terminal hair in a male-like distribution pattern. Androgens, testosterone and dihydrotestosterone (DHT) transform vellus to terminal hair in androgen sensitive areas of the body. Hyperandrogenism is the key endocrine abnormality of PCOS, which is responsible for 70% of the patients with hirsutism. Since our knowledge about the pathogenesis of hyperandrogenism in PCOS is increased, newer treatment options are added to our conventional hirsutism treatment. Reduction of ovarian androgen production and amelioration of hyperandrogenemia with suppression of adrenal androgen production, increasing the binding of androgens to specific plasma-binding proteins, and blocking androgen action at the level of the target tissue, are essential in such cases.

Combination estrogen-progestin therapy

Although a new alternative therapy method is presented at any moment, combination estrogen-progestin therapy remains the predominant treatment for hirsutism. The main mechanism of combined oral contraceptive action is the inhibition of folliculogenesis. Mid-cycle surge and secretion of FSH and LH are suppressed by the action of estrogen and progestin components of the oral contraceptive. Thus, this interaction leads to suppression of folliculogenesis and decreases androgen production. The estrogenic components also increase the levels of sex hormone–binding globulin (SHBG), which results in a dose-related decrease in concentrations of free testosterone in the serum that can bind to the androgen receptor. Selection of the most favorable product among the available combined oral contraceptives is very important in clinical practice. At this time, all available combined oral contraceptives contain the same estrogen, ethinyl estradiol, the daily dose of which ranges from 15 to 50 mg. The dose of estrogen influences the activity of the pituitary–ovarian axis and consequently, the ovarian activity. It has been shown that the dose of ethinyl estradiol in combination with the same dose and type of gestagen, correlates with the final concentration of SHBG. A daily dose of 30–35 mg of ethinyl estradiol guarantees sufficient suppression of ovarian follicular activity as well as effective stimulation of SHBG production. Oral contraceptive therapy decreases dehydroepiandrosterone sulfate (DHEAS) levels, possibly by way of reducing adrenocorticotropic hormone (ACTH) levels. It has also been shown that progestins inhibit 5α-reductase activity, act as antagonists at the androgen receptor, and increase the metabolic clearance rate of both testosterone and DHT. Nevertheless, each progestin has a different suppressive effect on SHBG levels and additionally, has a divergent androgenic potential. With increasing antiestrogenic activity, the stimulatory effect of combined oral contraceptive on SHBG synthesis is decreased. It was shown that although the same dose of ethinyl estradiol had been used, a greater change in SHBG levels were observed when high androgenic (levonorgesterol, LNG) gestagens were given compared to low androgenic (desogestrel, DSG) gestagens for six months (270% versus 80% respectively).[43] Similarly, the effect of combined oral contraceptive on the lipid spectrum is contingent on the type of gestagen. Low androgenic gestagens such as DSG, gestodene or dienogest should be chosen. However, it is also known that the changes remain within reference limits in a vast majority of healthy users, and have no clinically significant effect on the risk of cardiovascular diseases. Combined oral contraceptives may worsen glucose tolerance in healthy users. There are a few short-term studies assessing the effects of different combined oral contraceptives on glucose tolerance. Based on available data, it is speculated that the type of gestagen could play a role. In obese women, it has been shown that glucose levels increased after an oral glucose load by the use of combined oral contraceptives containing DSG or cyproterone acetate (CPA). However, this kind of relationship was not observed in non-obese women by use of norethindrone (NET), DSG or CPA. Although some studies demonstrate a deterioration in glucose tolerance following combined oral contraceptive use in healthy women, there is no evidence to show an increased risk of diabetes mellitus (DM) in the past or present users. Even in women with a history of gestational DM, combined oral contraceptive use did not alter the risk.

For these reasons, the choice of progestin type in oral contraceptives is crucial. Actually, progestins can be divided into two types: natural and synthetic. Synthetic progestins can be categorized into two groups: those that are structurally related to progesterone, and those that are structurally related to testosterone. Progestins structurally related to testosterone include norethindrone, norgestimate, norethindrone acetate, gestodene and levonorgestrel. Although newer progestins norgestimate and desogestrel are structurally related to testosterone, they are not androgenic. The newer, more potent and less androgenic progestins are considered by some gynecologists to be more beneficial. A novel progestin drospirenone (DRSP), an analogue of spironolactone has gained popularity, thanks to the peculiar characteristics of both, antimineralocorticoid and antiandrogenic activities with no androgenic, estrogenic, glucocorticoid, or antiglucocorticoid activity. The blockade of androgen receptors in the skin (sebaceous glands and hair follicles) represents an additional mechanism implicated in the positive effects of ethinyl estradiol/DRSP on the cosmetically unacceptable signs of hyperandrogenism in PCOS women (acne, seborrhea, and hirsutism). More recently, Guido et al.[44] showed that the free androgen index is significantly decreased after the third cycle and dehydroepiandrosterone sulfate and 17-hydroxyprogesterone are significantly decreased after six cycles following the use of the estro-progestin combination containing DRSP.[44] In the same study, SHBG increased approximately five times in the third cycle and this increment has been found to be greater than that reported in literature after administration of 17α-hydroxyprogesterone derivatives, such as CPA . These effects were explained by specific chemical properties of DRSP, which does not neutralize the stimulatory effect of ethinyl estradiol on SHBG synthesis and does not prevent androgen binding with it. Besides, they found that the mean Ferriman-Gallwey (F-G) score was decreased from 16.2 ± 5.8 (mean $\pm$ SEM) to 14.3 ± 5 within six cycles and this trend was maintained after 12 cycles of treatment after which, the mean F-G score reached to 13.5 ± 5. The authors did not observe any change in serum total cholesterol, triglycerides, and high- and low- density lipoprotein (HDL and LDL) concentrations and glycoinsulinemic homeostasis after the treatment in their study.[44]

Androgen receptor antagonists

Spironolactone
Spironolactone, an aldosterone antagonist, was traditionally used as a diuretic in the treatment of hypertension. Spironolactone has been used for the treatment of hirsutism since 1978. It has multiple antiandrogenic effects including, inhibition of ovarian and adrenal androgen production, blockade of DHT binding to skin androgen receptors, elevation of SHBG levels, increase in testosterone clearance from the body and decrease in 5α-reductase activity. The effectiveness of spironolactone in hirsute women is related to the dose. The dosage used for treatment of hirsutism varies between 50 and 300 mg/day. An initial dose of 100 mg/day may be sufficient for lean hirsute woman. Higher daily doses of 200 or 300 mg/day should be given for better treatment in some severely hirsute or obese women. Spironolactone may cause some side effects such as polydypsea, polyuria, nausea, headaches, fatigue, gastritis and ovulatory dysfunction, resulting in polymenorrhea, and hyperkalemia. Its common side effect is menstrual irregularity when used alone; for this reason, estrogen-progestin should be given in conjunction with spironolactone. Use of estrogen-progestin in conjunction with spironolactone may also be important to prevent pregnancy because of the risk of the compound causing feminization of a male fetus. Hyperkalemia is extremely rare in healthy patients and has been reported only in patients who are elderly, diabetic, or who have impaired renal function. To minimize the side effects, a starting dose of 25 mg/day should be increased over several weeks. Spironolactone should be given for at least 6 months to gain maximum improvement in hirsutism. The maintenance dose can then be dropped to 25–100 mg daily, with overweight women requiring

a higher amount. According to the Cochrane review published in 2003, spironolactone (100 mg/day) is a more effective treatment than finasteride (5 mg/day) and cyproterone acetate (12.5 mg/day) in reducing hair growth, but less effective than flutamide 500 mg/day in reducing F–G scores.[45]

Cyproterone acetate (CPA)
Cyproterone acetate is known as the first androgen receptor antagonist used to treat hirsutism. Actually, it is a progestational agent having antigonadotropic and antiandrogenic peripheral activity. It binds to the dihydrotestosterone receptor in the cytoplasm in the hair follicle, preventing its translocation into the nucleus to cause an androgenic effect. In addition to this activity, it inhibits 5α-reductase activity, reducing DHT production, and also inhibits the production of the gonadotropins. The reduced gonadotropin levels in turn reduce steroidogenesis.

Its side effects include irregular uterine bleeding, nausea, headache, fatigue, weight gain, and decreased libido. There are no data comparing CPA alone to placebo. In addition, there are no data comparing CPA alone to combination therapy using cyproterone acetate and ethinyl estradiol. Therefore, the answer to whether CPA is less effective without ethinyl estradiol is not known. Cyclical administration of CPA, 50–100 mg, on days 1–10 of the menstrual cycle combined with oral estrogen on days 1–21 produces a *therapeutic effect* in hirsutism Additionally, this method counters hypoestrogenism and irregular bleeding, and prevents pregnancy and the potential teratogenic complications that may result. The incidence of side effects of therapy with CPA compared to spironolactone, flutamide and GnRH analogues is not significantly different. There is insufficient data to compare side effects experienced with ketoconazole or finasteride therapy. Cyproterone acetate is not approved for marketing in the United States because of the concern that the drug has the propensity to cause breast cancer in beagle dogs and teratogenicity in rodents when administered in extremely high doses during pregnancy.[46] As we know, oral contraceptives have some adverse effects on lipid metabolism in healthy women and those with PCOS, but these effects generally depend on the dose of estrogen and the type and dose of progestin used. Cyproterone acetate, is a pregnane-derived progestogen and does not have androgenic activity. It has been shown that ethinyl estradiol–CPA combination was associated with increased serum HDL cholesterol, decreased LDL cholesterol and total cholesterol:HDL cholesterol ratio. On the other hand, the slight worsening effect of this combination on triglycerides, serum free fatty acid and glucose tolerance, has also been shown. It is postulated that the beneficial effects of ethinyl estradiol–CPA on lipid metabolism are generally due to the slight estrogen dominance of ethinyl estradiol–CA treatment.

Flutamide

Flutamide is a non-steroidal highly specific antiandrogen without any interactions with glucocorticoid, progesterone or estrogen receptors; it acts via the blockade of the androgen receptor, interference with cellular uptake of testosterone and DHT, and increase in androgen metabolism to inactive compounds, which have no intrinsic hormonal or antigonadotropin activity. Flutamide, 250 mg, 1–3 times daily, is a highly effective treatment for moderate to severe hirsutism. Flutamide, 250 mg/day was shown to decrease F–G scores by approximately 70% after 12 months of treatment Side effects include decreased appetite, amenorrhea, decreased libido, and dry skin. A rare but serious reported side effect is hepatotoxicity. No cases of fatal hepatotoxicity have been reported with flutamide at doses less than 500 mg/day, although there have been reports of a mild, transient hepatotoxicity with daily doses ranging from 375 to 500 mg. Lower dosages (250 or 375 mg per day) are currently preferred. At these dosages, the drug is generally safe and effective, although some patients may experience an increase in transaminase enzymes.

Since flutamide is an expensive drug and has potential fatal hepatotoxicity, it is not used routinely in the treatment of hirsutism. Recent studies have shown that lower doses of this drug (125 mg and 62.5 mg flutamide) are equally effective in reducing hirsutism after 3 and 6 months of treatment respectively. This approach may provide low cost therapy and decrease the risk of hepatotoxicity. Flutamide can be combined with other drug regimens to further improve hirsutism scores in women with PCOS. Compared to GnRHa treatment alone, the addition of 250 mg flutamide a day to a monthly GnRH-a injection, resulted in significantly lower F–G scores after 6 months treatment in 35 women with PCOS.[47]

Flutamide is usually reserved for resistant cases of hirsutism, and liver enzymes should be checked regularly in patients on the drug. Additionally, because of possible teratogenic effects, oral contraceptives must be used with this therapy.

Finasteride

Finasteride was released in 1992 for the treatment of prostatic disorders. It inhibits type 2, 5α-reductase activity and blocks dihydrotestosterone production without binding to the androgen receptor. Because finasteride interferes with conversion of testosterone to DHT, its routine use causes serum testosterone levels to rise. Also, as the inhibition of 5α-reductase can result in feminization of a male fetus, effective contraception must be used. Finasteride, at dosages ranging from 2.5–5.0 mg/day, has been shown to be effective in decreasing hirsutism symptoms in women with PCOS. However, finasteride may induce side effects such as reduced libido, depression, headaches, dry skin and gastrointestinal disorders. Since the withdrawal of treatment generally results in recurrence of symptoms within few months, long-term administration of finasteride is required. Therefore, in order to reduce the incidence of side effects and also costs of treatment, the lowest effective dosage of finasteride is preferred. It has been demonstrated in hirsute women that, 50% of the standard daily dose of finasteride (i.e. 2.5 mg) is as effective as the standard dose in the treatment of hirsutism. Both the 2.5 and 5 mg doses exhibited equivalent reductions in hirsutism scores after 6 and 12 months of treatment. Side effects and cost of medication were shown to decrease in the group receiving the lower dose.

The half-life of finasteride has been reported to range from 4.7–7.1 hours. Tartagni et al.[48] proposed an intermittent, low-dose finasteride regimen due to slow accumulation of finasteride with multiple doses and bioactivity of its metabolite that cause much longer activity than one would expect on the basis of the half-life of the drug. The authors compared intermittent, low-dose finasteride regimen consisting of 2.5 mg of drug, given every 3 days for 10 months, with those of a continuous 2.5 mg administration of finasteride and showed that, intermittent low-dose administration of finasteride (2.5 mg every 3 days) is as effective as continuous administration in improving the hirsutism in patients with PCOS. Moreover, the authors stated that the intermittent low-dose regimen has the advantage of being safer and less expensive compared with conventional continuous administration.[48] The vast majority of the studies showed that finasteride is as efficient as other drugs.

Metformin treatment

There has been increasing interest in insulin-sensitizing drugs, since the relationship between pathogenesis of hyperandrogenism and insulin resistance in hirsute women with PCOS has been showed. It has been postulated that both insulin itself and also insulin-stimulated growth factors, including IGF-I, increase the secretion of ovarian androgens. The activity of IGF-I is related to both, absolute circulating concentrations and those of its carrier proteins, which effectively reduce IGF potency. Women with PCOS may also have increased growth factor stimulation via increased circulating free IGF-I due to reduced IGFBPs. It has also been previously demonstrated that insulin increases serum total and free testosterone by stimulating ovarian androgen synthesis and lowering circulating SHBG levels. Therefore, insulin-sensitizing drugs may be effective in ameliorating hirsutism by means of reducing circulating insulin concentrations, leading to both, decreased free androgen concentrations and end-organ sensitivity to testosterone. Actually, a vast majority of the controlled studies using metformin showed modest reductions in circulating free androgens. However, some of the studies did not demonstrate any change in the circulating concentrations of IGF-I, IGFBP-3, or IGFBP-1 after metformin treatment.

Generally, hirsutism takes a long time to treat and therefore, metformin is more advantageous than other treatments owing to its beneficial effects on lipids and blood pressure. For that reason, metformin could be valuable in the prevention of cardiovascular disease, especially in obese women with PCOS. The mechanisms by which metformin improves the lipid profile are not clear. It has been suggested that metformin reduces lipid uptake or synthesis in the intestine and in the hepatocytes. Another contributory factor to the improvement of lipid profile during metformin treatment may be a decrease in release of FFAs from adipose tissue following weight loss, especially in patients who have abdominal obesity. Very recently, it has been shown that metformin significantly increased serum levels of HDL cholesterol, decreased the total cholesterol:HDL cholesterol ratio and decreased serum triglyceride levels. When one study compared metformin with ethinyl estradiol-CPA treatment, although both treatments have positive effects on HDL cholesterol and total cholesterol: HDL cholesterol ratio, ethinyl estradiol-CPA treatment was shown to increase serum levels of total cholesterol and triglycerides.[49]

Recently Harborne et al.[50] showed that metformin (500 mg, three times daily) treatment, for moderate to severe hirsutism, is potentially effective in women with PCOS. They also suggested that this treatment is more efficacious than the standard Dianette ethinyl estradiol, 35 mg plus CPA, 2 mg treatment according to the F-G scores and patient self-assessment after 12 months.[50] In this study, metformin treatment showed negligible effects on circulating total androgens, SHBG, free androgen index, or 17-α hydroxyprogesterone, although a significant increase in circulating DHEAS was observed. However, no change in the circulating concentrations of IGF-I, IGFBP-3, or IGFBP-1 was found after metformin treatment. The authors proposed that the beneficial effect of metformin may be due to a mechanism involving local growth factor action at the dermal papillae due to increased insulin sensitivity. There are few conflicting results regarding the efficiency of metformin in the treatment of hirsutism. Ibanez et al.[51] noted a marked drop in the hirsutism score after metformin treatment.[51] Morin-Papunen et al.[52] reported no change in hirsutism.[52] There has been one very small study reporting the effect of metformin on hirsutism as a primary end-point measure and using an objective measure of hair growth. The results suggested that metformin may show benefit compared with placebo.[53]

Whether metformin confers any additional benefit over antiandrogens is yet to be determined. Given the length of the hair cycle, long-term studies are warranted to clarify this issue.

Metformin in combination treatment
Hyperandrogenism, hyperinsulinemia and obesity are involved in the pathogenesis of PCOS, contributing in different ways to the clinical expression of this syndrome. The most favorable modality for long-term treatment should be in favor of SHBG production, the lipid profile and insulin sensitivity beyond the lowering effect of androgen synthesis. The above requirements are not easy to obtain together with a single form of treatment. Dietary-induced weight loss has many hormonal and metabolic benefits and may improve hirsutism and ovulation in obese PCOS women as mentioned previously. On the other hand, management with insulin sensitizers such as metformin without dietary restriction, produces the same effects. Moreover, the combination of a hypocaloric diet with metformin has synergistic effects.

The significant effect of combined oral contraceptives on SHBG, androgen production, skin androgenic symptoms and irregular menstrual cycle, might be successfully combined with the effects of metformin on glucose tolerance and insulin sensitivity. An additional benefit of combined oral contraceptives in combination therapy may be the need for effective contraception in women while on metformin. A small number of studies have been published related to combined treatment with combined oral contraceptives and metformin in patients with PCOS. It has been shown that the addition of metformin to ethinyl estradiol–CPA oral contraceptive treatment, caused a significant decrease in BMI and WHR, and in addition, improved the lipid profile and insulin sensitivity in non-obese women with PCOS, compared with ethinyl estradiol–CPA treatment alone, suggesting that at least some women with PCOS could benefit from the combination of oral contraceptives and metformin.[54] On the other hand, most recently, Cibula et al.[55] were not able to show an expected improvement in insulin sensitivity while on combined treatment, and the trends in fasting insulin and glucose concentrations were comparable in both combined oral contraceptive, and combined oral contraceptive + metformin groups. Besides a few positive trends, combined treatment with metformin did not cause added beneficial effects on lipids, insulin sensitivity, SHBG or testosterone. According to the authors, due to the unsatisfactory improvement of endocrine and metabolic parameters, the available data do not offer enough evidence to advocate the standard use of combined oral contraceptives in combination with metformin in the long-term treatment of PCOS. However, it might be argued that the value of metformin could be different in specific subgroups of PCOS patients, especially in obese ones.[55]

Another plausible combination treatment in the treatment of PCOS is the combination of insulin sensitizers and antiandrogens, that may produce further benefits due to the different spectrum of actions. Gambineri et al.[56] showed that the combination of these drugs have an additive effect in reducing testosterone concentrations and a synergistic effect in increasing HDL cholesterol and SHBG levels, despite the fact that their data emphasized the dominant role of a hypocaloric diet in improving insulin resistance and hyperinsulinemia. Moreover, with respect to placebo, combination treatment with these drugs has been found to further reduce the hirsutism score, and further improve menstrual abnormalities after six months of therapy.[56]

Ibanez and Zegher[57] focused on the additive effect of combined oral contraceptives on a continuous treatment with metformin and flutamide in adolescent girls with PCOS. The only significant change following the addition of a combined oral contraceptive was an increase in SHBG and consequently, a decrease in the free androgen index. The most important point in the use of the combined oral contraceptive as a part of combination treatment is to decide which progestin must be chosen to achieve the best response. Recently, Ibanez et al.[57] carried out an open-labelled study among young non-obese women with PCOS. All patients took a combination of flutamide (62.5 mg/day), metformin (850 mg/day) and ethinyl estradiol–gestodene for 8–15 months before randomization. Then they were randomized for replacement of the gestodene by drospirenone. After a six-month treatment, it was found that low-dose flutamide–metformin reduced total and abdominal fat excess more effectively if the contraceptive co-therapy contained drospirenone, instead of gestodene as the progestin. The authors concluded that drospirenone allows flutamide to exert its anti-androgen actions in contrast to gestodene. However, there have been no significant differences in BMI, F-G score, and serum levels of glucose, insulin, SHBG and testosterone after the six-month treatment between the two groups.[57]

Very recently, the same authors published a new article related to this topic. They constituted two groups to show the additive effects of metformin (850 mg/d) over 3 months in young patients with hyperinsulinemic hyperandrogenism. In the first group, all patients started flutamide (62.5 mg/d) and a monophasic oral contraceptive (Yasmin) at month zero and were randomized to receive either additional placebo or metformin for 3 months. In the second group, all participants received full combination therapy for a mean duration of 17 months and they were randomized for discontinuation of either placebo or metformin during the subsequent 3 months. In the first group, the addition of metformin was found to have consistently beneficial effects on interleukin-6 (IL-6) and body adiposity, whereas the body weight remained unchanged. Maintenance of metformin addition showed detectably beneficial effects on circulating IL-6 and adiponectin, as well as on body adiposity in the second group. Therefore, the authors concluded that metformin treatment proves to be a pivotal component of a prime combination therapy that attenuates the dysadipocytokinemia, the lean mass deficit, and the central adiposity of young patients with PCOS.[58]

Conclusion

The selection of therapy for PCOS generally depends on the physical symptoms and patients' desire for childbearing. For obese women with PCOS, weight loss should be considered as a first option. For infertile patients, clomiphene citrate is the first-line option. If clomiphene fails to induce ovulation and pregnancy, treatment with metformin alone, or in combination with clomiphene can be the second resort. In resistant women, other treatment modalities such as laparoscopic electrocautery or ovulation induction with gonadotropins have been proposed as alternative therapies. Gonadotropin treatment requires a high degree of skill, extensive hormone and ultrasound monitoring, since follicular response tends to be initially slow, but explosive at later stages of stimulation, which may be in association with multiple pregnancies and ovarian hyperstimulation syndrome (OHSS). IVF should be considered as a last option. Medical treatment of hirsutism and acne in polycystic ovary syndrome generally aims to reduce androgen levels, attenuate their effects by lowering androgen production, augmenting androgen binding to specific plasma-binding proteins, and blocking androgen action at the level of the target tissue. The effects of drugs used to treat hirsutism are very similar. Some authors have reported beneficial effects of metformin on hirsutism when used either alone or in combination with dietary restriction or antiandrogenic medications. More randomized, controlled studies in a larger population are needed to determine the effect of metformin on hirsutism in women with PCOS. Chronic anovulation and oligomenorrhea should be treated to prevent future complications.

References

1. Legro RS. Diabetes prevalence and risk factors in polycystic ovary syndrome. *Obstet Gynecol Clin North Am* 2001; 28: 99–109.
2. Guzick D. Polycystic ovary syndrome: symptomatology, pathophysiology, and epidemiology. *Am J Obstet Gynecol* 1998; 179: 89–93.
3. Farhi D, Nosanchuk J, Silverberg S. Endometrial adenocarcinoma in women under 25 years of age. *Obstet Gynecol* 1986; 68: 741–745.
4. Balen AH, Conway GS, Kaltsas G, Techatrasak K, Manning PJ, West C, Jacobs HS. Polycystic ovary syndrome: the spectrum of the disorder in 1741 patients. *Hum Reprod* 1995; 10: 2107–2111.
5. Norman RJ, Noakes M, Wu R, Davies MJ, Moran L, Wang JX. Improving reproductive performance in overweight/obese women with effective weight management. *Hum Reprod Update* 2004; 10: 267–280.
6. Huber-Buchholz MM, Carey DG, Norman RJ. Restoration of reproductive potential by lifestyle modification in obese polycystic ovary syndrome: role of insulin sensitivity and luteinizing hormone. *J Clin Endocrinol Metab* 1999; 84: 1470–1474.
7. Kriplani A, Agarwal N. Effects of metformin on clinical and biochemical parameters in polycystic ovary syndrome. *J Reprod Med* 2004; 49: 361–367.
8. Glueck CJ, Wang P, Fontaine R, Tracy T, Sieve-Smith L. Metformin-induced resumption of normal menses in 39 of 43 (91%) previously amenorrheic women with the polycystic ovary syndrome. *Metabolism* 1999; 48: 511–519.
9. Glueck CJ, Wang P, Fontaine R, Tracy T, Sieve-Smith L. Metformin to restore normal menses in oligo-amenorrheic teenage girls with polycystic ovary syndrome (PCOS). *J Adolesc Health* 2001; 29: 160–169.
10. Kashyap S, Wells GA, Rosenwaks Z. Insulin-sensitizing agents as primary therapy for patients with polycystic ovarian syndrome. *Hum Reprod* 2004; 19: 2474–2483.
11. Tuomilehto J, Lindstrom J, Eriksson JG, Valle TT, Hamalainen H, Ilanne-Parikka P, et al. Finnish Diabetes Prevention Study Group. Prevention of type 2 diabetes mellitus by changes in lifestyle among subjects with impaired glucose tolerance. *N Engl J Med* 2001; 344: 1343–1350.
12. Knowler WC, Barrett-Connor E, Fowler SE, Hamman RF, Lachin JM, Walker EA, Nathan DM. Diabetes Prevention Program Research Group. Reduction in the incidence of type 2 diabetes with lifestyle intervention or metformin. *N Engl J Med* 2002; 346: 393–403.
13. UK Prospective Diabetes Study (UKPDS) Group. Effect of extensive blood glucose control with Metformin on complications in overweight patients with type 2 diabetes (UKPDS 34). *Lancet* 1998; 352: 854–865.
14. Clark AM, Thornley B, Tomlinson L, Galletley C, Norman RJ. Weight loss in obese infertile women results in improvement in reproductive outcome for all forms of fertility treatment. *Hum Reprod* 1998; 13: 1502–1505.
15. Farquhar CM. The role of ovarian surgery in polycystic ovary syndrome. Best Practice & Research Clinical Obstetrics and Gynaecology, 2004; 18: 789–802.
16. Bayram N, van Wely M, Kaaijk EM, Bossuyt PM, van der Veen F. Using an electrocautery strategy or recombinant follicle stimulating hormone to induce ovulation in polycystic ovary syndrome: randomised controlled trial. BMJ, 2004; 328: 192.
17. Farquhar CM, Williamson K, Brown PM, Garland J. An economic evaluation of laparoscopic ovarian diathermy versus gonadotrophin therapy for women with clomiphene citrate resistant polycystic ovary syndrome. *Hum Reprod* 2004; 19: 1110–1115.
18. Attia GR, Rainey WE, Carr BR. Metformin directly inhibits androgen production in human thecal cells. *Fertil Steril* 2001; 76: 517–524.
19. Nestler JE, Jakubowicz DJ, Evans WS, Pasquali R. Effects of metformin on spontaneous and clomiphene induced ovulation in the polycystic ovary syndrome. *N Engl J Med* 1998; 338: 1876–1880.
20. Lord JM, Flight IH, Norman RJ. Metformin in polycystic ovary syndrome: systematic review and meta-analysis. *BMJ* 2003; 327: 951–953.
21. Sahin Y, Yirmibes U, Kelestimur F, Aygen E. The effects of metformin on insulin resistance,

clomiphene-induced ovulation and pregnancy rates in women with polycystic ovary syndrome. *Eur J Obstet Gynecol Reprod Biol* 2004; 113: 214–220.

22. Pasquali R, Gambineri A, Biscotti D, Vicennati V, Gagliardi L, Colitta D, et al. Effect of long-term treatment with metformin added to hypocaloric diet on body composition, fat distribution, and androgen and insulin levels in abdominally obese women with and without the polycystic ovary syndrome. *J Clin Endocrinol Metab* 2000; 85: 2767–2774.

23. Palomba S, Orio F Jr, Falbo A, Manguso F, Russo T, Cascella T, et al. Prospective parallel randomized, double-blind, double-dummy controlled clinical trial comparing clomiphene citrate and metformin as the first-line treatment for ovulation induction in nonobese anovulatory women with polycystic ovary syndrome. *J Clin Endocrinol Metab* 2005; 90: 4068–4074.

24. Dale PO, Tanbo T, Haug E, Abyhalin T. The impact of insulin resistance on the outcome of ovulation induction with low-dose follicle stimulating hormone in women with polycystic ovary syndrome. *Hum Reprod* 1998; 13: 567–570.

25. De Leo V, Marca A, Ditto A, Morgante G, Cionci A. Effects of metformin on gonadotropin-induced ovulation in women with PCOS. *Fertil Steril* 1999; 72: 282–285.

26. Yarali H, Yildiz BO, Demirol A, Zeyneloglu HB, Yigit N, Bukulmez O, Koray Z. Co-administration of metformin during rFSH treatment in patients with clomiphene citrate-resistant polycystic ovarian syndrome: a prospective randomized trial. *Hum Reprod* 2002; 17: 289–294.

27. Christin-Maitre S, Hugues JN. Recombinant FSH Study Group. A comparative randomized multicentric study comparing the step-up versus step-down protocol in polycystic ovary syndrome. *Hum Reprod* 2003; 18: 1626–1631.

28. Imani B, Eijkemans MJ, Faessen GH, Bouchard P, Giudice LC, Fauser BC. Prediction of the individual follicle-stimulating hormone threshold for gonadotropin induction of ovulation in normogonadotropic anovulatory infertility: an approach to increase safety and efficiency. *Fertil Steril* 2002; 77: 83–90.

29. Hugues JN, Cedrin-Durnerin I, Avril C, Bulwa S, Herve F, Uzan M. Sequential step-up and step-down dose regimen: an alternative method for ovulation induction with follicle-stimulating hormone in polycystic ovarian syndrome. *Hum Reprod* 1996; 11: 2581–2584.

30. Laml T, Obruca A, Fischl F, Huber JC. Recombinant luteinizing hormone in ovarian hyperstimulation after stimulation failure in normogonadotropic women. *Gynecol Endocrinol* 1999; 13: 98.

31. Nugent D, Vandekerckhove P, Hughes E, Arnot M, Lilford R. Gonadotrophin therapy for ovulation induction in subfertility associated with polycystic ovary syndrome. *Cochrane Database Syst Rev* 2000; 4: CD000410.

32. Van Wely M, Westergaard LG, Bossuyt PM, Van der Veen F. Human menopausal gonadotropin versus recombinant follicle stimulation hormone for ovarian stimulation in assisted reproductive cycles. *Cochrane Database Syst Rev* 2003; 1: CD003973.

33. van Wely M, Bayram N, van der Veen F. Recombinant FSH in alternative doses or versus urinary gonadotrophins for ovulation induction in subfertility associated with polycystic ovary syndrome: a systematic review based on a Cochrane review. *Hum Reprod* 2003; 18: 1143–1149.

34. Gerli S, Casini ML, Unfer V, Costabile L, Mignosa M, Di Renzo GC. Ovulation induction with urinary FSH or recombinant FSH in polycystic ovary syndrome patients: a prospective randomized analysis of cost-effectiveness. *Reprod Biomed Online* 2004; 9: 494–499.

35. Balen A, Tan S, MacDougall J, Jacobs H. Miscarriage rates following in-vitro fertilization are increased in women with polycystic ovaries and reduced by pituitary desensitization with buserelin. *Hum Reprod* 1993; 8: 959–964.

36. Homburg R, Levy T, Berkovitz D. Gonadotropin-releasing hormone agonist reduces the miscarriage rate for pregnancies achieved in women with polycystic ovarian syndrome. *Fertil Steril* 1993; 59: 527–531.

37. Al-Inany H, Aboulghar M. Gonadotrophin-releasing hormone antagonists for assisted conception. *Cochrane Database Syst Rev* 2001; 4: CD001750.

38. Hwang JL, Seow KM, Lin YH, Huang LW, Hsieh BC, Tsai YL, et al. Ovarian stimulation by concomitant administration of cetrorelix acetate and hMG following Diane-35 pre-treatment for patients with polycystic ovary syndrome: a prospective randomized study. *Hum Reprod* 2004; 19: 1993–2000.

39. Hu Y, Cortvrindt R, Smitz J. Effects of aromatase inhibition on in vitro follicle and oocyte development analyzed by early preantral mouse follicle culture. *Mol Reprod Dev* 2002; 61: 549–559.

40. Damario MA, Barmat L, Liu HC, Davis OK, Rosenwaks Z. Dual suppression with oral contraceptives and gonadotrophin releasing-hormone

agonists improves in-vitro fertilization outcome in high responder patients. *Hum Reprod* 1997; 12: 2359–2365.

41. Stadtmauer LA, Toma SK, Riehl RM, Talbert LM. Metformin treatment of patients with polycystic ovary syndrome undergoing in vitro fertilization improves outcomes and is associated with modulation of the insulin-like growth factors. *Fertil Steril* 2001; 75: 505–509.

42. Fedorcsak P, Dale PO, Storeng R, Tanbo T, Abyholm T. The impact of obesity and insulin resistance on the outcome of IVF or ICSI in women with polycystic ovarian syndrome. *Hum Reprod* 2001; 16: 1086–1091.

43. Wiegratz I, Kutschera E, Lee JH, Moore C, Mellinger U, Winkler UH, Kuhl H. Effect of four different oral contraceptives on various sex hormones and serum-binding globulins. *Contraception* 2003; 67: 361–366.

44. Guido M, Romualdi D, Giuliani M, Suriano R, Selvaggi L, Apa R, Lanzone A. Drospirenone for the treatment of hirsute women with polycystic ovary syndrome: a clinical, endocrinological, metabolic pilot study. *J Clin Endocrinol Metab* 2004; 89: 2817–2823.

45. Farquhar C, Lee O, Toomath R, Jepson R. Spironolactone versus placebo or in combination with steroids for hirsutism and/or acne. *Cochrane Database Syst Rev* 2003; 4: CD000194.

46. Miller JA, Jacobs HS. Treatment of hirsutism and acne with cyproterone acetate. *Clin Endocrinol Metab* 1986; 15: 373–389.

47. De Leo V, Fulghesu AM, la Marca A, Morgante G, Pasqui L, Talluri B, et al. Hormonal and clinical effects of GnRH agonist alone, or in combination with a combined oral contraceptive or flutamide in women with severe hirsutism. *Gynecol Endocrinol* 2000; 14: 411–416.

48. Tartagni M, Schonauer MM, Cicinelli E, Petruzzelli F, De Pergola G, De Salvia MA, Loverro G. Intermittent low-dose finasteride is as effective as daily administration for the treatment of hirsute women. *Fertil Steril* 2004; 82: 725–752.

49. Rautio K, Tapanainen JS, Ruokonen A, Morin-Papunen LC. Effects of metformin and ethinyl estradiol-cyproterone acetate on lipid levels in obese and non-obese women with polycystic ovary

syndrome. *Eur J Endocrinol* 2005; 152: 269–275.

50. Harborne L, Fleming R, Lyall H, Sattar N, Norman J. Metformin or antiandrogen in the treatment of hirsutism in polycystic ovary syndrome. *J Clin Endocrinol Metab* 2003; 88: 4116–4123.

51. Ibanez L, Valls C, Potau N, Marcos MV, de Zegher F. Sensitization to insulin in adolescent girls to normalize hirsutism, hyperandrogenism, oligomenorrhea, dyslipidemia, and hyperinsulinism after precocious pubarche. *J Clin Endocrinol Metab* 2000; 85(10): 3526–3530.

52. Morin-Papunen LC, Koivunen RM, Ruokonen A, Martikainem HK. Metformin therapy improves the menstrual pattern with minimal endocrine and metabolic effects in women with polycystic ovary syndrome. *Fertil Steril* 1998; 69: 691–696.

53. Kelly CJ, Gordon D. The effect of metformin on hirsutism in polycystic ovary syndrome. *Eur J Endocrinol* 2002; 147: 217–221.

54. Elter K, Imir G, Durmusoglu F. Clinical, endocrine and metabolic effects of metformin added to ethinyl estradiol-cyproterone acetate in non-obese women with polycystic ovarian syndrome: a randomized controlled study. *Hum Reprod* 2002; 17: 1729–1737.

55. Cibula D, Fanta M, Vrbikova J, Stanicka S, Dvorakova K, Hill M, et al. The effect of combination therapy with metformin and combined oral contraceptives (COC) versus COC alone on insulin sensitivity, hyperandrogenaemia, SHBG and lipids in PCOS patients. *Hum Reprod* 2005; 20: 180–184.

56. Gambineri A, Pelusi C, Genghini S, Morselli-Labate AM, Cacciari M, Pagotto U, Pasquali R. Effect of flutamide and metformin administered alone or in combination in dieting obese women with polycystic ovary syndrome. *Clin Endocrinol* 2004; 60: 241–249.

57. Ibanez L, de Zegher F. Flutamide-metformin plus an oral contraceptive (OC) for young women with polycystic ovary syndrome: switch from third- to fourth-generation OC reduces body adiposity. *Hum Reprod* 2004; 19: 1725–1727.

58. Ibanez L, de Zegher F. Flutamide-metformin plus ethinylestradiol-drospirenone for lipolysis and antiatherogenesis in young women with ovarian hyperandrogenism: the key role of metformin at the start and after more than one year of therapy. *J Clin Endocrinol Metab* 2005; 90: 39–43.

Frequently Asked Questions

1. What is the rationale for the use of insulin sensitizers in management of PCOS?

When administered to insulin-resistant patients, these compounds act to increase target tissue responsiveness to insulin, thereby reducing the compensatory hyperinsulinemia, which plays a pivotal pathologic role in PCOS. In general, clinical studies have shown that metformin administration to women with PCOS led to a significant improvement in insulin sensitivity, serum insulin and androgen levels, accompanied by decreased LH and increased SHBG concentrations, and thereby an increased frequency of spontaneous ovulation, menstrual cyclicity, and ovulatory response to clomiphene.

2. Which insulin sensitizing drug is preferred?

If a decision to use insulin-sensitizing agents has been made, metformin is the first-choice drug. The safety profile of pioglitazone and rosiglitazone remains to be established, so these agents should be considered as second-choice therapeutic options when the administration of metformin is contraindicated.

3. Is the use of metformin during pregnancy safe?

Metformin crosses the placenta and is classified as a category B drug for use in pregnancy. However, the safety profile of metformin has been sufficiently established for the use of this drug during gestation. Its use throughout pregnancy is advised by some authors to reduce the risk of abortion and gestational diabetes mellitus.

4. If a cost-effective and evidence-based treatment approach to anovulatory patients with PCOS is considered, what should be the order of treatment options?

Lifestyle modifications
Metformin
Metformin and clomiphene
Laparoscopic ovarian drilling

FSH injections
Assisted reproduction

5. If any combined oral contraceptive (COC) is planned to be used in a patient with PCOS, what should be the drug of choice?

The effectiveness of all preparations is similar in suppressing folliculogenesis, ovarian androgen production and endometrial proliferation. However, the COCs including a progesterone without androgenic and glucocorticoid activity should be preferred.

6. Which protocol of ovarian stimulation is more effective and beneficial in anovulatory patients with PCOS?

A low dose step-up protocol using u-FSH has the advantage of a more controlled stimulation, resulting in the development of fewer multiple follicles and therefore, a decreased risk of OHSS, cycle cancellation and multiple pregnancies. The low dose step-up protocol was also reported to result in a higher rate of ovulation when compared to the low dose step-down protocol.

7. If an exaggerated ovarian response to gonadotropins is encountered, what measures should be undertaken to reduce the risk of OHSS?

– Reduction of the hCG dose from 10 000 IU to 5000 or 3000 IU
– The induction of final maturation of the follicles and oocytes may be with triggered by recombinant LH after the administration of a GnRH-a
– Retrieval of all the oocytes and cryopreservation of the embryos thus produced
– Coasting
– Oocyte retrieval, in vitro maturation and fertilization of immature oocytes

8. What are the treatment strategies for hirsutism?

Suppression of ovarian androgen production
Suppression of adrenal androgen production

Increased binding of androgens to specific plasma-binding proteins,
Blocking androgen action at the level of the target tissue

9. Are insulin sensitizers effective in ameliorating hirsutism?

Insulin-sensitizing drugs may be effective in ameliorating hirsutism by reducing circulating insulin concentrations, leading to both, decreased free androgen concentrations and end-organ sensitivity to testosterone. Some authors have reported beneficial effects of metformin on hirsutism when used either alone or in combination with dietary restriction or antiandrogenic medications.

27
Polycystic Ovary Syndrome in the Menopausal Years

Yair Frenkel, Howard J Carp

Summary

The polycystic ovary syndrome (PCOS) is a relatively common condition affecting 10% of women of childbearing age. However, there is little information available as to the subsequent behaviour of the condition after menopause, or as to the appropriate management of patients. PCOS is associated with enlarged polycystic ovaries, and metabolic disturbances including hyperandrogenism, insulin resistance raised serum triglycerides and low-density lipoproteins, and decreased levels of high-density lipoprotein. Clinically, the syndrome presents with obesity and anovulation. The enlarged ovaries persist into the menopausal years; however, there does not seem to be any difference in the incidence of menopausal symptoms. The metabolic changes predispose to diabetes in menopause, and to the development of atherosclerosis, including hypertension and coronary heart disease. The chronic anovulation associated with PCOS may raise the incidence of endometrial cancer. The relative risk of developing postmenopausal endometrial cancer is 5.3 times higher in the presence of PCOS, which is not statistically significant. However, high circulating levels of androstendione are associated with a statistically significant odds ratio of 2.8 (95%CI 1.5–5.2) for developing endometrial cancer. PCOS women do not seem to be at an increased risk for breast cancer after menopause despite years of an unopposed estrogen effect.

Introduction

Polycystic ovaries (PCOS) were first described by Stein and Leventhal in 1935.[1] Most of the literature on polycystic ovaries refers to the management of young women desiring fertility. Indeed, it is the most common endocrine disorder in women, affecting almost 10% of women of childbearing age.[2] There is a dearth of information on the possible effects of PCOS in the menopausal and postmenopausal years. Does PCOS affect general health? What is the ultrasonic image of the postmenopausal ovary in PCOS? Is there a connection between PCOS, its hormonal and metabolic changes and menopause?

PCOS is associated with menstrual irregularity, anovulation, hyperandrogenemia, acne, hirsutism, and obesity. There are metabolic alterations including insulin resistance and altered lipid levels including raised serum triglycerides and low-density lipoprotein (LDL), and low serum concentrations of high-density lipoprotein (HDL). All these are risk factors that might affect the menopausal patient. These metabolic changes expose women to cardiovascular risks, and long-term anovulation exposes them to oncological risks due to the effect of unopposed estrogen. PCOS may have a range of clinical presentations, from normal menstruation with only an ultrasonographic picture of PCOS to amenorrhea accompanied with obesity, acne, hirsutism and the metabolic changes described above. The severe form of the condition may predispose to long-term effects resulting from the long duration of hormonal and metabolic changes.[3] Various features of PCOS and menopause are discussed below.

Clinical Discussion

Ultrasound in PCOS

Birdsall and Farquhar[4] have ultrasonographically scanned two groups of women. One group consisted of 142 pre-and postmenopausal women undergoing coronary angiography. The second (control) group consisted of 18 postmenopausal women not undergoing angiography. The 142 coronary angiography women had a mean age of 53.2 years (range 36–60). Ninety-four women were postmenopausal and 48 were pre-menopausal. In the pre-menopausal group, PCOS was detected in 25/48 (52%) women. The ovarian volume was larger in pre-menopausal PCOS women (9.19 ± 3.49cc) than normal ovaries in pre-menopausal women, (5.34 ± 2.39cc) (p = 0.0001), and the number of follicles was greater (9.66 ± 0.99 compared to 2.68 ± 1.51 respectively; p = 0.0001). The study group consisted of 94 postmenopausal women and polycystic ovaries were found in 35/94 (37.2%) women. The ovarian volume was larger in PCOS women than non-PCOS women (6.38cc and 3.7cc respectively, p = 0.0001). There were more follicles in the PCOS ovaries (9.01 vs. 1.7 in non PCOS ovaries, p = 0.0001). However, the uterine size and endometrial thickness were similar in both groups. The PCOS women were more hirsute (Ferriman-Gallwey scores of 5.3 ± 3.9 vs. 3.4 ± 2.5, p = 0.005). Testosterone and free testosterone levels were higher in PCOS women compared to non-PCOS women (1.25 ± 0.59 vs. 0.96 ± 0.54 nmol/l, p = 0.02 and 28.3 ± 14.3 vs. 21.8 ± 13.7 pmol/l, p = 0.03 respectively). Triglycerides were also higher in PCOS patients compared to non-PCOS patients (1.99 ± 1.28 vs. 1.48 ± 0.81 mmol/l, p = 0.02). There was no difference in luteinizing hormone (LH), follicle stimulating hormone (FSH), sex hormone binding globulin (SHBG), fasting glucose, fasting insulin, fasting C-peptide, cholesterol, HDL, LDL, apolipoprotein A1, lipoprotein A, ferritin or fibrinogen levels between both groups.

The control (non coronary angiography) group consisted of 18 postmenopausal women with a mean age of 56.9 years (range 51–65). Polycystic ovaries were found in 8/18 (44%) women in the control group. PCOS women had larger ovaries (5.0cc compared to 3.17 cc, p = 0.03), which contained more follicles (8.6 vs. 2.1, p = 0.0001), and had higher serum testosterone concentrations (1.3 vs. 0.83 nmol/l, p = 0.04). Hence, postmenopausal women with PCOS seem to have the same features as before the menopause, i.e enlarged ovaries and more follicles. In the first decade after the menopause, the ovaries might not yet be completely devoid of follicles. There is also hyperandrogenemia resulting in hirsutism. Hypertriglyceridemia may also occur with the attendant metabolic effects.

Post menopausal symptoms in PCOS

Dahlgren et al.[5] found that after menopause, the concentrations of estrone, testosterone, testosterone/SHBG ratio and androstendione are significantly higher in postmenopausal PCOS women than in non-PCOS women, (estrone: 0.21 ± 0.04 nmol/L vs. 0.17 ± 0.04) p ≤ 0.05; testosterone: 2.3 ± 1.0 n mol/L vs. 1.5 ± 0.8, p ≤ 0.05; testosterone/SHBG ratio: 0.07 ± 0.04 vs. 0.04 ± 0.03, p ≤ 0.05; androstendione: 4.1 ± 2.0 vs. 2.7 ± 1.0, p ≤ 0.05). Thirty three per cent of PCOS women had experienced sporadic episodes of hot flushes compared to 27% in non-PCOS women, and 21% of PCOS women suffered from menopausal symptoms compared to 22% non-PCOS women who reported constant symptoms. Vaginal dryness was reported by 14% of PCOS women and 17% of non-PCOS women. 17% of PCOS women used hormone replacement therapy (HRT) as opposed to 2% in non-PCOS women. Six per cent of PCOS women used local treatment with estriol for urogenital atrophy compared to 9% of non-PCOS women. The fact that a similar proportion of PCOS and non-PCOS women used HRT after menopause indicates that there is probably, no difference in menopausal symptoms between women with and without PCOS.

Metabolic effects and consequences

Hyperinsulinemia and insulin resistance are characteristic features of obese and non-obese women with PCOS. Up to 60% of lean women with PCOS exhibit fasting hyperinsulinemia.[6] Kalish et al.[7] in a cross sectional study examined the association between insulin resistance and testosterone (total and bioavailable), estradiol and SHBG in 845 healthy postmenopausal women. Endogenous levels of bioavailable estradiol were significantly associated with insulin resistance. Androgenicity (high bioavailable testosterone and low SHBG) was also associated with insulin resistance. Androgenicity and upper abdominal adiposity were also associated with insulin resistance. A population-based cohort study of 362 postmenopausal women not using HRT,[8] has shown that the free androgen index (FAI) (total testosterone/sex hormone binding globulin ratio), which is an estimate of free testosterone, is strongly associated with the hyperinsulinemic and hyperglycemic components of the metabolic syndrome in postmenopausal women. Free testosterone is positively associated with fasting hyperglycemia and post challenge insulin levels and a higher ratio of insulin/glucose, which indicates that free testosterone, is associated with greater insulin resistance. Elevated free testosterone predicts incident type 2 diabetes as well as higher insulin levels.[9] Hence, androgen influences insulin sensitivity and glucose metabolism.

In addition to the contribution of hyperandrogenism and insulin resistance to the increased risk of non-insulin dependent diabetes mellitus (NIDDM), there are additional factors such as obesity that aggravate the condition. Dahlgren et al.[5] showed a higher prevalence of hypertension and NIDDM in a group of 33 perimenopausal patients treated previously for PCOS compared to 132 age matched controls in a retrospective cohort study. In a subsequent study, a higher prevalence of hypertension and diabetes mellitus was reported[10] in 28 PCOS women in peri and post menopause, matched by age and BMI to 56 controls. Cibula et al.[11] have reported similar results in a group of 28 women aged 45–59 with PCOS, compared with 752 matched controls. The diagnosis of NIDDM was established in 32% of women with PCOS and in 8% of controls ($p \leq 0.001$).

Obesity is common in PCOS women in whom the atherogenic lipid profile,[12] and enhanced plasminogen activator inhibitor type 1 (PAI-1) production[13] increase the risk of atherosclerosis, and subsequent hypertension and coronary heart disease. Guzick et al.[14] compared 16 PCOS women after 40 years of age with 16 age matched controls. The PCOS women had a significantly greater intima-media thickness and a higher prevalence of plaques measured by carotid artery ultrasonography. While the blood pressure is usually normal in young PCOS women, hypertension has been reported to be three times more common in menopausal women with PCOS.[5] In Cibula et al's study,[11] hypertension was diagnosed in 50% of PCOS women and in 39% of the controls, but the figures did not reach statistical significance.

Coronary artery disease (CAD) is more common in PCOS. Dahlgren et al.[5] reported an 11-fold increase in the relative risk of myocardial infarction in postmenopausal women aged 50 to 60 yrs with a history of PCOS who underwent a previous wedge resection. Cibula et al.[11] reported CAD in 21% of PCOS women compared to 5% in controls ($p \leq 0.001$). The increased risk of myocardial infarction is attributed to long-standing insulin resistance with or without type 2 diabetes, obesity, hyperlipidemia, hypertension, hyperandrogenism and impaired fibrinolysis. The macrovascular disease presented in the coronary arteries may be manifested by angina, acute myocardial infarction, congestive heart failure, sudden death, stroke, and peripheral and renal vascular disease.

Cardiovascular disease is the leading cause of death in women. Therefore, active treatment is indicated for obesity, hyperinsulinemia, and hyperlipidemia in order to decrease the incidence of hypertension and cardiovascular disease. Both, metformin and troglitazone decrease hyperinsulinemia. Both the drugs are used in infertility management and could possibly be used in menopause to normalize steroidogenesis and relieve the endothelial cell dysfunction associated with estrogen deficiency.[15] Troglitazone has been shown to ameliorate androgen excess and its manifestations, attenuate insulin resistance, and reduce elevated concentrations of plasminogen activator inhibitor type 1 (PAI-1), thereby improving the function of the fibrinolytic system.[16] Metformin reduces LDL, triglycerides, and blood pressure, lowers elevated concentrations of serum insulin and improves glucose tolerance.[17]

Breast cancer

A PCOS phenotype with infertility, obesity (especially abdominal obesity with a high waist to hip ratio, WHR), might be associated with breast carcinoma. Therefore, a higher incidence of breast carcinoma is expected in postmenopausal PCOS patients. Indeed, Coulam et al.[18] reported a three-fold risk of breast cancer in PCOS postmenopausal patients in a retrospective cohort study. (RR = 3.6, 95% CI 1.2–8.30). The risk was similar in pre- or perimenopausal women. However, other studies have not found an increased risk. Gammon et al.[19] in a population based case control study, interviewed 4730 women with breast carcinoma and 4688 controls. The age adjusted OR was 0.38 (C.I. 0.04–3.65). Anderson et al.[20] reported results of a cohort study comprising 472 women with a history of PCOS. The age adjusted RR for breast carcinoma was 1.2 (95% CI 0.7–2). Multivariate analysis adjusting for the various risk factors for breast carcinoma (menarchal age, menopausal age, age

at first pregnancy, parity, oral contraceptive use, HRT use, BMI, WHR, benign breast disease, and a family history of breast carcinoma) lowered the RR to 1 (95% CI 0.5–1.8). Parazzini et al.[21] studied 2569 women with incident breast carcinoma and 2588 controls. The OR for breast carcinoma in women with a history of PCOS was 0.8 (95% CI 0.3–2.4). The data confirm that there is no association between PCOS and breast carcinoma, despite the presence of risk factors. This apparent paradox of risk factors and no increased risk of breast cancer is understandable considering the results of the estrogen without progesterone arm of the Women's Health Initiative (WHI) study.[22] This arm of the study showed that estrogen alone is not a risk factor for breast carcinoma. Therefore, the ovulation disturbances in PCOS and its associated unopposed estrogen is not a risk factor for breast carcinoma. However, unopposed estrogen might affect the endometrium and predispose to endometrial carcinoma.

Endometrial carcinoma

Clinical and epidemiological studies have indicated an association between long-term anovulation and endometrial cancer due to the unopposed estrogen effect. Obesity, a characteristic of PCOS, has a dual effect: (a) it increases the risk of endometrial cancer due to increased conversion of androgens to estrogen in the adipose tissue of postmenopausal women. (b) lowers SHBG levels resulting in higher levels of free estradiol in the circulation.[23] Coulam et al.[18] in a cohort follow-up study of 1270 patients (summarizing 12816 women years of risk), found a RR of 5.3 (95% CI 0.6–19.0) for endometrial cancer in postmenopausal women. The endometrium was the only site at increased risk. All other malignant neoplasms were within the expected ranges. Gibson.[24] emphasized that unopposed estrogen, obesity, insulin resistance or frank diabetes, and hyperandrogenism, (all characteristics of PCOS) are all well-known risk factors for endometrial carcinoma. Additionally, Potischman et al.[25] found that high circulating levels of androstendione are associated with an

OR of 2.8 (95%CI 1.5–5.2) for developing endometrial cancer.

Conclusions

PCOS affects the life of many women. It does not affect menopause per se, but might affect general health after reaching the menopausal age. Diabetes mellitus, hypertension, cardiovascular disease and endometrial carcinoma are possible adverse consequences. Appropriate treatment is recommended to avoid these adverse events.

References

1. Stein IF, Leventhal ML. Amenorrhea associated with bilateral polycystic ovaries. *Am J Obstet Gynecol* 1935: 29: 181–191.
2. Yen SSC. Chronic anovulation caused by peripheral endocrine disorders. In Yen S.S.C. and Jaffe R. (eds), Reproductive Endocrinology. Physiology, Pathophysiology and Clinical Management. 2nd edition. Saunders, Philadelphia, 1986 pp. 441–499.
3. Farquhar CM, Birdsall M, Manning P, Mitchell JM, France JT. The prevalence of polycystic ovaries on ultrasound scanning in a population of randomly selected women. *Aust NZ J Obstet Gynaecol* 1994: 34: 1–67.
4. Birdsall MA, Farquhar CM. Polycystic ovaries in pre and post-menopausal women. *Clin Endocrinol* 1966; 44: 269–276.
5. Dahlgren E, Johansson S, Lindstedt G, Kuntsson F, Oden A, Janson PO et al. Women with polycystic ovary syndrome wedge resected in 1956 to 1965: A long-term follow-up focusing on natural history and circulating hormones. *Fertil Steril* 1992; 57: 505–513.
6. Conway GS, Jacobs HS. Clinical implications of hyperinsulinaemia in women. *Clin Endocrinol* 1993; 39: 623–632.
7. Kalish GM, Barrett-Connor E, Laughlin GA, Gulanski BA. Association of endogenous sex hormones and insulin resistance among postmenopausal women: results from the Postmenopausal Estrogen/Progestin Intervention trail. *J Clin Endocrinol Metab* 2003; 88: 1646–1652.
8. Golden SH, Ding J, Szklo M, Schmidt MI, Duncan BB, Dobs A. Glucose and insulin components of the metabolic syndrome are associated with hyperandrogenism in postmenopausal women. The atherosclerosis risk in communities study. *Am J Epidemiol* 2004; 160: 540–548.
9. Oh JY, Barrett-Connor E, Wedick NM. Wingard DL. Endogenous sex hormones and the development of type 2 diabetes in older men and women; The Bancho Bernardo Study. *Diabetes Care* 2002; 25: 55–60.
10. Dahlgren E, Janson PO, Johnsson S, Lapidus L, Lindstedt G, Tengborn L. Hemostatic and metabolic variables in women with polycystic ovary syndrome. *Fertil Steril* 1994; 61: 942–947.
11. Cibula D, Cifkova R, Fanta M, Poledne R, Zivny J, Skibova J. Increased risk of non-insulin dependent diabetes mellitus, arterial hypertension and coronary artery disease in perimenopausal women with a history of the polycystic ovary syndrome. *Hum Reprod* 2000; 15: 785–789.
12. Rajkhowa M, Neary RH, Kumpatla P, Game FL, Jones PW, Obhrai MS, Clayton RN. Altered composition of high-density lipoproteins in women with the polycystic ovary syndrome. *J Clin Endpcrinol Metab* 1997; 82: 3389–3394.
13. Atiomo WU, Bates SA, Condon JE, Shaw S, West JH, Prentice AG. The plasminogen activator system in women with polycystic ovary syndrome. *Fertil Steril* 1998; 69: 236–241.
14. Guzick DS, Talbott EO, Sutton-Tyrrell K, Herzog HC, Kuller LH, Wolfson SK. Carotid atherosclerosis in women with polycystic ovary syndrome: initial results from a case control study. *Am J Obstet Gynecol* 1996; 174: 1224–1232.
15. Bush DE, Jones CE, Bass KM, Walters GK, Bruza JM, Ouyang P. Estrogen replacement reverses endothelial dysfunction in postmenopausal women. *Am J Med* 1998; 104: 552–558.
16. Ehrmann DA, Schneider DJ, Sobel BE, Cavaghan MK, Imperial J, Rosenfield RL, Polonsky KS. Troglitazone improves defects in insulin action, insulin secretion, ovarian steroidogenesis, and fibrinolysis in women with polycystic ovary syndrome. *J Clin Endocrinol Metab* 1997; 82: 2108–2116.
17. Nestler JE, Jakubowicz DJ, Evans WS, Pasquali R. Effects of metformin on spontaneous and clomiphene-induced ovulation in PCOSS. *N Engl J Med* 1998; 338: 1876–1880.
18. Coulam CB, Annegers JF, Kranz JS. Chronic anovulation syndrome and associated neoplasia. *Obstet Gynecol* 1983; 61: 403–407.
19. Gammon MD, Thompson WD. Polycystic ovaries and the risk of breast cancer. *Am J Epidemiol* 1991; 134: 818–824.

20. Anderson KE, Sellers TA, Chen PL, Rich SS, Hong CP, Folsom AR, Association of Stein – Leventhal syndrome with the incidence of postmenopausal breast carcinoma in a large prospective study of women in Iowa. *Cancer* 1977; 79: 494–499.

21. Parazzini F, La Vecchia C, Franceschi S, Talamini R, Negri E, Crosignani PG. Association of Stein-Leventhal Syndrome with the incidence of postmenopausal breast carcinoma in a large prospective study of women in Iowa. *Cancer* 1997; 80: 1360–1361.

22. Women's health initiative steering committee. Effects of conjugated equine estrogen in postmenopausal women with hysterectomy: the women's health initiative randomized controlled trial. *JAMA* 2004; 291: 1701–1712.

23. Nisker JA, Hammond GL, Davidson BJ. Frumar AM, Takaki NK, Judd HL, Siiteri PK. Serum sex hormone-binding globulin capacity and the percentage of free estradiol in postmenopausal women with and without endometrial carcinoma. A new biochemical basis for the association between obesity and endometrial carcinoma. *Am J Obstet Gynecol* 1980; 138: 637–642.

24. Gibson M. Reproductive health and polycystic ovary syndrome. *Am J Med* 1995; 98 (1A): 67S–75S.

25. Potischman N, Hoover RN, Brinton LA, Siiteri P, Dorgan JF, Swanson CA et al. Case-control study of endogenous steroid hormones and endometrial cancer. *J Nat Cancer Instit* 1996; 88: 1127–1135.

Insulin-Sensitizing Drugs

28

Should Patients with Polycystic Ovary Syndrome be Treated with Metformin?

Richard Fleming, Naveed Sattar

Summary

There are two distinct reasons for treating women with polycystic ovary syndrome (PCOS) with metformin – the relatively short-term benefits to be found in treatment for reasons of fertility, and the longer term approach to their metabolic health. Insulin resistance is an important 'upstream' driver for reproductive and metabolic abnormalities in women with PCOS, particularly the obese. These women exhibit varying degrees of visceral adiposity, glucose intolerance, dyslipidemia, haematological abnormalities, low grade inflammation, and endothelial dysfunction. They are at increased risk (ca 50%) of type 2 diabetes and coronary heart disease, and investigations should include determination of a fasting glucose value.

The use of metformin in PCOS is becoming increasingly widespread, although clinical practice is ahead of the evidence in both metabolism and reproduction. Reproductive data from controlled studies (usually short-term) indicate modest effects on ovulation, hirsutism and perhaps, benefits in pregnancy complications. Reliable data on metabolic changes are sparse, but include modest reductions in body mass index (BMI), insulin, tissue plasminogen activator antigen (t-PA), low density lipoprotein (LDL)-cholesterol and C-reactive protein (CRP), with increases in high density lipoprotein (HDL)-cholesterol and improved endothelial structure and function. It is thus probable that longer treatment with metformin in PCOS will attenuate the development of diabetes and vascular risk in PCOS, but prospective clinical trial data are absent.

Given the benefits obtainable by exercise in lowering diabetes and vascular risk, as well as reproductive and wider health benefits, future studies should address how physical activity levels can be enhanced in women with PCOS.

Introduction

Patients with PCOS present at clinics, complaining of infertility, menstrual disturbance or hirsutism, with or without acne, and are therefore, seen by gynecologists, primary care physicians, endocrinologists and dermatologists. However, there appear to be substantial variations in the features of the disorder, depending upon the source of the patients studied, including the primary complaint, ethnic origins and degrees of obesity. It is noteworthy that it has been accepted for some years that abnormal insulin metabolism is a major underlying feature of PCOS, but no aspect of it is included in the most recent consensus definition (Rotterdam Consensus).[1] It is therefore, even more surprising that one of the most common therapeutic approaches is through the route of oral antihyperglycemic medication in the form of metformin. It is true to say that metformin is used in women with PCOS for many indications: from infertility to pregnancy outcome, from hirsutism to cycle regulation, and for long-term prevention of undiagnosed and theoretical morbidities. In none of these indications is metformin licensed, and the prospect of change in that situation is remote.

This chapter will discuss the role of insulin resistance in PCOS, the range of metabolic perturbances that increase the risk of future vascular disease, and also, the effects upon fertility. The real and potential role of metformin, and its evidence base in resolving these issues will be addressed, and current evidence of the benefits of lifestyle intervention will be overviewed.

Clinical Discussion

Insulin resistance in PCOS and its roles

A link between perturbed insulin action and PCOS was first highlighted in 1980.[2] Peripheral insulin resistance is most evident in obese patients, but it has been proposed that obesity and PCOS have separate and synergistic relationships with insulin resistance.[3] Lean women with PCOS rarely demonstrate frank insulin resistance, but they do show insulin hypersecretion.[4]

The etiological mechanism(s) underpinning insulin resistance and reproductive abnormalities in women with PCOS are unclear. There are several factors potentially implicated including:

- Genetic contributions to both reproductive and metabolic features, with the possibility that the same genetic factor (s) are simultaneously responsible for both.[3]
- Defects in adipose tissue lipolytic cascades.[5]
- Inflammation mediators leading to insulin resistance.[6]
- Fetal programming effects.[7]
- Primary ovarian hypersensitivity to insulin, and/or androgens, at least in some functional aspects, leading firstly to an altered hormonal milieu, and over time, to alterations in body fat distribution (central > peripheral) with positive feedback towards greater insulin resistance.

Research to clarify the potential mechanisms, in general, requires larger studies than published so far. The heterogeneity of PCOS also allows the possibility that differing factors underpin different phenotypes in PCOS women. Furthermore, different ethnic populations, combined with different environmental and clinical perspectives (gynecologists/endocrinologists/vascular biologists) across the world, render it a phenomenon whose complexity will take much effort to resolve.

Despite insulin resistance in the adipose tissue and skeletal muscle, the ovary (and adrenals) may remain relatively sensitive to insulin for at least some of insulin's actions, and both, insulin and insulin-like growth factor 1 (IGF-1) have stimulatory effects, enhancing thecal and stromal androgen production within the ovary. Androgens are carried in the circulation bound to sex hormone binding globulin (SHBG) with high affinity. Thus, clinical manifestations of androgen activity (hirsutism, acne and alopecia) depend upon the SHBG activity as well as the total circulating androgen concentrations (Figure 28.1), and insulin resistance is associated with reduced circulating SHBG.

Fertility abnormalities in PCOS are mostly due to reduced ovulation frequency, possibly secondary to the fundamental observation in the ovary of an increased density of primary follicles in relation to the primordial follicle pool.[8,9,10] After a long growth phase to antral stages, excess small follicles appear to lead to reduced incidence of follicular maturation and ovulation, and also to the definitive and diagnostic hyperandrogenemia.[11] The hyperinsulinemia is probably also responsible for increased adrenal androgen output. There is also a possible increase in early pregnancy loss, and an increased frequency of pregnancy complications. These are diverse phenomena, which are not clearly related except by an unidentified concept relating energy metabolism and steroid metabolism. The incidence and degrees of all these phenomena appear to be promoted by obesity.

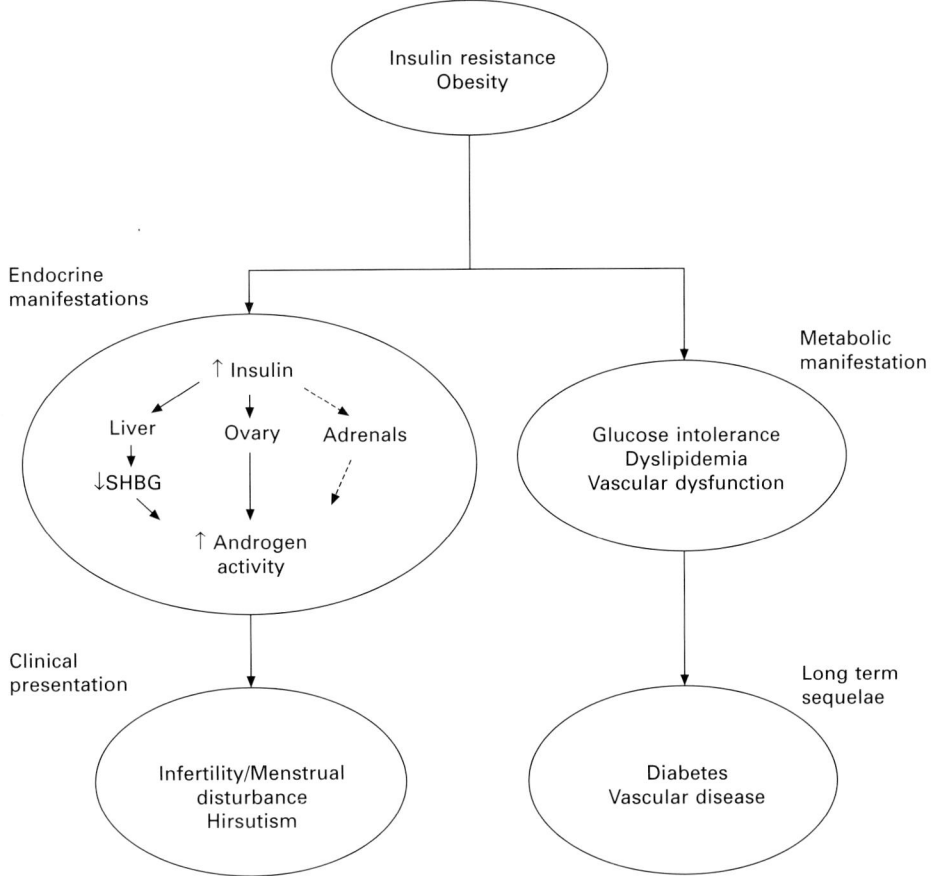

Figure 28.1   The postulated consequences linked to insulin resistance in women with PCOS.

Insulin resistance and metabolic features in women with PCOS

The association between PCOS and insulin resistance and the metabolic syndrome, underlies the use of metformin for this disorder. Insulin resistance is linked to a spectrum of metabolic abnormalities, which eventually lead to diabetes and cardiovascular disease. These include lipid perturbances, hemostatic alterations, low grade chronic inflammation, high blood pressure, endothelial dysfunction, body fat redistribution and glucose intolerance. The evidence collated below indicates that many such pathways are indeed altered in young women with PCOS.

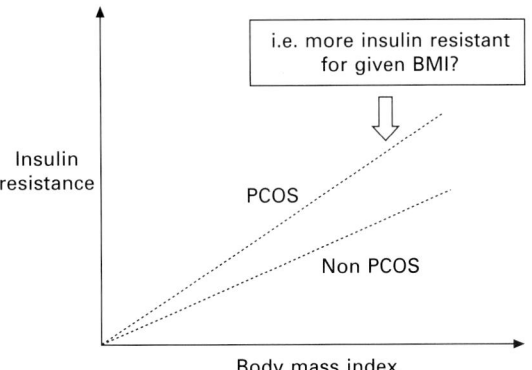

Figure 28.2   Women with PCOS are more insulin resistant and consistent with this, they have a greater prevalence of metabolic syndrome for a given BMI.

Circulating lipids and lipoproteins

The lipoprotein profile in obese women with PCOS is characterised by elevated plasma triglycerides, and reduced high density lipoprotein cholesterol (HDL-C) concentrations, as seen in subjects with type 2 diabetes.[12] It is well recognized that insulin resistance can lead to elevations in triglycerides by promoting hepatic synthesis of very low density lipoprotein (VLDL) particles and by impairing its catabolism by a reduction in lipoprotein lipase activity, yielding reduced circulating HDL-cholesterol concentrations.

Circulating LDL cholesterol is only modestly elevated in women with PCOS, but this may be misleading since LDL does not exist as homogenous particles. LDL particles that are small and dense (LDL-III), are more atherogenic than large buoyant LDL species (LDL-I and LDL-II), and their preponderance in the circulation (even with normal LDL-cholesterol concentrations) is strongly associated with increased coronary heart disease (CHD) and type 2 diabetes. Increased small, dense LDL is now considered to be an integral part of the metabolic syndrome, and women with PCOS show a shift to small, dense LDL relative to BMI matched controls – probably secondary to increased hepatic lipase activity in women with PCOS, an enzyme critical to the generation of small dense LDL species.[13]

However, in terms of *absolute* CHD risk, the modest differences in lipid levels and ratios when considered in conjunction with other risk factors (young age, blood pressure usually normal), result in a low 10 year risk for CHD events. Current treatment guideline thresholds (based on 10 year risk), indicate that most women with PCOS should not be considered for primary prevention care of CHD. Our practice restricts lipid evaluations only to PCOS women with other significant risk factors; lipid measurements will rarely alter clinical practice.

Hemostatic factors

There is increasing evidence that elevated plasma levels of hemostatic factors, (fibrinogen, factor VII, von Willebrand factor, fibrin D-dimer, and tissue plasminogen activator antigen (t-PA), are independently linked to the risk of coronary heart disease (CHD), and are positively associated with insulin resistance.[14]

Evidence from modest numbers of cases of women with PCOS are conflicting about the incidence and degree of these perturbations.[15–17] In line with the non-PCOS population, t-PA concentrations in women with PCOS correlated directly with the degree of obesity, and inversely with insulin sensitivity.[16] Of note, neither lipid abnormalities nor hemostatic perturbances correlate with total testosterone concentrations in women with PCOS.[13,16]

Blood pressure

Patients with diabetes are at increased risk of hypertension and many already have hypertension by the time their diabetes is diagnosed. However, in women with PCOS, evidence for perturbation is unconvincing.[12] The current data are limited by small studies and weak methodology, so much more extensive studies are required before we can make any firm conclusions on blood pressure trends in women with PCOS.

Inflammation

Inflammation as a causal factor in the atherogenic process is currently a major topic. Surrogate markers of inflammation, such as C-reactive protein (CRP), predict the risk of CHD events in both men and women, independently of classical risk factors. At the cellular level, inflammation is involved in several stages of the atherosclerotic process, and elevations in CRP predict type 2 diabetes in men and in women.[17] Women with PCOS have been shown to have increased concentrations of circulating CRP,[6,16,18] possibly independent of BMI. Thus, low-grade chronic inflammation might be another mechanism contributing to the increased risk of CHD and type 2 diabetes in women with PCOS.

Other markers linked to low grade

inflammation, such as white blood cell elevations,[19] and serum interleukin-18 levels,[20] have also been shown to be elevated in women with PCOS. Whilst these observations are of potential interest, much more work is required to dissect any pathogenic role of inflammation in PCOS. It should be remembered that insulin resistance could lead to low grade inflammation rather than the reverse, and that obesity is a major factor promoting low grade inflammation in general. Finally, whether inflammatory mediators (i.e. CRP, IL-6, TNF-alpha) are truly causally related to diabetes and CHD remains to be proven.

Obesity and central body fat distribution

Obesity is common in PCOS, with perhaps 60% having a BMI greater than 25 kg/m^2. It is recognized that visceral distribution of body fat is of greater consequence to the metabolic effects of insulin resistance than obesity alone. Central obesity and insulin resistance lead to an altered lipolytic response to insulin, with attenuated suppression of free fatty acids release from adipose tissue. It is also speculated that an increased flux of free fatty acids from central sites enters the portal circulation, increasing the availability of substrate to the liver for triglyceride production, leading to greater hepatic fat accumulation and potentially provoking greater gluconeogenesis. Women with PCOS show greater central fat accumulation,[21,22] and insulin resistance is probably, largely determined by this increased truncal-abdominal fat mass. This may be a critical factor in the genesis of the metabolic syndrome and also PCOS.

Metabolic syndrome criteria and PCOS

A recent, modified definition of the metabolic syndrome was proposed[23] using thresholds for five easily measured variables linked to insulin resistance: waist circumference, triglycerides, HDL-cholesterol, fasting plasma glucose concentration and blood pressure. Three of these criteria are diagnostic. There are now many studies using the 'ATPIII criteria' demonstrating that individuals with metabolic syndrome are at elevated risk for type 2 diabetes (several folds higher) and CHD events (~70–200% higher). As a large proportion of women with PCOS are overweight, we would predict that they would show a high incidence of metabolic syndrome.

We noted previously that PCOS may be the gynecological presentation of the metabolic syndrome in young women.[24] Using ATPIII criteria, one study[25] revealed a 15% prevalence of metabolic syndrome in a cohort of PCOS women with a mean BMI of 25.8 kg/m^2, which compared to a 3.5% prevalence in healthy controls with a mean BMI of 24.6 kg/m^2. Similar data have recently been reported in a series of more than 100 consecutive patients,[26] where it was also noted that those with metabolic syndrome had higher free testosterone and lower SHBG. Overall, these reports confirm impressions from individual risk factor studies described above and demonstrate that both obesity and PCOS status separately influence the likelihood of having metabolic syndrome. In other words, women with PCOS may accrue more metabolic abnormalities with increasing BMI compared to normal women.

The role and importance of ethnicity in these discussions was revealed by a recent European study,[27] with a much smaller proportion (<5%) of the PCOS population qualifying for metabolic syndrome criteria.

Whether clinicians should routinely ascertain metabolic syndrome status in their patients with PCOS is debatable, although it may justify the use of metformin in some cases. The recent consensus statement (Rotterdam, 3) suggested that metabolic syndrome features (waist circumference, triglyceride levels, HDL-cholesterol levels, blood pressure, fasting glucose levels) *should* be routinely recorded in their patients with PCOS, but did not recommend insulin measurement. The best use of metabolic syndrome criteria presently, might be to facilitate targeting of more comprehensive lifestyle advice to those overweight or obese women with PCOS who also have elements of the metabolic syndrome. Future studies should seek to address this issue.

Glucose intolerance and diabetes in PCOS

The excess risk of type 2 diabetes in women with PCOS, compared with age-matched normal women is strongly contributed to by obesity.[28] One large report[29] showed that the prevalence of glucose intolerance was significantly higher in PCOS women compared with control women (odds ratio = 2.76).

Overall, there is a two to four fold increase risk of glucose intolerance/type 2 diabetes in women with PCOS compared with age-and weight-matched controls. This increase is consistent with the array of risk factors discussed above, along with the metabolic syndrome and visceral fat accumulation independent of total obesity.

A diagnosis of diabetes has clinical ramifications, and all women with PCOS should have at least a fasting glucose performed as part of their baseline tests. We would suggest restricting oral glucose tolerance tests (OGTTs) for PCOS women who have other risk factors such as obesity (BMI > 30 kg/m^2), or fasting glucose >5.5 mmol/l, or a relevant family history.[30]

Atherosclerotic risk in women with PCOS

Angiographic studies have linked androgenic and metabolic features of PCOS including polycystic ovaries to a greater likelihood of coronary lesions.[31,32] Talbott et al.[33] using carotid intima media thickness (IMT) measurements, noted that women (> 45y) with a history of PCOS had significantly greater mean IMT than did controls. Younger women showed no difference.

There are now two concordant studies reporting coronary calcification measurements assessed by electron beam tomography in women with PCOS.[34,35]

CHD event risk in PCOS

A possible link between PCOS and CHD over a follow-up period of three decades, in a cohort of 786 women with PCOS was examined through death certificate data of 70 women.[36] The small number of CHD deaths (n = 15), did not determine an increased CHD risk in women with PCOS: the odds ratio (compared with national data) was 1.5 (95% CI 0.7–2.9). Stronger indications were derived from the prospective study of 82,439 female nurses linking a history of menstrual regularity (at ages 20–35 yr) in 1982 to subsequent CHD end points over 14 years follow-up.[37] This study revealed an association of irregular menses with an increased risk for nonfatal or fatal CHD [age-adjusted relative risks (RR), 1.25 and 1.67, respectively]. As up to 90% of women with very irregular cycles are likely to have PCOS, the data suggest PCOS is associated with a 50% increased risk for CHD compared to age, BMI-matched women without PCOS. This excess CHD risk is in keeping with a greater prevalence of metabolic syndrome and IGT or type 2 diabetes in women with PCOS (Figure 28.3). Future studies should address to what extent this excess risk is accounted for using a comprehensive panel of traditional risk factors including presence of diabetes, and direct measures of blood pressure and cholesterol especially, HDL-cholesterol.

Mechanisms to decrease diabetes and vascular risk in women with PCOS

There is no study examining effects of lifestyle or insulin sensitizing agents on diabetes or CHD end-points in women with PCOS. The evidence base is also sparse concerning the effects of intervention on surrogate vascular end-points, such as endothelial function measures or carotid IMT. There are many short-term data on changes in insulin measures and related reproductive hormonal changes, in particular, with metformin. Few robustly designed studies have addressed changes in CHD risk factors with interventions, and further data are required.

Lifestyle modification

Some of the best evidence demonstrates substantial metabolic and reproductive benefits attainable by lifestyle improvements in PCOS, as seen in the general population. In women with PCOS, a reduction in BMI of around 5–10% by dint of dietary therapy, leads to improvements in

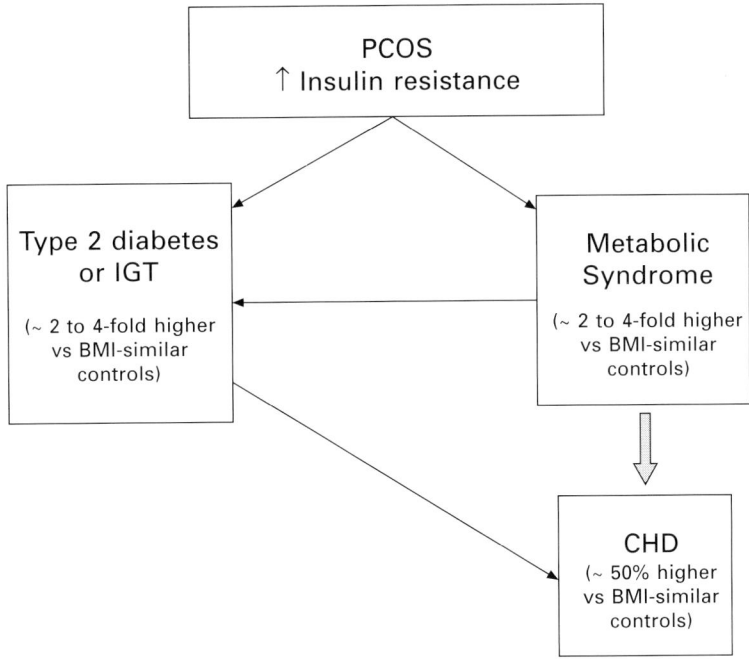

Figure 28.3   In line with greater insulin resistance, women with PCOS have greater prevalence of metabolic syndrome, and associated with this, around a 2 to 4-fold increased risk of impaired glucose tolerance/type 2 diabetes relative to age and BMI matched healthy controls. Data on risk for CHD events is currently sparse but suggest around a 50% higher CHD risk relative to controls with adjustment for age, BMI, smoking, parity, and menopausal status. Whether adjustment for all traditional risk factors completely accounts for this excess risk remains to be determined.

ovarian function and some metabolic risk factors.[38,39] The most exciting evidence in support of lifestyle modification derives from a non-PCOS population, showing that intensive intervention, with a 7% weight loss and at least 150 minutes of physical activity per week, can substantially reduce (by 58%) the development of diabetes in subjects at risk.[40] This work should provoke more robust dietary and exercise intervention studies in women with PCOS. It could be argued that due to their greater accumulation of risk factors for a similar weight gain, women with PCOS have more to gain from increasing physical activity levels than their non-PCOS counterparts. Critically, since many women with PCOS wish to improve fertility, lifestyle measures will be physiologically far better for subsequent pregnancy outcomes than approaches requiring medication alone.

Metformin: ovarian function and metabolism

Metformin, the oral biguanide antihyperglycemic drug has been used for many years in Europe and is now also widely employed worldwide. It has primary effects on increasing peripheral glucose uptake in response to insulin, with some reduction in basal hepatic glucose production. It also lowers adipose tissue lipolysis and improves insulin sensitivity in muscle. It does not provoke hypoglycemia, and it is now the first line therapy in overweight patients with diabetes.

Most of the studies on metformin use in PCOS have addressed effects on reproductive parameters (ovulation rate), with some attention to insulin and lipid metabolism. The ovulation rate summaries for placebo and metformin arms from the major reviews are shown in Table 28.1 One important point to recognize in all these studies

Table 28.1 Summaries of evidence on ovulation rates with metformin from recent reviews

Reviews	No. of studies included (n)	Ovulation rates (%) Placebo	Metformin
Harborne et al.[30]	7	21%	41%
Lord et al.[42]	7	24%	46%
Costello et al.[43]	9	35%	56%

is the short term nature of the observation period. Insulin is known to promote the actions of LH, leading to increased androgen production from ovarian tissue, and metformin treatment has shown to lead to a rapid, if modest, reduction in androgen secretion in most studies. However, as noted above, one of the prime features of PCOS is abnormal primordial-to-primary follicle development, and so far, little attention has been paid to these events with any clinical intervention in PCOS.

However, there is evidence from one study of protracted metformin treatment[41] suggesting that the number of follicles recruited to grow at this earliest stage, may indeed be attenuated by such treatment, which may be related to reduced insulin and/or androgen drive at the earliest stages of development. This in turn suggests that, to explore a role for metformin in correcting the over-production of follicles by women with PCOS, the investigations should only start after 6 months of treatment or more – not during the first 6 months.

Ovulation rates and patients who benefit most

Restricted to short-term observations as we are, the first three reviews[23,42,43] suggest that metformin doubles ovulation rates from low basal levels. On average, one additional ovulation is attained every five months with metformin treatment, which is a modest benefit in a clinical setting, and it has rarely been shown to increase pregnancy rates. However, more encouraging results, in a relatively lean cohort, were obtained on comparison with the effect of laparoscopic

ovarian diathermy, showing that metformin was at least as effective.[44]

Sub-group analyses[45] and direct investigation[46] suggest that metformin may be more effective in lean women with the least metabolic disturbance, suggesting that the therapy is insufficient to correct the metabolic disturbance induced by obesity in the short term, at least at current doses.

First line fertility treatment?

In standard fertility treatment, metformin has been shown to increase the response rate to clomiphene citrate (the erstwhile first line therapy), leading to an increased pregnancy rate with this first line approach.[47] As metformin alone may lead to spontaneous ovulation, particularly in the leaner patient with PCOS, and that any pregnancy is more likely to be a singleton, there is a valid case supporting the use of metformin as first line therapy. However, there is no direct evidence to support this concept, and it should be tested prospectively.

Metformin in assisted conception

Standard assisted conception treatment involves stimulation of ovarian function with exogenous gonadotropins, and because metformin appears to improve some aspects of follicular growth, its potential role has been explored in some interesting trials. Many of the trials lack acceptable levels of control, but useful evidence is emerging.

The main observations in the randomized control studies[48,49] indicate that relatively short-term metformin treatment does not influence total follicular responses to exogenous FSH, evidenced by numbers of follicles, duration and dose of FSH and numbers of oocytes. However, there does appear to be an increased pregnancy rate (particularly in the leaner patients), and a very important reduction in the rate of ovarian hyperstimulation syndrome (OHSS). This latter observation, if confirmed by extended trials would be reason enough to use the drug in these circumstances, because women with PCOS are at an increased risk of OHSS.

Metformin in pregnancy

Large observational studies[50] have suggested that metformin may confer a number of protective advantages through pregnancy in women with PCOS by reducing complications such as, gestational diabetes, and even early pregnancy loss. This effect was explored prospectively in a randomized program,[51] in which secondary end-point evaluations of late pregnancy problems were abundant in the placebo arm and virtually absent from the metformin arm.

Overall, these studies suggest that women with PCOS in the fertility clinic may derive benefit and improved safety from treatment with metformin at all stages. Whilst it is critically important that these studies are confirmed in more extensive trials, it is also important to establish the mechanisms by which the drug confers these benefits. There may be an underlying issue of energy metabolism, but the connections with a number of observations are tenuous, and in reproductive terms, the link with androgen metabolism may prove to be the critical element.

Metformin in PCOS outside fertility issues

In terms of metabolic and anthropometric effects, current evidence supports a reduction in BMI by around 4% over a few months compared to placebo (representing ~2–3 kg reduction) in women with PCOS.[52] More data are required but a weight-reducing effect would be consistent with the documented effects of metformin in large prospective studies of patients at elevated risk for diabetes (~2kg reduction relative to placebo at 6 months).[40] In addition, a role for different doses of metformin has been minimally explored, and where it has, perhaps more consistent effects upon weight loss, can be determined with a higher dose schedule.[52]

Biochemical changes

Biochemical changes in these short-term studies reveal decreased total and free androgen levels with metformin by approximately 20% relative

to placebo, and a decline in fasting insulin levels to a mean of 5.4 mIU/L (95% CI –8.11 to –2.63). Reduction in LDL-cholesterol and t-PA antigen and increases in HDL-cholesterol have been frequently recorded with metformin in PCOS, but larger trials are required to confirm these effects. A reduction in CRP with metformin use in PCOS has been recorded,[18] although this was not confirmed in a further study by the Glasgow group.[52]

The recent demonstration of improvements in both endothelial structure and function in young, normal-weight women with PCOS after 6 months' metformin therapy is a critical observation.[53]

Finally, it has been reported that a combination of diet and metformin for 6 months[54] has been shown to decrease the prevalence of metabolic syndrome in women with PCOS.

Summary of the effects of metformin

Overall, the metabolic and reproductive changes noted with metformin use in women with PCOS are consistent with its known effect in patients with type 2 diabetes. However, effects are generally modest, and larger trials, with longer duration of use and more comprehensive controls are required. Ideally, these should include direct vascular measures and, if sufficiently powered, document risk reduction for development of diabetes.

It is important to note that metformin is not licensed for any of these indications and, from the evidence presented above, it is certainly not a 'cure' for all reproductive and metabolic derangements in women with PCOS. Despite this, once established on metformin treatment, women with a history of PCOS are reluctant to discontinue treatment.[55]

In view of metformin's generally modest benefits in women with PCOS, the relative merits of metformin combined with lifestyle changes, in particular, exercise, would be very important to examine further, and such studies are being developed. It is interesting that both exercise and metformin up-regulate AMP-activated protein kinase activity, a metabolic switch regulating efficient glucose and fatty acid metabolism. It should also be noted that lifestyle intervention was more successful than metformin alone in reducing risk of diabetes in the Diabetes Prevention Program (DPP), once again emphasizing the critical role for lifestyle intervention.

Future research: reproduction in women with PCOS

In the fertility arena, there is a need for a coordinated program of investigations using multi center prospective methods. The influence of obesity and metformin dose on ovarian function has yet to be explored to the degree that is needed to fully elucidate the effects. As the life history of ovarian follicular development is so protracted, and PCOS appears to be associated with abnormalities from the very beginning, examinations of the effects of treatment at this level are required. Other potential areas of benefit, including pregnancy complications, should be examined on a large, multi center scale.

There is evidence to support the use of metformin, in association with other approaches, from the very beginning of treatment of women with PCOS, and this prospect should be explored in the research arena.

Conclusion

Insulin resistance is an important feature in many women with PCOS, particularly the obese, and insulin hypersecretion is potentially universal. It is clear that women with PCOS have both reproductive and metabolic consequences, and they exhibit visceral adiposity, dyslipidemia, low grade inflammation, abnormalities in clotting and glucose intolerance. They are at an increased risk for type 2 diabetes or IGT (about 2–4 fold relative to weight matched controls) and CHD events.

The best estimate for increased CHD risk is currently around 50% higher relative to non-PCOS women of similar age and BMI. Since CHD risk is generally low in young women, the absolute CHD risk in PCOS is low, and there is little demand for further investigation, in the absence of other significant risk factors.

The use of metformin in PCOS is increasingly undertaken even in the absence of demonstrable insulin resistance, but its reproductive and metabolic effects are modest in the relatively short term studies available. Although data are relatively sparse, metformin seems to achieve modest improvements in LDL-cholesterol, HDL-cholesterol, in t-PA and CRP, and endothelial function, at least in some circumstances. It is probable that longer term treatment with metformin in PCOS will attenuate the progress to diabetes, and perhaps, vascular risk in PCOS, and also lead to improved ovarian follicular development.

Finally, the proven benefits of exercise in lowering diabetes and vascular risk, together with wider health benefits, suggest that future studies should urgently address how best to enhance physical activity levels in women with PCOS. The latter approach has the potential to be the cheapest and physiologically the best mechanism to decrease the metabolic and vascular risk in this risk population.

In the fertility arena, metformin may prove to be of considerable benefit, but mainly in association with other forms of treatment, and the results of recent studies are generally supportive of its extended use, perhaps from the very first stages of treatment.

References

1. The Rotterdam ESHRE/ASRM-Sponsored PCOS consensus workshop group. Revised 2003 consensus on diagnostic criteria and long-term health risks related to polycystic ovary syndrome (PCOS). *Hum Reprod* 2004; 19: 41–47.
2. Burghen GA, Givens JR, Kitabchi AE. Correlation of hyperandrogenism with hyperinsulinemia in polycystic ovarian disease. *J Clin Endocrinol Metab* 1980; 50: 113–116.
3. Dunaif A, Thomas A. Current concepts in the polycystic ovary syndrome. *Annu Rev Med* 2001; 52: 401–419.
4. Vrbikova J, Cibula D, Dvorakova K, et al. Insulin sensitivity in women with polycystic ovary syndrome. *J Clin Endocrinol Metab* 2004; 89: 2942–2945.

5. Ek I, Arner P, Ryden M, Holm C, et al. A unique defect in the regulation of visceral fat cell lipolysis in the polycystic ovary syndrome as an early link to insulin resistance. *Diabetes* 2002; 5: 484–492.

6. Kelly CC, Lyall H, Petrie JR, Gould GW, Connell JM, Sattar N. Low grade chronic inflammation in women with polycystic ovarian syndrome. *J Clin Endocrinol Metab* 2001; 86(6): 2453–2455.

7. Cresswell JL, Barker DJ, Osmond C, Egger P, Phillips DI, Fraser RB. Fetal growth, length of gestation, and polycystic ovaries in adult life. *Lancet* 1997; 350 (9085): 1131–1135.

8. Hughesdon PE Morphology and morphogenesis of the Stein-Leventhal ovary so called 'hyperthecosis'. *Obstet Gynecol Survey* 1982; 37: 59–77.

9. Webber LJ, Stubbs S, Stark J, Trew GH, Margara R, Hardy K, Franks S. Formation and early development of follicles in the polycystic ovary. *Lancet* 2003; 362(9389): 1017–1021.

10. Maciel GA Baracat EC, Benda JA, Markham SM, Hensinger K, Chang RJ, Erickson GF. Stockpiling of transitional and classic primary follicles in ovaries of women with polycystic ovary syndrome. *J Clin Endocrinol Metab* 2004; 89: 5321–5327.

11. Jonard S, Dewailly D. The follicular excess in polycystic ovaries, due to intra-ovarian hyperandrogenism, may be the main culprit for the follicular arrest. *Hum Reprod Update* 2004; 10: 107–117.

12. Wild RA. Polycystic ovary syndrome: a risk for coronary artery disease? *Am J Obstet Gynecol* 2002; 186: 35–43.

13. Pirwany IR, Fleming R, Greer IA, Packard CJ, Sattar N. Lipids and lipoprotein subfractions in women with PCOS: relationship to metabolic and endocrine parameters. *Clin Endocrinol (Oxf)* 2001; 54(4): 447–453.

14. Meigs JB, Mittleman MA, Nathan DM, et al. Hyperinsulinemia, hyperglycemia, and impaired hemostasis the Framingham Offspring Study. *JAMA* 2000; 283: 221–228.

15. Atiomo WU, Bates SA, Condon JE, Shaw S, West JH, Prentice AG. The plasminogen activator system in women with polycystic ovary syndrome. *Fertil Steril* 1998; 69(2): 236–241.

16. Kelly CJ, Lyall H, Petrie JR, et al. A specific elevation in tissue plasminogen activator antigen in women with polycystic ovarian syndrome. *J Clin Endocrinol Metab* 2002; 87: 3287–3290.

17. Sattar N, Perry CG, Petrie JR. Type 2 diabetes as an inflammatory disorder. *British Journal of Diabetes and Vascular Disease* 2003; 3: 36–41.

18. Morin-Papunen L, Rautio K, Ruokonen A, Hedberg P, Puukka M, Tapanainen JS. Metformin reduces serum C-reactive protein levels in women with polycystic ovary syndrome. *J Clin Endocrinol Metab* 2003; 88 (10): 4649–4654.

19. Orio F Jr, Palomba S, Cascella T, et al. The increase of leukocytes as a new putative marker of low-grade chronic inflammation and early cardiovascular risk in polycystic ovary syndrome. *J Clin Endocrinol Metab* 2005; 90: 2–5.

20. Escobar-Morreale HF, Botella-Carretero JI, Villuendas G, Sancho J, San Millan JL. Serum interleukin-18 concentrations are increased in the polycystic ovary syndrome: relationship to insulin resistance and to obesity. *J Clin Endocrinol Metab* 2004; 89(2): 806–811.

21. Holte J, Bergh T, Berne C, Berglund L, Lithell H. Enhanced early insulin response to glucose in relation to insulin resistance in women with polycystic ovary syndrome and normal glucose tolerance. *J Clin Endocrinol Metab* 1994; 78: 1052–1058.

22. Yildirim B, Sabir N, Kaleli B. Relation of intra-abdominal fat distribution to metabolic disorders in nonobese patients with polycystic ovary syndrome. *Fertil Steril* 2003; 79: 1358–1364.

23. Expert Panel on Detection, Evaluation, and Treatment of High Blood Cholesterol in Adults. Executive summary of the third report of The National Cholesterol Education Program (NCEP) Expert Panel on detection, evaluation, and treatment of high blood cholesterol in adults (Adult Treatment Panel III). *JAMA* 2001; 285: 2486–2497.

24. Hopkinson ZE, Sattar N, Fleming R, Greer IA. Polycystic ovarian syndrome: the metabolic syndrome comes to gynaecology. BMJ 1998; 317: 329–332.

25. Talbott EO, Zborowski JV, Rager JR, Boudreaux MY, Edmundowicz DA, Guzick DS. Evidence for an association between metabolic cardiovascular syndrome and coronary and aortic calcification among women with polycystic ovary syndrome. *J Clin Endocrinol Metab* 2004; 89(11): 5454–5461.

26. Apridonidze T, Essah PA, Iuorno MJ, Nestler JE. Prevalence and characteristics of the metabolic syndrome in women with polycystic ovary syndrome. *J Clin Endocrinol Metab* 2005; 90(4): 1929–1935.

27. Vrbikova J, Cifkova R, Jirkovska A, Lanska V, Platilova H, Zamrazil V, Starka L. Cardiovascular risk factors in young Czech females with polycystic ovary syndrome. *Hum Reprod* 2003; 18(5): 980–984.

28. Bonora E, Kiechl S, Willeit J, Oberhollenzer F, Egger G, Meigs JB, et al. Bruneck study. Population-based incidence rates and risk factors for type 2 diabetes in white individuals: the Bruneck study. *Diabetes* 2004; 53: 1782–1789.

29. Legro RS, Kunselman AR, Dodson WC, Dunaif A. Prevalence and predictors of risk for type 2 diabetes mellitus and impaired glucose tolerance in polycystic ovary syndrome: a prospective, controlled study in 254 affected women. *J Clin Endocrinol Metab* 1999; 84: 165–169.

30. Harborne L, Fleming R, Lyall H, Norman J, Sattar N. Descriptive review of the evidence for the use of metformin in polycystic ovary syndrome. *Lancet* 2003; 361(9372): 1894–1901.

31. Wild RA, Grubb B, Hartz A, Van Nort JJ, Bachman W, Bartholomew M. Clinical signs of androgen excess as risk factors for coronary artery disease. *Fertil Steril* 1990; 54: 255–259.

32. Birdsall MA, Farquhar CM, White HD. Association between polycystic ovaries and extent of coronary artery disease in women having cardiac catheterization. *Ann Intern Med* 1997; 126: 32–35.

33. Talbott EO, Guzick DS, Sutton-Tyrrell K, McHugh-Pemu KP, Zborowski JV, Remsberg KE, Kuller LH. Evidence for association between polycystic ovary syndrome and premature carotid atherosclerosis in middle-aged women. *Arterioscler Thromb Vasc Biol* 2000; 20(11): 2414–2421.

34. Talbott EO, Zborowski JV, Boudreaux MY, McHugh-Pemu KP, Sutton-Tyrrell K, Guzick DS. The relationship between C-reactive protein and carotid intima-media wall thickness in middle-aged women with polycystic ovary syndrome. *J Clin Endocrinol Metab* 2004; 89(12): 6061–6067.

35. Christian RC, Dumesic DA, Behrenbeck T, Oberg AL, Sheedy PF 2nd, Fitzpatrick LA. Prevalence and predictors of coronary artery calcification in women with polycystic ovary syndrome. *J Clin Endocrinol Metab* 2003; 88(6): 2562–2568.

36. Wild S, Pierpoint T, Jacobs H, McKeigue P. Long-term consequences of polycystic ovary syndrome: results of a 31 year follow-up study. *Hum Fertil (Camb)* 2000; 3: 101–105.

37. Solomon CG, Hu FB, Dunaif A, et al. Menstrual cycle irregularityand risk for future cardiovascular disease. *J Clin Endocrinol Metab* 2002; 87: 2013–2017.

38. Kiddy DS, Hamilton-Fairley D, Bush A, Short F, Anyaoku V, Reed MJ, Franks S. Improvement in endocrine and ovarian function during dietary treatment of obese women with polycystic ovary syndrome. *Clin Endocrinol (Oxf)* 1992; 36(1): 105–111.

39. Clark AM, Thornley B, Tomlinson L, Galletley C, Norman RJ. Weight loss in obese infertile women results in improvement in reproductive outcome for all forms of fertility treatment. *Hum Reprod* 1998; 13(6): 1502–1505.

40. Knowler WC, Barrett-Connor E, Fowler SE, Hamman RF, Lachin JM, Walker EA, Nathan DM; Diabetes Prevention Program Research Group. Reduction in the incidence of type 2 diabetes with lifestyle intervention or metformin. *N Engl J Med* 2002 7; 346(6): 393–403.

41. Fleming R, Harborne L, MacLaughlin DT, Ling D, Norman J, Sattar N, Seifer DB. Metformin reduces serum mullerian-inhibiting substance levels in women with polycystic ovary syndrome after protracted treatment. *Fertil Steril* 2005; 83: 130–136.

42. Lord JM, Flight IH, Norman RJ. Metformin in polycystic ovary syndrome: systematic review and meta-analysis. *BMJ* 2003; 327: 951–953.

43. Costello MF, Eden JA. A systematic review of the reproductive system effects of metformin in patients with polycystic ovary syndrome. *Fertil Steril* 2003; 79: 1–13.

44. Palomba S, Orio F Jr, Nardo LG, et al. Metformin administration versus laparoscopic ovarian diathermy in clomiphene citrate-resistant women with polycystic ovary syndrome: a prospective parallel randomized double-blind placebo-controlled trial. *J Clin Endocrinol Metab* 2004; 89: 4801–4809.

45. Fleming R, Hopkinson ZE, Wallace AM, Greer IA, Sattar N. Ovarian function and metabolic factors in women with oligomenorrhea treated with metformin in a randomized double blind placebo-controlled trial. *J Clin Endocrinol Metab* 2002; 87(2): 569–574.

46. Maciel GA, Soares Junior JM, Alves da Motta EL, Abi Haidar M, de Lima GR, Baracat EC Nonobese women with polycystic ovary syndrome respond better than obese women to treatment with metformin. *Fertil Steril* 2004; 81: 355–360.

47. Nestler JE, Jakubowicz DJ, Evans WS, Pasquali R. Effects of metformin on spontaneous and clomiphene-induced ovulation in the polycystic ovary syndrome. *N Engl J Med* 1998; 338: 1876–1880.

48. Kjøtrød SB, von Düring V, Carlsen SM. Metformin treatment before IVF/ICSI in women with polycystic ovary syndrome; a prospective, randomized, double blind study, *Hum Reprod* 2004; 19: 1315–1322.

49. Tang T, Barth JH, Balen AH. The use of metformin for women with PCOS undergoing IVF treatment. *Hum Reprod* 2005; 20: i7, O-021.

50. Glueck CJ, Goldenberg N, Wang P, Loftspring M, Sherman A. Metformin during pregnancy reduces insulin, insulin resistance, insulin secretion, weight, testosterone and development of gestational diabetes: prospective longitudinal assessment of women with polycystic ovary syndrome from preconception throughout pregnancy. *Hum Reprod* 2004; 19(3): 510–521.

51. Vanky E, Salvesen KA, Heimstad R, Fougner KJ, Romundstad P, Carlsen SM. Metformin reduces pregnancy complications without affecting androgen levels in pregnant polycystic ovary syndrome women: results of a randomized study. *Hum Reprod* 2004; 19(8): 1734–1740.

52. Harborne LR, Sattar N, Norman JE, Fleming R. Metformin and weight loss in obese women with polycystic ovary syndrome: comparison of doses. *J Clin Endocrinol Metab* 2005; 90: 4593–4598.

53. Orio F Jr, Palomba S, Cascella T, et al. Improvement in endothelial structure and function after metformin treatment in young normal-weight women with polycystic ovary syndrome: results of a 6-month study. *J Clin Endocrinol Metab* 2005; 90: 6072–6076.

54. Glueck CJ, Papanna R, Wang P, Goldenberg N, Sieve-Smith L. Incidence and treatment of metabolic syndrome in newly referred women with confirmed polycystic ovarian syndrome. *Metabolism* 2003; 52(7): 908–915.

55. Muth S, Norman J, Sattar N, Fleming R. Women with polycystic ovary syndrome (PCOS) often undergo protracted treatment with metformin and are disinclined to stop: indications for a change in licensing arrangements? *Hum Reprod* 2004; 19: 2718–2720.

29

Do Insulin Sensitizing Drugs Increase Ovulation Rates in Women with PCOS?

Galia Biran, Amir Ravhon, David Levran, Ariel Weissman

Summary

Insulin resistance with resultant hyperinsulinemia is a prominent feature of PCOS, and it is seen in both, obese and lean PCOS patients. Hyperinsulinemia contributes to anovulation and infertility in women with PCOS. At present, insulin resistance is not a diagnostic criterion and there is little evidence to support its formal assessment outside the context of a research set-up. Metformin, the most frequently studied insulin sensitizing agent in PCOS, appears to be most promising as a short-term measure to improve ovulatory function (with or without ovulation-inducing agents) in PCOS patients seeking fertility.

Introduction

Since the first description of the polycystic ovary syndrome (PCOS) by Stein and Leventhal, the diagnostic criteria of this syndrome have been under constant debate. Recently, the PCOS Consensus Workshop Group held in Rotterdam in 2003, determined the necessity for two of three characteristics to define the syndrome:

1. oligo- and/or anovulation
2. clinical and/or biochemical signs of hyperandrogenism
3. demonstration of polycystic ovaries by ultrasound.[1]

As implied by the broad definition criteria, the clinical implications of PCOS are diverse. Insulin resistance is a common endocrine feature of PCOS although it has not yet been included as a diagnostic criterion. The prevalence of insulin resistance among PCOS patients differs according to the diagnostic modality used to define insulin resistance and it is more common among obese than lean PCOS patients.[2] Since the hyperinsulinemia that accompanies insulin resistance has a pathophysiological role in hyperandrogenism and anovulation that characterize PCOS, insulin-sensitizing drugs, as a treatment modality for PCOS- associated infertility, have been extensively studied since the mid-90's. Of the available insulin sensitizing drugs, metformin is the most comprehensively studied agent in this context, and is therefore, discussed in this chapter. Troglitazone was withdrawn from the market in March 2000 due to liver toxicity. Rosiglitazone and pioglitazone are classified as "class C" drugs by the FDA due to evidence of teratogenicity in animals, and are thus, not recommended for the treatment of infertile patients.[3,4] Another insulin-sensitizing agent, *D*-chiro-inositol that mediates insulin action, has been only briefly studied and is therefore, not reviewed in this chapter.[5]

Metformin, a biguanide, lowers glucose levels without increasing insulin secretion, or causing hypoglycemia.[6] The precise mechanism of action of metformin is controversial, but recent studies support the fact that metformin decreases hepatic glucose production, and that this mechanism is the primary route through which metformin exerts its anti-hyperglycemic effect. Metformin may also be propitious in improving insulin sensitivity at the post-receptor level and decreasing intestinal glucose absorption.[7,8] Contraindications for metformin treatment are: disturbed renal or liver function, congestive heart failure, acute or chronic metabolic acidosis, alcoholism and dehydration. It is recommended that kidney and liver function tests should be performed before initiation of metformin treatment.[9,10] Adverse effects include gastrointestinal complaints, such as nausea, diarrhea and or abdominal cramping, which occur in up to 50% of treated patients. These symptoms usually subside with continued treatment. Ten to 30% of patients on long-term metformin therapy may develop mild vitamin B12 deficiency due to malabsorption. The most serious adverse effect is lactic acidosis, that has been reported to occur only in 1 per 30000 patient-years of use.[7,11]

Metformin has been approved for the treatment of non-insulin-dependent diabetes mellitus, but has not yet been licensed for treatment of PCOS-related infertility or other PCOS indications.[12] Metformin is a "category B" drug for pregnant women.

It is not yet apparent which PCOS patients will benefit the most from metformin treatment. In the light of current inaccuracies and lack of firm diagnostic criteria for insulin resistance, some physicians recommend metformin as the first line of treatment for all PCOS patients.[13] This chapter will delineate the different aspects of metformin treatment to PCOS patients who wish to conceive.

Clinical Discussion

Metformin alone

Costello and Eden[14] analyzed the results of several uncontrolled studies and found that metformin restored regular menses in approximately 62% and ovulation in 61% of PCOS women with oligomenorrhea or amenorrhea. In controlled trials, these authors reported ovulation rates of 56% and 35% for metformin and placebo, respectively. Carmina and Lobo[2] observed that in patients randomly allocated to metformin or placebo for 3 months, the menstruation/ovulation rates were 67%/58% and 25%/17%, respectively. Nestler et al.[15] reported that 34% of obese PCOS patients achieved ovulation after a month of metformin treatment compared to 4% in the placebo group. Glueck et al.[16] described resumption of menses in 91% of the PCOS women after 6 months of metformin treatment.[16] Morin-Papunen et al.[17] found an improvement in the menstrual cycle pattern in 68.8% of PCOS patients following metformin treatment for 4 to 6 months. Valazquez et al.[18] reported that 95.7% of 22 PCOS patients treated with metformin for 6 months achieved regular menstrual cycles that proved to be related to ovulation in 86.7% of cases. In a randomized double-blind placebo controlled trial, Moghetti et al.[19] detected improvement not only in menstrual cyclicity, but also in metabolic parameters after metformin treatment.

Women with PCOS, who desire to conceive, have traditionally been treated with clomiphene citrate (CC) as a first-line medical therapy for induction of ovulation. Problems with CC include low pregnancy rates relative to the ovulation rates, a slight risk of ovarian hyperstimulation syndrome (OHSS) and a 5% to 10% risk of multiple pregnancies.

Metformin administration to PCOS patients may achieve the main goal for treatment of anovulatory infertility: induction of mono-ovulatory cycles in order to avoid multiple pregnancies.[14] It may also be useful in restoring normal endocrinological and clinical parameters of PCOS.

Improvement in menstrual cyclicity and ovulation rates appears to be independent of the mild weight reduction occasionally observed with metformin treatment.[20] Although obesity, which is prevalent in at least 60% of PCOS patients, aggravates the PCOS-related hyperinsulinemia, insulin resistance and hyperinsulinemia are also present in lean PCOS patients. Lean PCOS patients respond favorably to metformin treatment. Moreover, Kumari et al.[21] compared the response of 17 lean and 17 obese PCOS patients and found that 41% of the obese and 100% of the lean subjects resumed menstrual cycles after 3 months of metformin treatment. Ovulation and pregnancy rates were also higher in the lean group.

As most studies on this issue have been performed on small populations, it is difficult to draw conclusions regarding the fecundity rate in PCOS patients treated with metformin alone. In a Cochrane review published in 2003,[4] Lord et al.[4] found that metformin is effective in achieving ovulation in women with PCOS, with an odds ratio of 3.88 (95% confidence interval 2.25 to 6.69, p < 0.0001) for metformin compared with placebo (Figure 29.1). The clinical pregnancy rate reported by trials comparing metformin with placebo did not show evidence of benefit (odds ratio 2.76, 95% confidence interval 0.85 to 8.98, P = 0.09). The duration of metformin treatment required before adding another ovulation induction drug to the treatment protocol has still not been well established.[4,22]

Metformin and clomiphene citrate (CC)

Lord et al.[4] reported an odds ratio of 4.41 (95% confidence interval 2.37 to 8.22, p < 0.0001) for achieving ovulation in the metformin combined with clomiphene in comparison to clomiphene group alone (Figure 29.2). Significantly higher clinical pregnancy rates were achieved with CC and metformin compared with CC alone (odds ratio 4.40, 95% confidence interval 1.96 to 9.85, P = 0.0003). These Cochrane reviewers concluded that the combination of metformin and CC regimen is significantly more beneficial than CC alone.[4]

The combination of metformin and CC may be administered in three modes: the first involves initiation of metformin treatment and if ovulation and/or pregnancy are not achieved, CC should be added. Nestler et al.[15] reported that 90% of 20 patients who received combined metformin and CC ovulated (after failure to ovulate with metformin alone) compared to 8% of 25 patients on combined placebo and CC therapy. A significant proportion of women with PCOS fail to ovulate on standard dosages of CC and are thus, termed "CC resistant". The second method of combined therapy entails initiation of CC with the addition of metformin to CC-resistant patients. The supplementation of metformin to CC resulted in ovulation rates of 75%, compared to 27% in the placebo and CC group.[23] This higher rate of ovulation was also associated with a higher

Comparison: Metformin versus placebo or no treatment (clinical outcomes)
Outcome: Ovulation rate

Study	Treatment n/N	Control n/N	Peto odds ratio (95% fixed)	Weight %	Peto odds ratio (95% CI fixed)
Fleming 2002	37/45	30/47		35.4	2.51 (1.01 to 6.25)
Jakubowicz 2001	8/28	0/28		13.4	9.89 (2.24 to 43.61)
Nestler 1996	5/11	1/13		9.0	6.89 (1.12 to 42.33)
Nestler 1996	12/35	1/26		19.6	5.96 (1.74 to 20.38)
Ng 2001	3/9	3/9		8.1	1.00 (0.15 to 6.72)
Vandermoten 2001	1/12	1/15		3.7	1.26 (0.07 to 21.72)
Yarali 2002	6/16	1/16		10.9	5.88 (1.13 to 30.61)
Total (95% CI)	72/156	37/154		100.0	3.88 (2.25 to 6.69)

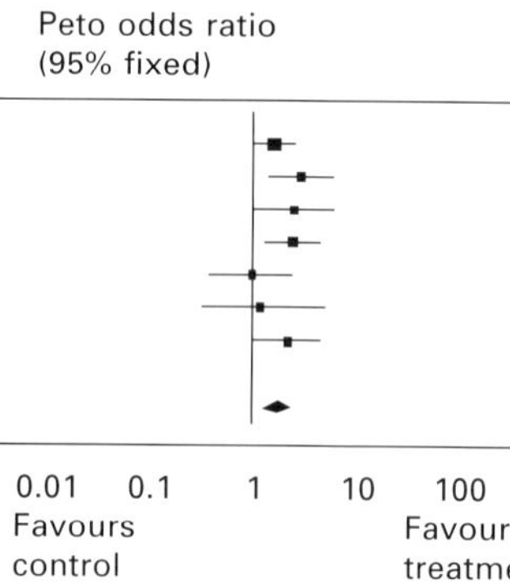

Test for heterogeneity: x^2 = 6.05, df = 6, P = 0.42
Test for overall effect: z = 4.89, P < 0.00001

0.01   0.1   1   10   100
Favours control   Favours treatment

Figure 29.1   Metformin compared with placebo or no treatment: ovulation rate.
[Adopted from Lord JM, Flight IH, Norman RJ. Insulin-sensitising drugs (metformin, troglitazone, rosiglitazone, pioglitazone, D-chiro-inositol) for polycystic ovary syndrome. Cochrane Database Syst Rev 2003; CD003053].

pregnancy rate in the metformin and CC groups. Analogous to this finding, Batukan and Baysal.[24] reported a 58% ovulation rate with metformin and CC, compared to 28% in the CC alone group in CC-resistant patients. Not only did ovulation rates increase with the metformin and CC regimen compared to CC and placebo, but pregnancy rates were also reported to be higher in the CC-resistant patients.[25]

As many infertile couples seek a rapid resolution to their problems, some physicians choose a third approach that comprises combined CC and metformin together as the first line of treatment. In a meta-analysis published in 2004, Kashyap et al.[8] found that metformin and CC

may be superior to CC alone or combined with placebo with regard to ovulation (relative risk 3.04, 95% confidence interval 1.77 to 5.24) and pregnancy (relative risk 3.65, 95% confidence interval 1.11 to 11.9).

Metformin and ovulation induction with gonadotropins

Only a few studies have addressed the use of metformin in patients with PCOS undergoing ovulation induction with follicle stimulating hormone (FSH) or human menopausal gonadotropin (hMG). De Leo et al.[26] compared 19 cycles of ovulation induction with FSH alone

Comparison: Metformin combined with ovulation induction agent versus ovulation induction agent alone (clinical outcomes)
Outcome: Ovulation rate

Study	Treatment n/N	Control n/N	Peto odds ratio (95% CI fixed)	Weight %	Peto odds ratio (95% CI fixed)
Polycystic ovary syndrome and clomifene senstive					
Subtotal (95% CI)	0/0	0/0		0.0	Not estimable
Test for heterogeneity: x^2 = 0.0, df = 0					
Test for overall effect: z = 0.0 P = 1					
Polycystic ovary syndrome and clomitene resistant					
Kocak 2002	21/27	4/28		35.0	12.36 (4.32 to 35.39)
Malkawi 2002	11/16	3/12		17.9	5.41 (1.24 to 23.51)
Subtotal (95% CI)	32/43	7/40		52.9	9.34 (3.97 to 21.97)
Test to heterogeneity: x^2 = 0.80, df = 1 p = 0.37					
Test for overall effect: z = 5.12 P < 0.00001					
Polycystic ovary syndrome and clomifene sensitivity not defined					
El-Biely 2001	35/45	29/45		47.1	1.90 (0.77 to 4.70)
Subtotal (95% CI)	35/45	29/45		47.1	1.90 (0.77 to 4.70)
Test for heterogeneity: x^2 = 0.0, df = 0					
Test for overall effect: z = 1.39 P = 17					
Total (95% CI)	67/88	36/85		100.0	4.41 (2.37 to 8.22)
Test for heterogeneity: x^2 = 7.07, df = 2 P = 0.029					
Test for overall effect: z = 4.68 P < 0.00001					

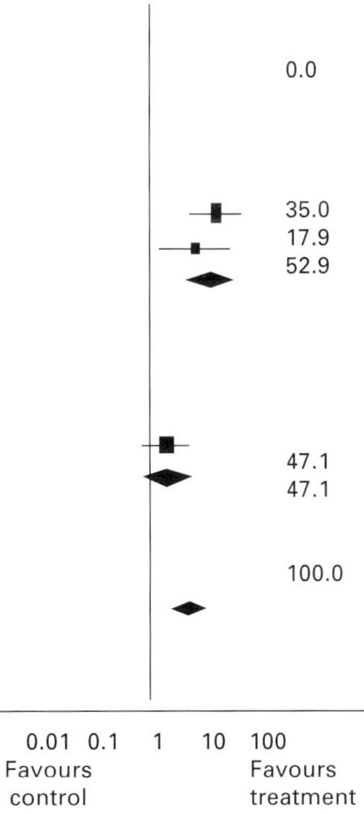

0.01 0.1 1 10 100
Favours control   Favours treatment

Figure 29.2 Metformin combined with clomiphene compared with clomiphene alone: ovulation rate.
[Adopted from Lord JM, Flight IH, Norman RJ. Insulin-sensitising drugs (metformin, troglitazone, rosiglitazone, pioglitazone, D-chiro-inositol) for polycystic ovary syndrome. Cochrane Database Syst Rev 2003; CD003053]

to 18 cycles with a combination of FSH and metformin, and found that the number of follicles >15 mm diameter on the day of human chorionic gonadotropin (hCG) administration was lower in the latter group as were the number of canceled cycles, and plasma estradiol (E2) levels. Yarali et al.[27] reported higher pregnancy rates (with comparable ovulation rates): 31.3% for patients treated with low dose gonadotropins and metformin, compared to 6.3% in the group that received gonadotropins and placebo. This difference was not statistically significant due to the small patient population involved. Palomba et al.[28] randomized PCOS patients receiving gonadotropins for ovulation induction to co-administration with metformin or placebo. No significant difference was found in cancellation rates. The number of dominant follicles and peak E2 levels were significantly lower in the metformin group. No difference in pregnancy rates was observed between the groups.

Metformin and IVF

The information available on inclusion of metformin in controlled ovarian hyperstimulation (COH) prior to in vitro fertilization (IVF) is rather limited. A study by Stadtmauer et al.[29] evaluated metformin treatment during IVF cycles in CC-resistant PCOS patients. They retrospectively compared 30 IVF cycles with metformin to 30 IVF cycles without metformin using the same dose of gonadotropins in both the groups. The total number of follicles was increased in the non-metformin treated group. Metformin significantly decreased the number of ovarian follicles < 14 mm in diameter, decreased peak E2 levels and the need for coasting. In another study by the same authors,[30] PCOS patients who experienced an exaggerated ovarian response during IVF treatment and required 'coasting' were compared to patients who received and did not receive metformin treatment. Metformin treatment significantly decreased serum peak E2 levels on day of hCG administration and increased the mean number of mature oocytes, fertilized oocytes and cleaving embryos. No significant differences were

found regarding pregnancy and severe OHSS rates.

Kjotrod et al.[31] compared a group of PCOS patients treated with metformin prior to IVF until the day of hCG administration to a group of PCOS patients undergoing IVF without metformin. No statistically significant differences were found between the groups in terms of the number of retrieved oocytes, fertilization rates, mean cleavage rates and good quality embryos. Pregnancy rates were also comparable between the groups. In contrast, Tang et al.[32] have recently reported the results of a randomized placebo-controlled double-blind study in which PCOS patients undergoing IVF were randomized to metformin, or placebo treatment. No significant differences were observed between the groups regarding total dose of FSH, number of oocytes retrieved and fertilization rates. Surprisingly, despite similar clinical, endocrine and embryological characteristics, pregnancy rates per cycle (38.5% vs. 16.3%, p = 0.023) and per transfer (44.4% vs. 19.1%, p = 0.022) were significantly higher in patients treated with metformin.[32]

Conclusions

Current evidence indicates that metformin monotherapy, or in combination with CC is a safe and effective treatment for anovulation associated with PCOS. It also ameliorates the metabolic syndrome associated with PCOS. More data is however, needed in order to clarify the role of metformin in combination with gonadotropin therapy or prior to IVF. Metformin is becoming the primary drug of choice for ovulation induction in PCOS.

References

1. Revised 2003 consensus on diagnostic criteria and long-term health risks related to polycystic ovary syndrome (PCOS). *Hum Reprod* 2004; 19: 41–47.
2. Carmina E, Lobo RA. Does metformin induce ovulation in normoandrogenic anovulatory women? *Am J Obstet Gynecol* 2004; 191: 1580–1584.
3. Cheang KI, Nestler JE. Should insulin-sensitizing

drugs be used in the treatment of polycystic ovary syndrome? *Reprod Biomed Online* 2004; 8: 440–447.

4. Lord JM, Flight IH, Norman RJ. Insulin-sensitising drugs (metformin, troglitazone, rosiglitazone, pioglitazone, D-chiro-inositol) for polycystic ovary syndrome. *Cochrane Database Syst Rev* 2003; CD003053.

5. Nestler JE, Jakubowicz DJ, Reamer P, Gunn RD, Allan G. Ovulatory and metabolic effects of D-chiro-inositol in the polycystic ovary syndrome. *N Engl J Med* 1999 29; 340: 1314–1320.

6. Barbieri RL. Induction of ovulation in infertile women with hyperandrogenism and insulin resistance. *Am J Obstet Gynecol* 2000 Dec; 183: 1412–1418.

7. Hundal RS, Inzucchi SE. Metformin: new understandings, new uses. *Drugs* 2003; 63: 1879–1894.

8. Kashyap S, Wells GA, Rosenwaks Z. Insulin-sensitizing agents as primary therapy for patients with polycystic ovarian syndrome. *Hum Reprod* 2004; 19: 2474–2483.

9. Harborne L, Fleming R, Lyall H, Norman J, Sattar N. Descriptive review of the evidence for the use of metformin in polycystic ovary syndrome. *Lancet* 2003 May 31; 361: 1894–1901.

10. Norman RJ, Wang JX, Hague W. Should we continue or stop insulin sensitizing drugs during pregnancy? *Curr Opin Obstet Gynecol* 2004; 16: 245–250.

11. McCarthy EA, Walker SP, McLachlan K, Boyle J, Permezel M. Metformin in obstetric and gynecologic practice: a review. *Obstet Gynecol Surv* 2004; 59: 118–127.

12. Muth S, Norman J, Sattar N, Fleming R. Women with polycystic ovary syndrome (PCOS) often undergo protracted treatment with metformin and are disinclined to stop: indications for a change in licensing arrangements? *Hum Reprod* 2004; 19: 2718–2720.

13. Goldenberg N, Glueck CJ, Loftspring M, Sherman A, Wang P. Metformin-diet benefits in women with polycystic ovary syndrome in the bottom and top quintiles for insulin resistance. *Metabolism* 2005; 54: 113–121.

14. Costello MF, Eden JA. A systematic review of the reproductive system effects of metformin in patients with polycystic ovary syndrome. *Fertil Steril* 2003; 79: 1–13.

15. Nestler JE, Jakubowicz DJ, Evans WS, Pasquali R. Effects of metformin on spontaneous and clomiphene-induced ovulation in the polycystic ovary syndrome. *N Engl J Med* 1998 25; 338: 1876–1880.

16. Glueck CJ, Wang P, Fontaine R, Tracy T, Sieve-Smith L. Metformin-induced resumption of normal menses in 39 of 43 (91%) previously amenorrheic women with the polycystic ovary syndrome. *Metabolism* 1999; 48: 511–519.

17. Morin-Papunen LC, Koivunen RM, Ruokonen A, Martikainen HK. Metformin therapy improves the menstrual pattern with minimal endocrine and metabolic effects in women with polycystic ovary syndrome. *Fertil Steril* 1998; 69: 691–696.

18. Velazquez E, Acosta A, Mendoza SG. Menstrual cyclicity after metformin therapy in polycystic ovary syndrome. *Obstet Gynecol* 1997; 90: 392–395.

19. Moghetti P, Castello R, Negri C, Tosi F, Perrone F, Caputo M, et al. Metformin effects on clinical features, endocrine and metabolic profiles, and insulin sensitivity in polycystic ovary syndrome: a randomized, double-blind, placebo-controlled 6-month trial, followed by open, long-term clinical evaluation. *J Clin Endocrinol Metab* 2000; 85: 139–146.

20. Homburg R. Should patients with polycystic ovarian syndrome be treated with metformin? A note of cautious optimism. *Hum Reprod* 2002; 17: 853–856.

21. Kumari AS, Haq A, Jayasundaram R, Abdel-Wareth LO, Al Haija SA, Alvares M. Metformin monotherapy in lean women with polycystic ovary syndrome. *Reprod Biomed Online* 2005; 10: 100–104.

22. Lord JM, Flight IH, Norman RJ. Metformin in polycystic ovary syndrome: systematic review and meta-analysis. *BMJ*, 2003 25; 327: 951–953.

23. Vandermolen DT, Ratts VS, Evans WS, Stovall DW, Kauma SW, Nestler JE. Metformin increases the ovulatory rate and pregnancy rate from clomiphene citrate in patients with polycystic ovary syndrome who are resistant to clomiphene citrate alone. *Fertil Steril* 2001; 75: 310–315.

24. Batukan C, Baysal B. Metformin improves ovulation and pregnancy rates in patients with polycystic ovary syndrome. *Arch Gynecol Obstet* 2001; 265: 124–127.

25. Kocak M, Caliskan E, Simsir C, Haberal A. Metformin therapy improves ovulatory rates, cervical scores, and pregnancy rates in clomiphene citrate-resistant women with polycystic ovary syndrome. *Fertil Steril* 2002; 77: 101–106.

26. De Leo V, la Marca A, Ditto A, Morgante G, Cianci A. Effects of metformin on gonadotropin-induced ovulation in women with polycystic ovary syndrome. *Fertil Steril* 1999; 72: 282–285.

27. Yarali H, Yildiz BO, Demirol A, Zeyneloglu HB, Yigit N, Bukulmez O, et al. Co-administration of metformin during rFSH treatment in patients with clomiphene citrate-resistant polycystic ovarian syndrome: a prospective randomized trial. *Hum Reprod* 2002; 17: 289–294.

28. Palomba S, Falbo A, Orio F, Jr., Manguso F, Russo T, Tolino A, et al. A randomized controlled trial evaluating metformin pre-treatment and co-administration in non-obese insulin-resistant women with polycystic ovary syndrome treated with controlled ovarian stimulation plus timed intercourse or intrauterine insemination. *Hum Reprod* 2005; 20: 2879–2886.

29. Stadtmauer LA, Toma SK, Riehl RM, Talbert LM. Metformin treatment of patients with polycystic ovary syndrome undergoing in vitro fertilization improves outcomes and is associated with modulation of the insulin-like growth factors. *Fertil Steril* 2001; 75: 505–509.

30. Stadtmauer LA, Toma SK, Riehl RM, Talbert LM. Impact of metformin therapy on ovarian stimulation and outcome in 'coasted' patients with polycystic ovary syndrome undergoing in-vitro fertilization. *Reprod Biomed Online* 2002; 5: 112–116.

31. Kjotrod SB, von During V, Carlsen SM. Metformin treatment before IVF/ICSI in women with polycystic ovary syndrome; a prospective, randomized, double blind study. *Hum Reprod* 2004; 19: 1315–1322.

32. Tang T, Barth BJ, Balen AH. The use of metformin for women with PCOS undergoing IVF treatment. Abstract O-021. Presented at the 21st Annual ESHRE Meeting, Copenhagen, Denmark, June 19–22, 2005. *Hum Reprod* 2005; 20 (Suppl. 1): i7–i8.

30

Insulin-Sensitizing Drugs in the Treatment of Women with PCOS – The Promise of Metformin

Samuel Hernandez Ayup, Pedro Galache Vega, Roberto Santos Halliscak, Maria Lidia Arenas Montezco, Victor Alfonso Batiza Resendiz, Jose Sepulveda Gonzalez, Pablo Diaz Spindola

Summary

Polycystic Ovary Syndrome (PCOS) is characterized by anovulation, infertility and hyperandrogenism with clinical manifestations of irregular menstrual cycles, hirsutism, and acne. This condition affects about 4 to 10% of women of reproductive age. One of the commonest presenting complaints of women with PCOS is anovulatory infertility. Hyperinsulinemic insulin resistance is commonly associated with hyperandrogenemia and menstrual dysfunction. The recognition of insulin resistance as a principal factor in the pathogenesis of PCOS, has led the use of insulin-lowering agents, also called "insulin/sensitizing drugs" for its treatment to produce regular ovulation and menstruation. The most extensively studied insulin-lowering agent in the treatment of PCOS is metformin, an oral antihyperglycemic agent used initially in the treatment of type 2 diabetes mellitus. Metformin theoretically decreases hepatic gluconeogenesis and reduces the androgen level. It has been effective in the treatment of PCOS-related anovulation and infertility, as well as in decreasing the risk of early spontaneous miscarriage, and decreasing the risk of development of type 2 diabetes. The most important and promising therapeutic profile of metformin is related to the role of this agent in controlling an important etiologic factor in the pathogenesis of PCOS-hyperinsulinemia.

Introduction

Polycystic Ovary Syndrome (PCOS) is one of the most common endocrinopathies affecting 4 to 10% of women of reproductive age.[1,2] Stein and Leventhal initially observed the association between amenorrhea, hirsutism, infertility and polycystic ovaries in the first half of the 20th century.[3] Since then, a broad range of clinical and laboratory findings have been associated with PCOS. The findings include elevated serum luteinizing hormone (LH), elevated LH/FSH ratio, elevated serum testosterone and/or dehydroepiandrostenedione sulphate (DHEAS), and more recently recognized findings, hyperinsulinemia and hyperlipidemia[4].

Since PCOS was identified, amenorrhea, infertility and hirsutism appeared as signs and symptoms related to this syndrome. In 2003, The Rotterdam ESHRE/ASRM diagnostic criteria for the diagnosis of PCOS included any of the following two features: oligo/anovulation, clinical and biochemical signs of hyperandrogenism, ultrasound evidence of polycystic ovaries, following the exclusion of other pathologies such as congenital adrenal hyperplasia, androgen producing tumors or Cushing's syndrome. PCOS is one of the most common endocrine disorders, accounting for 75% of anovulatory infertility.[5]

PCOS and insulin resistance

Women with PCOS are known to exhibit insulin resistance with compensatory hyperinsulinemia.[6] The insulin resistance associated with PCOS exists in obese and non-obese patients; PCOS patients also have higher insulin levels than weight-matched controls.[7] The mechanism appears to be related to excessive serine phosphorylation of the insulin receptor, causing a low response after insulin binds its receptor and producing an increment in plasma insulin levels.[8] In addition to this, it is proposed that a single defect can produce both insulin resistance and hyperandrogenism in some PCOS patients.[9] Evidence strongly suggests that a defect in insulin-like growth factor-1 (IGF-I) action in PCOS patients augments not only ovarian and adrenal steroidogenesis, but also pituitary LH release.[10]

Clinical Discussion

Metformin and PCOS

The recognition of insulin resistance as a principal factor in the pathogenesis of PCOS has led to the use of insulin-lowering agents, also called "insulin-sensitizing drugs" for its treatment. The most extensively studied insulin-lowering agent in the treatment of PCOS is metformin. Metformin is an oral antihyperglycemic agent that was used initially in the treatment of type 2 diabetes mellitus. Metformin therapy improves insulin sensitivity, as shown by a reduction in fasting plasma glucose and insulin concentration. Its beneficial effects on glycemic control in diabetic patients are primarily the result of inhibition of hepatic glycogenolysis, leading to a decreased hepatic glucose output and, to a lesser extent, increased peripheral glucose uptake. Several other actions, such as increased intestinal use of glucose

and decreased fatty acid oxidation, may contribute to the action of metformin. Unlike sulfonylureas and insulin, metformin use does not result in increased serum insulin levels. It also decreases ovarian androgen production.[11]

One of the problems that patients with PCOS exhibit is, infertility due to anovulation. Clomiphene citrate is the primary agent used for ovulation induction in infertile patients with PCOS. Clomiphene citrate induces ovulation in ~80% of the patients but achieves pregnancy in only 35% of these patients.[12] Previous studies involving larger numbers of women have shown an approximate 30% ovulation rate in PCOS subjects treated with either troglitazone or metformin. One of the fist references to the use of metformin as a treatment for PCOS was made in 1994 by Velazquez and co-workers.[13] In this study, 26 obese women with PCOS were treated with 1500 mg of metformin daily for 8 weeks. Metformin improved insulin sensitivity, lowered serum LH, total and free testosterone concentrations by 50% and caused an elevation in serum follicle stimulating hormone (FSH) and sex hormone-binding globulin (SHBG). Moreover, three spontaneous pregnancies occurred, and menstrual cycles were normalized in another 7 women who continued the treatment.[13]

These initial observations were followed by several studies investigating the effect of metformin on women with PCOS. While most of the studies suffered from low power and lacked control groups, they showed improvements in ovulation and/or a reduction in androgens following metformin treatment in obese women with PCOS.

Ovulation induction with metformin and clomiphene citrate

Not all patients ovulate with just the use of an insulin-sensitizing drug and/or weight loss; hence, drugs for ovulation induction are used to treat them. The first drug administered usually was clomiphene citrate. An enhanced rate of ovulation was observed after treatment with a combination of metformin and clomiphene citrate compared with metformin alone in women with this disorder.[14]

However, there are clomiphene citrate-resistant patients who will not respond to CC. Based on the theory that insulin resistance and hyper-insulinemia impede ovulation, it is reasonable to propose the use of an insulin-sensitizing drug, such as metformin in combination with exogenous gonadotropins such as human menopausal gonadotropin (hMG) or recombinant follicle stimulating hormone (r-FSH), to increase ovulation and pregnancy rates in clomiphene citrate-resistant patients.[15]

Ovulation induction with metformin and gonadotropins

Ovulation induction (OI) is indicated in patients with infertility due to anovulation, which maybe a unique or combined problem in 30 to 40% of the infertile couples. Anovulatory patients who belong to group I of the WHO (World Health Organization), (including patients with hypogonadotropic hypogonadism) or the anovulatory group II of the WHO, in which the majority of the women have PCOS, may be candidates for the clinical applications of OI.[16]

Since knowledge of the mechanisms of the human reproduction, from follicular development and its hormonal regulation has improved, better schemes of OI have emerged. Today, there exists a diversity of drugs used for OI, presenting several choices for the treatment for these patients.[17]

As we know, the ovaries of PCOS patients show a slow response to treatment using ovulation inducing drugs. This impaired response could be due to the unfavorable endocrine environment to which ovarian follicles are exposed.[18] Insulin resistance, a frequent feature of women with PCOS, produces compensatory hyperinsulinemia, which contributes to this unfavorable environment (ovarian hyperandrogenism), and plays an important role in the pathogenesis of PCOS.[19] Hyperinsulinemia produces hyperandrogenism by favoring androgen production by the ovarian theca cells, increasing 17β-estradiol conversion (granulosa cells), and reducing serum sex hormone binding globulin (SHBG) levels, thus increasing the circulating active androgen levels (free testosterone).[20]

There is evidence that metformin improves the follicular environment, reducing the levels of ovarian androgens by improving hyperinsulinemia.[21] Once PCOS patients do respond to stimulation drugs, they tend to develop multiple follicles and ovarian hyperstimulation syndrome (OHSS).

However, De Leo et al.[22] in a randomized prospective trial, evaluated 20 patients to find out whether pre-treatment with metformin improves FSH-induced ovulation in women with clomiphene-resistant polycystic ovary syndrome (PCOS). The women were divided randomly into groups A and B (10 subjects each). Group A underwent two cycles of FSH stimulation and then received metformin for a month before undergoing a third cycle. Group B received 1,500 mg of metformin for at least a month before a single cycle of FSH stimulation. There was no difference between the groups in the age, time of infertility, body mass index (BMI) hormonal profile data. The number of follicles > 15 mm in diameter on the day of human chorionic gonadotropin (hCG) administration was significantly lower in cycles performed after metformin treatment (2.5 ± 0.7 vs. 4.5 ± 1; $p < 0.001$). Plasma levels of estradiol were significantly lower in FSH + metformin treated cycles (450 ± 130 pg/ml vs. 720 ± 150 pg/ml; $p < 0.001$) compared to those treated with FSH alone. The cycles cancelled due to excessive follicular growth were higher in the FSH alone group (6/19 vs. 0/18; $p > 0.03$). There were no differences in the pregnancy rate (2 pregnancies in each group). The authors concluded that by reducing hyperinsulinism, metformin determines a reduction in intraovarian androgens. This leads to a reduction in E2 levels and favors orderly follicular growth in response to exogenous gonadotropins.

Another proposed mechanism by which metformin improves hyperinsulinemia, is by reducing the activity of the ovarian cytochrome P450c-17α hydroxylase, an enzyme regulated by insulin in PCOS patients. This enzyme, found in small amounts in granulosa cells, plays an important role in androgen synthesis, providing the substrate for aromatization and leading homogeneous development of follicles and atresia of the small follicles.[23] Palomba et al.[24] performed a prospective, randomized study to assess the effect of pre-treatment and co-administration of metformin in infertile PCOS women treated with highly purified urinary FSH (hpFSH). Seventy insulin-resistant primary infertile women with PCOS were randomized to receive metformin cloridrate (850 mg twice daily; group A) or placebo tablets (two tablets daily; group B) for 3 months. Three trials of controlled ovarian stimulation (COS) using highly purified urinary FSH (hpFSH) were performed, followed by timed intercourse (TI) or intrauterine insemination (IUI). No difference between the groups was detected in ovulation, cycle cancellation, pregnancy, abortion, live birth, multiple pregnancy and OHSS rates. The mono-ovulatory cycle rates were significantly (P = 0.002) more frequent in group A (metformin + hpFSH) than in group B (placebo+hpFSH), whereas the days of stimulation for non-cancelled cycles and the number of vials of gonadotropins used were significantly (P < 0.001) higher in group A than in group B. The authors concluded that the pre-treatment and co-administration of metformin in non-obese insulin-resistant PCOS patients induces a more physiological growth of follicles and a reduced risk of high order multiple pregnancies.[24]

Treatment with recombinant FSH (r-FSH)

It has been shown that in women with PCOS, initial suboptimal ovarian responsiveness to FSH stimulation during ovulation induction may be, in part, due to insulin resistance within the granulosa cell,[25] but there is also evidence that women with PCOS exhibited dose-dependent granulosa cell hyper-responsiveness to FSH, the duration of which is transitory.[26] These *in vivo* results are essentially identical with other *in vitro* findings.[27]

Because of this hyper-responsiveness, patients diagnosed as clomiphene citrate-resistant PCOS and with a normal glucose tolerance test and infertility, were treated with metformin and r-FSH in a low-dose step-up protocol. It is easy to understand this protocol option in these patients because it yields a high rate of monofollicular growth and ovulation,[28,29] avoiding the great concern of severe ovarian hyperstimulation syndrome and high-order multiple pregnancies and yields a high rate of monofollicular growth and ovulation.

In the prospective, randomized, double blind, placebo-controlled study of Yarali et al.[28] the authors found a marked and significant increase in spontaneous ovulation rate to 38%, despite a lack of improvement in insulin resistance with metformin, suggesting that the mode of action of metformin to restore spontaneous ovulation may not be mediated directly through an improvement in insulin resistance. Rather, metformin may act directly within the ovary by modulating the sensitivity of ovarian follicles to circulating insulin, perhaps by augmenting the post-receptor mechanism of action of insulin within the follicular apparatus.[30]

However, there was no significant statistical difference in ovulation rates during treatment with exogenous gonadotropins between control and treated groups (75% and 94%, respectively), or in the pregnancy rates for the same groups (6.3% and 31.3% respectively; p > 0.05).

Metformin treatment, for a month prior to ovulation induction with FSH, results in a lowering of the number of ovarian follicles >15 mm on the day of hCG administration and a lowering in the plasma estradiol.[22] These findings indicated that metformin reduces the risk of ovarian hyperstimulation syndrome in these patients.

In PCOS, the mechanism responsible for follicular arrest, which suggests inadequate FSH stimulation and/or a relative unresponsiveness of granulosa cells, remains unknown, although ovarian response to gonadotropin therapy has resulted in ovulation. Our previous *in vitro* studies have demonstrated that granulosa cells from women with PCOS exhibit greater estradiol (E_2) release after FSH stimulation compared with that observed in normal granulosa cells, which indicates that the inherent capacity of these cells to respond to FSH is retained. However, the time course of response was characterized by an inability to sustain peak levels in contrast to that of normal cells, which implied suboptimal granulosa cell function.[31]

Other studies, employing larger numbers of subjects, have shown that PCOS granulosa cells were extremely sensitive to insulin, whether in the presence or absence of gonadotropin stimulation.[32] These apparent contradictory *in vitro* experiments have been attributed to differences in the population of granulosa cells studied.

That insulin resistance in this disorder may be linked to anovulation is suggested by the resumption of ovulation in individuals who have sustained a reduction in hyperinsulinemia by treatment with insulin-lowering drugs or dietary weight loss.[33]

During both, low and high-dose insulin infusions, E_2 responses to r-hFSH were unaltered compared with that observed in the absence of insulin.[34] Granulosa cell responsiveness to exogenous FSH was enhanced by insulin after improved insulin sensitivity induced by pioglitazone. These findings are consistent with the possibility that PCOS granulosa cells are insulin resistant. Insulin resistance in the granulosa cell may be, at least in part, responsible for decreased E_2 responsiveness to FSH. In PCOS women, reduced follicle responsiveness may be overcome with progressive increases in the dose or duration of FSH.

In contrast, inhibition of aromatase activity by troglitazone was demonstrated in luteinized granulosa cells obtained from women undergoing *in vitro* fertilization. Troglitazone (Tro) directly inhibits aromatase activity in human granulosa cells, probably via the nuclear receptor system peroxisome proliferator activated receptor-gamma (PPAR-γ) RXR heterodimer. The findings may provide a biochemical basis for the decrease in the blood concentrations of estrogens, which is observed after the in vivo administration of troglitazone.[35] An effect of insulin administration on basal E_2 secretion before r-hFSH stimulation was not found.[36]

This is in contrast with previous results obtained in PCOS women undergoing a 6-h hyperinsulinemic clamp at a comparable dose of insulin infusion. In that study, postinfusion serum E_2 levels were significantly increased compared with values measured before the clamp despite the absence of changes in circulating gonadotropin concentrations. In the current study, initiation of the insulin infusion preceded administration of r-hFSH by 2 h, which may have been insufficient time to observe a change in serum E_2 as a result of insulin action. In the recent report of the PCOS/Troglitazone Study Group involving 305 subjects, ovulation rates were significantly lower in women with obesity with markedly increased basal insulin levels, which is consistent with our findings.[37]

The failure of ovulation in our subjects may have been due to the comparatively few numbers of women treated, a relatively low dose of pioglitazone (30 mg/d), the presence of significant obesity as reflected in the mean body mass index of 40 kg/m^2 or a combination of all. In addition, the mean fasting insulin levels in our subjects were more than 3-fold greater than the control group.

Conclusions

- We conclude that in clomiphene citrate-resistant PCOS women with normal glucose tolerance: (i) metformin may markedly restore spontaneous ovulation with no improvement in insulin resistance; and (ii) metformin has no significant effect on ovarian response during the low-dose step-up protocol using rFSH.
- There is convincing evidence that metformin improves the regularity of menstrual cycles in women with PCOS. Furthermore, metformin is effective in ovulation induction, either alone or in combination with other fertility enhancing medications. However, these beneficial affects have only been demonstrated in lean and obese women with insulin resistance and at present, there is no systematic published report examining the use of metformin in women with PCOS who are not insulin resistant.
- Metformin treatment reduces hyperinsulinemia and hyperandrogenemia in PCOS patients, independently of changes in body weight. In

a large number of subjects, these changes are associated with striking, sustained improvements in menstrual abnormalities and resumption of ovulation. Lower plasma insulin, lower serum androstenedione, and less severe menstrual abnormalities are baseline predictors of the clinical response to metformin.

- Previous studies have reported conflicting data on the effect of metformin on insulin resistance and endocrine parameters in patients with PCOS. Although some studies reported an improvement in insulin resistance,[13,19,21,38–40] others failed to observe any statistically significant effect.[30,41–43]. The effect of metformin on endocrine parameters has also been variable[44]. The three studies reporting no effect of metformin on insulin resistance have not provided data on restoration of ovulation.[41–43] However, in 15 obese patients with PCOS, despite no change in fasting insulin concentration, a significant improvement in spontaneous ovulation was reported with metformin.[30]

- Some studies report that in PCOS, the role of insulin on granulosa cell function is minimal or, alternatively, the granulosa cell is resistant to the action of insulin, while others report that PCOS granulosa cells are extremely sensitive to insulin whether in the presence or absence of gonadotropin stimulation. These apparent contradictory *in vitro* experiments could be attributed to differences in the population of granulosa cells studied. Relevant human studies to assess effect of insulin on granulosa cell responsiveness to FSH in PCOS have not been performed.

- Thus, in PCOS women, resumption of ovulatory function in response to medical or dietary therapy appears to correlate with improved insulin sensitivity and reduced levels of circulating insulin, which suggests that insulin resistance and compensatory hyperinsulinemia may inhibit normal follicular function. However, the mechanism by which insulin resistance disrupts granulosa cell function remains unclear.

- Multiple follicular development, resulting in high rates of multiple pregnancy and OHSS, is the major drawback of conventional protocols. Co-administration of metformin with r-FSH in a low-dose step-up protocol is the treatment of choice in clomiphene citrate-resistant cases and yields a high rate of monofollicular growth and ovulation.[28,29]

- Administration of pioglitazone to women with PCOS is associated with increased granulosa cell responsiveness to FSH stimulation during insulin infusion compared with that observed without pioglitazone therapy.

- These findings are consistent with the possibility that PCOS granulosa cells may be insulin resistant. Reversal of insulin resistance by pioglitazone was accompanied by a uniformly robust response to r-hFSH, characterized by an E_2 increment that was more rapid, of greater magnitude, and of longer duration than that of the response observed without treatment.

- These findings underscore the synergistic relationship between insulin and FSH relative to E_2 release from the granulosa cell in PCOS, which may have clinical implications regarding ovulation induction and the risk of ovarian hyperstimulation.

We should stress that the exact molecular biological mechanism(s) of action of metformin on the ovary, if present, is not known. The mechanism by which FSH and insulin may interact within the granulosa cell has not been extensively studied. Previous histochemical analysis of human ovaries have demonstrated that insulin receptor mRNA and protein expression in granulosa cells of PCOS follicles was similar to that found in antral follicles from normal ovaries.

There are few well-designed studies to evaluate the effect of metformin on ovarian response when co-administered with exogenous gonadotropins, specifically r-FSH, using the low-dose step-up protocol.

While the scientific value of many of these studies is questionable and solid evidence of the efficiency and safety is not complete, the honorable intent of lowering high insulin levels in this way, prompts the bottom line of this debate, to strike a note of cautious optimism that insulin-sensitizing agents will be of some clinical usefulness both, in the short-term, aiding infertility treatment and, possibly, in the prevention of the long-term sequelae for this troublesome and very prevalent condition. Hard evidence of its ability to improve results of ovulation induction is scanty but promising. The promise afforded by the use of metformin must be followed up in larger, randomized, controlled studies to give us more complete assurance of their efficiency and safety.[45]

References

1. Asuncion M, Calvo RM, San Millan JL, Sancho J, Avila S, Escobar-Morreale HF. A prospective study of the prevalence of the polycystic ovary syndrome in unselected Caucasian women from Spain. *J Clin Endocrinol Metab* 2000; 85: 2434–2438.

2. Franks S. Polycystic ovary syndrome. *N Engl J Med* 1995; 333: 853–861.

3. Stein IF and Leventhal ML. Amenorrhea associated with bilateral polycystic ovaries. *Am J Obstet Gynecol* 1935; 29: 181–191.

4. Pirwany JR, Yates RWS, Cameron LT and Fleming R, Effects of the insulin sensitizing drug metformin on ovarian function follicular growth and ovulation rate in obese women with oligomenorrhoea. *Human Reprod* 1999; 14(12): 2963–2968.

5. Hull MGR. Epidemiology of infertility and polycystic ovarian disease: endocrinologic and demographic studies. *Gynecol Endocrinol* 1987; 1: 235–245.

6. Coffler MS, Patel K, Dahan MH, Yoo RY, Malcom PJ and Chang RJ. Enhanced granulosa cell responsiveness to follicle-stimulating hormone during insulin infusion in women with polycystic ovary syndrome treated with pioglitazone. *J Clin Endocrinol Metab* 2003; 88 (12): 5624–5631.

7. McKenna TJ. Pathogenesis and treatment of polycystic ovary syndrome. *N Engl J Med* 1988; 318: 558–562.

8. Ciampelli M and Lanzone A. Insulin and polycystic ovary syndrome: a new look at on old Subject. *Gynecol Endocr* 1998; 12: 277–292.

9. Dunaif A. Insulin resistance and the polycystic ovary syndrome: mechanism and implications for pathogenesis. *Enocr Rev* 1997; 18(6): 774–800.

10. Book CB and Dunaif A. Selective insulin resistance in the polycystic ovary syndrome. *J Clin Endocrinol Metab* 1999; 84(9): 3110–3116.

11. Seli E and Duleba A. Should patients with polycystic ovarian syndrome be treated with metformin? *Human Reprod* 2002;19(9): 2230–2236.

12. Macgregor AH, Johnson JE and Bunde CA. Further clinical experience with clomiphene citrate. *Fertil Steril* 1968; 19: 616–622.

13. Velazquez EM, Mendoza S, Hamer T and Sosa F. CJG Metformin therapy in polycystic ovary syndrome reduces hyperinsulinemia, insulin resistance, hyperandrogenemia, and systolic blood pressure, while facilitating normal menses and pregnancy. *Metabolism* 1994; 43: 647–654.

14. Raja A, Hashmi SN, Sultana N and Rashid H. Presentation of polycystic ovary syndrome and its management with clomiphene alone and in combination with metformin. *J Ayub Med Coll Abbottabad* 2005 Apr-Jun; 17(2): 50–53.

15. Kashyap S, Wells GA and Rosenwaks Z. Unsulin-sensitizing agents as primary therapy for patients with polycystic ovarian syndrome. *Human Reprod* 2004; 19(11): 2474–2483.

16. Yen- Jaffe – Barbieri. Clinical handout of physiopathology, physiology and reproductive endocrinology 4th edition. Panamerican, 2002.

17. Shoham Z and Howles CM. Female Infertility Therapy. Current practice. Jacobs Howard. *Editorial Martin Dunitz* 2001.

18. Buyalos RP and Lee CT. Polycystic ovary syndrome: pathophysiology and outcome with *in vitro* fertilization. *Fertil Steril* 1996; 65: 1–10.

19. Nestler JE, Jakubowicz WS, Evans WS and Pasquali R. Effects of metformin on spontaneous and clomiphene-induced ovulation in the polycystic ovary syndrome. *N Engl J Med* 1998; 338: 1876–1880.

20. Palomba S, Falbo A, Russo T and Zullo F. Ovulation induction in anovulatory patients with polycystic ovary syndrome. Current Drug Therapy 2006; 1: 23–29.

21. Diamanti-Kandarakis E, Kouli C and Tsianateli T. Therapeutic effects of metformin on insulin resistance and hyperandrogenism in polycystic ovary syndrome. *Eur J Endocrinol* 1998; 138: 269–274.

22. De Leo V, La Marca A, Ditto A, Morgante G and Cianci A. Effects of metformin on gonadotropin-induced ovulation in women with polycystic ovary syndrome. *Fertil Steril* 1999; 72(2): 282–285.

23. Gray SA, Mannan MA and O'Shaughnessy PJ. Development of cytochrome P450 17 alpha-hydroxylase (P450c17) mRNA and enzyme activity in neonatal ovaries of normal and hypogonadal mice. *J Mol Endocrinol* 1996; 17(1): 55–60.

24. Palomba S et al. A randomized controlled trial evaluating metformin pre-treatment and co-administration in non-obese insulin-resistant women with polycystic ovary syndrome treated with controlled ovarian stimulation plus timed intercourse or intrauterine insemination. *Hum Reprod* 2005; 20(10): 2879–2886.

25. Van Der Meer M, Hompes PG, De Boer JA, Schats R and Schoemaker J. Cohort size rather than follicle-stimulating hormone threshold level determines ovarian sensitivity in polycystic ovary syndrome, 1998; 83: 423–426.

26. Coffler MS, Patel KS, Dahan MH, Malcom PJ, Kawashima T, Deutsch R and Chang RJ. Evidence for abnormal granulosa cell responsiveness to follicle stimulating hormone in women with polycystic ovary syndrome. *J Clin Endocrinol Metab* 2003; 88: 1742–1747.

27. Erickson GF, Magoffin DA, Cragun JR and Chang RJ. The effects of insulin and insulin-like growth factor-I and -II on estradiol production by granulosa cells of polycystic ovaries. *J Clin Endocrinol Metab* 1990; 70: 894–902.

28. Yarali H, Yildiz BO, Demirol A, Zeyneloglu HB, Yigit N, Bukulmez O and Koray Z. Co-administration of metformin during rFSH treatment in patients with clomiphene citrate-resistant polycystic ovarian syndrome: a prospective randomized trial. *Hum Reprod* 2002 17(2): 289–294.

29. White DM, Polson DW, Kiddy D. et al. Induction of ovulation with low-dose gonadotropins in polycystic ovary syndrome: an analysis of 109 pregnancies in 225 women. *J Clin Endocrinol Metab* 1996; 81: 3821–3824.

30. Pirwany IR, Yates RW, Cameron IT and Fleming R. Effects of the insulin sensitizing drug metformin on ovarian function, follicular growth and ovulation rate in obese women with oligomenorrhoea. *Hum Reprod* 1999 14(12): 2963–2968.

31. Erickson GF, Magoffin DA, Cragun JR and Chang RJ. The effects of insulin and insulin-like growth factor-I and -II on estradiol production by granulosa cells of polycystic ovaries. *J Clin Endocrinol Metab* 1990; 70: 894–902.

32. Willis D, Mason H, Gilling-Smith C and Franks S. Modulation by insulin of follicle-stimulating hormone and luteinizing hormone actions in human granulosa cells of normal and polycystic ovaries. *J Clin Endocrinol Metab* 1996; 81: 302–309.

33. Butzow TL, Lehtovirta M, Siegberg R, Hovatta O, Koistinen R, Seppala M and Apter D. The decrease in luteinizing hormone secretion in response to weight reduction is inversely related to the severity of insulin resistance in overweight women. *J Clin Endocrinol Metab* 2000; 85: 3271–3275.

34. Mickey S, Coffler, Ketan Patel Michael H, Dahan Richard Y, Yoo Pamela J and Malcom R. Jeffrey Chang. Enhanced Granulosa Cell Responsiveness to Follicle-Stimulating Hormone during Insulin Infusion in Women with Polycystic Ovary Syndrome Treated with Pioglitazone. The Journal of Clinical Endocrinology & Metabolism Vol. 88, No. 12 5624–5631.

35. Mu YM, Yanase T, Nishi Y, Waseda N, Oda T, Tanaka A, et al. Insulin sensitizer, troglitazone, directly inhibits aromatase activity in human ovarian granulosa cells. *Biochem Biophys Res Commun* 2000; 271(3): 710–713.

36. Patel KS, Coffler MS, Dahan MH, Yoo RY, Malcom PJ, Chang RJ. Suppression of increased pituitary LH secretion in polycystic ovary syndrome (PCOS) by hyperinsulinemia. 2003. *Proc Soc Gyn Invest* (Abstract 250990).

37. Azziz R, Ehrmann D, Legro RS, Whitcomb RW, Hanley R, Fereshetian AG, et al. Troglitazone improves ovulation and hirsutism in the polycystic ovary syndrome: a multicenter, double-blind, placebo-controlled trial. *J Clin Endocrinol Metab* 2001; 86: 1626–1632.

38. Kolodziejczyk B, Duleba AJ and Spaczynski RZ et al. Metformin therapy decreases hyperandrogenism and hyperinsulinemia in women with polycystic ovary syndrome. *Fertil Steril* 2000; 73: 1149–1154.

39. Glueck CJ, Wang P and Fontaine R. et al. Metformin-induced resumption of normal menses in 39 of 43 (91%) previously amenorrheic women with the polycystic ovary syndrome. *Metabolism* 1999; 48: 511–519.

40. Moghetti P, Castello R and Negri C. et al. Metformin effects on clinical features, endocrine and metabolic profiles, and insulin sensitivity in polycystic ovary syndrome: a randomized, double-blind, placebo-controlled 6-month trial, followed by open, long-term clinical evaluation. *J Clin Endocrinol Metab* 2000; 85: 139–146.

41. Crave JC, Fimbel S and Lejeune H. et al. Effects of diet and metformin administration on sex hormone-binding globulin, androgens, and insulin in hirsute and obese women. *J Clin Endocrinol Metab* 1995; 80: 2057–2062.

42. Ehrmann DA, Cavaghan MK and Imperial J. et al. Effects of metformin on insulin secretion, insulin action, and ovarian steroidogenesis in women with

polycystic ovary syndrome. *J lin Endocrinol Metab* 1997; 82: 524–530.

43. Acbay O and Gundogdu S. Can metformin reduce insulin resistance in polycystic ovary syndrome? *Fertil Steril* 1996; 65: 946–949.

44. Taylor AE. Insulin-lowering medications in polycystic ovary syndrome [In Process Citation]. *Obstet Gynecol Clin North Am* 2000; 27: 583–595.

45. Homburg R. Should patients with polycystic ovarian syndrome be treated with metformin?: A note of cautious optimism. *Hum Reprod* 2002; 17: 853–856.

31

Effects of Metformin and Rosiglitazone Alone, and in Combination, in Women with Polycystic Ovary Syndrome

Sawaek Weerakiet

Summary

Polycystic Ovary Syndrome (PCOS) is a common female endocrinological disorder of which, insulin resistance is accepted as the central pathophysiology. It is rational to treat PCOS women with insulin-sensitizing agents. Metformin, a biguanide hypoglycemic drug, has been used in PCOS for 10 years. It has substantial efficacy in ovulation induction both, in the unselected, and CC-resistant PCOS women. Metformin, as the first-line of treatment, may be better than CC for induction of ovulation and pregnancy in non-obese PCOS women. Moreover, metformin decreases miscarriage, gestational diabetes mellitus (GDM) and pregnancy induced hypertension (PIH) rates in pregnant women with PCOS.

On the metabolic parameter, it can decrease fasting glucose, low-density lipoprotein cholesterol (LDL-C), inflammatory and coagulation markers, and can improve the endothelial structure and function. Rosiglitazone, which is a new insulin sensitizer and acts as a perioxisome proliferator activated receptor (PPAR) agonist, has been used in PCOS for a shorter period of time. Rosiglitazone is rather, more effective in ovulation induction than placebo, but not more effective than metformin. Importantly, rosiglitazone has an outstanding effect on glucose metabolism. However, its effect on lipid metabolism is inconclusive. Like metformin, rosiglitazone can improve the inflammatory and coagulation markers, as well as the endothelial parameters.

Further studies on the effect of rosiglitazone on ovulation induction and metabolic parameters, alone, or in combination with metformin, are required.

Rationale

Polycystic Ovary Syndrome (PCOS) is a common female reproductive endocrinological disorder, characterized by menstrual irregularities and hyperandrogenism.[1] To date, it is well-accepted that insulin resistance (IR) and the resultant hyperinsulinemia are the major causes of the pathogenesis of PCOS.[2] Insulin exerts its effects through several mechanisms and results in an increase in androgen levels. Increased insulin stimulates the ovarian theca cells via its own receptors to produce more androgens and enhances the effect of luteinizing hormone (LH) on the production of ovarian androgens.[3] Also, excess insulin decreases the synthesis of sex hormone binding globulin (SHBG), and insulin – like growth factor binding protein (IGFBP) from the liver, leading to an increase in free androgen levels[4] and free insulin-like growth factors (IGF) 1 and 2 respectively.[5] Both, free IGF-1 and IGF-2 enhance androgen production from the theca cells.[6]

Insulin resistance and hyperinsulinemia are the major causes for the development of impaired glucose tolerance (IGT) and the metabolic syndrome (MS).[7] Therefore, women with PCOS are at a risk of IGT[8] and MS,[9] which consequently, are also important risk factors of cardiovascular disease (CVD).[10]

To correct the clinical reproductive problems and theoretically, to prevent IGT, MS and subsequent CVD in PCOS women, improving IR and lowering insulin levels are the aims of treatment. Insulin-sensitizing agents, which are widely used for diabetes mellitus (DM) treatment, have been used in PCOS. Metformin and rosiglitazone are the two agents that are discussed in this chapter.

Introduction

Metformin and rosiglitazone are important insulin-sensitizing drugs used to treat diabetic patients. Metformin, a biguanide agent, has been used for more than two decades.[11] It has been accepted as a good, safe and effective hypoglycemic drug. Rosiglitazone however, a member of thiazolidinediones, is a newer insulin sensitizer and has been used for a shorter period of time.[12] It is also an excellent quality hypoglycemic drug. These two agents are different in their nature, mechanisms of action and adverse effects, therefore, they are discussed separately.

Metformin

Mechanisms of action

Metformin has several mechanisms of action. It mainly reduces hepatic glucose production by the inhibition of gluconeogenesis and, in part, by the inhibition of glycogenolysis. In addition, metformin can enhance glucose uptake, and glycogen and lipid synthesis in the skeletal muscle cells and adipocytes.[13] Additionally, metformin improves insulin sensitivity by decreasing the

release of free fatty acids from adipose tissues. Subsequently, the deterioration in β-cell function following long-term exposure to free fatty acids, can be improved.[14] Metformin also decreases gastrointestinal glucose absorption[13]. The actions of metformin are summarized in Table 31.1.

Table 31.1 Summary of mechanisms of action of metformin and rosiglitazone

---

A : Metformin
1. Inhibits hepatic glucose production
   - Inhibits gluconeogenesis
   - Inhibits glycogenolysis
2. Enhances the biological actions of insulin on skeletal muscles and adipocytes
   - Glucose transport
   - Glycogen synthesis
   - Lipid synthesis
3. Increases insulin sensitivity and improves pancreatic β-cell function
   - Decreases free fatty acids
4. Decreases gastrointestinal glucose absorption

B : Rosiglitazone
- increases insulin sensitivity in the liver
  - Increases lipid uptake
  - Increases energy expenditure
  - Decreases gluconeogenesis
- Increases insulin sensitivity in the skeletal muscles
  - Increases glucose uptake
  - Increases energy expenditure
- Increases insulin sensitivity in the adipose tissues
  - Increases glucose uptake
  - Increases lipid uptake
  - Increases energy expenditure

Doses of metformin vary between 1500-2550-mg/day. Important adverse effects include gastrointestinal symptoms, such as diarrhea, nausea and abdominal discomfort. To eliminate these adverse effects, metformin should be started in low doses and taken with meals. Development of hypoglycemia during metformin treatment is rare. Lactic acidosis, a serious adverse effect, is very rare and almost always, develops in patients having predisposing conditions.[13]

Rosiglitazone

Mechanisms of action

Rosiglitazone acts as a perioxisome proliferator activated receptor agonist, a nuclear receptor, in various tissues. It has effects on several gene transcriptions in insulin-responsive tissues and organs,[15] leading to an improvement in insulin sensitivity. As a result, glucose uptake is increased in the adipose tissues and skeletal muscles. Lipid uptake and energy expenditure are increased in the adipose tissues and the liver as well.[12,15] Moreover, an improvement in insulin sensitivity results in a decrease in hepatic gluconeogenesis and an increase in muscular glucose oxidation.[15] The actions of rosiglitazone are also summarized in Table 31.1.

Table 31.2 Summary of the effects of metformin and rosiglitazone on the metabolic parameters

	Metformin	Rosiglitazone
Fasting insulin	Decreased	Decreased
Fasting glucose	Decreased	Decreased
2h post load glucose	Unchanged	Decreased
Triglyceride	Unchanged	Inconclusive
Total cholesterol	Unchanged	Inconclusive
HDL-C	Unchanged	Inconclusive
LDL-C	Decreased	Inconclusive
Body weight	Decreased	Increased
BMI	Decreased	Increased
WHR	Decreased	Decreased
Blood pressure	Decreased	Decreased
PAI-1	Decreased	Decreased
CRP	Decreased	Decreased
ET-1	Decreased	Decreased
Endothelial		
Function	Improved	Improved
Structure	Improved	Improved

BMI: body mass index;
WHR: waist to hip ratio;
PAI-1: plasminogen activator inhibitor 1
CRP: C-reactive protein;
ET-1: endothelin-1.

Doses of rosiglitazone used in clinical practice are 4–8 mg/day and can be divided as 2 mg or 4 mg, twice a day.[12] The adverse effects are commonly weight gain, peripheral edema and a slight decrease in hemoglobin with no clinical consequence.[12] Hepatotoxicity is very rare. However, in long-term use, liver function should be monitored.[12]

Rosiglitazone is categorized as a class C drug by the FDA, therefore, it should not be used during pregnancy.[12]

Metformin and Rosiglitazone actions in PCOS

Both, metformin and rosiglitazone can reduce IR and subsequently, decrease insulin secretion. Many studies have shown that the administration of metformin[16–18] and rosiglitazone[19–22] decreases insulin levels. The improvement in insulin sensitivity has a positive effect on hepatocytes, resulting in the production of more SHBG and IGFBP. As a result, there are decreases in free testosterone as well as free IGF-1 concentrations, leading to lower androgen levels owing to lesser stimulation of the theca cells. In addition, the increased insulin sensitivity after metformin treatment can reduce the activity of CYP-17, leading to reduced ovarian androgen production.[23] Besides the action on insulin sensitivity, both metformin,[24] and rosiglitazone,[25] have a direct effect on the theca cells resulting in decreased androgen production.

Hence, metformin and rosiglitazone can reduce androgen production by several mechanisms, which can resume reproductive function and restore normal metabolism. Figure 31.1 summarizes the several pathways of metformin and rosiglitazone actions in reducing androgen production in PCOS.

Clinical Discussion

Having been used for two decades in the general population and for 10 years in PCOS patients, there is a lot of information about metformin both, in the reproductive and metabolic aspects. Since rosiglitazone has recently been used in PCOS, there is therefore, lesser information with regard to its use in pregnancy for instance.

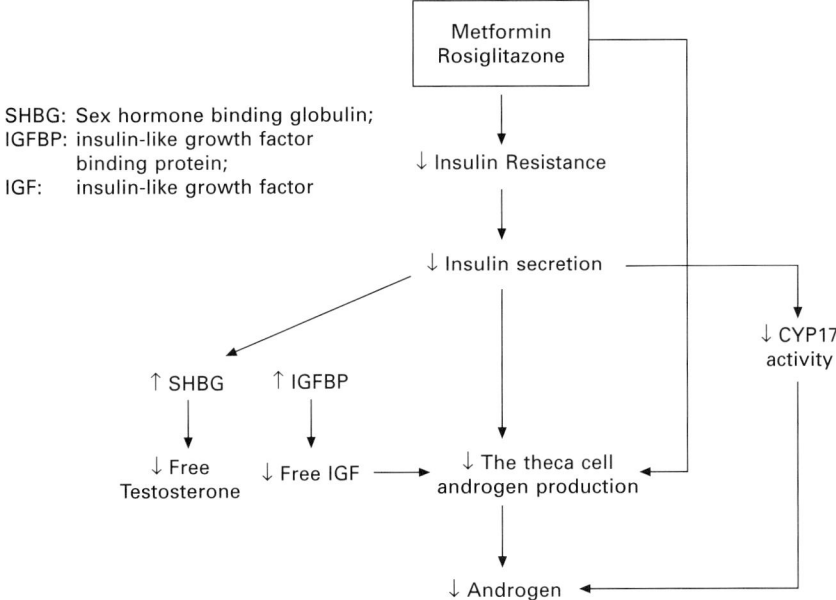

Figure 31.1   The actions of metformin and rosiglitazone in the reduction androgen production in women with PCOS.

Effects on ovulation induction and pregnancy

Metformin has a high efficacy in the induction of ovulation in PCOS women. Initial studies on the effect of metformin treatment on ovulation induction in PCOS women revealed that in unselected PCOS women, the ovulation rate is significantly higher in the metformin group than in the placebo groups.[26] The combination of metformin and clomiphene citrate (CC) seems to improve the ovulation rate in this group of patients[26]. Interestingly, the large randomized controlled trial, comparing the efficacy of metformin plus CC vs. CC alone in obese unselected PCOS women,[17] has shown that 80–90% ovulation rates were achieved following the use of metformin and CC in combination, and were significantly much higher than the placebo plus CC use. In addition, the pregnancy rate was also significantly greater in the metformin plus CC group than the placebo plus CC group.[27]

The following studies were aimed at evaluating the efficacy of metformin on ovulation induction and pregnancy in CC-resistant PCOS women. It appears that metformin enhances the effect of CC in this group of women. As a result, the ovulation and pregnancy rates are significantly higher in metformin plus CC than placebo plus CC groups.[26,27] Some prospective observatory studies also demonstrated the beneficial effect of metformin, in which ovulation rates of 40–50% were achieved with metformin alone, and two-thirds of the remaining patients could be ovulated with the addition of CC. The overall pregnancy rates were 40–60% within 6 months of treatment.[28,29] Recently, a report from Taiwan,[30] showed that metformin, 1,500 mg per day for 12 days (ultra-short regimen), prior to the administration of CC, 150 mg daily for 5 days, could improve ovulation and pregnancy rates (42.5% and 15% respectively vs. 12.5% and 0%, respectively) compared with controls without metformin in CC-resistant PCOS women.

The effect of rosiglitazone on ovulation and pregnancy was first reported by Cataldo and colleagues[31] in 2001. They reported one case of an infertile PCOS woman who experienced a regular cycle and conceived after rosiglitazone treatment for 6 months. There are several reports of the efficacy of rosiglitazone on ovulation and menstruation. Improvement in menstruation can be achieved after rosiglitazone treatment alone in obese women with PCOS.[21,22] In addition, rosiglitazone can not only enhance the effect of CC on ovulation induction, resulting in an increase in ovulatory menstrual cycles,[32] but can also improve ovulation in CC-resistant PCOS women. Ghazeeri et al.[33] reported an ovulation rate of 33% following the use of rosiglitazone alone, compared to 77% when used with a combination with CC.

Most recent evidence comparing the efficacies of rosiglitazone and metformin has shown that rosiglitazone is not superior to metformin in ovulation induction in PCOS women. Although ovulation and regular menstrual cycle rates are higher in PCOS women following the administration of rosiglitazone alone compared to placebo, these rates are significantly lower compared to those obtained using metformin alone.[34] Moreover, the addition of rosiglitazone to metformin does not improve the efficacy of metformin. The ovulation and cumulative ovulation rates, and the frequencies of menstrual bleeding are comparable between the PCOS women using rosiglitazone plus metformin and those using metformin alone.[34]

Metformin and miscarriage

The beneficial effect of metformin on the reduction of miscarriage rate in pregnant women with PCOS has been established.[35–37] Glueck and colleagues[35] reported that the abortion rate was reduced from 73% in the previous pregnancy to 10% in the current pregnancy in the same PCOS women with the administration of metformin throughout pregnancy.[35] A recent randomized controlled trial showed that metformin, when used as the first-line drug, resulted in a lower abortion rate compared to laparoscopic ovarian drilling,[36] and CC use.[37] This fact implies that metformin may have a higher impact on some factors that increase uterine receptivity and decrease the incidence of miscarriage.

Plasminogen activator inhibitor 1 (PIA-1), glycodelin and IGFBP-1 appear to be the important factors involved in spontaneous abortion. Substantially, metformin can reduce IR and lead to decreased PAI-I levels, lowering the abortion rate.[38] Furthermore, metformin increases glycodelin, which is a protein with an inhibitory effect on the endometrial immune system, and IGFBP-1, and which enhances the adhesion process between the maternal and the fetal interface, in the luteal phase resulting from improved insulin sensitivity in PCOS women.[39] It has been reported that, in PCOS women with first trimester spontaneous abortions, the levels of these two substances were lower in comparison to women with a normal pregnancy.[39] Although there is no information in the early pregnancy period, metformin may have a positive effect on the early pregnancy outcome through an increase in these two proteins.

Metformin and gestational diabetes mellitus (GDM)

It appears that GDM is more prevalent in PCOS women than controls[40] and PCOS is a significant risk factor for GDM.[40,41] Glueck and colleagues[42] have shown that metformin treatment throughout pregnancy could reduce the prevalence of GDM from 31% in women who did not take metformin in previous pregnancies, to 3% in current pregnancies. Although metformin seems to prevent the development of GDM, it should not be routinely used for this purpose because there is limited evidence on the safety of this drug during pregnancy. Prospective randomized controlled trials with a statistically adequate population size are required to substantiate the safety metformin treatment during pregnancy.

Metformin and pregnancy induced hypertension (PIH)

PCOS appears to increase the risk for PIH, including pre-eclampsia and gestational hypertension, which is associated with IR.[40,41] Metformin can reduce the risk of PIH by decreasing IR. Glueck and colleagues[43] demonstrated that the reduction in the rate of development of pre-eclampsia in 97 PCOS women following metformin use was higher than that observed in 252 community based controls (5.2% vs. 3.6% respectively, p = NS). However, metformin should not be used in pregnant PCOS women as a routine medication. Further studies in this regard are necessary.

Safety of metformin used for ovulation induction and pregnancy

The possibility of teratogenicity and a negative impact on the fetal outcome, remain the central core of the problem in using metformin throughout pregnancy. Previously, Coetzee and Jackson,[44] experienced in the treatment of diabetes mellitus with insulin sensitizing agents, including metformin in pregnancy, reported that metformin was not teratogenic and had no the effect on the fetal outcome. In addition, metformin is classified as a class B drug by the FDA. Some authors have conducted studies that demonstrated a decrease in the miscarriage,[35] GDM, and pre-eclampsia rates,[43] following metformin use.

In contrast, because there are only few studies, and the number of PCOS samples studied are insufficient to conclude the safety of metformin treatment during pregnancy, metformin should be discontinued if a diagnosis of pregnancy is made.[27,45]

Effect on glucose metabolism and the metabolic syndrome in PCOS

Glucose metabolism

Results of the effect of metformin on glucose, fasting glucose, in particular, levels in PCOS women, are contradictory. However, the Cochrane meta-analysis review showed that metformin could reduce the fasting glucose levels and the area under the glucose curve (AUC) in PCOS women when compared with placebo.[27]

Rosiglitazone may have an excellent effect on glucose metabolism. Although a reduction in the fasting glucose level after rosiglitazone treatment has been controversially reported,[20,34] it has no clinical significance because the fasting glucose levels in PCOS are not too high, and mostly within normal range. Moreover, rosiglitazone has the same efficacy as metformin on glucose regulation, both fasting glucose levels and AUC of glucose calculated by glucose levels during the oral glucose tolerance test (OGTT).[34] Surprisingly, the combination of rosiglitazone and metformin appears to have a lesser efficacy than that of either drug.[34] Importantly, the effect of rosiglitazone on the reduction of 2-h post load (2-h PL) glucose levels, which is the main abnormal glucose metabolism finding in PCOS women, is better.[7] This efficacy depends on doses and duration of treatment.[20] Rosiglitazone, when adinistered at a dose of 4 to 8 mg/day for 6 months, can reduce the abnormal 2-h PL glucose levels to normal.[20]

Lipid metabolism

The effect of metformin on the other components of MS, including dyslipidemia, obesity and hypertension, has been reported as well. According to the meta-analysis, metformin only has an effect on LDL-C, but not on total cholesterol, HDL-C and triglyceride levels. Metformin reduces the LDL-C levels when compared with placebo.[27]

The effect of rosiglitazone on lipid metabolism in PCOS women is inconclusive. Some,[46] but not all authors,[20] showed the difference in lipid levels compared between before and after treatment. However, this reduction in lipid levels may not have any clinical significance because the levels of all lipid components were in the normal range.[20,46]

Obesity

Weight reduction, which can restore normal physiologic events, is the treatment of choice in PCOS women.[47] The effect of metformin on weight loss has been interesting. Metformin alone cannot change body weight and the degree of obesity, assessed by both body mass index and waist to hip ratio (WHR) as compared with the placebo.[27] It has recently been reported that protracted metformin treatment accompanied with life style modifications, may benefit a weight reduction in PCOS women with morbid obesity.[48]

Unlike metformin, rosiglitazone has an adverse effect on body weight. Body weight and BMI in PCOS women may increase following rosiglitazone use.[20,34] A comparison of the effect of using metformin or rosiglitazone alone, or a combination of rosiglitazone and metformin in PCOS women, has shown that women using rosiglitazone alone have a significant increase in BMI after treatment, whereas there is no change in the other two groups.[34] However, this change has no clinical significance as well. In contrast, reduction in WHR, which is associated with reduction in IR, has been reported by some.[34]

Blood Pressure

According to the meta-analysis, metformin treatment can decrease both, the systolic and diastolic blood pressure in PCOS women as compared with placebo.[27] Rosiglitazone can also reduce the systolic blood pressure with the same efficacy as metformin. However, rosiglitazone does not have a synergistic effect with metformin in decreasing the blood pressure.[34]

Effect on coagulation and inflammatory markers, hemocystein, endothelial structure and function.

PAI-1, which is a potent fibrinolytic inhibitor, and C-reactive protein (CRP), which is an inflammatory marker, are associated with IR and hyperinsulinemia. The higher PAI-1 and CRP levels have been implicated as risk factors for cardiovascular disease (CVD).[49] It has been reported that PAI-1 and CRP levels were higher in PCOS than the control women.[18,50]

Homocystein is an intermediate in the process of synthesis of cystein from metionine. Hyperhomocysteinemia is accepted as a risk factor for CVD. This situation may be a cause of vascular injury, leading to an abnormal coagulation process.[51] There have been reports of the higher levels of hemocystein in PCOS women than controls.

Impairment of the endothelial structure and function, as well as an increase in the markers of endothelial injury, which are accepted as the early signs of CVD, have been observed in PCOS.[52,53] Markers of endothelial structure, function and endothelial injury include carotid-intima media thickness (IMT), the brachial flow mediated dilation (FMD), baseline diameter (BAD), diameter after reactive hyperemia (DARH), and plasma endothelin-1 (ET-1).

Treating PCOS women with metformin can improve insulin sensitivity leading to decrease in PAI-1,[18] and ET-1 to baseline both, in obese,[53] and non-obese PCOS women.[52] Also, metformin can reduce CRP in PCOS women.[54] Recent data revealed an improvement in the endothelial structure and function following metformin treatment for 6 months. BAD, DARH, and IMT were significantly decreased, and FMD was significantly increased as compared with the baseline levels.[52]

Rosiglitazone has a positive effect on the inflammation and endothelial functions. Tarkun and colleagues[55] demonstrated that CRP was significantly reduced, and the endothelium-dependent vascular functions were significantly improved from the baseline following a daily 4 mg rosiglitazone treatment for one year.

Unlike the favorable treatment effect of insulin-sensitizing agents on PAI-1 and ET-1, both metformin and rosiglitazone result in an increase in hemocystein[46]. This unfavorable effect of insulin-sensitizing agents on increasing hemocystein may result from their interference with Vitamin B12 and folic acid pathways, leading to elevated hemocystein levels.[56] The addition of Vitamin B12 and folic acid to the treatment protocol, results in a decrease in hemocystein levels.[56]

Effect on hirsutism

There are several studies on the effect of metformin on hirsutism.[57–59] Some studies with prolonged metformin treatment in which hirsutism was not the main aim of the studies, showed controversial results.[58,59] Kelly and Gordon,[57] demonstrated an improvement in hirsutism evaluated by the Ferriman-Gallwey (F-G) score, hair growth velocity and patient self assessment after metformin treatment for 14 months compared with base-line values. The F–G scores were decreased from 17.7 ± 1.4 to 15.8 ± 1.4 (p = 0.025). Hair growth velocity was reduced from 0.76 ± 0.2 to 0.67 ± 0.2 mm/day. Clinically, the significance of these reductions in hirsutism measurement is questionable, because only a 10% reduction is achieved. Metformin may not be the drug of choice for the treatment of hirsutism.

There have been reports of the effect of rosiglitazone on hirsutism.[55,60] Rosiglitazone can significantly decrease the F-G scores after 6–12 months of treatment.[55,60] Moreover, rosiglitazone seems to be more effective than metformin in hirsutism treatment.[60]

Case studies

Case 1

A 35 year-old, para 1, woman complained of infertility for 2 years. She had irregular menstruation after menarche at age 18. She had a few cycles in the last few years and always had acne and seborrhea. Physical examination revealed obesity with a BMI of 27.8 kg/m^2 and WHR of 0.85. Other physical and pelvic examinations were unremarkable. Normal uterus and polycystic ovary appearance of both the ovaries were found by transvaginal ultrasound (TVS) examination. Polycystic ovary syndrome with infertility was the diagnosis after some hormonal tests for ruling out other diseases. CC was the first-line of treatment. CC-resistance was diagnosed after 150 mg × 5 days CC for 3 cycles without ovulation. A 75 g OGTT and endometrial biopsy were performed without abnormal detection. Metformin was used to induce ovulation.

The protocol was as follows: the first week, 500 mg of metformin, once a day with meals;

the second week, 500 mg, twice a day and the 3rd and 4th week, 500 mg three times a day. TVS for monitoring follicle development was done at the end of the 4th week. If a dominant follicle was observed, metformin treatment was continued until the follicle was mature. Timing of sexual intercourse (TSI) or an intrauterine insemination (IUI), 36 hrs after administration of 5,000 units of hCG injection, was advised. If there was no dominant follicle, metformin was still continued and CC, 50 mg a day for 5 days was added, TVS repeated 10 days later, and TSI or IUI selected if a dominant follicle appeared.

Three cycles of treatment were carried out with the addition of CC in the last 2 cycles. She conceived after IUI in the last cycle. There was no complication during pregnancy and she had a term singleton delivery.

Case 2

A 28-year single woman complained of amenorrhea accompanied with acne and seborrhea for 10 years. Physical examination revealed acanthosis nigricans, obesity with a BMI of 32 kg/m^2 and WHR of 0.85, and slightly increased blood pressure of 140/90 mmHg. Transabdominal sonography showed polycystic appearance of both the ovaries. The diagnosis of PCOS was made after diseases mimicking PCOS were excluded. Type 2 DM was diagnosed with an abnormal 75 g OGTT; 94 mg/dl and 211 mg/dl at 0 and 120 minutes respectively. Metformin was the drug of choice. Titrated doses up to 1500 mg were given daily for 3 months. With repeated OGTT, the fasting glucose decreased to 84 mg/dl, whereas the 2 h post load glucose remained high at 202 mg/dl. A maximum dose of metformin, 2,550 mg daily was given for 3 months. This did not improve the 2 h PL glucose, which was still greater than 200 mg/dl. During the treatment, progestin was added for induction of menstruation. Metformin was stopped and rosiglitazone was started. Glucose levels were controlled within the normal range tested by OGTT after 3 months of treatment. Rosiglitazone was continued. Menstruation occurred around every 2 months.

Recent Advances

With the evidence that metformin can improve ovulation and pregnancy rates, it has been suggested to be the first-line of treatment for ovulation induction in PCOS women.[45] On the other hand, CC, which is accepted as the first-line drug for ovulation induction in PCOS, is highly effective in ovulation induction, but yields low pregnancy rates.[36] Most recently, Palombo and colleagues[37] performed an RCT to compare between metformin and CC as the first-line of treatment for ovulation induction in PCOS.[37] They found that although there were no differences in the cumulative ovulation rate, the pregnancy rate per ovulatory cycle was higher in the metformin than the CC-group (15.1% vs. 7.2% respectively, $P = 0.0009$). Therefore, there maybe a trend for using metformin for ovulation induction in PCOS women. Not only is metformin used in CC-resistant PCOS women, but it may be used as the first line of treatment in infertile PCOS women as well.

Conclusion

Metformin, a biguanide hypoglycemic drug, has commonly been studied in PCOS. The high efficacy of metformin in ovulation induction has been established in CC-resistant PCOS women. Recent data reveals that it may be better than CC as the first-line of treatment in ovulation induction in non-obese PCOS. Also, metformin has positive effects on pregnancy outcomes in PCOS women, decreasing miscarriage, GDM and PIH rates. Metformin has a positive effect on several metabolic parameters, which are risk factors for CVD.

Rosiglitazone is a new hypoglycemic drug that has been studied in PCOS women only recently. It has an excellent effect on glucose metabolism. However, with limited data, rosiglitazone has not been shown to be more effective than metformin in ovulation induction and other metabolic parameters. In addition, it does not have a synergistic effect with metformin when compared to metformin alone.

Further studies to document the safety of metformin treatment throughout pregnancy should be performed. Research of the effects of rosiglitazone in PCOS should be continued to prove its efficacy in several aspects.

References

1. Franks S. Polycystic ovary syndrome. *N Engl J Med* 1995; 333: 853–861.
2. Dunaif A. Insulin action in the polycystic ovary syndrome. *Endocrinol Metab Clin North Am* 1999; 28: 341–359.
3. Bergh C, Olsson JH, Selleskog U, Hillensjo T. Steroid production in cultured thecal cells obtained from human ovarian follicles. *Hum Reprod* 1993; 8: 519–524.
4. Dunaif A. Insulin resistance and the polycystic ovary syndrome: mechanism and implications for pathogenesis. *Endocr Rev* 1997; 18: 774–800.
5. LeRoith D, Werner H, Beitner-Johnson D, Roberts CT, Jr. Molecular and cellular aspects of the insulin-like growth factor I receptor. *Endocr Rev* 1995; 16: 143–163.
6. Voutilainen R, Franks S, Mason HD, Martikainen H. Expression of insulin-like growth factor (IGF), IGF-binding protein, and IGF receptor messenger ribonucleic acids in normal and polycystic ovaries. *J Clin Endocrinol Metab* 1996; 81: 1003–1008.
7. Weerakiet S, Srisombut C, Bunnag P, Sangtong S, Chuangsoongnoen N, Rojanasakul A. Prevalence of type 2 diabetes mellitus and impaired glucose tolerance in Asian women with polycystic ovary syndrome. *Int J Gynaecol Obstet* 2001; 75: 177–184.
8. Glueck CJ, Papanna R, Wang P, Goldenberg N, Sieve-Smith L. Incidence and treatment of metabolic syndrome in newly referred women with confirmed polycystic ovarian syndrome. *Metabolism* 2003; 52: 908–915.
9. Haffner SM. Insulin resistance, inflammation, and the prediabetic state. *Am J Cardiol* 2003; 92: 18J–26J.
10. Reaven GM. Banting lecture 1988. Role of insulin resistance in human disease. *Diabetes* 1988; 37: 1595–1607.
11. Bailey CJ, Turner RC. Metformin. *N Engl J Med* 1996; 334: 574–579.
12. O'Moore–Sullivan TM, Prins JB. Thiazolidinediones and type 2 diabetes: new drugs for an old disease. *Med J Aust* 2002; 176: 381–386.

13. Kirpichnikov D, McFarlane SI, Sowers JR. Metformin: an update. *Ann Intern Med* 2002; 137: 25–33.

14. Patane G, Piro S, Rabuazzo AM, Anello M, Vigneri R, Purrello F. Metformin restores insulin secretion altered by chronic exposure to free fatty acids or high glucose: a direct metformin effect on pancreatic beta-cells. *Diabetes* 2000; 49: 735–740.

15. Lee CH, Olson P, Evans RM. Minireview: lipid metabolism, metabolic diseases, and peroxisome proliferator-activated receptors. *Endocrinology* 2003; 144: 2201–2207.

16. Morin-Papunen LC, Koivunen RM, Ruokonen A, Martikainen HK. Metformin therapy improves the menstrual pattern with minimal endocrine and metabolic effects in women with polycystic ovary syndrome. *Fertil Steril* 1998; 69: 691–696.

17. Nestler JE, Jakubowicz DJ, Evans WS, Pasquali R. Effects of metformin on spontaneous and clomiphene-induced ovulation in the polycystic ovary syndrome. *N Engl J Med* 1998; 338: 1876–1880.

18. Velazquez EM, Mendoza SG, Wang P, Glueck CJ. Metformin therapy is associated with a decrease in plasma plasminogen activator inhibitor-1, lipoprotein (a), and immunoreactive insulin levels in patients with the polycystic ovary syndrome. *Metabolism* 1997; 46: 454–457.

19. Cataldo NA, Abbasi F, McLaughlin TL, Basina M, Fechner PY, Giudice LC, Reaven GM. Metabolic and ovarian effects of rosiglitazone treatment for 12 weeks in insulin-resistant women with polycystic ovary syndrome. Hum Reprod 2006; 21(1): 109–120.

20. Dereli D, Dereli T, Bayraktar F, Ozgen AG, Yilmaz C. Endocrine and metabolic effects of rosiglitazone in non-obese women with polycystic ovary disease. *Endocr J* 2005; 52: 299–308.

21. Belli SH, Graffigna MN, Oneto A, Otero P, Schurman L, Levalle OA. Effect of rosiglitazone on insulin resistance, growth factors, and reproductive disturbances in women with polycystic ovary syndrome. *Fertil Steril* 2004; 81: 624–629.

22. Sepilian V, Nagamani M. Effects of rosiglitazone in obese women with polycystic ovary syndrome and severe insulin resistance. *J Clin Endocrinol Metab* 2005; 90: 60–65.

23. Nestler JE, Jakubowicz DJ. Lean women with polycystic ovary syndrome respond to insulin reduction with decreases in ovarian P450c17 alpha activity and serum androgens. *J Clin Endocrinol Metab* 1997; 82: 4075–4079.

24. Attia GR, Rainey WE, Carr BR. Metformin directly inhibits androgen production in human thecal cells. *Fertil Steril* 2001; 76: 517–524.

25. Seto-Young D, Paliou M, Schlosser J, et al. Direct thiazolidinedione action in the human ovary: insulin-independent and insulin-sensitizing effects on steroidogenesis and insulin-like growth factor binding protein-1 production. *J Clin Endocrinol Metab* 2005; 90: 6099–6105.

26. Costello MF, Eden JA. A systematic review of the reproductive system effects of metformin in patients with polycystic ovary syndrome. *Fertil Steril* 2003; 79: 1–13.

27. Lord JM, Flight IH, Norman RJ. Insulin-sensitising drugs (metformin, troglitazone, rosiglitazone, pioglitazone, D-chiro-inositol) for polycystic ovary syndrome. *Cochrane Database Syst Rev* 2003; CD003053.

28. Heard MJ, Pierce A, Carson SA, Buster JE. Pregnancies following use of metformin for ovulation induction in patients with polycystic ovary syndrome. *Fertil Steril* 2002; 77: 669–673.

29. Weerakiet S, Tingthanatikul Y, Sophonsritsuk A, Choktanasiri W, Wansumrith S, Rojanasakul A. Efficacy of metformin on ovulation induction in Asian women with polycystic ovary syndrome. *Gynecol Endocrinol* 2004; 19: 202–207.

30. Hwu YM, Lin SY, Huang WY, Lin MH, Lee RK. Ultra-short metformin pretreatment for clomiphene citrate-resistant polycystic ovary syndrome. *Int J Gynaecol Obstet* 2005; 90: 39–43.

31. Cataldo NA, Abbasi F, McLaughlin TL, Lamendola C, Reaven GM. Improvement in insulin sensitivity followed by ovulation and pregnancy in a woman with polycystic ovary syndrome who was treated with rosiglitazone. *Fertil Steril* 2001; 76: 1057–1059.

32. Shobokshi A, Shaarawy M. Correction of insulin resistance and hyperandrogenism in polycystic ovary syndrome by combined rosiglitazone and clomiphene citrate therapy. *J Soc Gynecol Investig* 2003; 10: 99–104.

33. Ghazeeri G, Kutteh WH, Bryer-Ash M, Haas D, Ke RW. Effect of rosiglitazone on spontaneous and clomiphene citrate-induced ovulation in women with polycystic ovary syndrome. *Fertil Steril* 2003; 79: 562–566.

34. Baillargeon JP, Jakubowicz DJ, Iuorno MJ, Jakubowicz S, Nestler JE. Effects of metformin and rosiglitazone, alone and in combination, in nonobese women with polycystic ovary syndrome and normal indices of insulin sensitivity. *Fertil Steril* 2004; 82: 893–902.

35. Glueck CJ, Phillips H, Cameron D, Sieve-Smith L, Wang P. Continuing metformin throughout pregnancy in women with polycystic ovary syndrome appears to safely reduce first-trimester spontaneous abortion: a pilot study. *Fertil Steril* 2001; 75: 46–52.

36. Palomba S, Orio F, Jr., Nardo LG, et al. Metformin administration versus laparoscopic ovarian diathermy in clomiphene citrate-resistant women with polycystic ovary syndrome: a prospective parallel randomized double-blind placebo-controlled trial. *J Clin Endocrinol Metab* 2004; 89: 4801–4809.

37. Palomba S, Orio F, Jr., Falbo A, et al. Prospective parallel randomized, double-blind, double-dummy controlled clinical trial comparing clomiphene citrate and metformin as the first-line treatment for ovulation induction in nonobese anovulatory women with polycystic ovary syndrome. *J Clin Endocrinol Metab* 2005; 90: 4068–4074.

38. Palomba S, Orio F, Jr., Falbo A, Russo T, Tolino A, Zullo F. Plasminogen activator inhibitor 1 and miscarriage after metformin treatment and laparoscopic ovarian drilling in patients with polycystic ovary syndrome. *Fertil Steril* 2005; 84: 761–765.

39. Jakubowicz DJ, Essah PA, Seppala M, et al. Reduced serum glycodelin and insulin-like growth factor-binding protein-1 in women with polycystic ovary syndrome during first trimester of pregnancy. *J Clin Endocrinol Metab* 2004; 89: 833–839.

40. Mikola M, Hiilesmaa V, Halttunen M, Suhonen L, Tiitinen A. Obstetric outcome in women with polycystic ovarian syndrome. *Hum Reprod* 2001; 16: 226–229.

41. Weerakiet S, Srisombut C, Rojanasakul A, Panburana P, Thakkinstian A, Herabutya Y. Prevalence of gestational diabetes mellitus and pregnancy outcomes in Asian women with polycystic ovary syndrome. *Gynecol Endocrinol* 2004; 19: 134–140.

42. Glueck CJ, Wang P, Kobayashi S, Phillips H, Sieve-Smith L. Metformin therapy throughout pregnancy reduces the development of gestational diabetes in women with polycystic ovary syndrome. *Fertil Steril* 2002; 77: 520–525.

43. Glueck CJ, Bornovali S, Pranikoff J, Goldenberg N, Dharashivkar S, Wang P. Metformin, pre-eclampsia, and pregnancy outcomes in women with polycystic ovary syndrome. *Diabet Med* 2004; 21: 829–836.

44. Coetzee EJ, Jackson WP. The management of non-insulin-dependent diabetes during pregnancy. *Diabetes Res Clin Pract* 1985; 1: 281–287.

45. Norman RJ. Editorial: Metformin—comparison with other therapies in ovulation induction in polycystic ovary syndrome. *J Clin Endocrinol Metab* 2004; 89: 4797–4800.

46. Kilicdag EB, Bagis T, Zeyneloglu HB, et al. Homocysteine levels in women with polycystic ovary syndrome treated with metformin versus rosiglitazone: a randomized study. *Hum Reprod* 2005; 20: 894–899.

47. Guzick DS, Wing R, Smith D, Berga SL, Winters SJ. Endocrine consequences of weight loss in obese, hyperandrogenic, anovulatory women. *Fertil Steril* 1994; 61: 598–604.

48. Harborne LR, Sattar N, Norman JE, Fleming R. Metformin and weight loss in obese women with polycystic ovary syndrome: comparison of doses. *J Clin Endocrinol Metab* 2005; 90: 4593–4598.

49. Talbott EO, Zborowskii JV, Boudraux MY. Do women with polycystic ovary syndrome have an increased risk of cardiovascular disease? Review of the evidence. *Minerva Ginecol* 2004; 56: 27–39.

50. Kelly CC, Lyall H, Petrie JR, Gould GW, Connell JM, Sattar N. Low grade chronic inflammation in women with polycystic ovarian syndrome. *J Clin Endocrinol Metab* 2001; 86: 2453–2455.

51. Audelin MC, Genest J, Jr. Homocysteine and cardiovascular disease in diabetes mellitus. *Atherosclerosis* 2001; 159: 497–511.

52. Orio F, Jr., Palomba S, Cascella T, et al. Improvement in endothelial structure and function after metformin treatment in young normal-weight women with polycystic ovary syndrome: results of a 6-month study. *J Clin Endocrinol Metab* 2005; 90: 6072–6076.

53. Diamanti-Kandarakis E, Spina G, Kouli C, Migdalis I. Increased endothelin-1 levels in women with polycystic ovary syndrome and the beneficial effect of metformin therapy. *J Clin Endocrinol Metab* 2001; 86: 4666–4673.

54. Morin-Papunen L, Rautio K, Ruokonen A, Hedberg P, Puukka M, Tapanainen JS. Metformin reduces serum C-reactive protein levels in women with polycystic ovary syndrome. *J Clin Endocrinol Metab* 2003; 88: 4649–4654.

55. Tarkun I, Cetinarslan B, Turemen E, Sahin T, Canturk Z, Komsuoglu B. Effect of rosiglitazone on insulin resistance, C-reactive protein and endothelial function in non-obese young women with polycystic ovary syndrome. *Eur J Endocrinol* 2005; 153: 115–121.

56. Kilicdag EB, Bagis T, Tarim E, et al. Administration of B-group vitamins reduces circulating homocysteine in polycystic ovarian syndrome patients treated with metformin: a randomized trial. *Hum Reprod* 2005; 20: 1521–1528.

57. Kelly CJ, Gordon D. The effect of metformin on hirsutism in polycystic ovary syndrome. *Eur J Endocrinol* 2002; 147: 217–221.

58. Pasquali R, Gambineri A, Biscotti D, et al. Effect of long-term treatment with metformin added to hypocaloric diet on body composition, fat distribution, and androgen and insulin levels in abdominally obese women with and without the polycystic ovary syndrome. *J Clin Endocrinol Metab* 2000; 85: 2767–2774.

59. Moghetti P, Castello R, Negri C, et al. Metformin effects on clinical features, endocrine and metabolic profiles, and insulin sensitivity in polycystic ovary syndrome: a randomized, double-blind, placebo-controlled 6-month trial, followed by open, long-term clinical evaluation. *J Clin Endocrinol Metab* 2000; 85: 139–146.

60. Yilmaz C, Karakoc A, Toruner F, et al. The effects of rosiglitazone and metformin on menstrual cyclicity and hirsutism in polycystic ovary syndrome. *Gynecol Endocrinol* 2005; 21: 154160.

Frequently Asked Questions

1. What is the rationale for treatment with metformin and rosiglitazone in PCOS?

Most PCOS women possess insulin resistance as the main etiology for the pathogenesis of the disorder. Insulin-sensitizing agents, metformin or rosiglitazone can improve IR, decrease androgen production and subsequently, resolve clinical manifestations of the disorder.

2. Can metformin and rosiglitazone be used for ovulation induction?

Yes, metformin can successfully be used for ovulation induction. Data from the meta-analysis revealed the high efficacy of metformin on ovulation induction in CC-resistant PCOS.

With the little information available, rosiglitazone seems to be more effective than placebo for ovulation induction, though not superior in efficacy to metformin.

3. Can metformin and rosiglitazone prevent GDM and PIH in the pregnant women with PCOS?

Because metformin and rosiglitazone can improve IR, theoretically, they should prevent GDM and PIH. It has been reported that metformin, used throughout pregnancy, can reduce the prevalence of GDM and PIH in PCOS women. However, there is a controversy with regard to this issue among authors. Since there is insufficient data about the teratogenic effect of the drug, metformin should not be used in pregnancy and should be discontinued after pregnancy is diagnosed following use for ovulation induction.

Rosiglitazone is classified as a class C drug. It is not appropriate to use during pregnancy. No data are available on these issues.

4. Can metformin and rosiglitazone be used continuously to prevent diabetes mellitus and the metabolic syndrome (MS)?

As we know PCOS women are at risk for type 2 DM, MS and consequently, cardiovascular disease. Weight reduction with life style changes is a first-line of treatment that must be considered. Insulin sensitizers should be an adjuvant therapy, a secondary choice. Metformin alone can prevent type 2 DM, but is not superior to life style modification and exercise in the general populations at risk. In PCOS women, it has been reported that metformin can improve IR and subsequently, reduce fasting glucose, LDL-C and improve the endothelial structure and function. However, there is no data with regard to continuous treatment with metformin for the prevention of type 2 DM and MS.

Likewise, there is no data on rosiglitazone with regard to this issue. The efficacy, and cost-benefit of using rosiglitazone to prevent the metabolic disease should be further assessed.

32

Pioglitazone and Metformin in Obese Women with Polycystic Ovary Syndrome Not Optimally Responsive to Metformin

Marzieh Salehi, Charles J Glueck

Summary

The association of reproductive and metabolic manifestations of polycystic ovary syndrome (PCOS) was first described by Archard and Thiers in 1920s, as 'diabetes des femmes a barbe' or diabetes of the bearded women.[1] However, it was not until 1980, when Burghen et al.[2] demonstrated the relationship between circulating insulin levels and testosterone levels in non-diabetic women with PCOS. For the last two decades, it has become evident that insulin resistance is a prominent feature of PCOS that can play a pathogenic role in ovarian androgen overproduction and long-term metabolic consequences, including impaired glucose tolerance/diabetes, defects in fibrinolysis, and dyslipidemia. Therefore, it is reasonable to postulate that attenuation of insulin resistance or hyperinsulinemia ameliorates hyperandrogenemia, as well as some of the metabolic abnormalities associated with this condition. This hypothesis, in fact, has been tested by many investigators over the last decade by lowering insulin levels by weight loss,[3] metformin[4–6] and thiazolidinediones,[7,8] which resulted in improved ovulatory cycles and lower androgen levels. Recently, co-administration of metformin and thiazolidinediones has been tested in PCOS, of which combined metformin and pioglitazone therapy will be discussed in this chapter.[9,10]

Introduction

Reproductive features of PCOS (Fig. 32.1)

The cardinal features of PCOS are disordered gonadotropin secretion,[11] elevated ovarian and adrenal androgen production[12] and polycystic ovaries. An enhanced gonadotropin releasing hormone (GnRH) secretion, which fails to respond to the negative feedback of estradiol and progesterone, leads to an increased luteinizing hormone (LH) secretion,[13,14] while follicular stimulating hormone (FSH) levels are in the midfollicular range.[11] As a result, ovarian androgen production is enhanced and multiple ovarian follicles are seized at the pre-ovulatory stage. A primary defect in ovarian steroidogenesis cannot be excluded as cultured PCOS theca cells demonstrate an increased androgen production basally and in response to LH, which remains unchanged even in propagated long-term culture.[15,16]

Furthermore, insulin resistance or hyper-insulinemia contributes to hyperandrogenemia, though the causal relationship has been debated for many years. Insulin directly stimulates ovarian or adrenal steroidogenesis.[5,17] Infusion of insulin failed to show any difference in mean serum gonadotropin concentrations, LH pulse frequency, or LH pulse amplitude in either PCOS or controls,[18,19] while insulin increased the sensitivity

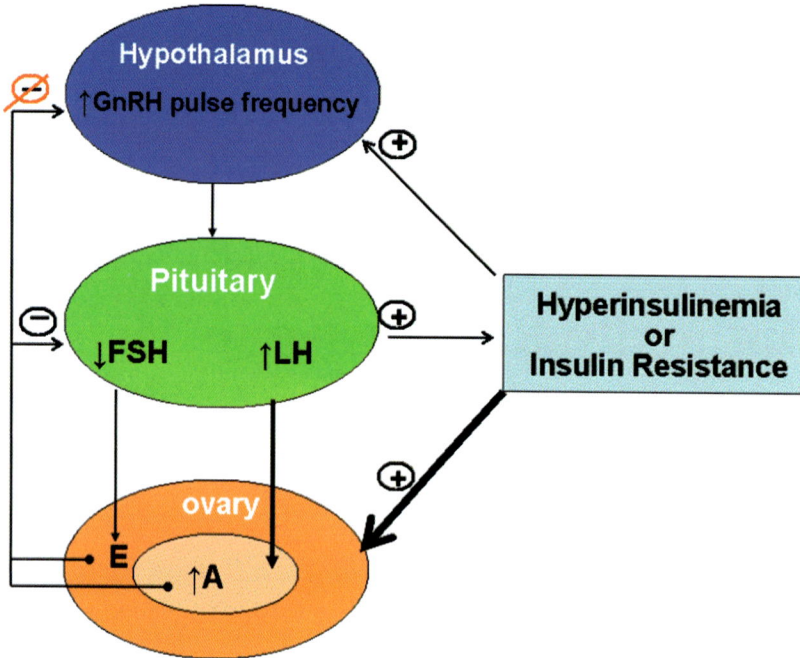

Figure 32.1   Schematic representation of the complex interactions between insulin resistance and the reproductive axis, leading to polycystic ovary syndrome: GnRH, gonadotropin releasing hormone; FSH, follicle-stimulating hormone; LH, luteinizing hormone; A, androgens, E, estradiol, (+), stimulatory effect, (−), inhibitory effect. Thick arrow emphasizes that most evidence supports the direct effect of insulin resistance on ovarian steroidogenesis. Note that GnRH secretion does not respond to the negative feedback of estradiol, enhancing LH secretion in this condition.

of gonadotrophs to GnRH during in vitro culture studies.[20] Nevertheless, administration of insulin lowering agents, such as diazoxide,[21] or insulin sensitizers, such as metformin[5] or thiazolidinediones,[8] lowered serum androgen levels, as well as circulatory LH concentrations in women with PCOS.

Metabolic features of PCOS

Insulin resistance is a key characteristic of PCOS, independent of obesity.[22] Obesity and PCOS have an additive deleterious effect on insulin sensitivity.[23] The molecular mechanisms of insulin resistance in PCOS are unique compared with those in other insulin resistant conditions, such as obesity and diabetes. Studies of skeletal muscle from women with PCOS have demonstrated a post-binding defect rather than a receptor defect

in insulin signal transduction.[24] The insulin signaling defect in PCOS appears to be a selective insulin resistance, affecting the metabolic but not the mitogenic actions of insulin.[25] Therefore, insulin may continuously enhance ovarian steroidogenesis despite the systemic insulin resistance due to defects in insulin-mediated glucose metabolism.[26] Insulin also contributes to increased adrenal androgen production in PCOS, by augmenting adrenal sensitivity to adrenocorticotropin hormone.[12]

Diabetes and its precursor, *glucose intolerance*, using World Health Organization criteria, are more prevalent (7% and 40%, respectively) in women with PCOS compared with that in the general population.[27] In vivo studies in PCOS have shown both reduced insulin-mediated glucose disposal determined by the hyperinsulinemic euglycemic clamp method,[28] and impaired beta cell function, which are independent of obesity.[29] Obesity has a synergistic negative influence on insulin action by exaggerating hepatic insulin resistance in PCOS.[23]

Obesity has been recognized as one of the prominent features of PCOS since the original description of this condition by Stein and Leventhal in 1935.[30] Even though obesity has been reported in as many as 50% in women with PCOS,[31] not all women with PCOS are obese and not all obese women have PCOS, possibly due to underlying genetic differences in etiology. Obese women with PCOS are more likely to develop type 2 diabetes (5 fold),[27] hypertriglyceridemia,[32] and a high systolic blood pressure[32] compared with nonobese women with PCOS.

Clinical Discussion

Applications of insulin sensitizer therapy to the treatment of PCOS

Considering the role of insulin resistance in the pathogenesis of PCOS, insulin sensitizers in addition to weight loss can improve both the metabolic and reproductive features of PCOS. Both, metformin and thiazolidinediones lower insulin levels; however, they do so by fundamentally different mechanisms of action, which potentially can be employed to confer additive effects when administration of metformin as single agent is not satisfactorily effective.

Metformin belongs to the family of biguanides that increases insulin-stimulated glucose utilization by up to 50% in subjects with type 2 diabetes,[33] or normoglycemic insulin resistance[34] without any risk of hypoglycemia. The mechanism of action of metformin is not entirely understood, but it seems to lower basal hepatic glucose production since the observed improved glucose tolerance following metformin treatment is associated with only a modest reduction in plasma insulin levels[35] and a modest improvement in the glucose disposal rate.[36] Insignificant reduction in body weight has been found in patients with diabetes who were treated with metformin, mostly due to reduced calorie intake.[37]

Thiazolidinediones, on the other hand, activate nuclear peroxisome proliferator-activated receptor gamma (PPAR-γ), which is largely expressed in fat tissues and muscles, and when activated, enhances the transcription of a host of factors that promote glucose disposal. Therefore, thiazolidinediones improve glucose uptake in adipose and muscle tissues, leading to lower insulin levels in nondiabetic, insulin-resistant subjects without any hypoglycemic risk when they are used as a monotherapeutic agent.[36]

1. Metformin

Metformin, an old 'drug' that was introduced in 1957 for lowering blood sugar in patients with type 2 diabetes, has become the first line of treatment in PCOS in addition to life style interventions because of its efficacy and safety profile.

Velazquez et al.[6] were the first to investigate the therapeutic effects of metformin in PCOS. Administration of metformin 1.5 g daily for 8 weeks to 26 obese women [mean body mass index (BMI) = 29.1 kg/m^2] resulted in lower testosterone levels, as well as higher sex-hormone binding globulins (SHBG). However, these changes were associated with weight loss and decreased insulin response to oral glucose administration.[6] Later, in a randomized controlled study, 24 obese women (BMI = 34.1 kg/m^2) with PCOS were assigned to metformin (1.5 g daily) or placebo.[17] After 4–8 wk of metformin therapy, significant reductions in serum insulin, unbound testosterone and LH levels, and increased SHBG concentrations were reported, independent of weight changes. Moreover, treated women showed a reduction in 17-hydroxy progesterone (17OHP) response to GnRH stimulation, a hallmark of ovarian hyperandrogenism. Similar results were obtained when lean women with PCOS were treated with metformin, confirming that metabolic changes following metformin therapy were weight independent.[5] Likewise, studies using the euglycemic clamp technique demonstrated that metformin improved the glucose utilization rate irrespective of changes in body weight.[4,38]

Metformin may improve hyperandrogenemia

in PCOS via three different pathways: (1) improving the deranged gonadotropin secretion or (2) reducing ovarian and/or adrenal androgen production or (3) enhancing circulatory levels of SHBG. The results of studies on metformin effect on gonadotropin secretion have not been consistent, ranging from no effect,[39,40] to a positive effect.[17,41] The androgen lowering effect of metformin, indeed, may occur independent of any alteration in the LH level,[42] indicating that the reduction in plasma levels of LH is not a primary event in the reduction of ovarian androgen production induced by metformin. Metformin can improve ovarian/adrenal steroidogenesis by enhancing insulin sensitivity considering the major pathophysiologic role of insulin resistance in glandular androgen production. However, a direct effect of metformin on ovarian steroidogenesis cannot be excluded. Ovarian theca-like tumor cells treated with metformin (50 μM and 200 μM) displayed reduced expression of steroidogenic acute regulatory protein, the rate-limiting step in steroid hormone production.[43] Moreover, metformin (various concentrations ranging from 0.001 μM to 1 μM) was able to decrease estradiol and progesterone production in cultured granulosa cells, as well as androstenedione production from theca cells.[44] Many studies,[5,17,45,46] though not all,[4,39,42,47] have shown increased SHBG levels following metformin therapy that can contribute to its androgen lowering effect. Altogether, the mechanism by which metformin results in decreased androgen levels is mainly through reduced ovarian steroidogenesis and partially due to SHBG changes.

Improvement in insulin resistance has generally been accompanied by a significant reduction in hyperandrogenemia, and an improvement in ovarian function and menstrual cycles. The two studies that did not find changes in insulin levels failed to show any improvements in circulating levels of androgens as well.[47,48] In the first of the two studies,[48] insulin sensitivity and androgen levels in 16 women with PCOS (BMI = 29.8 kg/m^2) did not change following a 10-week treatment with metformin, 1.7 g daily. In the second study,

14 women with PCOS (BMI = 39 kg/m^2) were treated with metformin 2.5 g daily for 3 months.[47] Insulin sensitivity, measured by intravenous glucose injection, remained unchanged following metformin therapy and the response of androgen levels to leuprolide was only slightly reduced.

The conflicting outcomes may stem from the interindividual variability in the efficacy of metformin or the heterogeneity of pathogenetic mechanisms in PCOS, given that only about 50–80% of women with PCOS respond to metformin.[10,49] Besides, extreme obesity may impede the insulin lowering effect of metformin given that a very large difference in body weight in individuals whose BMI exceed 30 kg/m^2 is associated only with small differences in insulin sensitivity.[50]

Many observational small-sized studies found an improvement in menstrual cyclicity following metformin therapy,[4,41,42] which was also confirmed by few randomized controlled studies.[39,51] However, not all women responded favorably to metformin. Metformin administration (1.5 g daily for 6 months) in a randomized control trial, resulted in an increased frequency of menstrual cycles by 50%, of which about 80% were ovulatory, determined by luteal progesterone levels. Subjects whose menstrual cyclicity did not improve on treatment were found to have lower insulin levels, higher androstenedione, and more severe menstrual abnormalities at baseline compared with those who responded to metformin.[39] A similar increased frequency of ovulation rates was reported in another randomized control study, in which 94 anovulatory women with polycystic ovaries were assigned to metformin (1.5 g daily for 12–14 weeks) or placebo. In the subgroup analysis, women who did not respond to metformin were found to have higher testosterone levels and lower SHBG levels, but similar glucose and insulin levels (fasting and in response to an oral glucose load) compared to those who responded. A review of most cohort and randomized controlled trials indicates that metformin improves ovulatory cycles by 50%, which was not improved further by extending the duration of therapy (>3 months). Likewise, metformin therapy benefits infertile women with

PCOS by regulating their menstrual cycles.[52] Metformin seems to have the most favorable impact on the hormonal profile and reproductive features of those women with PCOS, in whom insulin resistance plays a major pathogenetic role in anovulation. Effectiveness of metformin may depend upon the individual's body weight, leading to a higher therapeutic failure rate in women with PCOS who are morbidly obese.

2. Thiazolidinediones

Troglitazone, the first thiazolidinedione to be released for clinical use, enhanced insulin sensitivity and SHBG levels in PCOS women as well as decreased testosterone concentrations without any change in body weight, leading to resumption of ovulation and improved hirsutism. However, it was withdrawn in 2000 because of its hepatotoxicity.[7,8] Clinical data are emerging regarding the utility of newer thiazolidinediones, pioglitazone and rosiglitazone in PCOS, as the second-line treatment alternative to metformin, or as part of a combined regimen with other therapeutic agents, such as metformin, antiandrogen agents, or oral contraceptives. Pioglitazone-treated women are reported to have an improved hormonal profile comparable to that reported in metformin-treated women,[53] and superior to that found in the placebo group,[54] despite the weight gain in the pioglitazone group. Thiazolidinediones improve hyperandrogenemia and ovulation rates by direct effects on ovarian cells,[55] as well as by improving insulin sensitivity, which in turn, enhances ovarian[56]/adrenal[57] steroidogenesis and increases SHBG levels.[53,54]

Weight gain is one of the main adverse effects of thiazolidinedione treatment; nonetheless, pioglitazone modifies visceral fat to subcutaneous fat depots, offering favorable metabolic effects irrespective of the weight gain.[58]

3. Combination of metformin and thiazolidinediones with focus on pioglitazone

Combination therapy of metformin and thiazolidinediones can hypothetically enhance the endocrine effect of each of the two compounds, given that they have different mechanisms of action on insulin sensitivity.

Our group tested this hypothesis by administration of pioglitazone (45 mg daily) as an additional therapeutic agent to women who did not respond adequately to metformin therapy (2.5 g daily for 12 months).[10] Metformin-treated women whose weight, androgen profile (androstenedione, testosterone, and dehydroepiandrostenedione sulfate (DHEAS), indices of insulin secretion and insulin resistance and/or menstrual cyclicity, did not significantly improve compared to pre-treatment baseline values, were considered as non-responders. Non-responders (N = 13) were heavier and had lower fasting insulin and higher SHBG and androstenedione concentrations pre-treatment compared to responders (N = 26). On comparing the 12-month metformin therapy with the 10-month combination therapy (pioglitazone and metformin), the non-responder group displayed improved SHBG, DHEAS, fasting insulin, glucose, and HDL levels regardless of a steady weight. Subsequent comparison of endocrine changes during the 12-month metformin-only treatment program with metformin plus pioglitazone treatment in a larger group of non-responders (N = 41) showed similar results despite an increased body weight.[9] Approximately 80% of subjects were obese (BMI> 30 kg/m^2), of whom 45% had a BMI >40 kg/m^2. During metformin therapy, menstrual cyclicity mildly increased following 3 months of treatment and remained stable for the first year, and then increased further to about two-fold following 6 months treatment with metformin and pioglitazone. This level remained significantly elevated throughout the study period (Fig. 32.2).

Rosiglitazone, either alone, or in combination with metformin, like pioglitazone is useful as a second choice therapy in women with PCOS.[59–61]

Conclusion

To date, there is growing, yet insufficient understanding of the pathophysiology, long-term

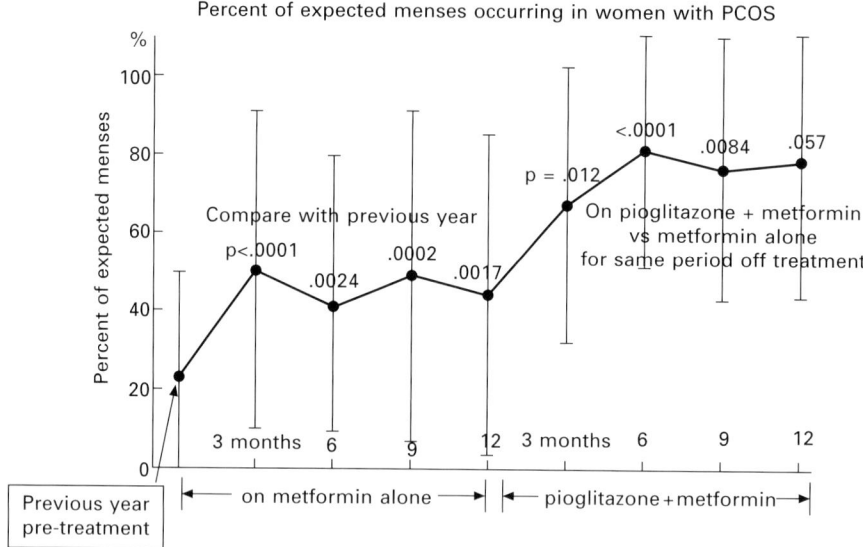

Figure 32.2   Frequency of menstrual cycles in women with PCOS who did not optimally respond to metformin therapy as a single agent.

health consequences and the right therapy for women with PCOS. Insulin resistance, as a result of genetic and lifestyle factors, is involved in the pathogenesis, metabolic and clinical features, and the long-term implications of PCOS in a majority of patients. Thus, therapeutic strategies targeting insulin resistance improve clinical features and may reduce the long-term sequelae of PCOS, including diabetes. In addition to lifestyle modifications, metformin has been used as the first line therapy in women with PCOS who are insulin resistant or have diabetes, and a second choice therapy for infertility, and in women with oligomenorrhea in order to regulate menstrual cyclicity. In obese women, who may not optimally respond to metformin, the addition of pioglitazone to metformin improves insulin resistance, and consequently menstrual cyclicity and androgen profile.

References

1. Achard EC, Thiers J. Le virilisme pilaire et son association à l'insuffisance glycotique (diabète des femmes à barbe). Bulletin de l'Académie Nationale de Médecine 1921; 86: 51–56.

2. Burghen GA, Givens JR, Kitabchi AE. Correlation of hyperandrogenism with hyperinsulinism in polycystic ovarian disease. *J Clin Endocrinol Metab* 1980; 50: 113–6.

3. Kiddy DS, Hamilton-Fairley D, Bush A, et al. Improvement in endocrine and ovarian function during dietary treatment of obese women with polycystic ovary syndrome. *Clin Endocrinol (Oxf)* 1992; 36: 105–11.

4. Morin-Papunen LC, Koivunen RM, Ruokonen A, Martikainen HK. Metformin therapy improves the menstrual pattern with minimal endocrine and metabolic effects in women with polycystic ovary syndrome. *Fertil Steril* 1998; 69: 691–696.

5. Nestler JE, Jakubowicz DJ. Lean women with polycystic ovary syndrome respond to insulin reduction with decreases in ovarian P450c17 alpha activity and serum androgens. *J Clin Endocrinol Metab* 1997; 82: 4075–4079.

6. Velazquez EM, Mendoza S, Hamer T, Sosa F, Glueck CJ. Metformin therapy in polycystic ovary syndrome reduces hyperinsulinemia, insulin resistance, hyperandrogenemia, and systolic blood pressure, while facilitating normal menses and pregnancy. *Metabolism* 1994; 43: 647–654.

7. Azziz R, Ehrmann D, Legro RS, et al. Troglitazone improves ovulation and hirsutism in the polycystic ovary syndrome: a multicenter, double blind, placebo-controlled trial. *J Clin Endocrinol Metab* 2001; 86: 1626–1632.

8. Dunaif A, Scott D, Finegood D, Quintana B, Whitcomb R. The insulin-sensitizing agent troglitazone improves metabolic and reproductive abnormalities in the polycystic ovary syndrome. *J Clin Endocrinol Metab* 1996; 81: 3299–3306.

9. Aregawi D, Salehi M, Agloria M, Winiarska M, Sieve L, Wang P, Glueck CJ. Success of metformin-pioglitazone in resolving endocrinopathy and insulin resistance-hyperinsulinemia in 41 women with polycystic ovary syndrome. *J Invest Med* 2006; In Press (Abstract).

10. Glueck CJ, Moreira A, Goldenberg N, Sieve L, Wang P. Pioglitazone and metformin in obese women with polycystic ovary syndrome not optimally responsive to metformin. *Hum Reprod* 2003; 18: 1618–1625.

11. Marshall JC, Eagleson CA. Neuroendocrine aspects of polycystic ovary syndrome. *Endocrinol Metab Clin North Am* 1999; 28: 295–324.

12. Rosenfield RL. Ovarian and adrenal function in polycystic ovary syndrome. *Endocrinol Metab Clin North Am* 1999; 28: 265–293.

13. Pastor CL, Griffin-Korf ML, Aloi JA, Evans WS, Marshall JC. Polycystic ovary syndrome: evidence for reduced sensitivity of the gonadotropin-releasing hormone pulse generator to inhibition by estradiol and progesterone. *J Clin Endocrinol Metab* 1998; 83: 582–590.

14. Daniels TL, Berga SL. Resistance of gonadotropin releasing hormone drive to sex steroid-induced suppression in hyperandrogenic anovulation. *J Clin Endocrinol Metab* 1997; 82: 4179–4183.

15. Nelson VL, Qin Kn KN, Rosenfield RL, et al. The biochemical basis for increased testosterone production in theca cells propagated from patients with polycystic ovary syndrome. *J Clin Endocrinol Metab* 2001; 86: 5925–5933.

16. Franks S, Gilling-Smith C, Watson H, Willis D. Insulin action in the normal and polycystic ovary. *Endocrinol Metab Clin North Am* 1999; 28: 361–378.

17. Nestler JE, Jakubowicz DJ. Decreases in ovarian cytochrome P450c17 alpha activity and serum free testosterone after reduction of insulin secretion in polycystic ovary syndrome. *N Engl J Med* 1996; 335: 617–623.

18. Patel K, Coffler MS, Dahan MH, et al. Increased luteinizing hormone secretion in women with polycystic ovary syndrome is unaltered by prolonged insulin infusion. *J Clin Endocrinol Metab* 2003; 88: 5456–5461.

19. Dunaif A, Graf M. Insulin administration alters gonadal steroid metabolism independent of changes in gonadotropin secretion in insulin-resistant women with the polycystic ovary syndrome. *J Clin Invest* 1989; 83: 23–29.

20. Adashi EY, Hsueh AJ, Yen SS. Insulin enhancement of luteinizing hormone and follicle-stimulating hormone release by cultured pituitary cells. *Endocrinology* 1981; 108: 1441–1449.

21. Nestler JE, Barlascini CO, Matt DW, et al. Suppression of serum insulin by diazoxide reduces serum testosterone levels in obese women with polycystic ovary syndrome. *J Clin Endocrinol Metab* 1989; 68: 1027–1032.

22. Dunaif A, Graf M, Mandeli J, Laumas V, Dobrjansky A. Characterization of groups of hyperandrogenic women with acanthosis nigricans, impaired glucose tolerance, and/or hyperinsulinemia. *J Clin Endocrinol Metab* 1987; 65: 499–507.

23. Dunaif A, Segal KR, Shelley DR, Green G, Dobrjansky A, Licholai T. Evidence for distinctive and intrinsic defects in insulin action in polycystic ovary syndrome. *Diabetes* 1992; 41: 1257–1266.

24. Dunaif A, Wu X, Lee A, Diamanti-Kandarakis E. Defects in insulin receptor signaling in vivo in the polycystic ovary syndrome (PCOS). *Am J Physiol Endocrinol Metab* 2001; 281: E392–399.

25. Book CB, Dunaif A. Selective insulin resistance in the polycystic ovary syndrome. *J Clin Endocrinol Metab* 1999; 84: 3110–3116.

26. Barbieri RL, Makris A, Randall RW, Daniels G, Kistner RW, Ryan KJ. Insulin stimulates androgen accumulation in incubations of ovarian stroma obtained from women with hyperandrogenism. *J Clin Endocrinol Metab* 1986; 62: 904–910.

27. Legro RS, Kunselman AR, Dodson WC, Dunaif A. Prevalence and predictors of risk for type 2 diabetes mellitus and impaired glucose tolerance in polycystic ovary syndrome: a prospective, controlled study in 254 affected women. *J Clin Endocrinol Metab* 1999; 84: 165–169.

28. Dunaif A, Segal KR, Futterweit W, Dobrjansky A. Profound peripheral insulin resistance, independent of obesity, in polycystic ovary syndrome. *Diabetes* 1989; 38: 1165–1174.

29. Dunaif A, Finegood DT. Beta-cell dysfunction independent of obesity and glucose intolerance in the polycystic ovary syndrome. *J Clin Endocrinol Metab* 1996; 81: 942–947.

30. Stein IF, Leventhal ML. Amenorrhea associated with bilateral polycystic ovaries. *Am J Obstet Gynecol* 1935; 29: 181–191.

31. Carmina E, Legro RS, Stamets K, Lowell J, Lobo RA. Difference in body weight between American and Italian women with polycystic ovary syndrome:

influence of the diet. *Hum Reprod* 2003; 18: 2289–2293.

32. Conway GS, Agrawal R, Betteridge DJ, Jacobs HS. Risk factors for coronary artery disease in lean and obese women with the polycystic ovary syndrome. *Clin Endocrinol (Oxf)* 1992; 37: 119–125.

33. Prager R, Schernthaner G, Graf H. Effect of metformin on peripheral insulin sensitivity in non insulin dependent diabetes mellitus. *Diabete Metab* 1986; 12: 346–350.

34. Widen EI, Eriksson JG, Groop LC. Metformin normalizes nonoxidative glucose metabolism in insulin-resistant normoglycemic first-degree relatives of patients with NIDDM. *Diabetes* 1992; 41: 354–358.

35. DeFronzo RA, Barzilai N, Simonson DC. Mechanism of metformin action in obese and lean noninsulin-dependent diabetic subjects. *J Clin Endocrinol Metab* 1991; 73: 1294–1301.

36. Inzucchi SE, Maggs DG, Spollett GR, et al. Efficacy and metabolic effects of metformin and troglitazone in type II diabetes mellitus. *N Engl J Med* 1998; 338: 867–872.

37. DeFronzo RA, Goodman AM. Efficacy of metformin in patients with non-insulin-dependent diabetes mellitus. The Multicenter Metformin Study Group. *N Engl J Med* 1995; 333: 541–549.

38. Diamanti-Kandarakis E, Kouli C, Tsianateli T, Bergiele A. Therapeutic effects of metformin on insulin resistance and hyperandrogenism in polycystic ovary syndrome. *Eur J Endocrinol* 1998; 138: 269–274.

39. Moghetti P, Castello R, Negri C, et al. Metformin effects on clinical features, endocrine and metabolic profiles, and insulin sensitivity in polycystic ovary syndrome: a randomized, double-blind, placebo-controlled 6-month trial, followed by open, long-term clinical evaluation. *J Clin Endocrinol Metab* 2000; 85: 139–146.

40. Unluhizarci K, Kelestimur F, Bayram F, Sahin Y, Tutus A. The effects of metformin on insulin resistance and ovarian steroidogenesis in women with polycystic ovary syndrome. *Clin Endocrinol (Oxf)* 1999; 51: 231–236.

41. Velazquez EM, Mendoza SG, Wang P, Glueck CJ. Metformin therapy is associated with a decrease in plasma plasminogen activator inhibitor-1, lipoprotein (a), and immunoreactive insulin levels in patients with the polycystic ovary syndrome. *Metabolism* 1997; 46: 454–457.

42. Pirwany IR, Yates RW, Cameron IT, Fleming R. Effects of the insulin sensitizing drug metformin on ovarian function, follicular growth and ovulation rate in obese women with oligomenorrhoea. *Hum Reprod* 1999; 14: 2963–2968.

43. Attia GR, Rainey WE, Carr BR. Metformin directly inhibits androgen production in human thecal cells. *Fertil Steril* 2001; 76: 517–524.

44. Mansfield R, Galea R, Brincat M, Hole D, Mason H. Metformin has direct effects on human ovarian steroidogenesis. *Fertil Steril* 2003; 79: 956–962.

45. Kowalska I, Kinalski M, Straczkowski M, Wolczyski S, Kinalska I. Insulin, leptin, IGF-I and insulin-dependent protein concentrations after insulin-sensitizing therapy in obese women with polycystic ovary syndrome. *Eur J Endocrinol* 2001; 144: 509–515.

46. Glueck CJ, Wang P, Fontaine R, Tracy T, Sieve-Smith L. Metformin-induced resumption of normal menses in 39 of 43 (91%) previously amenorrheic women with the polycystic ovary syndrome. *Metabolism* 1999; 48: 511–519.

47. Ehrmann DA, Cavaghan MK, Imperial J, Sturis J, Rosenfield RL, Polonsky KS. Effects of metformin on insulin secretion, insulin action, and ovarian steroidogenesis in women with polycystic ovary syndrome. *J Clin Endocrinol Metab* 1997; 82: 524–530.

48. Acbay O, Gundogdu S. Can metformin reduce insulin resistance in polycystic ovary syndrome? *Fertil Steril* 1996; 65: 946–949.

49. Kriplani A, Agarwal N. Effects of metformin on clinical and biochemical parameters in polycystic ovary syndrome. *J Reprod Med* 2004; 49: 361–367.

50. Kahn SE, Prigeon RL, McCulloch DK, et al. Quantification of the relationship between insulin sensitivity and beta-cell function in human subjects. Evidence for a hyperbolic function. *Diabetes* 1993; 42: 1663–1672.

51. Fleming R, Hopkinson ZE, Wallace AM, Greer IA, Sattar N. Ovarian function and metabolic factors in women with oligomenorrhea treated with metformin in a randomized double blind placebo-controlled trial. *J Clin Endocrinol Metab* 2002; 87: 569–574.

52. Kashyap S, Wells GA, Rosenwaks Z. Insulin-sensitizing agents as primary therapy for patients with polycystic ovarian syndrome. *Hum Reprod* 2004; 19: 2474–2483.

53. Ortega-Gonzalez C, Luna S, Hernandez L, et al. Responses of serum androgen and insulin resistance to metformin and pioglitazone in obese, insulin-resistant women with polycystic ovary syndrome. *J Clin Endocrinol Metab* 2005; 90: 1360–1365.

54. Brettenthaler N, De Geyter C, Huber PR, Keller U.

Effect of the insulin sensitizer pioglitazone on insulin resistance, hyperandrogenism, and ovulatory dysfunction in women with polycystic ovary syndrome. *J Clin Endocrinol Metab* 2004; 89: 3835–3840.

55. Seto-Young D, Paliou M, Schlosser J, et al. Direct thiazolidinedione action in the human ovary: insulin-independent and insulin-sensitizing effects on steroidogenesis and insulin-like growth factor binding protein-1 production. *J Clin Endocrinol Metab* 2005; 90: 6099–6105.

56. Coffler MS, Patel K, Dahan MH, Yoo RY, Malcom PJ, Chang RJ. Enhanced granulosa cell responsiveness to follicle-stimulating hormone during insulin infusion in women with polycystic ovary syndrome treated with pioglitazone. *J Clin Endocrinol Metab* 2003; 88: 5624–5631.

57. Guido M, Romualdi D, Suriano R, et al. Effect of pioglitazone treatment on the adrenal androgen response to corticotrophin in obese patients with polycystic ovary syndrome. *Hum Reprod* 2004; 19: 534–539.

58. Miyazaki Y, Mahankali A, Matsuda M, et al. Effect of pioglitazone on abdominal fat distribution and insulin sensitivity in type 2 diabetic patients. *J Clin Endocrinol Metab* 2002; 87: 2784–2791.

59. Baillargeon JP, Jakubowicz DJ, Iuorno MJ, Jakubowicz S, Nestler JE. Effects of metformin and rosiglitazone, alone and in combination, in nonobese women with polycystic ovary syndrome and normal indices of insulin sensitivity. *Fertil Steril* 2004; 82: 893–902.

60. Dereli D, Dereli T, Bayraktar F, Ozgen AG, Yilmaz C. Endocrine and metabolic effects of rosiglitazone in non-obese women with polycystic ovary disease. *Endocr J* 2005; 52: 299–308.

61. Stout DL, Fugate SE. Thiazolidinediones for treatment of polycystic ovary syndrome. *Pharmacotherapy* 2005; 25: 244–252.

33

Improvement in the Decreased Endogenous Dopaminergic Tone in Obese Insulin Resistant Women with Polycystic Ovary Syndrome following Pioglitazone or Metformin Administration

Carlos Ortega-González, Adalberto Parra

Summary

A deficiency of hypothalamic dopamine (DA) has been implicated in moderate hyperprolactinemia, frequently detected in a subset of obese women with polycystic ovary syndrome (PCOS) and insulin resistance (IR). Because of the known interplay between prolactin (PRL) and insulin, we investigated whether prolonged administration of insulin sensitizing drugs, pioglitazone or metformin could induce changes in the DA tone in 34 obese women with PCOS (21–35 years of age), and whether this was associated with modifications in IR. Patients were randomly allocated to receive pioglitazone (group 1, n = 17) 30 mg/day or metformin (group 2, n = 17) 850 mg three times a day for 6 months. Before, and 6 months after administration of the drugs, all the women were identically studied, including a clinical evaluation, a 2 hr oral glucose tolerance test (2h-OGTT) for serum glucose and insulin determinations, and a week later, a 2 hr intravenous metoclopramide test (10 mg bolus) for prolactin (PRL) determination. The area under the insulin curve (AUC-insulin), the indexes of insulin sensitivity [quantitative check index for insulin sensitivity (QUICKI) and fasting glucose insulin ratio] and homeostasis model assessment for insulin resistance (HOMA-IR), along with the AUC-PRL were calculated. Body weight and body mass index did not changed significantly during the study and the severity of the hirsutism significantly decreased. After 6 months of treatment, there were no significant differences in either group in basal PRL concentrations, however and the AUC-PRL significantly increased in a similar fashion in both the groups. On the contrary, fasting serum insulin concentrations and the AUC-insulin significantly decreased by the end of the trial. At baseline, AUC-PRL had a significant negative correlation with fasting insulin and HOMA-IR index, and a positive correlation with the QUICKI index. At the end of the study, AUC-PRL best correlated with the HOMA-IR index in a negative fashion. It is suggested that administration of either pioglitazone or metformin for 6 months induced an amelioration of the insulin resistance milieu in these obese women with PCOS and IR, which was associated with a significant improvement in their endogenous hypothalamic DA tone.

Rationale

It is known that the administration of dopamine (DA) or bromocriptine, a dopamine agonist, to women with polycystic ovary syndrome (PCOS) may decrease their serum luteinizing hormone (LH)[1,2] concentrations and also restore the cyclic ovarian function.[3] Also, in a subset of women with PCOS, mild to moderate hyperprolactinemia is frequently detected.[4] These findings have suggested that some women with PCOS may have a disruption of the neuroendocrine mechanisms, particularly, a deficiency of hypothalamic DA, which is normally responsible for the release of gonadotropins and prolactin (PRL).[5–7]

In addition, a stimulatory effect of PRL on pancreatic islet cell division and insulin secretion,[8] as well as the presence of PRL receptors in islets of Langerhans has been demonstrated.[9] Finally, DA has also been implicated in the regulation of insulin secretion.[9]

Introduction

Polycystic ovary syndrome (PCOS) is the most frequent endocrine disorder in women of reproductive age with an estimated frequency between 4% and 7%,[10] and is characterized by chronic anovulation and/or hyperandrogenism and/or polycystic ovaries by ultrasound in the absence of hypothyroidism, hyperprolactinemia, late-onset congenital virilizing adrenal hyperplasia and Cushing's syndrome.[11]

The existence of insulin resistance (IR) and secondary hyperinsulinemia, mainly in obese women with PCOS,[12] are considered as key factors responsible for the hyperandrogenism.[12,13] Because IR is a cardinal feature of PCOS, the long-term administration of insulin sensitizing drugs, such as metformin and thiazolidinediones (TZDs) has become a basic therapeutic approach in women with this disorder.[14] Up to now, there are no data on the possible influence of either drug on the hypothalamic DA tone in obese women with PCOS, which is an important aspect since a hypothalamic deficiency of DA,[7] has been implicated in mild hyperprolactinemia, frequently observed in women with PCOS.[4] The suggestion of an altered DA modulation of PRL secretion,[2,7,15] is supported by the recent finding of a low DA hypothalamic tone with increased PRL bioactivity in obese hyperinsulinemic women with PCOS.[16] This issue becomes more interesting because DA also influences insulin secretion;[17,18] PRL receptors have been unequivocally identified in islets of Langerhans,[9] and this hormone has a potent stimulatory effect on pancreatic islet β cell division.[8]

Therefore, we aimed to analyze whether prolonged administration of metformin or a TZD compound–pioglitazone- to obese women with PCOS and IR could induce changes in the hypothalamic DA tone and whether or not these changes could be correlated with modifications in insulin sensitivity.

Insulin resistance is most frequently, but not exclusively, associated with obesity, and the precise mechanisms involved in this central abnormality have not been fully elucidated. Importantly, women with PCOS and IR have a greater risk for carbohydrate intolerance and type 2 diabetes mellitus (type 2 DM)[19,20] among other metabolic abnormalities.[21] Although type 2 DM and PCOS share in common the existence of insulin resistance, hyperandrogenism of variable degree is always present in the latter making a crucial difference.

In a recent report,[16] an increased PRL bioactivity was found only in obese PCOS women with the highest basal and glucose-stimulated insulin concentrations. This finding may have clinical relevance, since PRL has a proven stimulatory effect on insulin secretion and pancreatic β cell proliferation.[8,9] Thus, hyperinsulinemia could be related not only to obesity but also to moderately elevated circulating concentrations of bioactive PRL. In this sense, it is interesting to note that the DA system has been reported to influence the regulation of insulin secretion.[17,18] In brief, PRL could play a role in the development of hyperinsulinemia in a subset of women with PCOS, especially in those who are overweight.

Under physiological conditions, basal production of pituitary PRL is mainly controlled by tonic inhibitory mechanisms mediated by DA.[22] Both basal serum PRL concentrations and its response to intravenous metoclopramide, a DA blocking agent, have been considered as an indirect way to evaluate the functional level of the hypothalamic DA tone in the clinical setting.[2,23-25] In fact, a decreased PRL response to intravenous metoclopramide has been interpreted as evidence of a decreased endogenous DA tone and thus, an increased production of pituitary PRL.

On the contrary, an increased response to metoclopramide would represent an increased endogenous DA tone and consequently, a decreased production of pituitary PRL.[2,25]

Materials and Methods

Our study was conducted after the protocol was approved by the Internal Review Board and the Human Ethical Committee of The Instituto Nacional de Perinatología, México City and written informed consent was obtained from all volunteers. The study was performed according to the Declaration of Helsinki (as amended, October 2000).

Subjects

Women with PCOS (n = 34), aged 21 to 35 years without any specific treatment, consulting for hirsutism (Ferriman-Gallwey [F-G] score, > 8) and/or infertility, were first seen in the outpatient Endocrinology and Sterility Clinics of the Instituto Nacional de Perinatología (México City, México). The diagnosis of PCOS was made if at least two of the three following abnormalities were present: oligomenorrhea or amenorrhea, high serum androstenedione (> 2.9 ng/mL) and/or free testosterone (free T) (> 3.0 pg/mL) concentrations, and/or polycystic ovaries by ultrasound.[11] All women had a body mass index (BMI) > 28 Kg/m^2, acanthosis nigricans, fasting insulin levels (> 16 mUI/mL) and a fasting glucose/insulin (G/I) ratio < 4.5.[26] Using specific

laboratory tests, the diagnosis of type 2 DM, hyperprolactinemia, thyroid disorders, late-onset congenital adrenal hyperplasia and Cushing's syndrome were excluded. Six months prior to the study, none of the women had been taking any drugs known to interfere with PRL secretion. Unsuspected pregnancy was ruled out in all participant women prior to entry into the study.

Protocol of study

Patients were randomly allocated to receive either pioglitazone (n = 17) (group 1) (Zactos ®, Eli Lilly de México, S.A. de C.V., México) 30 mg/day, single oral dose, during 24 weeks or metformin (n = 17) (group 2) (Ficonax ®, Laboratorios Pisa, S.A. de C.V., México City) 850 mg three times daily during 24 weeks. No changes in their daily caloric intake or physical exercise pattern were recorded throughout the study. Pioglitazone or metformin were started after the results of the basal (biochemical and hormonal) studies were available (usually 2 weeks).

Clinical and hormonal evaluation

At basal conditions and six months after initiation of treatment, all patients underwent a similar evaluation, which included: height, weight, BMI, waist/hip (W/H) ratio and hirsutism (F-G) score. Following a 10- to 12 hour overnight fast, between 0800 and 0830 h, a 2 h-oral glucose tolerance test (OGTT) was performed (75 g oral glucose load) and non-heparinized blood samples were obtained at 0, 30, 60, 90 and 120 minutes for the duplicate determinations of serum glucose and insulin concentrations. A week later and after a 10-to 12 hour overnight fast, between 08.00 and 08.30 h, three basal non-heparinized blood samples were obtained at 15- minute intervals (30, 15, and zero minutes before metoclopramide injection) and thereafter, at 60, 90 and 120 min following a single 10 mg intravenous bolus of metoclopramide (an antidopaminergic drug) (Pramotil ®, Laboratorios Pisa, S.A. de C.V.,

México City). All blood samples were centrifuged at 1000 g within the next 30 minutes and the serum was kept frozen at $-20°$ C until assayed.

Methods

BMI was calculated using the equation: weight (kg)/height (meters^2) and the waist and hip circumferences were measured to the nearest centimeter with a soft tape according to WHO criteria. Hirsutism was recorded using the F-G score, obtained by a single observer (COG); a score > 8 was considered as positive for hirsutism.

PRL and insulin concentrations were measured in duplicate using commercially available immunoradiometric and radioimmunoassay kits, respectively, (Diagnostic Products Corporation, Los Angeles, CA, USA). The intra- and interassay coefficients of variation were < 6.0% and < 7.8%, respectively for both the hormones. Plasma glucose was measured by a glucose oxidase method (GOD-PAP, Diagnostica Merck, México City, México) using an automatic enzymatic autoanalyzer (Vitalab Scientific, Dieren, The Netherlands). The intra- and interassay coefficients of variation were < 2.5% and < 3.9%, respectively.

Based on serum glucose and insulin concentrations, both fasting and during the 2h-OGTT, the following parameters were calculated:

(a) Homeostasis model assessment for insulin-resistance (HOMA-IR)[27] = fasting serum insulin (µU/mL) × fasting serum glucose (mmol/L)/22.5.

(b) Insulin sensitivity index (QUICKI)[28] = (1/ [log (I_0) + log (G_0)]), where I_0 = fasting serum insulin (µU/mL) concentration and G_0 = fasting serum glucose (mg/dL) concentration.

(c) Fasting glucose-insulin (G/I) ratio[13,26] = fasting serum glucose concentration (mg/dl)/fasting serum insulin concentration (µU/mL).

(d) Area under the glucose curve (AUC -glucose) and area under the insulin curve (AUC-insulin) using a trapezoidal method.[29]

Additionally, the area under the prolactin curve (AUC-PRL) during the 2-h intravenous metoclopramide test was calculated also using a trapezoidal method.[29]

Statistical analysis

Descriptive statistics and frequencies for all variables were performed. Within and between group differences among the variables studied were assessed by using one-way ANOVA and the paired Student's t test. Correlations between variables were analyzed using the Pearson's correlation coefficient. Statistics were analyzed using the SPSS software, version 11.0. Values in the text and figures represent mean ± S.E.M.

A 'P' value < 0.05 was statistically significant.

Results

Before treatment, women in both groups, pioglitazone and metformin treatment groups, had a similar age (28.8 ± 0.9 and 28.6 ± 0.7 years, respectively), BMI (32.3 ± 1.1 and 34.4 ± 1.7 kg/m^2, respectively), and W/H ratio (0.88 ± 0.02 and 0.86 ± 0.01, respectively). No extrapyramidal signs were recorded in any patient during the intravenous metoclopramide test and significant changes in serum transaminase levels were not recorded during the trial. Following completion of the study, BMI and W/H ratio did not changed significantly and the F-G score showed a similar decrease in both groups (10.4 ± 0.62 and 11.0 ± 0.85, respectively) (P = 0.04), (Table 33.1).

Intravenous metoclopramide test

Fasting serum PRL concentrations (mean value of three basal samples: –30, –15 and 0 minutes) in groups 1 and 2 were similar before (9.3 ± 1.1 ng/mL and 7.3 ± 1.3 ng/mL, respectively) and after 6 months of treatment (10.6 ± 1.1 ng/mL and 7.9 ± 0.7 ng/mL, respectively) with pioglitazone and metformin respectively.

The AUC-PRL before initiation of the drug administration subsequently increased after 6 months of treatment with either pioglitazone (P = 0.007) or metformin (P = 0.003). No significant

Table 33.1   Demographic and biochemical parameters in obese PCOS women at baseline and at the end of study (Mean + S.E.M.)

	Group 1 Pioglitazone			Group 2 Metformin		
	Baseline	6 Months	P value*	Baseline	6 Months	P value*
n	17	17		17	17	
Age (years)	28.8 ± 0.9					
Body weight (Kg)	79.1 ± 2.6	82.3 ± 3.0	> 0.05	83.8 ± 4.0	81.8 ± 4.0	> 0.05
BMI (Kg/m^2)	32.3 ± 1.1	34.0 ± 1.2	> 0.05	34.4 ± 1.7	32.3 ± 1.7	> 0.05
Waist/Hip ratio	0.88 ± 0.02	0.86 ± 0.02	> 0.05	0.86 ± 0.01	0.85 ± 0.01	> 0.05
Ferriman-Gallwey Score	15.4 ± 0.87	10.4 ± 0.62	> 0.05	16.4 ± 0.95	11.0 ± 0.85	> 0.05
Fasting Glucose (mg/dL)	92.5 ± 2.55	90.8 ± 2.1	> 0.05	94.7 ± 3.0	91.0 ± 2.5	> 0.05
Fasting Insulin (μUI/mL)	31.1 ± 1.1	12.0 ± 1.8	0.001	31.1 ± 1.6	18.9 ± 4.0	0.013
Fasting Glucose/Insulin ratio	3.02 ± 0.14	9.84 ± 1.20	0.002	3.15 ± 0.16	9.41 ± 1.69	0.002
HOMA-IR index	7.03 ± 0.29	2.69 ± 0.41	0.001	7.31 ± 0.57	4.41 ± 1.0	0.026
QUICKI index	0.29 ± 0.001	0.34 ± 0.007	0.001	0.29 ± 0.002	0.33 ± 0.01	0.002
Fasting Prolactin (ng/mL)	9.35 ± 1.13	10.68 ± 1.16	> 0.05	7.36 ± 1.29	7.87 ± 0.70	> 0.05

*P values represent intragroup differences for 6 months compared to corresponding baseline.

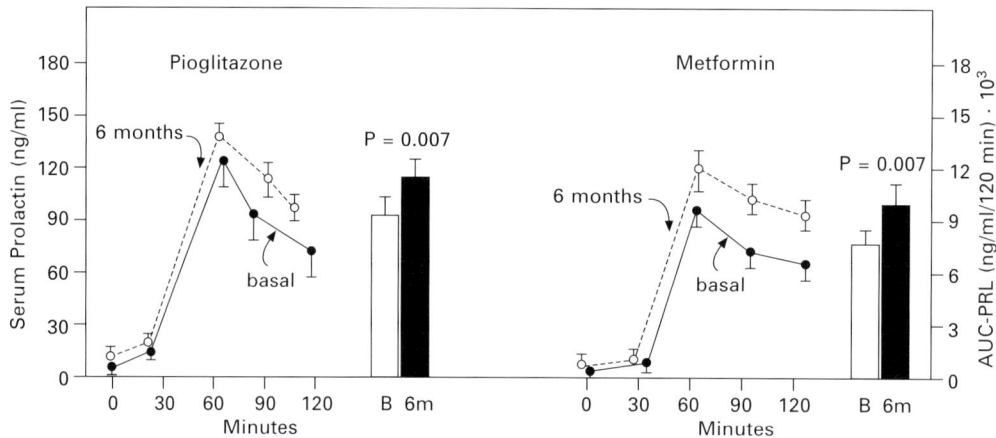

Figure 33.1   Effect of pioglitazone (PIO) and metformin (MET) on serum prolactin concentrations during the intravenous metoclopramide test, before (continuous line) and six months after (dotted line) administration of either drug. The area under the prolactin curve (AUC-PRL) was also calculated for each drug before (open bars) and after (black bars) six months of its administration. Values represent mean ± SEM.

differences were observed between the groups (Fig 33.1).

2h-oral glucose tolerance test

At baseline, fasting serum insulin concentrations were similarly above the normal in both groups, with a marked decrease thereafter (Fig. 33.2). Also, the AUC-insulin significantly decreased after six months of treatment with either drug (Fig. 33.3) without significant differences between the two groups. Before treatment, fasting serum glucose concentrations were normal in both groups, without significant intra – or intergroup

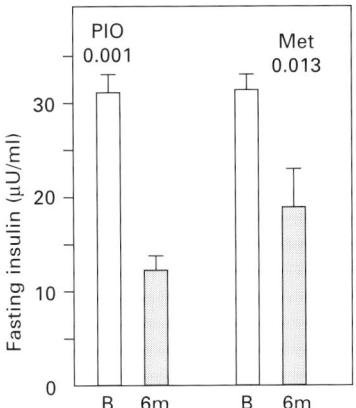
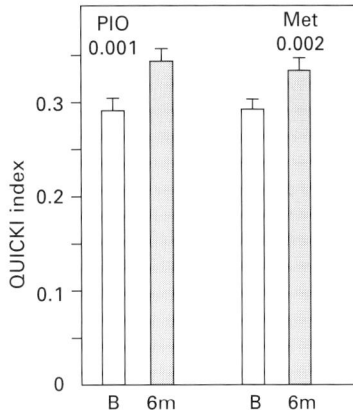

Figure 33.2   Effect of pioglitazone (PIO) and metformin (MET) on fasting serum insulin concentrations and on the quantitative insulin sensitivity check index (QUICKI). Open bars: Before drug administration. Black bars: six months after administration of either drug. Values represent mean ± SEM.

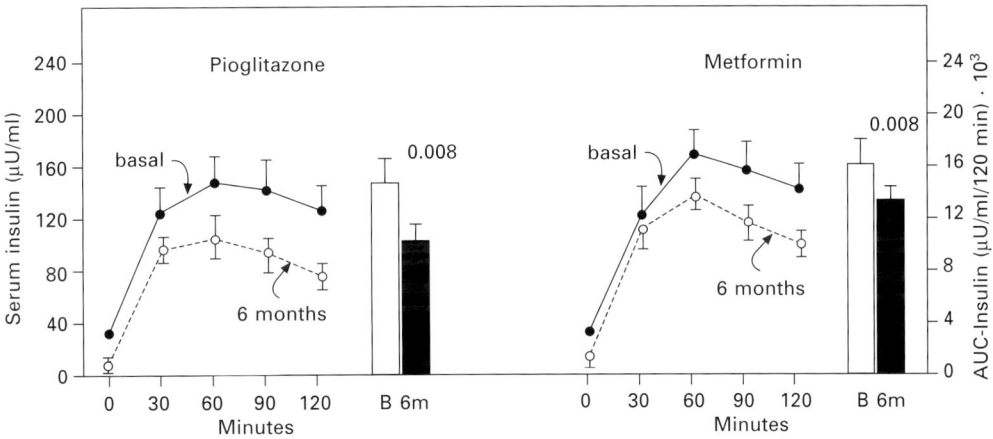

Figure 33.3   Effect of pioglitazone (PIO) and metformin (MET) on serum insulin concentrations during a 2 hour- oral glucose tolerance test, before (continuous line) and after (dotted line) six months after administration of either drug. The area under the insulin curve (AUC-insulin) was also calculated for each drug, before (open bars) and after (black bars) six months of its administration. Values represent mean ± SEM.

differences by the end of the study. The AUC-glucose during the 2h-OGTT showed a mild decrease in both groups by the end of the trial, with a borderline statistical significance ($P = 0.05$) (Data not shown). After 6 months of treatment with either drug the indices of insulin sensitivity, QUICKI (Fig. 33.2) and G/I ratio (Fig. 33.4) showed a similar and marked increment above the pretreatment values, but without significant differences between the groups. On the contrary,

the insulin resistance index (HOMA-IR) at baseline was nearly identical in both groups with a subsequent decrease in both groups, although more pronounced in group one (Fig. 33.4).

Correlations

After 6 months of treatment with either drug the AUC-PRL and the AUC-insulin underwent opposite changes. At baseline, AUC-PRL had a

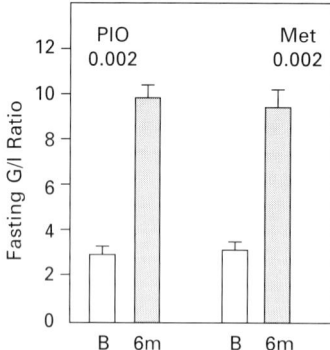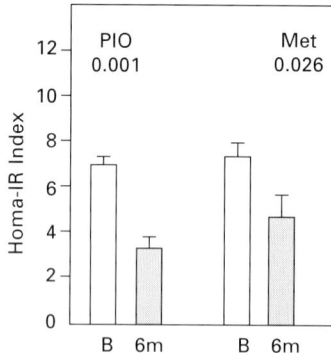

Figure 33.4   Effect of pioglitazone (PIO) and metformin (MET) on fasting glucose-insulin ratio (fasting G/I) and
on Homeostasis Model of Assessment of Insulin Resistance (HOMA-IR index). Open bars: Before drug
administration. Black bars: six months after administration of either drug. Values represent mean ± SEM.

significant negative linear correlation with fasting
insulin ($r = -0.436$, $P = 0.05$) and HOMA-IR
index ($r = -0.470$, $P = 0.05$) and a positive
linear correlation with QUICKI index ($r = 0.452$,
$P = 0.05$). At the end of the study, AUC-PRL
best correlated with the HOMA- IR index ($r = -0.360$, $P = 0.03$).

Clinical Discussion

A major feature of our results was the
demonstration that administration of both insulin
sensitizing drugs, pioglitazone and metformin
to obese, non-diabetic, PCOS women with severe
IR was associated with a significant increase in
AUC-PRL. This finding suggests that the
decreased endogenous DA tone present at baseline
(leading to an increased pituitary PRL production)
in these obese PCOS women, as has already been
reported,[16] subsequently increased (and
consequently, the pituitary PRL production
decreased) in association with the administration
of drugs, pioglitazone and metformin.
Interestingly, this increased endogenous DA tone
occurred in the face of a significant decrease
both, in fasting insulin concentrations and in the
AUC-insulin during a 2h-OGTT without any
noticeable diminution in body weight.
Consequently, the AUC-PRL showed a negative
correlation with HOMA-IR index, which is an
index of IR ($r = -0.360$, $P = 0.034$).

Our results are in accordance with the proposal
of the existence of a low hypothalamic DA content
in obese women with PCOS leading to disruption
of the neuroendocrine mechanisms modulating
PRL synthesis and/or release.[5–7,30] This would
explain the moderate fasting hyperprolactinemia
seen in a subset of these women,[4] and also the
recovery of their cyclic ovarian function with
the use of bromocriptine (a dopamine agonist).
The improvement in the endogenous DA
hypothalamic tone associated with the use of either
drug could be the consequence either of an
increase in the DA concentrations in the
hypophyseal portal circulation, or to a recovered
sensitivity of the lactotrophs exposed to normal
concentrations of DA. However, the precise
mechanism(s) involved in this improvement in
the hypothalamic DA tone could not be elucidated
from our study. Nevertheless, such a finding
cannot be ascribed to an indirect effect of any
drug, since all women studied were naïve to any
specific treatment. Neither could it be related to
a decrease in the obesity degree[31] inasmuch as
body weight and BMI remained essentially
unchanged throughout the study. A possible
criticism of the general interpretation of our results
is the lack of significant differences in fasting
PRL concentrations between the baseline and the
6 months post drug studies, in the face of
significant changes in the endogenous DA tone.
This could have at least two explanations. Firstly,
the mean basal (fasting) PRL concentration was
obtained from only three fasting blood samples,

which are not truly representative of the 24-h basal PRL secretion, and secondly, the endogenous DA tone was decreased, but not completely abolished, in the baseline study.[25]

The existing evidence of the interplay between PRL and insulin, and the known influence of DA in the regulation of insulin secretion,[8,9,17,18] along with the findings of the present study (including the opposite changes observed in AUC-PRL and AUC-insulin and the negative correlations between AUC-PRL and the indices of IR suggest that: (1) changes in the hypothalamic DA tone occurred in parallel with the improvement in insulin resistance seen in these obese women with PCOS in response to either pioglitazone or metformin administration, and (2) the increased endogenous hypothalamic DA tone (leading to a decreased pituitary PRL secretion), in association with the administration of either drug, may be a factor participating in the improvement of the IR status in these women.

In primary cultures of rat preadipocytes, chronically exposed to sex hormones, androgens (testosterone and dihydrotestosterone) had an inhibitory effect upon preadipocyte differentiation while estrogens (17 β-estradiol) had a stimulatory effect on preadipocyte differentiation, with a clear evidence for sex and site-related specifications.[32] Furthermore, these modulatory effects of androgens and estrogens on preadipocyte differentiation are mediated via their own receptors inducing down-regulation or up-regulation, respectively, of the insulin-like growth factor (IGF) receptor and the peroxisome proliferator activated receptor γ2 (PPARγ2) expression. In this respect, one should keep in mind that, untreated women with PCOS have precisely low estrogen and high androgen serum concentrations. Thus, we would like to hypothesize that the latter hormonal milieu would facilitate the fat tissue accumulation, leading to increase IR and hyperinsulinemia favored by the increased endogenous PRL synthesis and/or release, secondary to the decreased endogenous hypothalamic DA tone present in a subset of obese PCOS women. This hyperinsulinemia would in turn, up-regulate the IGF receptors and

PPARγ2 expression with the subsequent increase in preadipocyte differentiation and renewed increase in fat depot, creating a self-feeding vicious cycle.

Conclusion

In summary, the use of insulin sensitizing drugs such as pioglitazone and metformin, by augmenting the hypothalamic DA tone and thus, reducing the pituitary PRL production, could contribute to the amelioration of IR and hyperinsulinemia in obese women with PCOS and therefore, the exaggerated accretion of fat deposits.

References

1. Leblanc H, Lacheling GCL, Abu-Fadil S, Yen SSC. Effects of dopamine infusion on pituitary hormone secretion in humans. *J Clin Endocrinol Metab* 1976; 43: 668–674.
2. Quigley ME, Judd SJ, Gilliand GB, Yen SSC. Effects of a dopamine antagonist on the release of gonadotropin and prolactin in normal women and in women with hyperprolactinemic anovulation. *J Clin Endocrinol Metab* 1979; 52: 231–234.
3. Polson DW, Mason HD, Franks S. Bromocriptine treatment of women with clomiphene-resistant polycystic ovary syndrome. *Clin Endocrinol* 1987; 26: 197–203.
4. Luciano AA, Chapler FK, Sherman BM. Hyperprolactinemia in polycystic ovary syndrome. *Fertil Steril* 1984; 41: 719–725.
5. Taylor AE, Mc Court B, Martin KA, et al. Determinants of abnormal gonadotropin secretion in clinically defined women with polycystic ovary syndrome. *J Clin Endocrinol Metab* 1997; 82: 2248–2256.
6. Rosenfield RL. Is polycystic ovary syndrome a neuroendocrine or an ovarian disorder? *Clin Endocrinol* 1997; 47: 423–424.
7. Velardo A, Pantalioni M, Zironi C, Zizzo G, Marrama P. Evidence of altered dopamine modulation of prolactin and thyrotropin secretion in patients with polycystic ovary syndrome. *Horm Res* 1991; 35: 4–7.
8. Sinha YN, Sorenson RL Differential effects of glycosylated and nonglycosylated prolactin on islet cell division and insulin secretion. *Proc Soc Exp Biol Med* 1993; 203: 123–126.

9. Sorenson RL, Stout LE. Prolactin receptors and JAK 2 in islets of Langerhans: an immunohistochemical analysis. *Endocrinology* 1995; 136: 4092–4098.

10. Lobo RA. What are the key features of importance in polycystic ovary syndrome? *Fertil and Steril* 2003; 80: 259–261.

11. The Rotterdam ESHRE/ASRM-sponsored PCOS consensus workshop group. Revised 2003 consensus on diagnostic criteria and long-term health risks related to polycystic ovary syndrome (PCOS). *Hum Reprod* 2004; 19: 41–47.

12. Burghen GA, Givens JR, Kitabchi AE. Correlation of hyperandrogenism with hyperinsulinemia in polycystic ovarian disease. *J Clin Endocrinol Metab* 1980; 50: 113–116.

13. Dunaif A. Insulin resistance and the polycystic ovary syndrome: mechanism and implications for pathogenesis. *Endocr Rev* 1997; 18: 774–800.

14. Baillargeon JP, Iuorno MJ, Nestler JE. Comparison of metformin and thiazolidinediones in the management of polycystic ovary syndrome. *Curr Opin Endocrinol Diab* 2002; 9: 303–311.

15. Shoupe D, Lobo RA. Evidence for altered catecholamine metabolism in polycystic ovary syndrome. *Am J Obstet Gynecol* 1984; 150: 566–571.

16. Hernández I, Parra A, Méndez I, et al. Hypothalamic dopaminergic tone and prolactin bioactivity in women with polycystic ovary syndrome. *Arch Med Res* 2000; 31: 216–222.

17. Cincotta AH, Meier AH. Bromocriptine (Ergoset) reduces body weight and improves glucose tolerance in obese subjects. *Diabetes Care* 1996; 19: 667–670.

18. Uvnas-Moberg K, Ahlenius S, Alster P, Hillegaart V. Effects of selective serotonin and dopamine agonists on plasma levels of glucose, insulin and glucagon in the rat. *Neuroendocrinol* 1996; 63: 269–274.

19. Solomon CG, Hu FB, Dunaif A, et al. Long or highly irregular menstrual cycles as a marker for risk of type 2 diabetes mellitus. JAMA, 2001; 286: 2421–2426.

20. Legro RS. Diabetes prevalence and risk factors in polycystic ovary syndrome. *Curr Opin Endocrinol Diab* 2002; 9: 451–458.

21. Legro RS. Polycystic ovary syndrome and cardiovascular disease: a premature association? *Endocr Rev* 2003; 24: 302–312.

22. Ben-Jonathan N. Dopamine: a prolactin-inhibiting hormone. *Endocr Rev* 1985; 6: 564–589.

23. Parra A, Barrón J, Sinibaldi J, Coria I, Espinosa de los Monteros A. Differences in the metoclopramide-induced prolactin release related to age at first full-term pregnancy or nulliparity *Hum Reprod* 1997; 12: 214–219.

24. Birnbacher R, Scheibenreiter S, Blau N, Bieglmayer C, Frisch H, Waldhauser F. Hyperprolactinemia, a tool in treatment control of tetrahydrobiopterin deficiency: endocrine studies in an affected girl. *Ped Res* 1998; 43: 472–477.

25. Parra A, Ramírez-Peredo J, Larrea F, et al. Decreased dopaminergic tone and increased basal bioactive prolactin in men with human immunodeficiency virus infection. *Clin Endocrinol (Oxf)* 2001; 54: 731–738.

26. Parra A, Ramírez A, Espinosa de los Monteros A. Fasting glucose/insulin ratio. An index to differentiate normo from hyperinsulinemic women with polycystic ovary syndrome. *Rev Inves Clin (Méx)* 1994; 46: 363–368.

27. Albareda M, Rodríguez-Espinosa J, Murugo M, de Leyva A, Corcoy R. Assessment of insulin sensitivity and beta -cell function from measurements in the fasting state and during and oral glucose tolerance test. *Diabetologia* 2000; 43: 1507–1511.

28. Katz A, Nambi SS, Mather K, et al. Quantitative insulin sensitivity check index: a simple, accurate method for assessing insulin sensitivity in humans. *J Clin Endocrinol Metab* 2000; 85: 2402–2410.

29. Tai MM. A mathematical model for the determination of total area under glucose tolerance and other metabolic curves. *Diabetes Care* 1994 ; 17: 152–154.

30. Taylor AE, Mc Court B, Martin KA, et al. Determinants of abnormal gonadotropin secretion in clinically defined women with polycystic ovary syndrome. *J Clin Endocrinol Metab* 1997; 82: 2248–2256.

31. Takemoto M, Morishita H, Higuchi K, Yoshida J, Aono T. Effects of body weight on responses of serum prolactin to metoclopramide and thyrotrophin releasing hormone in secondary amenorrhoeic women. *Hum Reprod* 1994; 9: 800–805.

32. Dieudonne MN, Pecquery RM, Leneven MC, Giudicelli Y. Opposite effects of androgens and estrogens on adipogenesis in rat preadipocytes: evidence for sex and site related specificities and possible involvement of insulin like growth factor 1 receptor and peroxisome proliferators activated receptor γ2. *Endocrinol* 2000; 141: 649–656.

Frequently Asked Questions

1. Which is the putative mechanism by which hyperprolactinemia could affect insulin secretion in women with PCOS?

An increase in the PRL bioactivity has been found in some women with PCOS, which represents an added stimulatory factor to insulin secretion and beta cell proliferation thus, further contributing to the hyperinsulinemia.

2. What would be the biological consequence of a decreased dopaminergic tone in the subgroup of women with PCOS?

High serum concentrations of PRL.

3. How would you interpret a decreased serum PRL response during the metoclopramide test?

It indicates the existence of a decreased endogenous dopaminergic tone and therefore, a greater endogenous release of PRL.

4. Why is the treatment with bromocriptine in some women with PCOS beneficial, and favors the recovery of regular menstrual cycles and ovulation?

Since bromocriptine is a dopaminergic agonist, it contributes to a decrease in hyperprolactinemia and simultaneously, improves the hypothalamic imbalance of neurotransmitters that also affects the pulsatile pituitary release of LH.

Induction of Ovulation

34

Aromatase Inhibitors for Ovulation Induction in Polycystic Ovary Syndrome

Malek Mansour Aghssa, Hedie Asheghan, Shahin Khazali, Maryam Bagheri

Summary

Clomiphene citrate has been used as the first line treatment for anovulatory infertility in PCOS patients for more than 40 years. The use of aromatase inhibitors for ovulation induction was proposed by Mitwally and Casper in 2001. It appears that aromatase inhibitors are as effective as clomiphene citrate in inducing ovulation, do not have any antiestrogenic side effects, result in lower serum estrogen concentrations, and are associated with better pregnancy rates with a lower incidence of multiple pregnancies than clomiphene citrate.

Our aim is to review the latest data on the use of aromatase inhibitors for this purpose and to share our experience of the use of Letrozole in 1092 anovulatory infertile patients.

Introduction

Ovulation induction (OI) drug therapy is the most widely used method for the management of patients with anovulatory infertility.[1,2] Patients eligible for ovulation induction belong either to World Health Organization (WHO) group I, which includes women with hypogonadotropic hypogonadism, or to WHO group II, in which the vast majority of the women have polycystic ovary syndrome (PCOS). Patients belonging to WHO group II constitute the majority of patients with anovulatory infertility and they are much more difficult to treat.[3,4] These women account for 90% of the cases of oligomenorrhea and around 30% of those with amenorrhea.[5,6]

Until recently, clomiphene citrate was the first choice of treatment in PCOS women.[7,8] Low dose follicle stimulating hormone (FSH) protocols were the second line of treatment. Laparoscopic ovarian drilling could be used as an alternative but not as a first choice treatment in clomiphene resistant patients. Other treatments such as pulsatile gonadotropin releasing hormone (GnRH) and GnRH agonists were hardly used in PCOS. However, in obese women with PCOS weight loss and exercise is the recommended first line of therapy.[9]

Clomiphene citrate (CC) has been widely used in the treatment of infertility since its introduction into clinical practice in 1960s.[10,11] CC results in a 60 to 80% ovulation rate and a disappointing 10 to 20% pregnancy rate per cycles.[12–18] Twenty to 25% of women are resistant to CC and do not ovulate. Furthermore, there is a discrepancy between ovulation and conception rates during CC treatment and a higher than expected incidence of miscarriage in conception cycles.[11,19–21] Peripheral anti estrogenic effects are frequently cited as a possible explanation for the relatively low pregnancy rates with CC despite the high rate of ovulation observed.[22] Prolonged endometrial estrogen receptor depletion results in the significant thinning of the endometrium. CC accumulates in the body because of its long half life,[22–26] and may have a negative effect on the quality and quantity of cervical mucus,[27] and on endometrial development.[28]

Gonadotropin preparations such as human menopausal gonadotropin (hMG) or pure FSH have been used as a second line treatment for ovulation induction in WHO group II patients. In women with PCOS, because of the high sensitivity of the ovaries to gonadotropin stimulation, treatment with hMG or pure FSH is difficult to control and characteristically induces several ovulatory follicles, leading to the risk of multiple pregnancies and ovarian hyperstimulation syndrome (OHSS).[29] Therefore, a simple oral treatment that could be used without the risk of hyperstimulation and with minimal monitoring would be the preferred therapy.[30]

It may be possible to mimic the action of CC without the depletion of estrogen receptors by administration of an aromatase inhibitor in the early part of the menstrual cycle. Aromatase inhibitors are agents that suppress the biosynthesis of estrogen and therefore, reduce the negative feedback effect on the hypothalamic pituitary system. This results in an increased secretion of FSH that can lead to follicle selection and maturation.[9,31] This was first postulated by Mitwally and Casper.[30] A group of new, highly selective aromatase inhibitors has been approved for use in post menopausal women with breast cancer to suppress estrogen production. These aromatase inhibitors have a relatively short half life compared with CC and therefore, would be eliminated from the body rapidly.[32–33] In addition, because estrogen receptor down regulation does not occur, no adverse effects on estrogen target tissues as observed in CC treated cycles, would be expected.[30]

Letrozole (Femara, Novartis), has been recently used for ovulation induction in anovulatory PCOS women resistant to clomiphene or with inadequate endometrial thickness during CC treatment.[9,30] The main impetus for the development of aromatase inhibitors as ovulation induction agents was to avoid the peripheral antiestrogenic

effects of clomiphene citrate.[34] The half-life of letrozole is approximately 48 hours, thus resulting in complete clearance in about 10 days after taking the last tablet and in a reduction of letrozole concentrations below the therapeutic level by 6 to 8 days.[35] Administration of letrozole from days 3 to 7 suppresses ovarian estradiol (E2) secretion and reduces estrogen- negative feedback at the pituitary and mediobasal hypothalamus. Increased FSH secretion from the anterior pituitary stimulates growth of multiple ovarian follicles.[22,35] Later in the follicular phase, the effect of the aromatase inhibitors is reduced and E2 levels increase as a result of follicular growth.[35,36]

Because aromatase inhibitors do not affect estrogen receptors centrally, the increased E2 levels result in normal negative feedback on FSH secretion and follicles smaller than the dominant follicle become atretic, with resultant mono follicular development in most cases.[34]

Letrozole may have several advantages over clomiphene. Because letrozole is more rapidly eliminated than clomiphene and does not cause estrogen receptor depletion, it is likely that letrozole may not cause the adverse endometrial effects observed with clomiphene, ultimately resulting in improved pregnancy rates.[35,36] A major advantage of aromatase inhibitors for ovulation induction is mono-ovulation. A drug that consistently results in mono-ovulation is very desirable, especially in patients with PCOS who are often hyper-responsive to gonadotropins. Both these advantages allow gynecologists who lack access to ultrasonography to participate in the management of PCOS.[34]

Anastrozole is another third generation aromatase inhibitor. To date, letrozole has been studied much more extensively than anastrozole. Some evidence suggests that compared to anastrozole, letrozole results in higher endometrial thickness, higher ovulation rates and higher pregnancy rates.[37]

Clinical Discussion

Our experience with aromatase inhibitors in PCOS patients

We started prescribing letrozole for PCOS patients

resistant to CC shortly after Mitwally and Casper proposed the use of aromatase inhibitors for this purpose in 2001.[30] Initially, a daily dose of 2.5 mg was used starting from day 3 of the cycle for 5 days. This was later increased to higher doses of 5, 7.5 and rarely 10 mg/day in non-responsive cases after a course of low dose letrozole, or in CC resistant patients where non-responsiveness to lower doses was anticipated.

In 240 cases, we used letrozole 2.5 mg/day from the third day of the menstrual period for five days and we had 72 (30%) pregnancies. In the 236 patients who did not conceive, and also did not have regular periods with the low dose letrozole, the dose of letrozole was increased to 5 mg/ day from day three for five days. 92 patients (38.9%) got pregnant and 64 patients (27.1%) did not have regular periods. Therefore, in these 64 patients, we increased the letrozole dose to 7.5 mg/ day for five days. We had 24 (37.5%) pregnancies in these patients. If the patients still did not have regular periods and did not get pregnant, the dose of letrozole was increased to 10 mg per day for five days. We had 6 pregnancies with 10 mg letrozole. This was the maximum dose of letrozole, which was given to PCOS patients. In patients who were resistant to the maximum dose of letrozole, we decided to add metformin (Glucophage, Merck) with a dose of 1500 mg per day to the regimen. Among 552 cases that were given a combination of metformin and letrozole, we had 174 (31.5%) pregnancies.

Allocation of patients to dose or regimen groups was not randomized and was decided by one clinician in all the cases, based on personal experience. The same clinician saw all the patients during their treatment course and evaluated the side effects and complications. There was no set protocol in place and therefore, inclusion and exclusion criteria changed with time as the team gained more experience with the medication.

Table 34.1 summarizes the outcome in groups on different doses of letrozole or a combination of letrozole and metformin.

In total, 1102 patients took different doses of letrozole with or without Glucophage and 368 (33.4%) conceived. Pregnancy rates ranged between 30-60% in different dose groups.

No serious side effects were noted, even with the higher doses, and none of the patients withdrew from treatment because of adverse effects.

Table 34.2 summarizes the complications in pregnancies

Among 368 pregnancies, subsequent to different doses of letrozole, the number of miscarriages, in the first and second trimesters were 99 (27.3%). Fetal anomaly was noted in only one patient who had esophageal atresia. There was no other fetal abnormality to the best

Table 34.1 Summary of the outcomes following treatment with different doses of letrozole, or the combination of letrozole and metformin

Dose	2.5 mg/day	5 mg/day	7.5 mg/day	10 mg/day	Letrozole+ Glucophage	**TOTAL**
No of patients	240	236	64	10	552	**1102**
Pregnancies	72	92	24	6	174	**368**
Pregnancy rate (%)	30	38.5	37.5	60	31.5	**33.4%**

Table 34.2 Pregnancy complications

Total number of Pregnancies %	Miscarriage	Ectopic Pregnancies	Twin	Triplets	Fetal Anomalies
368	99	3	2	0	1
	27.3%	0.8%	0.5%	0%	0.2%

of our knowledge. We had 2 twin pregnancies and no triplets. There was no difference between our treated group from general population in the frequency of pre-eclampsia, preterm labor, ectopic pregnancy and intrauterine growth retardation (IUGR).

Conclusion

Letrozole is a very effective drug for PCOS patients resistant to clomiphene citrate. The promising pregnancy rates with letrozole in our experience, has made us rethink about our treatment policies. We have replaced CC with letrozole in our practice as the first line treatment and have seen encouraging results. The drug doses can safely be increased to up to 10 mg per day. In combination with metformin it gives very good results. It is very well accepted by patients and has few side effects. The biggest advantage in our experience is the high number of patients and close and intimate relationship between the clinician and patients, which resulted in an accurate and complete follow-up.

The anomaly rates in our patients were comparable to general population and we did not have a higher incidence of IUGR, preterm labour, ectopic pregnancies or multiple gestations, suggesting that letrozole is safe to use for this purpose. However, further studies must be performed to confirm this.

Our results should be interpreted with caution and should be regarded as a preliminary report from personal experience, hence not fitting into any of the conventional standards of a research project. However, we believe that our results highlight the need for well- designed randomized controlled trials to study different aspects of treatment with letrozole and its safety.

References

1. ESHRE Capri Workshop. Guidelines of the diagnosis, treatment and management of infertility. *Hum Reprod* 1996; 11: 1775–1807.
2. Collins JA, Hughes EG. Pharmacological interventions for the induction of ovulation. *Drugs* 1995; 50(3): 480–494.
3. ESHRE Capri Workshop. Female infertility: treatment options for complicated cases. *Hum Reprod* 1997; 12(6): 1191–1196.
4. Lenton EA. Ovulation induction and ovarian stimulation. In: Rodriguez-Armas O, Hedon B, Daya S, editors. Infertility and Contraception. Parthenon Publishing Group; 1998: p 128.
5. Adamson GD, Baker VL. Subfertility: causes, treatment and outcome. *Best Pract Res Clin Obstet Gynaecol* 2003; 17(2): 169–185.
6. Hamilton-Fairley D, Taylor A. Anovulation. *BMJ* 2003; 327: 546–548.
7. Shoham Z, Weissman A. Polycystic ovarian disease: Obesity and insulin resistance. In: Kempers RD, Cohen J, Haney AF, Younger JB. eds. Fertility and medicine. Amesterdam, New York, Oxford. Shannon, Singapore, Tokyo: *Elsevier* 1998; 263–272.
8. Franks S. Polycystic ovary syndrome. *N Eng J Med* 1995; 333: 853–861.
9. Ioannis E. Messinis. Ovulation induction: a mini review Human. *Rep* 2005; 20: 2688–2697.
10. Greenblatt RB, Barfield WE, Jugck EC, Ray AW. Induction of ovulation with MRL/41: preliminary report: *JAMA* 1961; 178: 101–104.
11. Hull MGR. The causes of infertility and relative effectiveness of treatment. In: Templeton AA, Drife JO. (editors). Infertility. London: *Springer- Verlag* 1992; 33–62.
12. Dickey RP, Taylor SN, Curole DN, Rye PH, Pyrzak R. Incidence of spontaneous abortion in clomiphene pregnancies. *Hum Reprod* 1996; 11(12): 2623–2628.
13. Garcia J, Jones GS, Wentz AC. The use of clomiphene citrate. *Fertil Steril* 1977; 28(7): 707–717.
14. Gorlitsky GA, Kasa NG, Speroff L. Ovulation and pregnancy rates with clomiphene citrate. *Obstet Gynecol* 1978; 51: 265–269.
15. Gysler M, March CM, Mishell DR, Bailey EJ. A decade's experience with an individualized clomiphene treatment regimen including its effects on the postcoital test. *Fertil Sterit* 1982; 37: 161–167.
16. Hammond MG. Montoring techniques for improved pregnancy rates during clomiphene ovulation induction. *Fertil Steril* 1984; 42: 499–508.
17. MacGregor AH, Johnson JE, Bundle CA. Further clinical experience with clomiphene citrate. *Fertil Steril* 1968; 19: 616–622.
18. Homburg R. Management of infertility and prevention of ovarian hyperstimulation in women with polycystic ovary syndrome. *Clin Obstet Gynecol* 2004; 18: 773–778.

19. Franks S, Adams J, Mason H, Poison D. Ovulatory disorders in women with polycystic ovary syndrome. *Clin Obstet Gynecol* 1985; 12: 605–632.

20. Kistner R. Induction of ovulation with clomiphene citrate (clomid). *Obstet Gynecol Surv* 1965; 20: 873–900.

21. Rabau E, Serr D, Mashiach S, Insler V, Salomy M, Lunenfeld B. Current concepts in the treatment of anovulation. *Br Med J* 1967; 4: 446–449.

22. Young SL, Opsahl MS, Fritz MA. Serum concentrations of enclomiphene and zuclomiphene across consecutive cycles of clomiphene citrate therapy in anovulatory infertile women. *Fertil Steril* 1999; 71: 639–644.

23. Eden JA, Place J, Carter GD, Jones J, Alaghband Zadeh J, Pawson ME. The effect of clomiphene citrate on follicular pahse increase in endometrial thickness and uterine volume. *Obstet Gynecol* 1989; 73: 187–190.

24. Gonen Y, Casper RF. Sonographic determination of a possible adverse effect of clomiphene citrate on endometrial growth. *Hum Reprod* 1990; 5: 670–674.

25. Opsahl MS, Robins ED, O Conner DM, Scott RT, Fritz MA. Charac teristics of gonadotropin response. Follicular development and endo.

26. Mikkelson TJ, Kroboth PD, Cameron WJ, Dittert LW, Chungi V, Manberg PJ. Single- dose pharmacokinetics of clomiphene citrate in normal volunteers. *Fertil Steril* 1986; 46: 392–396.

27. Randall JM, Templeton A, Cervical mucus score and in vitro sperm mucus interaction in spontaneous and clomiphene citrate cycles. *Fertil Steril* 1991; 56: 456–458.

28. Gonen Y, Casper RF. Sonographic determination of an adverse effect of clomiphene citrate on endometrial growth. *Hum Reprod* 1990; 5: 670–674.

29. Kettel IM, Roseff SJ, Berga SL, Mortola JF, Yen SCC. Hypothalamic pituitary- ovarian response to clomiphene citrate in women with polycystic ovary syndrome. *Fertil Steril* 1993; 59: 532–538.

30. Mitwally MF, Casper RF. Use of an aromatase inhibitor for induction of ovulation in patients with an inadequate response to clomiphene citrate. *Fertil Steril* 2001; 75(2): 305–309.

31. Mitwally MF, Casper RF. Aromatase inhibitors in ovulation induction. *Semin Reprod Med* 2004; 22(1): 61–78.

32. Lipton A, Demers LM, Harvey HA, Kambic KB, Grossberg H, Brady C, Adlercruetz H, Trunet PF, Santen RJ. Letrozole (CGS 20267). A phase I study of a new potent oral aromatase inhibitor of breast cancer. *Cancer* 1995; 75(8): 2132–2138.

33. Iveson TJ, Smith IE, Ahern J, Smithers DA, Trunet PF, Dowsett M. Phase I study of the oral nonsteroidal aromatase inhibitor CGS 20267 in postmenopausal patients with advanced breast cancer. *Cancer Res* 1993; 53(2): 266–270.

34. Casper RF. Letrozole: ovulation or superovulation? *Fertil Steril* 2003; 80(6): 1335–1337.

35. Casper RF, Mitwally MF. Review: aromatase inhibitors for ovulation induction. *J Clin Endocrinol Metab* 2006; 91(3): 760–771.

36. Fisher SA, Reid RL, Van Vugt DA, Casper RF. A randomized double-blind comparison of the effects of clomiphene citrate and the aromatase inhibitor letrozole on ovulatory function in normal women. *Fertil Steril* 2002; 78(2): 280–285.

37. Al-Omari WR, Sulman WR, Al-Hadithi N. Comparison of two aromatase inhibitors in women with clomiphene-resistant polycystic ovary syndrome. *Int J Gynaecol Obstet* 2004; 85: 289–291.

35

The Development, Mechanism of Action and Use of Aromatase Inhibitors for Ovulation Induction in Polycystic Ovary Syndrome

Mohamed FM Mitwally, Robert F Casper

Summary

Polycystic Ovary Syndrome (PCOS) is the most common reproductive endocrine disorder in women. Anovulation and infertility are hallmarks of this condition. We have recently proposed the use of aromatase inhibitors as a simple, cost-effective, oral method for inducing ovulation in women with PCOS. The advantages of aromatase inhibitors over existing ovulation induction agents include a high incidence of monofollicular ovulation leading to reduced multiple pregnancies and decreased risk of ovarian hyperstimulation syndrome. In addition, aromatase inhibitors have no antiestrogenic effects on the endometrium or cervical mucus. All of these benefits result in the need for minimal or no cycle monitoring when used alone. The addition of aromatase inhibitors to exogenous gonadotropins has also been shown to reduce the dose of follicle stimulating hormone (FSH) required for controlled ovarian hyperstimulation for intrauterine insemination and other assisted reproductive technologies. Further research is required to document the safety of aromatase inhibitors in terms of pregnancy outcome, and when clinical safety is established, we believe that aromatase inhibitors will become the first line treatment for ovulation induction in PCOS.

Introduction

Polycystic ovary syndrome is the most common reproductive endocrine disorder, affecting about 4.7% of White women and 3.4% of African-American women.[1] A higher prevalence of up to 7% has been reported by others.[2] Irving Stein and Michael Leventhal first described the syndrome in a group of patients presenting with amenorrhea, bilateral polycystic ovaries, and masculinizing changes.[3] However, the syndrome has been known in the literature for almost 15 centuries since the description of a bearded and hairy female in 1857.[4]

The two hallmarks of the syndrome include lack of consistent ovulation presented as irregular or long menstrual periods and excessive androgen action (hyperandrogenism) manifested as skin problems, excessive hair growth (hirsutism) and acne, excessive deposition of fat in the waist region (truncal obesity) and increased muscularity. In 1990, a consensus conference at the National Institutes of Health, agreed on three diagnostic criteria for PCOS based on majority opinion: clinical or biochemical evidence of hyperandrogenism, chronic anovulation, and exclusion of other known disorders.[5] Most recently, in the Rotterdam Consensus Conference, the diagnostic criteria were revised to include any two of the following: oligo- or anovulation, clinical and/or biochemical signs of hyperandrogenism, polycystic ovaries (diagnosed by transvaginal ultrasound), and exclusion of other etiologies such as congenital adrenal hyperplasia, androgen-secreting tumors, and Cushing's syndrome.[6] This revision acknowledged that women with PCOS could present with regular cycles, polycystic ovaries, and clinical or biochemical hyperandrogenism.[7] Conversely, women with PCOS could present with polycystic ovaries by ultrasonography and ovulatory dysfunction, but no evidence of hyperandrogenism. At this time, it is unclear whether these diverse phenotypes are dictated by multiple genetic alterations, or by limited genetic alterations buffered by lifestyle choices and environmental factors.

The main pathophysiological processes in women with PCOS include a combination of aberrant gonadotropin secretion,[8] hyperandrogenism,[9] and insulin resistance.[10] Obviously, a single underlying factor cannot explain the whole group of abnormalities seen in PCOS.

Ovulation induction in PCOS

The diagnosis of PCOS is frequently encountered in a great proportion of infertile couples attending infertility clinics. These couples may belong to one of two categories. In the first category, failure to achieve pregnancy is solely due to the lack of ovulation when the woman has PCOS. In this case, restoration of ovulation is obviously the treatment needed to achieve pregnancy. In the second category of infertile couples, anovulation due to PCOS is accompanied by other infertility factors such as male factor infertility, and infertility due to tubal obstruction or dysfunction. In this case, the woman may require ovarian stimulation, not only to restore ovulation, but also to achieve the development of multiple ovarian follicles (superovulation) with intrauterine insemination (IUI) or development of a larger number of ovarian follicles (controlled ovarian hyperstimulation) in conjunction with assisted

reproduction e.g. in vitro fertilization and embryo transfer (IVF-ET)

It is obvious that infertile women with PCOS, who do not suffer from other infertility factors, require restoration of ovulation as the mainstay of their infertility treatment. Several approaches have been suggested to achieve ovulation including encouraging resumption of spontaneous ovulation by improving insulin action through non-pharmacological approaches (exercise, diet modifications and weight loss). Pharmacological approaches include the use of insulin sensitizers such as metformin and glitazones (rosiglitazone and pioglitazone). These approaches have the major advantage of monofollicular development in most cases, which avoids the risk of multiple pregnancy and severe ovarian hyperstimulation syndrome, the two major complications associated with ovarian stimulation. However, these approaches that aim at ameliorating insulin resistance often require a long duration of treatment. This is usually a problem, particularly in routine infertility practice that deals with frustrated infertile couples who are usually too anxious to conceive to adhere to a treatment plan for several months. This is true, particularly when the female age is an important infertility factor due to the tendency for delaying childbirth these days, particularly in industrialized countries. For these reasons, the use of ovulation induction agents, such as the antiestrogen clomiphene citrate (CC) or gonadotropins, has been much more frequently used for treatment of infertility in women with PCOS.

In the last few years, we have reported the success of using aromatase inhibitors (AIs) for infertility treatment in couples with various infertility factors, including women with PCOS. We believe that AIs will have several advantages in treating infertility in women with PCOS including:

1   Restoration of ovulation by induction of monofollicular ovulation
2   Reducing the dose of gonadotropins needed for controlled ovarian hyperstimulation and the development of more than one mature ovarian follicle

3   Initiating the development of multiple ovarian follicles followed by retrieval of immature oocytes and in-vitro maturation

4   Improving the outcome of assisted reproduction by use in conjunction with gonadotropins

We believe that the above-mentioned roles of AIs can be achieved by applying AIs in different protocols that would suit each application.

Clinical Discussion

Aromatase inhibitors

Aromatase enzyme and development of aromatase inhibitors

Aromatase is a microsomal member of the cytochrome P450 hemoprotein-containing enzyme complex superfamily (P450 arom, the product of the CYP19 gene). It is the enzyme that catalyzes the rate-limiting step in the production of estrogens, that is, the conversion of androstenedione and testosterone via three hydroxylation steps into estrone and estradiol respectively.[11] The aromatase enzyme is present in many tissues, such as the ovaries, the brain, adipose tissue, muscle, liver, breast tissue, and in malignant breast tumors. The main sources of circulating estrogens are the ovaries in premenopausal women and adipose tissue in postmenopausal women.[12]

Aromatase is a good target for selective inhibition without affecting other steroidogenesis pathways because estrogen production is a terminal step in the biosynthetic sequence of steroid hormones. A large number of AIs have been developed over the last 30 years with the most recent, third generation AIs licensed mainly for breast cancer treatment in postmenopausal women.[13] AIs have been classified in different ways into steroidal and non-steroidal, and according to the stage of development into first, second and third generation groups. The first AI to be used clinically was aminoglutethimide, which induces a medical adrenalectomy by inhibiting many other enzymes involved in steroid biosynthesis.[14] Although aminoglutethimide is

an effective hormonal agent in postmenopausal breast cancer, its use is complicated by the need for concurrent corticosteroid replacement, in addition to side effects like lethargy, rashes, nausea and fever that results in 8–15% of patients stopping treatment.[15] The lack of specificity and unfavorable toxicity profile of aminoglutethimide, led to the search for more specific AIs. In addition, the earlier AIs were not able to completely inhibit aromatase activity in premenopausal patients.

The third-generation AIs commercially available, include two nonsteroidal preparations, anastrozole and letrozole, and a steroidal agent, exemestane. Anastrozole, ZN 1033, (Arimidex®) and letrozole, CGS 20267, (Femara®) are available for clinical use in North America, Europe and other parts of the world for treatment of postmenopausal breast cancer. These triazole (antifungal) derivatives are reversible, competitive AIs with considerably greater intrinsic potency than that of aminoglutethimide (more than 1000 times), and at doses of 1–5 mg/day, inhibit estrogen levels by 97% to >99% down to concentrations below detection by most sensitive immunoassays. AIs are completely absorbed after oral administration with a mean terminal $t_{1/2}$ of approximately 45 hrs (range, 30–60 hr) with clearance from the systemic circulation mainly by the liver. Mild gastrointestinal disturbances account for most of the adverse events, although these have seldom limited therapy. Other adverse effects such as asthenia, hot flushes, headache, and back pain have been reported based on studies in postmenopausal women.[16]

Use of aromatase inhibitors for infertility treatment in women with PCOS

Mechanism of ovarian stimulation by aromatase inhibitors and restoration of ovulation

We postulated that it would be possible to block estrogen negative feedback, without depletion of estrogen receptors as occurs with CC, by the administration of an aromatase inhibitor in the early part of the menstrual cycle. This will lead to lowering the levels of both circulating estrogen (produced mainly by the ovarian follicles and peripheral conversion of androgens in fat and other tissues) and locally produced estrogen in the brain, which exert a negative feedback on gonadotropin release.[17,18] Inhibition of aromatization will block estrogen production from all sources and release the hypothalamic/pituitary axis from estrogenic negative feedback (Figure 35.1). The resultant increase in gonadotropin secretion will stimulate growth of ovarian follicles. Withdrawal of estrogen centrally also increases activins, which are produced by a wide variety of tissues including the pituitary gland,[19] and stimulate synthesis of FSH by a direct action on the cells of the pituitary gland (gonadotrophs).[20]

The selective non-steroidal AIs have a relatively short half-life (~45 hours) compared to CC, and would be ideal for ovulation induction without the drawback of persistent antiestrogenic effect seen with CC since AIs are eliminated from the body rapidly.[21] Because AIs do not deplete estrogen receptors, as does CC, normal central feedback mechanisms remain intact. As the dominant follicle grows and estrogen levels rise, normal negative feedback occurs centrally resulting in suppression of FSH (Figure 35.1B) and atresia of the smaller growing follicles. A single dominant follicle, and mono-ovulation, should occur in most cases (Figure 35.1).

In women with PCOS, relative oversuppression of FSH may be the result of excessive androgen produced from the ovary, being converted to estrogen by aromatization in the brain. The AIs suppress estrogen production in both, the ovaries and the brain. In the case of PCOS, therefore, AIs should result in a robust increase in FSH release and subsequent follicle stimulation and ovulation. The actual FSH release is likely to be blunted by the high levels of circulating inhibin found in PCOS patients[22,23,24] that would not be altered by aromatase inhibition. In addition, as pointed out above, aromatase inhibition does not antagonize ER in the brain, and the initiation of

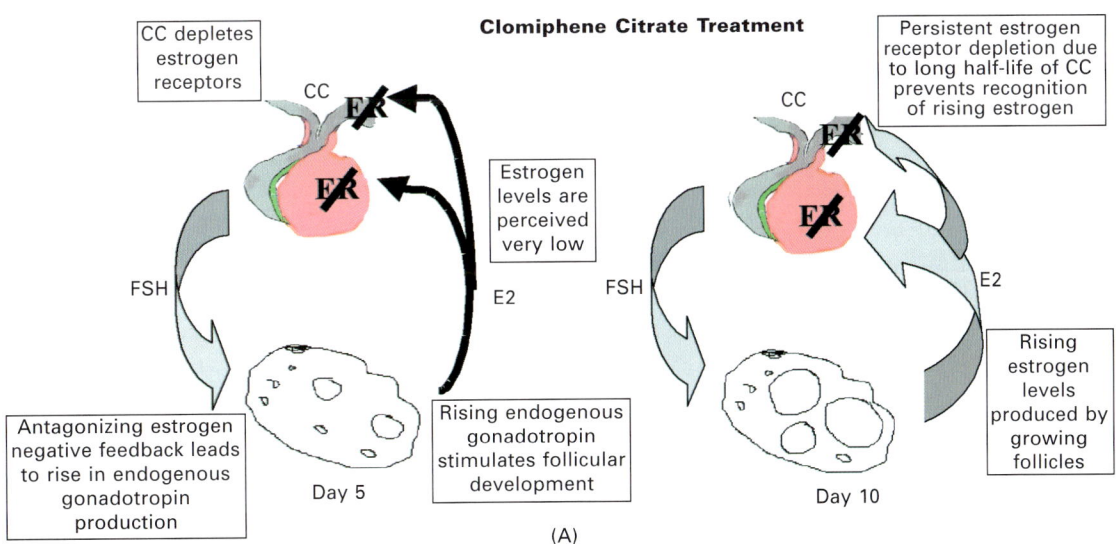

(A)

Figure 35.1 (A) CC: (Day 5) Administration of CC from days 3 to 7 results in estrogen receptor (ER) depletion at the level of the pituitary and mediobasal hypothalamus. As a result, estrogen negative feedback centrally is interrupted and FSH secretion increases from the anterior pituitary leading to multiple follicular growth. (Day 10) By the late follicular phase, because of the long tissue retention of CC, there continues to be ER depletion centrally and increased estradiol (E2) secretion from the ovary is not capable of normal negative feedback on FSH. The result is multiple dominant follicle growth and multiple ovulation.

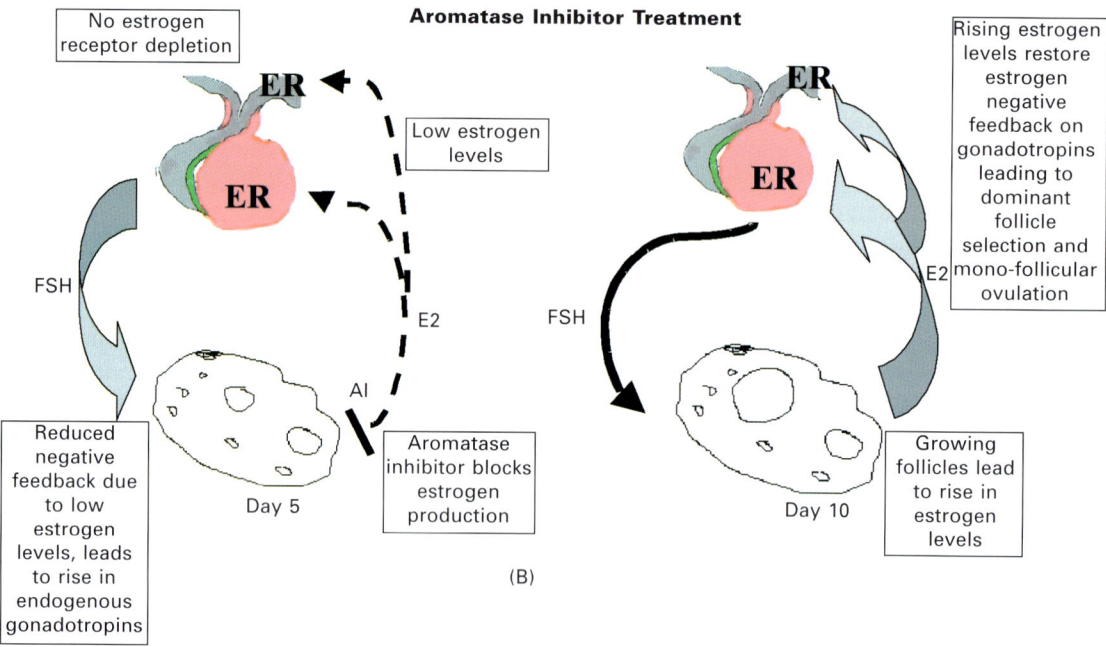

Figure 35.1(B) AI: (Day 5) Administration of an aromatase inhibitor (AI) from days 3 to 7 results in suppression of ovarian estradiol (E2) secretion and reduction in estrogen negative feedback at the pituitary and mediobasal hypothalamus. Increased FSH secretion from the anterior pituitary results in stimulation of multiple ovarian follicle growth. (Day 10) Later in the follicular phase, the effect of the AI is reduced and E2 levels increase as a result of follicular growth. Because AIs do not affect estrogen receptors (ER) centrally, the increased E2 levels result in normal negative feedback on FSH secretion and follicles less than dominant follicle size undergo atresia, with resultant monofollicular ovulation in most cases.
(From Casper RF. Letrozole: ovulation or superovulation? Fertil steril 2003; 80(6):1335-1337. Copyright The American Society for Reproductive Medicine)

follicle growth accompanied by increasing concentrations of both estradiol and inhibin, results in a normal negative feedback loop that limits response to FSH, thereby avoiding the risk of multiple ovulation and ovarian hyperstimulation syndrome.

Peripheral mechanism of action
A second hypothesis that may add to the mechanism of action of the AIs in ovarian stimulation involves an increased follicular sensitivity to FSH. This could result from temporary accumulation of intraovarian androgens, since conversion of androgen substrate to estrogen is blocked by aromatase inhibition. Recent data support a stimulatory role for androgens in early follicular growth in primates.[25]

Testosterone was found to augment follicular FSH receptor expression in primates suggesting that androgens promote follicular growth and estrogen biosynthesis indirectly by amplifying FSH effects.[26] It is likely that women with PCOS already have a relative aromatase deficiency in the ovary leading to increased intraovarian androgens[27] that leads to the development of multiple small follicles responsible for the polycystic morphology of the ovaries. The androgens, as described above, may also increase FSH receptors, making these PCOS ovaries exquisitely sensitive to an increase in FSH either through exogenous administration of gonadotropins (hence the high risk of OHSS), or through endogenous increases in FSH as a result of decreased central estrogen feedback induced by aromatase inhibition. In the latter case, a relatively small rise in FSH, because of a normal inhibin/estrogen feedback loop as described above, generally leads to monofollicular ovulation, thus avoiding the occurrence of OHSS.

Another part of the peripheral hypothesis involves ER in the endometrium. It is possible that aromatase inhibition, with suppression of estrogen concentrations in the circulation and in peripheral target tissues, results in upregulation of ER in the endometrium leading to rapid endometrial growth once estrogen secretion is restored. Estrogen has been shown to decrease the level of its own receptor by stimulating ubiquitination of ER, resulting in rapid degradation of the receptors. In the absence of estrogen, ubiquitination is decreased allowing upregulation of the ER and increasing sensitivity to subsequent estrogen administration.[28] This could increase endometrial sensitivity to estrogen resulting in more rapid proliferation of endometrial epithelium and stroma and improved blood flow to the uterus and endometrium.[29] As a result, normal endometrial development and thickness should occur by the time of follicular maturation, even in the face of the observed lower than normal estradiol concentrations in the AI treated cycle.

Superovulation and controlled ovarian hyperstimulation

As explained earlier, administration of an AI early in the menstrual cycle will result in a "temporary" increase in gonadotropin secretion. The rapid clearance of AIs as a result of their short half life, the reversible inhibition of the aromatase enzyme (by the non-steroidal reversible group), and the absence of estrogen receptor down-regulation, all lead to the preservation of the negative feedback between the ovary and hypothalamus/pituitary unit mediated by estrogen.

We believe that multiple ovarian follicular development (superovulation and controlled ovarian hyperstimulation) can be achieved by administering AIs in regimens that include "longer and higher" doses. We call this "the extended,

step-up protocol. By maintaining aromatase inhibition for a longer duration, we believe there will be longer and higher levels of endogenous gonadotropin production leading to multiple follicular development. However, this waits to be tested in controlled research studies. The major concern with these regimens is the potential accumulation of the AIs in the body close to the period of ovulation, fertilization and early embryo development. There is lack of safety data on the effect of AIs on the final stages of follicular development, ovulation and early embryonic development. Until these data are available, the concomitant use of the AIs with gonadotropins is a safer clinical approach to achieve adequate superovulation and controlled ovarian hyperstimulation. Also, it will be safer to try extended step up regimens in situations such as in-vitro maturation or in-vitro fertilization when the embryos can be frozen for transfer in a later menstrual cycle.

In-vitro maturation

The use of AIs for in vitro maturation is an exciting avenue that involves a brief endogenous gonadotropin stimulation of multiple ovarian follicles followed by retrieval of immature oocytes. Currently, there are no available data for such an application.

Improving the outcome of assisted reproduction

Based on our prior results with the combination of an AI with FSH, we believe that the combination of the two agents should be favorable for assisted reproduction, to decrease the dose of gonadotropins required (a benefit that is of major significance in poor responders rather than in women with PCOS).

Despite recent developments in ovarian stimulation and assisted reproductive technologies, there has not been a corresponding increase in implantation rates. Very high levels of estrogen (an inevitable outcome of multiple ovarian follicular development during ovarian stimulation, particularly in PCOS women) may explain some of the adverse effects of ovarian stimulation on the outcome of infertility treatment, including deleterious effects on the endometrium, the embryo, and other possible targets. This possibility has led to the suggestion of a step-down protocol for IVF in order to lower estradiol concentrations and improve successful implantation. However, an alternative approach is to use AIs to lower serum estrogen concentrations. This strategy may work similar to a step-down protocol without jeopardizing the potential number of oocytes retrieved. Another potential advantage in the use of AIs in women with PCOS undergoing assisted reproduction is a reduction in the risk of severe ovarian hyperstimulation syndrome, a life-threatening adverse effect complicating controlled ovarian hyperstimulation. Women with PCOS are more prone to suffer from this complication than other women without the condition. Such potential benefits of lowering estrogen levels during ovarian stimulation with AIs have been discussed recently.[30]

Advantages of aromatase inhibitors for induction of ovulation

There are several advantages of the use of AIs for induction of ovulation, summarized in Table 35.1.

Concerns about the use of aromatase inhibitors for induction of ovulation

Aromatase inhibitors' adverse effects
In clinical use, nonsteroidal AIs are generally well tolerated. The main side effects are hot flushes and gastrointestinal events (nausea and vomiting), and leg cramps.[31] These adverse effects were observed in older women with advanced breast cancer who were given the AIs on a daily basis over several months. Fewer adverse effects would be expected in the usually healthy younger women administered a short course of AI for induction of ovulation. In addition, our clinical experience with ovulation induction has been

Table 35.1   Advantages of the third generation aromatase inhibitors for induction of ovulation:

- Extremely potent in inhibiting the aromatase enzyme
- Very specific in inhibiting the aromatase enzyme without significant inhibition of the other steroidogenesis enzymes
- Orally administered
- 100% bioavailability after oral administration
- Rapid clearance from the body (short half-life, ~45 hours)
- No accumulation of the medications or their metabolites
- No significant active metabolites
- No significant interaction with other medications
- Well tolerated on daily administration for years
- Few adverse effects
- Very safe without significant contraindications
- Relatively inexpensive

fewer side effects such as hot flushes and premenstrual symptoms (PMS)-type symptoms with AIs compared to CC.

Low estrogen levels
Low intrafollicular estrogen levels associated with AIs use for ovulation induction are expected. The question whether low or very low intrafollicular estrogen is compatible with follicular development, ovulation, and corpus luteum formation, has been reviewed before.[32] Markedly reduced or even nearly absent intrafollicular concentrations of estrogen are known to be compatible with follicular "expansion," retrieval of fertilizable oocytes, and apparently normal embryo development.[32] However, the rapid clearance of the AIs, the reversible nature of enzyme inhibition, and elevated levels of FSH, which induce new expression of the aromatase enzyme, are factors that limit accumulation of androgens and likely result in increasing estrogen production resulting in relatively normal intrafollicular estrogen levels at the time of ovulation.

Pregnancy outcome with aromatase inhibitors
We recently reported the early clinical outcome

of pregnancies obtained through the use of AIs for ovulation induction or COH for IUI.[35] We described a cohort study comparing the outcome of pregnancies achieved after letrozole and other ovarian stimulation treatments with a control group of pregnancies spontaneously conceived without ovarian stimulation. In three tertiary referral centers over a 2-year period, there were 394 pregnancy cycles in 345 infertile couples (133 pregnancies with 2.5 mg or 5 mg letrozole alone, or with gonadotropins, 113 pregnancies with CC alone, or with gonadotropins, 110 pregnancies with gonadotropins alone, and 38 pregnancies achieved without ovarian stimulation). Pregnancies achieved after treatment with the aromatase inhibitor letrozole were associated with comparable miscarriage and ectopic pregnancy rates compared to all other groups including the spontaneous conceptions. In addition, letrozole use was associated with a significantly lower rate of multiple gestations compared to CC (4.3% versus 22% respectively), consistent with our hypothesis of an intact negative feedback loop centrally with aromatase inhibition.

A concern about the safety of letrozole for the fetus was recently raised in an abstract presentation at the 2005 ASRM meeting.[34] The authors reported the outcome of 170 infants of which 20 were lost to follow-up. As a result, 150 babies from 130 pregnancies were compared to a control group of over 36,000 infants born from low risk pregnant women in a community hospital. The control population was younger (mean age (SD) 30.5 ± 1.2 years) than the letrozole group (35.2 ± 4.7 years). The authors reported that the incidence of cardiac and "bone" anomalies was higher in the letrozole group than in the control group. We believe that both these differences are solely related to type I error.

A more recent study[35] did not find any significant increase in the rates of major and minor malformations in babies conceived after letrozole treatment. The study included a much larger group of babies born after letrozole treatment (911 babies, 514 babies born after letrozole treatment and 397 after clomiphene treatment). The study found 7 newborns in the CC group (1.8%) and only one in the letrozole group (0.2%) to have congenital cardiac anomalies (P: 0.02). The incidence of cardiac anomalies in the letrozole group was slightly lower than the rate of congenital cardiac anomalies reported among all births (0.4–1.2%) and the CC rates were slightly higher. Ventricular septal defect was the predominant cardiac anomaly (5 of 8 newborns with cardiac anomalies), similar to the findings in spontaneously conceived pregnancies.[36] These findings suggest that congenital cardiac anomalies are less frequent in the letrozole group than in the clomiphene group and general population, and refute the conclusion of the ASRM abstract[34] that had several methodological problems that, we believe, led to an erroneous conclusion. These problems included the erroneous choice of a control group predominantly composed of spontaneous conceptions, which are known to be associated with a lower risk of pregnancy complications and congenital malformations than an infertility population. Second, cardiac, and possibly skeletal abnormalities are likely to be diagnosed prepartum by ultrasound and transferred to a tertiary care hospital for delivery. Therefore, these abnormalities could be underrepresented in the 36,000 deliveries from the low risk hospital making calculation of a relative risk for the letrozole group impossible. Finally, for a drug to have a teratogenic effect, it must be present at the time of organogenesis. In the case of letrozole, and other AIs, the half-life of approximately 45 hours (range 30–60 hours) should allow rapid clearance of the drug from the body before the time of embryo implantation. Thus, the exposure to the drug predates the critical fetal development period, casting doubt on the biological plausibility of teratogenicity in the use of the drug for ovulation induction.

Conclusions

Polycystic ovary syndrome, the most common reproductive endocrine disorder, is responsible for the majority of cases of anovulatory infertility. Anovulation in PCOS has, for almost fifty years, been treated with the ovulation induction agent, clomiphene citrate despite the failure of clomiphene treatment in a significant proportion of infertile women. The absence of an effective alternative that is orally administered, inexpensive and safe, has resulted in the continuation of clomiphene use over several decades. We recently proposed the use of aromatase inhibitors as a simple, cost-effective oral method for inducing ovulation in women with PCOS. The advantages of aromatase inhibitors over existing ovulation induction agents include a high incidence of monofollicular ovulation, leading to reduced multiple pregnancies and decreased risk of ovarian hyperstimulation syndrome. In addition, aromatase inhibitors have no antiestrogenic effects on the endometrium or cervical mucus because of the absence of estrogen receptor depletion. All of these benefits result in the need for minimal, or no cycle monitoring when used alone. Aromatase inhibitors can also be used in conjunction with exogenous gonadotropins, to reduce the dose of gonadotropins required for controlled ovarian hyperstimulation for intrauterine insemination and other assisted reproductive technologies. The promising preliminary trials that showed the efficacy of aromatase inhibitors in infertility treatment, mandate the need for further research to document the safety of aromatase inhibitors in terms of pregnancy outcome. When clinical safety is established, we believe aromatase inhibitors will become the first line treatment for ovulation induction, especially in women with PCOS.

References

1. Knochenhauer ES, Key TJ, Kahsar-Miller M, Waggoner W, Boots LR, Azziz R. Prevalence of the polycystic ovary syndrome in unselected black and white women of the southeastern United States: a prospective study. *J Clin Endocrinol Metab* 1998; 83(9): 3078–3082.
2. Diamanti-Kandarakis E, Kouli CR, Bergiele AT, et al. A survey of the polycystic ovary syndrome in the Greek island of Lesbos: hormonal and metabolic profile. *J Clin Endocrinol Metab* 1999; 84: 4006–4011.
3. Stein IF, Leventhal ML. Amenorrhea associated with bilateral polycystic ovaries. *Am J Obstet Gynecol* 1935; 29: 181.
4. Laurence JZ. A short account of the bearded and hairy female. *The Lancet* 1857; 70: 48.
5. Zawadski JK, Dunaif A. Diagnostic criteria for polycystic ovary syndrome: towards a rational approach. In Dunaif A, Givens JR, Haseltine F, editors. Polycystic ovary syndrome. Boston: Blackwell Scientific, 1992; 377–384.
6. The Rotterdam ESHRE/ASRM-sponsored PCOS Consensus Workshop Group. Revised 2003 consensus on diagnostic criteria and long-term health risks related to polycystic ovary syndrome. *Fertil Steril* 2004; 81: 19–25.
7. Carmina E, Lobo RA. Polycystic ovaries in hirsute women with normal menses. *Am J Med* 2001; 111: 602–606.
8. Marshall JC, Eagleson CA. Neuroendocrine aspects of polycystic ovary syndrome. *Endocrinol Metab Cln North Am* 1999; 28: 295–324.
9. Rosenfield RL. Ovarian and adrenal function in polycystic ovary syndrome. *Endocrinol Metab Clin North Am* 1999; 28: 265–293.
10. Dunaif A, Segal KR, Futterweit W, Dobrjansky A. Profound peripheral insulin resistance, independent of obesity, in polycystic ovary syndrome. *Diabetes* 1989; 38(9): 1165–1174.
11. Cole PA, Robinson CH. Mechanism and inhibition of cytochrome P-450 aromatase. *J Med Chem* 1990; 33: 2933–2942.
12. Santen RJ, Manni A, Harvey H, Redmond C. Endocrine treatment of breast cancer in women. *Endocr Rev.* 1990; 11(2): 221–265.
13. Buzdar A, Howell A. Advances in aromatase inhibition: clinical efficacy and tolerability in the treatment of breast cancer. *Clin Cancer Res* 2001; 7: 2620–2635.
14. Santen RJ, Lipton A, Kendall J. Successful medical adrenalectomy with aminoglutethimide: role of altered drug metabolism. *J Am Med Assoc* 1974; 230: 1661–1665.
15. Newsome HH, Brown PW, Terz JJ, Lawrence W Jr. Medical and surgical adrenalectomy in patients with advanced breast carcinoma. *Cancer* 1977; 39(2): 542–546.
16. Winer EP, Hudis C, Burstein HJ et al. American Society of Clinical Oncology Technology Assessment on the use of aromatase inhibitors as adjuvant therapy for women with hormone receptor–positive breast cancer: Status Report 2002. *J Clin Oncol* 2002; 2015: 3317.

17. Kamat A, Hinshelwood MM, Murry BA, Mendelson CR. Mechanisms in tissue-specific regulation of estrogen biosynthesis in humans. *Trends Endocrinol Metab* 2002; 133: 122–128.

18. Naftolin F. Brain aromatization of androgens. *J Reprod Med* 1994; 39: 257.

19. Roberts V, Meunier H, Vaughan J et al. Production and regulation of inhibin subunits in pituitary gonadotropes. *Endocrinology* 1989; 124: 552–554.

20. Mason AJ, Berkemeier LM, Schmelzer CH, Schwall RH. Activin B: precursor sequences, genomic structure and in vitro activities. *Mol Endocrinol* 1989; 3: 1352–1358.

21. Sioufi A, Gauducheau N, Pineau V et al. Absolute bioavailability of letrozole in healthy post-menopausal women. *Biopharm Drug Dispos* 1997; 18: 779–789.

22. Roberts VJ, Barth S, El-Roeiy A, Yen SSC. Expression of inhibin/activin system messenger ribonucleic acids and proteins in ovarian follicles from women with polycystic ovarian syndrome. *J Clin Endocrinol Metab* 1994; 79: 1434–1439.

23. Anderson RA, Groome NP, Baird DT. Inhibin A and inhibin B in women with polycystic ovarian syndrome during treatment with FSH to induce mono-ovulation. *Clin Endocrinol Oxf* 1998; 48: 577–584.

24. Lockwood GM, Muttukrishna S, Groome NP, Matthews DR, Ledger WL. Mid-follicular phase pulses of inhibin B are absent in polycystic ovarian syndrome and are initiated by successful laparoscopic ovarian diathermy: a possible mechanism regulating emergence of the dominant follicle. *J Clin Endocrinol Metab* 1998; 83(5): 1730–1735.

25. Weil SJ, Vendola K, Zhou J et al. Androgen receptor gene expression in the primate ovary: cellular localization, regulation, and functional correlations. *J Clin Endocrinol Metab* 1998; 837: 2479–2485.

26. Weil S, Vendola K, Zhou J, Bondy CA. Androgen and follicle-stimulating hormone interactions in primate ovarian follicle development. *J Clin Endocrinol Metab* 1999; 848: 2951–2956.

27. Agarwal SK, Judd HL, Magoffin DA. A mechanism for the suppression of estrogen production in polycystic ovary syndrome. *J Clin Endocrinol Metab* 1996; 8110: 3686–3691.

28. Nirmala PB, Thampan RV. Ubiquitination of the rat uterine estrogen receptor: dependence on estradiol. *Biochem Biophys Res Commun* 1995; 213(1): 24–31.

29. Rosenfeld CR, Roy T, Cox BE. Mechanisms modulating estrogen-induced uterine vasodilation. *Vascul Pharmacol* 2002; 382: 115–125.

30. Mitwally MF, Casper RF, Diamond MP. The role of aromatase inhibitors in ameliorating deleterious effects of ovarian stimulation on outcome of infertility treatment. *Reprod Biol Endocrinol* 2005; 3: 54.

31. Goss PE. Risks versus benefits in the clinical application of aromatase inhibitors. *Endocr Relat Cancer* 1999; 6: 325–332.

32. Palter SF, Tavares AB, Hourvitz A, Veldhuis JD, Adashi EY. Are estrogens of import to primate/human ovarian folliculogenesis? *Endocr Rev* 2001; 22(3): 389–424.

33. Mitwally MF, Biljan MM, Casper RF. Pregnancy outcome after the use of an aromatase inhibitor for ovarian stimulation. *Am J Obstet Gynecol* 2005; 192(2): 381–386.

34. Biljan MM, Hemmings R, Brassard N. The outcome of 150 babies following the treatment with letrozole or letrozole and gonadotropins. *Fertil Steril* 2005; 84 (supp. 1); O-231, Abstract 1033.

35. Tulandi T, Martin J, Al-Fadhli R, Kabli N, Forman R, Hitkari J, Librach C, Greenblatt E, Casper RF. Congenital malformations among 911 newborns conceived after infertility treatment with letrozole or clomiphene citrate. *Fertil Steril* 2006; 85(6): 1761–1765.

36. Hoffman JI. Incidence of congenital heart disease: I. Postnatal incidence. *Pediatr Cardiol* 1995; 16(3): 103–113.

Frequently asked questions

1. Which aromatase inhibitors can be used for induction of ovulation in women with PCOS?

Likely, short acting reversible aromatase inhibitors such as anastrozole and letrozole are preferable, compared to irreversible inhibitors such as exemestane.

2. Which is the best regimen for administering aromatase inhibitors for ovulation induction in women with PCOS?

We have demonstrated that the single dose administration of letrozole on cycle day 3, results in equivalent ovulation rates and likely, similar pregnancy rates to daily administration for 5 days. The best regimen, however, has not yet been determined.

3. What is recommended when women with PCOS fail to respond to aromatase inhibitors?

Failure to respond to AIs alone suggests that adjunctive treatment with an insulin sensitizer may be required in the presence of documented insulin resistance. Alternatively, addition of exogenous FSH to an aromatase inhibitor may be required.

4. What is recommended when women with PCOS fail to get pregnant despite responding (achieving ovulation) to aromatase inhibitors?

Investigation of other potential causes of infertility such as tubal disorders, subtle male factor problems or endometriosis.

5. Can insulin sensitizers e.g. metformin be used with aromatase inhibitors?

Yes. See FAQ 3 above.

6. What do you recommend as regards monitoring ovulation induction with aromatase inhibitors in women with PCOS?

Minimal monitoring is required if AIs are used without exogenous gonadotropins since monofollicular ovulation usually occurs and adverse effects on the endometrial thickness are not seen, in contrast to CC.

7. Do we have to use hCG to trigger ovulation in PCOS women receiving aromatase inhibitors for induction of ovulation?

A spontaneous LH surge occurs to trigger ovulation. It is only necessary to use hCG if timing of ovulation, for example in intrauterine insemination, is necessary.

8. How should gonadotropins be used with aromatase inhibitors?

We recommend using gonadotropins sequentially with AIs. In other words, an AI is administered for 5 days, usually day 3 to 7 of the cycle and exogenous gonadotropins are then started on day seven of the menstrual period.

9. Do you recommend the use of LH-surge kits for detection of ovulation with the use of aromatase inhibitors for ovulation induction?

LH surge detection kits may be useful for timing of intercourse in cases where cycle monitoring by ultrasound and blood sampling is not convenient or available.

36

Clomiphene Citrate for Ovulation Induction in Women with Polycystic Ovary Syndrome

Gautam N Allahbadia, Rina Agrawal

Summary

Clomiphene Citrate (CC) is the traditional first-line treatment for chronic anovulation that characterizes polycystic ovary syndrome (PCOS). CC is accumulated in the body with a low clearance rate and long half-life (5 days). Significant plasma concentrations of the active zu isomer of CC can be detected up to 6 weeks after administration. However, 20–25% of PCOS women fail to ovulate with incremental doses of CC. In addition, clinical data reveals a discrepancy between ovulation rates (75–80%) and conception rates (30–40%) during CC treatment.[1] For these patients who do not respond to CC, there are a few limited adjunctive therapies including bromocriptine (in the presence of hyperprolactinemia or galactorrhea), insulin sensitizers (to treat hyperinsulinemia), oral contraceptives (for pretreatment suppression of luteinizing hormone (LH)), pulsatile gonadotropin releasing hormone (GnRH) (to preserve the physiological interactive feedback) and extended doses of CC that can be tried before moving on to gonadotropin therapy or laparoscopic ovarian drilling.[2]

Rationale

Ovulatory dysfunction is one of the most common causes of reproductive failure in subfertile and infertile couples. In the absence of other significant infertility factors, successful ovulation induction often, will restore normal fertility. Clomiphene Citrate (CC) is the best initial treatment for the large majority of anovulatory infertile women including the World Health Organization (WHO) Type 2 patients or the PCOS group. The first clinical trial of CC therapy demonstrated successful ovulation induction in 80% of women, half of whom achieved pregnancy following treatment.[3] In subsequent years, the results of CC treatment have not changed appreciably, despite the advent of modern immunoassays for steroid hormone assessment, advances in ultrasound technology for cycle monitoring, and the introduction of commercial test kits that allow detection of the midcycle luteinizing hormone (LH) surge in urine. The drug's effectiveness in ovulation induction can be attributed to its actions at the hypothalamic level. Depletion of hypothalamic estrogen receptors (ER) prevents correct interpretation of circulating estrogen levels. Reduced levels of estrogen act as a negative feedback to trigger normal compensatory mechanisms that alter pulsatile hypothalamic GnRH secretion to stimulate increased pituitary gonadotropin release that, in turn, drives ovarian follicular activity. In ovulatory women, CC treatment increases GnRH pulse frequency.[4] In anovulatory women with polycystic ovary syndrome (PCOS) in whom the GnRH pulse frequency is already abnormally high, CC treatment increases pulse amplitude, but not frequency.[5] In successful treatment cycles, one or more dominant follicles emerge and mature, generating a rising tide of estradiol (E2) that ultimately triggers the midcycle LH surge and ovulation.

Introduction

Clomiphene was originally developed by Merrell in 1956.[6] This first non-steroidal estrogen antagonist (MER-25) was clinically tested in women with endometriosis, breast cancer and endometrial hyperplasia.[6] Surprisingly, the application of this medication was followed by the recommencement of menstrual cycles in some patients.[7] Greenblatt and co-workers,[8] recognized the ovulation-inducing capacity of the next generation of closely related anti-estrogens (MRL/41), which was also called clomiphene citrate or clomiphene. Clomiphene citrate was approved in 1967, when it first became available by prescription in the USA, and has been marketed without interruption since its introduction. Clomiphene citrate is still considered to be the first-line treatment strategy in most cases of anovulatory infertility.[9–11] After more than 30 years, it is still the most applied drug for infertility treatment world-wide.[12–13] The beneficial effects are: low cost,[14,15] oral administration, minimal requirement for cycle monitoring; minimal side effects (hot flushes, nausea, dizziness, blurred vision, headaches), acceptable ovulation/pregnancy rates,[11] and low risk of ovarian hyperstimulation syndrome (OHSS) and multiple pregnancies, because of mono-ovulatory cycles.[16]

Two or 3 days following the administration of CC in the follicular phase of the ovarian cycle, the pulse frequency of LH increases, suggesting that the main action of the drug is to increase pulsatile secretion of gonadotropin releasing hormone (GnRH) by the hypothalamus.[17] Clomiphene could also have a direct estrogenic effect on the pituitary gonadotrophs, enhancing

sensitivity to GnRH. As a consequence of the effects mentioned above, there is an increase in plasma concentration of gonadotropins and in the number of follicles recruited. There is a resulting increase in plasma concentrations of estradiol before ovulation, and of progesterone during the luteal phase. Between 30 and 35% of patients who ovulate with clomiphene do so with a follicular rupture diameter that is larger than expected, as compared with spontaneous cycles.

Clomiphene induces ovulation at a high rate (70–90%) and, although the pregnancy rate is lower (30–40%),[18] in properly selected patients with no other causes of infertility, it can be as high as 60% after six cycles[19] and 97% after 10 cycles.[20] The reasons for the relatively low pregnancy rate are not clear, but may be related to the high LH levels, the antiestrogenic effects of clomiphene, and to adverse effects on the oocytes.[21,22] Although high in earlier studies, the miscarriage rate in the most recent studies is similar to that in the normal population.[19,20] The multiple pregnancy rate of 6–8% (mainly twins),[23] is rather low as compared to classical gonadotropin regimens,[24] but similar to that in the low-dose FSH protocols.[25] OHSS is a rare event.[23]

About 10–30% of the patients will be 'clomiphene resistant' i.e. will remain anovulatory even after 6 months of treatment.[9,10] Clomiphene citrate (CC) therapy has variable success rates in anovulatory women; however, it is the lowest in women with PCOS, particularly those with insulin resistance. Obese women with hyperandrogenemia are less likely to respond to clomiphene.[26] Insulin resistance is a cause of CC failure in patients with PCOS, not only in obese, but also in lean patients.[27,28] In addition, hyperinsulinemia might influence ovarian as well as adrenal steroidogenesis. Currently, there is increasing evidence that insulin sensitizers are particularly effective in inducing ovulation in patients with PCOS.[29] This is discussed in detail in another chapter in this textbook.

However, not all cases respond to insulin sensitizers.[30] Exploring other mechanisms to induce or augment ovulation in CC-resistant patients is a desirable goal in reproductive medicine. The potential insulin-sensitizing properties of N-Acetyl Cysteine (NAC) in patients with PCOS were recently explored.[31,32] N-Acetyl Cysteine (NAC) is commonly used as a safe mucolytic drug, and at higher doses, it increases the cellular levels of reduced glutathione, an antioxidant, which has been shown to influence insulin receptor activity.[33] It has been shown that NAC is able to improve insulin secretion in response to glucose. More recently, it has also been shown to have other diverse biological effects, notably: antiapoptotic,[34] antioxidant,[35] protection against focal ischemia,[36] inhibition of phospholipid metabolism, pro-inflammatory cytokine release, and protease activity.[37] N-Acetyl Cysteine (NAC) may exert the same effects at the ovarian level and these activities may be as important as its insulin-enhancing effects in inducing ovulation. A combination of CC and NAC has been reported to significantly increase both ovulation rate and pregnancy rate (PR) in women with CC-resistant PCOS when compared with the combination of CC and placebo (49.3% vs. 1.3% respectively and 21.3% vs. 0% respectively).[38] Hence, according to the authors, NAC as an adjuvant to CC is more effective than placebo in CC-resistant patients with PCOS. In addition, the anti apoptotic effects of NAC,[34] may be responsible for the significantly higher number of follicles in the NAC group compared to placebo, as it is well known that apoptosis is the main mechanism involved in follicular cohort atresia. Its protective effects against ischemic insults,[36] as well as its inflammatory-modulating capacity,[37] may be the contributory mechanisms that add to the positive reproductive effects of NAC.

When pregnancy is not achieved despite ovulation, the term 'clomiphene failure' is used. Important parameters for prediction of conception include patient age and cycle history.[39] In clomiphene resistance, some advocate a treatment period of >5 days with this drug.[40,41] Combinations with other drugs have also been used. Beneficial effects have been reported following co-administration of clomiphene with dexamethasone,[42] or when clomiphene was preceded by the oral contraceptive pill.[2]

Clinical Discussion

Clomiphene is preferably administered in 50 mg doses for 5 days from days 3–5 of a spontaneous or induced menstrual flow. Starting with higher doses fails to provide any advantages for the following two reasons. First, the administration of clomiphene at doses of 50 or 100 mg a day results in similar pregnancy rates. Second, the incidence of side-effects is dose-dependent, with adverse reactions first being observed with initial doses of 50 mg/day. Starting therapy with higher doses (100 mg/day) could result in more severe reactions. In hyper-reacting women (those who have developed ovarian cysts or hyperstimulation in previous cycles), lower doses (12.5–25 mg) may prevent hyperstimulation. In hypo-reacting patients, such as obese women, induction is started with a dose of 100 mg a day. The clomiphene dose may be increased progressively up to a maximum of 200 mg/day for 5 days. Fewer than 50% of hypo-reacting patients will ovulate at that dose. Approximately 50% of normal women ovulate with a dose of 50 mg, and an additional 20% will ovulate with 100 mg/day, the overall ovulation rate ranging from 70 to 85%.

Cycles induced with clomiphene in patients presenting with PCOS differ from those of ovulatory women, since the former show higher estrogen and progesterone concentrations.[5] The early administration of clomiphene could theoretically produce multiple follicular maturation, generating a higher incidence of multiple pregnancies. Nevertheless, no differences have been observed in ovulation, pregnancy, or miscarriage rates with clomiphene administered from days 2, 3, 4 or 5 of the cycle in the usual protocols for ovulation induction. Following the final dose of clomiphene on day 9 of the cycle, the LH surge may occur at any time between 5 and 12 days after the last dose. It occurs most frequently at 6–7 days after the last dose, especially with clomiphene from days 5–9 of the cycle. This observation is important in the planning of coitus. Couples are told they must have sexual intercourse for a week, starting on day 5 after the last clomiphene tablet.

Only 40–50% of ovulatory patients become pregnant. The discrepancy observed between the ovulation index and the fecundity index could be due to many factors. These include the coexistence of a male factor, the existence of other causes of infertility or an antiestrogenic effect of clomiphene on some effectors of the reproductive tract. This effect is known to arise in cervical mucus and its interaction with spermatozoa, in tubal transport of ova, and in the function and synchronization of the endometrium.[43]

Up to six cycles of clomiphene citrate administration with intercourse or intrauterine insemination (IUI) are common treatment algorithms in several countries for patients with anovulation and unexplained infertility, before human menopausal gonadotropin (hMG)/follicle stimulating hormone (FSH) stimulation or in vitro fertilization (IVF) treatment is initiated.[14,15] Compared with clomiphene citrate, gonadotropin treatment results in higher pregnancy rates; however, the cost of treatment and the need for more elaborate cycle monitoring is significantly increased. In a randomized trial, Lopez and co-workers[44] compared clomiphene citrate versus low-dose recombinant FSH as first line therapy in infertile women with polycystic ovary syndrome (PCOS).[44] The cumulative pregnancy rates after three treatment cycles were 43% for FSH and 24% for clomiphene citrate (P = 0.06).[44] Williams and co-workers[45] reported similar fecundity rates and cumulative pregnancy rates for clomiphene citrate/hMG/IUI cycles compared with more expensive ovarian stimulation/IUI protocols with the use of hMG/ IUI.[45] The cost of the clomiphene citrate/hMG/IUI protocol was US$662, which was about one-third that of an hMG/IUI protocol, which amounted to US$1854.50. The data of Ecochard and co-workers[46] and of Check and co-workers[47] indicate that clomiphene citrate is an effective alternative to hMG. Therefore, clomiphene citrate is still used by several clinics wishing to avoid the heavy cost of hMG or recombinant gonadotropins.

The administration of clomiphene is contraindicated during pregnancy, since it can cause congenital abnormalities. It is also contraindicated in chronic liver disease, since it is mainly cleared through the liver, and in the presence of functional ovarian cysts, which could grow larger. It is also contraindicated when there is a history of visual disorders (blurred vision and scotomas) during or after previous therapy with clomiphene. Its use in women who are infertile through non-ovulatory factors, remains controversial. Furthermore, it is not recommended in ovulatory patients because its administration may paradoxically cause disorders leading to a decrease in fertility. Such disorders include a reduction in the amount and quality of cervical mucus, abnormal development or dysfunction of the endometrium, reduction in adhesion proteins (integrins, mainly subunit b_3), decline in glandular density and an increase in vacuolated cells in the endometrium of ovulatory women.[43,48]

Two epidemiologic studies published early in the last decade suggested that the risk of ovarian cancer might be significantly increased in women exposed to ovulation inducing drugs,[49,50] but subsequent studies have failed to corroborate those findings.[51–54] A recent pooled analysis of eight case-control studies concluded that neither fertility drugs use nor use for more than 12 months was associated with invasive ovarian cancer.[55] Patients with concerns should be counseled that no causal relationship between ovulation inducing drugs and ovarian cancer has been established and no change in prescribing practices is warranted. In any case, prolonged treatment with CC is generally futile and should therefore be avoided.

Case studies

Case 1

Boothroyd and Yazdani[56] recently reported two cases of trichorionic pregnancy resulting from the use of metformin alone and in combination with clomiphene. A 30-year-old nulligravid woman was diagnosed with polycystic ovary syndrome (PCOS) at the age of 20 with a history of progressive oligomenorrhea associated with weight gain and hyperandrogenism. A combined oral contraceptive pill containing 2 mg of cyproterone as progestin was prescribed and the patient embarked on a weight loss program under the care of a dietician. She had a history of major depression requiring treatment with lithium and serotonin reuptake inhibitors. Her weight at the time that she reported for treatment was 93 kg (BMI-35 kg/m^2). Following cessation of lithium and the combined oral contraceptive pill, she commenced 50 mg clomiphene per day for five days. She had four ovulatory cycles on this dose but failed to conceive. Metformin, 500 mg three times a day, was introduced. The patient took another 3 cycles of clomiphene for 5 days each in the dose of 50 mg, and a chemical pregnancy resulted from the sixth cycle. She continued to diet and weighed 73 kg by the completion of her sixth cycle of clomiphene. Following seven clomiphene cycles she proceeded to a laparoscopy, where both tubes were found to be patent and a single spot of endometriosis (2–3 mm in diameter) was cauterized on the left ovary. She declined ovarian drilling. Ovulation induction with FSH was planned, but the patient conceived in the cycle following the laparoscopy while taking 500 mg metformin three times a day. The pregnancy was confirmed as trichorionic. Spontaneous demise of one fetus occurred at 7 weeks gestation. The patient developed pre-eclampsia and was delivered of twins by lower segment caesarean section at 30 weeks gestation.[56]

Case 2

A 31-year-old primigravid woman presented with oligo-ovulation due to lean PCOS.[56] She gave a history of postmenarchal oligomenorrhea and secondary amenorrhea following the cessation of a combined oral contraceptive pill at the age of 29. Her BMI was 23.6 kg/m^2. There was no evidence of galactorrhea, hirsutism, cortisol, or growth hormone (GH) excess on clinical examination. Investigation by her referring gynecologist showed marginal elevation of

prolactin (PRL) (less than twice the upper limit of the reference range) and a 6-mm adenoma on pituitary magnetic resonance imaging (MRI). She was commenced on cabergoline, but suppression of PRL secretion was not associated with ovulation in the following three months. While the patient was on this treatment, further investigation confirmed LH hypersecretion, marginal elevation of the free androgen index, and classic polycystic ovaries on ultrasound. In August 2003, ovulation induction with 5 days of clomiphene (50 mg per day) was unsuccessful. Clomiphene was poorly tolerated and the patient declined further doses. A laparoscopy in November 2003 was normal. Ovarian drilling was declined. She progressed to 50 IU recombinant FSH per day ovulation induction, resulting in an excessive ovarian response with a serum estradiol of 13,000 pmol/L after seven 50-IU injections. Cabergoline and FSH treatment were ceased. In March 2004, she was commenced on metformin and conceived a singleton pregnancy after her second clomiphene cycle (75 mg clomiphene, days 3–7; 500 mg metformin three times daily) resulting in a missed abortion at 7 weeks of gestation. This was the patient's first documented ovulatory cycle. In July 2004, she recommenced 75 mg clomiphene daily for 5 days while continuing 500 mg metformin three times daily. She conceived, and the pregnancy was confirmed as trichorionic. She elected to proceed with selective fetal reduction to twins and was delivered of healthy twins by elective caesarean section at 37 weeks gestation. The authors concluded that it was not possible to make proscriptive recommendations from these two cases.[56] However, women undertaking ovulation induction need to be counseled about the possible risks of higher-order multiple pregnancy from metformin therapy.

Recent Advances

A new strategy for the use of clomiphene in combination with GnRHa for ovulation induction has been proposed recently.[57,58] The physiological rationale supporting this association is mainly based on the ability of GnRHa to reduce high concentrations of LH generated by clomiphene. Antagonists, contrary to the action of GnRHa, competitively block GnRH receptors at the pituitary level, preserving the post-receptor mechanism of the latter intact. Nevertheless, it is necessary to conduct further studies on an adequate number of patients, in order to validate the basis of these new schemes.

A study using the down-regulation of the hypothalamus-pituitary-ovarian axis with oral contraceptives in patients with clomiphene-resistant PCOS showed that the LH surge can be prevented or reduced in the cycle following the discontinuation of oral contraceptives.[2] This observation enabled researchers to design the 'minimal stimulation study', using clomiphene at 100 mg/day for 8 days starting on day 3 of the cycle in a group of 36 candidates for IVF. These patients had undergone down-regulation with oral contraceptives 2 months prior to ovulation induction. No LH surge was observed in this group of patients. The average number of mature oocytes recovered was 3.2, with a 90% fertilization rate, an average number of 2.5 embryos transferred, and a 32.8% pregnancy rate per aspiration. These outcomes were similar to those obtained in IVF stimulated cycles, and this schedule has the advantages of being cheap and simple, while presenting low risks for the patients.[59]

Conclusion

Clomiphene citrate continues to be the most commonly used drug to induce ovulation in the treatment of normogonadotropic anovulatory infertility with normal estrogen concentrations. Its popularity is due to its low cost, scarce adverse reactions and easy monitoring. However, its ability to promote follicular stimulation is limited and it can induce high LH concentrations. Clomiphene may impair fertility through its adverse effects on cervical mucus and in causing various endometrial dysfunctions. This, together with other adverse aspects in reproductive function, limits the use of clomiphene in the development

of an optimum scheme in IVF programs.

However, if clomiphene is administered in 50 mg doses, side-effects are avoided and efficacy is similar to that of a 100 mg dose, although daily dosages of 200 mg/day over 5 days can induce ovulation in approximately 70% of the treated patients. Consequently, clomiphene citrate is the recommended drug for the treatment of infertility associated with PCOS, where the main objective is to obtain development of a single follicle and a reduction in multiple pregnancies. CC treatment generally, should be limited to the minimum effective dose and to no more than six ovulatory cycles. Failure to conceive after successful CC-induced ovulation is indication for further evaluation to exclude other possible contributing causes of infertility. Combination therapies involving CC and other agents (metformin, glucocorticoids, exogenous gonadotropins), may be effective when treatment with CC alone fails to induce ovulation. Alternative strategies for the CC-resistant woman include treatment with aromatase inhibitors or exogenous gonadotropins and, in selected patients, ovarian drilling. CC treatment should be monitored [transvaginal sonography, basal body temperature (BBT), serum progesterone concentrations, urinary LH excretion] to ensure its effectiveness in ovulation induction. Side effects of CC treatment are generally mild and well tolerated, the principal risk of CC treatment being an increased incidence of multifetal gestation (10%).

References

1. Yen SS. Chronic anovulation caused by peripheral endocrine disorders. In Yen SS and Jaffe RB (eds.) Reproductive Endocrinology; Physiology, Pathophysiology, and Clinical Management, 3rd edn. Philadelphia, Saunders, 1991, pp. 576–630.
2. Branigan ME and Estes A. Using oral contraceptives as a treatment for clomid-resistant patients. *Fertil Steril* 1999; 71: 544–546.
3. Greenblatt RB. Chemical induction of ovulation. *Fertil Steril* 1961; 12: 402–404.
4. Kerin JF, Liu JH, Phillipou G, Yen SS. Evidence for a hypothalamic site of action of clomiphene citrate

in women. *J Clin Endocrinol Metab* 1985; 61: 265–268.

5. Kettel LM, Roseff SJ, Berga SL, Mortola JF, Yen SS. Hypothalamic- pituitary-ovarian response to clomiphene citrate in women with polycystic ovary syndrome. *Fertil Steril* 1993; 59: 532–538.

6. Kistner RW. Observations on the use of a nonsteroidal estrogen antagonist. I. Cystic disease of the breast. *Am J Obstet Gynecol* 1961; 81: 233–242.

7. Kistner RW, Smith OW. Observations on the use of a nonsteroidal estrogen antagonist: MER-25. II. Effects in endometrial hyperplasia and Stein–Leventhal syndrome. *Fertil Steril* 1961; 12: 121–141.

8. Greenblatt RB, Barfield WE, Jungck EC. Induction of ovulation with MRL/41. Preliminary report. *JAMA* 1961; 178: 101–104.

9. Hughes E, Collins J and Vandekerckhove P. Clomiphene citrate for ovulation induction in women with oligo-amenorrhoea. *Cochrane Database Syst* 2000, Rev 2: CD000056.

10. Hughes EG, Collins J and Vandekerckhove P (2000b) Clomiphene citrate for unexplained subfertility in women. The Cochrane Database System Reviews, 2000; CD000057.

11. Practice Committee of the American Society for Reproductive Medicine 2004 Effectiveness and treatment for unexplained infertility. *Fertil Steril* 2004; 82 (Suppl. 1): S160–163.

12. Luteinizing hormone-releasing hormone and its analogues: a review of biological properties and clinical uses. *J Endocrinol Invest* 1988; 11(7): 535–557.

13. Nasseri S, Ledger WL. Clomiphene citrate in the twenty-first century. *Hum Fertil (Camb)* 2001; 4(3): 145–151.

14. Karande VC, Korn A, Morris R. Prospective randomized trial comparing the outcome and cost of in vitro fertilization with that of a traditional treatment algorithm as first-line therapy for couples with infertility. *Fertil Steril* 1999; 71: 468–475.

15. Philips Z, Barraza-Llorens M, Posnett J. Evaluation of the relative cost-effectiveness of treatments for infertility in the UK. *Hum Reprod* 2000; 15: 95–106.

16. ESHRE Capri Workshop Group 2003. Mono-ovulatory cycles: a key goal in profertility programmes. *Hum Reprod Update* 2003; 9: 263–274.

17. Sir T, Alba F, Devoto L, Rossmanith W. Clomiphene citrate and LH pulsatility in PCO syndrome. *Horm Metab Res* 1989; 21: 583–586.

18. Messinis IE. Clomiphene citrate. In Tarlatzis B (ed) Ovulation induction. *Elsevier, Paris* 2002; pp 87–97.

19. Messinis IE and Milingos SD. Current and future status of ovulation induction in polycystic ovary syndrome. *Hum Reprod Update* 1997; 3: 235–253.

20. Hammond MG, Halme JK and Talbert LM. Factors affecting the pregnancy rate in clomiphene citrate induction of ovulation. *Obstet Gynecol* 1983; 62: 196–202.

21. Wramsby H, Fredga K and Liedholm P. Chromosome analysis of human oocytes recovered from preovulatory follicles in stimulated cycles. *New Engl J Med* 1987; 316: 121–124.

22. Homburg R, Armar NA, Eshel A, Adams J and Jacobs HS. Influence of serum luteinising hormone concentrations on ovulation, conception, and early pregnancy loss in polycystic ovary syndrome. *Br Med J* 1988; 297: 1024–1026.

23. Adashi EY. Ovulation induction: clomiphene citrate. In Adashi EY, Rock JA and Rosenwaks Z (eds) Reproductive Endocrinology, Surgery and Technology. Lippincott–Raven, Philadelphia/New York, USA, 1996; pp 1181–1206.

24. Wang CF and Gemzell C. The use of human gonadotropins for the induction of ovulation in women with polycystic ovarian disease. *Fertil Steril* 1980; 33: 479–486.

25. Franks S and White D. Low-dose gonadotrophin treatment in polycystic ovary syndrome: the step-up protocol. In Tarlatzis B (ed) Ovulation Induction. Elsevier, Paris, 2002; pp 98–107.

26. Imani B, Eijkemans MJ, te Velde ER, Habbema JD and Fauser BC. Predictors of patients remaining anovulatory during clomiphene citrate induction of ovulation in normogonadotropic oligoamenorrheic infertility. *J Clin Endocrinol Metab* 1998; 83: 2361–2365.

27. Holte J, Bergh T, Berne C, Berglund L, Lithell H. Enhanced early insulin response to glucose in relation to insulin resistance in women with polycystic ovary syndrome and normal glucose tolerance. *J Clin Endocrinol Metab* 1994; 78: 1052–1058.

28. Moghetti P, Castello R, Negri C, Tosi F, Perrone F, Caputo M, et al. Metformin effects on clinical features, endocrine and metabolic profiles, and insulin sensitivity in polycystic ovary syndrome: a randomized, double-blind, placebo-controlled 6-month trial, followed by open, long-term clinical evaluation. *J Clin Endocrinol Metab* 2000; 85: 139–146.

29. Nestler JE. Obesity, insulin, sex steroids and ovulation. *Int J Obes Relat Metab Disord* 2000; 24 (Suppl 2): S71–73.

30. Malkawi HY, Qublan HS, Hamaideh AH. Medical vs. surgical treatment for clomiphene citrate-resistant women with polycystic ovary syndrome. *J Obstet Gynaecol* 2003; 23: 289–293.

31. Weidmann P, de Courten M and Bohlen L. Insulin resistance, hyperinsulinemia and hypertension. *J Hypertens Suppl* 1993; 11 (Suppl 5): S27–38.

32. Fulghesu AM, Ciampelli M, Muzj G, Belosi C, Selvaggi L, Ayala GF, et al. N-acetyl-cysteine treatment improves insulin sensitivity in women with polycystic ovary syndrome. *Fertil Steril* 2002; 77: 1128–1135.

33. Ammon HP, Muller PH, Eggstein M, Wintermantel C, Aigner B, Safayhi H, et al. Increase in glucose consumption by acetylcysteine during hyperglycemic clamp. A study with healthy volunteers. *Arzneimittelforschung* 1992; 42: 642–645.

34. Odetti P, Pesce C, Traverso N, Menini S, Maineri EP and Cosso L, et al. Comparative trial of N-acetyl-cysteine, taurine, and oxerutin on skin and kidney damage in long-term experimental diabetes. *Diabetes* 2003; 52: 499–505.

35. De Mattia G, Bravi MC, Laurenti O, Cassone-Faldetta M, Proietti A, De Luca O, et al. Reduction of oxidative stress by oral N-acetyl-Lcysteine treatment decreases plasma soluble vascular cell adhesion molecule-1 concentrations in non-obese, non-dyslipidaemic, normotensive, patients with non-insulin-dependent diabetes. *Diabetologia* 1998; 41: 1392–1396.

36. Sekhon B, Sekhon C, Khan M, Patel SJ, Singh I and Singh AK. N-Acetyl cysteine protects against injury in a rat model of focal cerebral ischemia. *Brain Res* 2003; 971: 1–8.

37. Lappas M, Permezel M, Rice GE. N-Acetyl-cysteine inhibits phospholipid metabolism, proinflammatory cytokine release, protease activity, and nuclear factor-kappaB deoxyribonucleic acid-binding activity in human fetal membranes in vitro. *J Clin Endocrinol Metab* 2003; 88: 1723–1729.

38. Rizk AY, Bedaiwy MA, Al-Inany HG. N-acetyl-cysteine is a novel adjuvant to clomiphene citrate in clomiphene citrate–resistant patients with polycystic ovary syndrome. *Fertil Steril* 2005; 83: 367–370.

39. Imani B, Eijkemans MJ, te Velde ER, Habbema JD and Fauser BC. Predictors of changes to conceive in ovulatory patients during clomiphene citrate induction of ovulation in normogonadotropic oligoamenorrheic infertility. *J Clin Endocrinol Metab* 1999; 84: 1617–1622.

40. O'Herlihy C, Pepperell RJ, Brown JB, Smith MA, Sandri L and McBain JC. Incremental clomiphene therapy: a new method for treating persistent anovulation. *Obstet Gynecol* 1981; 58: 535–542.

41. Fluker MR, Wang IY and Rowe TC. An extended 10-day course of clomiphene citrate (CC) in women with CC-resistant ovulatory disorders. *Fertil Steril* 1996; 66: 761–764.

42. Trott EA, Plouffe L Jr, Hansen K, Hines R, Brann DW and Mahesh VB. Ovulation induction in clomiphene-resistant anovulatory women with normal dehydroepiandrosterone sulfate levels: beneficial effects of the addition of dexamethasone during the follicular phase. *Fertil Steril* 1996; 66: 484–486.

43. Palomino AW, González R, Boric R et al. Expresión de integrinas de epitelio endometrial en ciclos estimulados con citrato de clomifeno. Libro IX Reunión de Resúmenes anual de la Sociedad Chilena de Fertilidad, 1998 p. 54.

44. Lopez E, Gunby J and Daya S. Ovulation induction in women with polycystic ovary syndrome: randomized trial of clomiphene citrate versus low-dose recombinant FSH as first line therapy. *Reproduction BioMedicine Online* 2004; 9: 382–390.

45. Williams RS, KiperSztok S, Hills D. A novel, simplified and cost effective protocol for superovulation and intrauterine insemination. *J Fla Med Assoc* 1997; 84: 316–319.

46. Ecochard R, Mathieu C, Royere D. A randomized prospective study comparing pregnancy rates after clomiphene citrate and human menopausal gonadotropin before intrauterine insemination. *Fertil Steril* 2000; 73, 90–93.

47. Check JH, Davies E, Adelson H. A randomized prospective study comparing pregnancy rates following clomiphene citrate and human menopausal gonadotrophin therapy. *Hum Reprod* 1992; 7: 801–805.

48. Sereepapong W, Suwajanakorn S, Triratanachat S et al. Effects of clomiphene citrate on the endometrium of regularly cycling women. *Fertil Steril* 2000; 73: 287–291.

49. Whittemore AS, Harris R, Itnyre J. Characteristics relating to ovarian cancer risk: collaborative analysis of 12 US case-control studies. II. Invasive epithelial ovarian cancers in white women. Collaborative Ovarian Cancer Group. *Am J Epidemiol* 1992; 136: 1184–1203.

50. Rossing MA, Daling JR, Weiss NS, Moore DE, Self SG. Ovarian tumors in a cohort of infertile women. *N Engl J Med* 1994; 331: 771–776.

51. Venn A, Watson L, Lumley J, Giles G, King C, Healy D. Breast and ovarian cancer incidence after infertility and in vitro fertilisation. *Lancet* 1995; 346: 995–1000.

52. Modan B, Ron E, Lerner-Geva L, Blumstein T, Menczer J, Rabinovici J, et al. Cancer incidence in a cohort of infertile women. *Am J Epidemiol* 1998; 147: 1038–1042.

53. Mosgaard BJ, Lidegaard O, Kjaer SK, Schou G, Andersen AN. Infertility, fertility drugs, and invasive ovarian cancer: a case-control study. *Fertil Steril* 1997; 67: 1005–1012.

54. Potashnik G, Lerner-Geva L, Genkin L, Chetrit A, Lunenfeld E, Porath A. Fertility drugs and the risk of breast and ovarian cancers: results of a long-term follow-up study. *Fertil Steril* 1999; 71: 853–859.

55. Ness RB, Cramer DW, Goodman MT, Kjaer SK, Mallin K, Mosgaard BJ, et al. Infertility, fertility drugs, and ovarian cancer: a pooled analysis of case-control studies. *Am J Epidemiol* 2002; 155: 217–224.

56. Boothroyd C and Yazdani A. Higher-order multiple pregnancy associated with metformin in women with polycystic ovary syndrome: two cases and review of the literature. *Fertil Steril* 2006 Jan; 85(1): 227.

57. Olivennes F, Ayoubi JM, Fanchin R. GnRH antagonist in single-dose applications. *Hum Reprod Update* 2000; 6: 313–317.

58. Reissmann T, Schally AV, Bouchard P. The LHRH antagonist cetrorelix: a review. *Hum Reprod Update* 2000; 6: 322–331.

59. Branigan EF, Estes MA. Minimal stimulation IVF using clomiphene citrate and oral contraceptive pill pretreatment for LH suppression. *Fertil and Steril* 2000; 73: 587–590.

37

Tamoxifen Citrate for Ovulation Induction in Polycystic Ovary Syndrome

Luciano G Nardo, Tarek A Gelbaya

Summary

Clomiphene citrate (CC) is widely used as first line treatment for ovulation induction in anovulatory women with polycystic ovary syndrome (PCOS). Tamoxifen citrate (TMX), another non-steroidal selective estrogen receptor modulator (SERM), is equally effective in resumption of ovulation in these women. In contrast to CC, TMX does not antagonise the endometrial development and has less of an anti-estrogenic effect on the cervical mucus. Despite the potential advantages of TMX over CC, current evidence shows similar pregnancy outcomes following ovulation induction with either compound. This may be due to the lack of studies with sufficient statistical power. Large randomized controlled trials are needed to confirm whether TMX might play a role in induction of ovulation in CC-resistant women with PCOS.

Rationale

Ovulation induction and pregnancy outcome remain a major challenge in infertile women with polycystic ovary syndrome (PCOS). Amongst several agents commercially available, clomiphene citrate (CC) continues to be the first line treatment for induction of ovulation in these women. While the efficacy of this pharmacological compound is relatively well known in terms of ovulation rate, safety and side effects, the pregnancy outcome is much lower than expected.[1] Another selective estrogen receptor modulator (SERM), tamoxifen citrate (TMX), has been reported to be equally effective in inducing ovulation and enhancing the pregnancy rate in anovulatory women with infertility.[2]

Introduction

Anovulation and oligo-ovulation account for 21% of female infertility.[3] The World Health Organization (WHO)[4] divides the causes of anovulation into three main categories:

- *Group 1:* Hypothalamic pituitary failure or hypogonadotropic hypogonadism (10% of ovulatory disorders).
- *Group 2:* Hypothalamic pituitary dysfunction or eugonadotropic (85% of ovulatory disorders).
- *Group 3:* Ovarian failure or hypergonadotropic hypogonadism (5% of ovulatory disorders).

Group 1 consists of women with low levels of endogenous estrogen production, non-elevated prolactin levels, normal or low follicle stimulating hormone (FSH) levels and no detectable space-occupying lesion in the hypothalamic pituitary region. Anovulation in these cases is often due to stress, weight loss or excessive exercise. Typically, these women do not have a withdrawal bleed after progestin treatment. Group 2 mainly consists of women with PCOS but may also include those with hyperprolactinemia (> 600 mU/l) and idiopathic anovulation. Group 3 consists of women with premature ovarian failure (i.e., premature menopause) characterised by high levels of FSH and low levels of estradiol.

PCOS, a complex endocrinopathy of uncertain etiology affecting women of reproductive age, represents the most common cause of anovulatory infertility. There is considerable heterogeneity of symptoms and signs in women with PCOS, and for an individual, these change over time. Women with PCOS have an increased risk of first-trimester pregnancy loss, impaired glucose tolerance, infertility and endometrial carcinoma. Their cardiovascular risk is also raised due to an increased risk of type 2 diabetes mellitus, hypertension and altered serum lipid profiles.[5,6]

The diagnostic criteria of PCOS have changed during the last decade. A recent consensus meeting between the European Society of Human Reproduction and Embryology (ESHRE) and the American Society for Reproductive Medicine (ASRM)[6] decided on the following criteria (mainly based upon experts' opinion). After exclusion of other etiologies such as congenital adrenal hyperplasia, androgen secreting tumours, hyperprolactinemia and Cushing' syndrome, two out of the three following factors are required to make a diagnosis of PCOS:

- Oligo- or anovulation,
- Clinical and/or biochemical signs of hyperandrogenism,
- Polycystic ovaries as seen on ultrasound scanning (USS).

While ovulation induction with CC is the first line treatment for anovulatory women at present, TMX has been less widely used for this purpose.[7–10] The recent National Institute for Clinical Excellence (NICE) report[4] regarded these SERMs equally effective for ovulation induction in anovulatory infertility.

Clinical Discussion

In anovulatory women, induction of ovulation aims to induce monofollicular ovulation. Without doubt, the underlying cause of anovulation as well as the efficacy, costs, risks and potential complications of each pharmacological strategy should be considered. The classification adopted by the WHO provides a practical guide to appropriate therapeutic intervention.

Ovulation induction with antiestrogens (CC or TMX) is mainly indicated in oligo-ovulatory or anovulatory normogonadotropic, normoprolactinemic and euthyroid women (WHO group 2). These subjects produce gonadotropins and estrogen (as demonstrated by spontaneous menses or withdrawal bleeding in response to progesterone challenge) and are therefore, able to respond to CC or TMX. In contrast, hypergonadotropic women (WHO group 3) with serum follicle stimulating hormone (FSH) concentrations ≥40 mIU/mL and markedly diminished follicular reserve, have little or no response to antiestrogens. Hypogonadotropic women (WHO group 1) with low FSH and low endogenous estrogen production are also unlikely to respond successfully to the antiestrogens.

Antiestrogen therapy

Clomiphene citrate is a triphenylethylene derivative distantly related to diethylstilbestrol. Like TMX and raloxifene, CC is a competitive inhibitor of estrogen binding to its site-specific receptors and has mixed agonist and antagonist activity depending upon the target tissue. CC is an anti estrogen that competes for receptor binding sites with endogenous estrogens. By blocking receptors in the hypothalamus and pituitary, CC interferes with the feedback mechanism of endogenous estrogens on the pituitary and hypothalamus, thus increasing FSH and luteinizing hormone (LH) secretion by the pituitary cells. The clomiphene-induced elevation of gonadotropins stimulates the production of ovarian follicles and induces ovulation. Nevertheless, other mechanisms involving changes in the insulin-like growth factor (IGF) system and sex hormone binding globulin (SHBG) levels may also take part in the folliculogenesis and ovulation.[11]

Clomiphene acts primarily as an anti estrogen in the uterus, cervix and vagina. The normal increase in uterine volume and endometrial thickening that occurs during spontaneous menstrual cycles is absent during CC-induced cycles despite higher estrogen levels.[12,13] Some researchers,[14,15] in disagreement with others,[16] have found an abnormal luteal phase endometrial pattern in these cycles. Of note, CC directly impairs implantation efficiency in mice.[17] Data on the effect of CC on cervical mucus are rather conflicting. In a meta-analysis, a detrimental effect was seen only with doses $\geq$ 100 mg/day.[18]

After analysing four placebo-controlled studies on CC in oligomenorrheic patients, a Cochrane review showed an odds ratio (OR) of 6.8 and 4.2 for ovulation and pregnancy respectively.[19] Despite inducing regular ovulation, the pregnancy rate per cycle falls significantly after six months of treatment.[20] Furthermore, pregnancy rates are lower among women who ovulate only with high doses of CC. It has been hypothesised that failure to conceive, particularly after high doses, may depend on the anti estrogenic effects of CC on the cervical mucus[21] and endometrium.[15]

The NICE guidelines state that the first line treatment for WHO group 2 women should be CC (or TMX) for up to twelve months[4] and the recommended daily dose of CC should be 50 mg to 100 mg with a maximum of 250 mg. However, CC-resistance (failure to ovulate following CC) is common, occurring in approximately 15% to 40% of women with PCOS.[22–24] It is well established that resistance is associated with an increased body mass index (BMI) and that weight loss improves the success rate of CC therapy.[22] Alternative and adjunctive treatments – TMX, dexamethasone, bromocriptine, metformin and rosiglitazone – have been sought for CC-resistant anovulatory women with PCOS.

Tamoxifen, like CC, is a non-steroidal triphenylethylene SERM. The endocrine profile of TMX-induced ovulatory cycles suggests that its mode of action is analogous to that of CC. Chosin and Taito[25] measured serial hormone levels in women receiving TMX. The authors found that FSH and LH rose gradually during or just a few days after TMX was administered. Thereafter, serum estradiol levels increased gradually during the follicular phase reaching a high pre-ovulatory peak concomitant with the LH surge.[25] Indeed, these changes are similar to those observed after CC. It therefore appears that the initial site and mode of action of TMX involve occupying estradiol-binding sites on the hypothalamo-pituitary axis and preventing the negative feed back of estradiol.

Tamoxifen has a mixed agonist and antagonist activity, depending on the target tissue. It provides some protection against menopausal bone loss, presumably due to its partial agonist activity.[26] However, the increase in bone density (about 1.2% in the lumbar spine at two years) is substantially less than that recorded after estrogen therapy (5% to 7% at two years).

Due to its antagonist properties, the clinical application of this SERM for the treatment of breast cancer is well established. Among women with estrogen receptor-positive breast cancer, TMX reduces the risk of recurrence and death when given as adjuvant therapy for early stage disease and can provide palliation in those with metastatic disease.[27,28] In contrast to CC, TMX does not antagonise endometrial development due to a lesser antiestrogenic effect at the uterine level.[29]

Wu[30] found lower a miscarriage rate with TMX compared with CC.[30] Animal data[31–34] have raised concerns about the safety of TMX administration in women trying to conceive. However, these studies failed to establish a cause-effect relationship. As yet, SERMs for ovulation induction have not been shown to be teratogenic.

The association between fertility drugs and cancer, especially borderline ovarian tumours, is another fascinating issue for debate. In one study, the risk appeared to be increased only in women who had undergone more than 12 cycles of CC therapy.[35] The apparent association between fertility drug use and epithelial ovarian neoplasia seems to be related to the fact that these drugs are more likely to be used in infertile anovulatory women. On the premises that pregnancy rates are low after six cycles of treatment and the risk of ovarian cancer is increased after 12 cycles,[35] the American College of Obstetricians and Gynecologists (ACOG) has recommended that CC treatment should not exceed 12 cycles, in any case.

Case studies

The estimates for numbers of women conceiving with CC therapy vary greatly between 15%[4] and 50%.[22] Approximately 7% of pregnancies resulting from CC-induced ovulation are twins and 0.5% are triplets.[23] Ovarian hyperstimulation syndrome (OHSS) is very rare following CC-therapy, but patient's awareness and the need for careful ultrasound monitoring are mandatory. The miscarriage rate following treatment with CC has been reported to be between 13% and 25%.[22] Whether this proportion is higher than in women who conceive spontaneously remains uncertain.[36]

The debate about correlation between SERMs and spontaneous miscarriage is unsolved. While some researchers found a higher, but not statistically significant, miscarriage rate in the TMX group compared with the CC group,[8] conversely, others noted a lower miscarriage rate after TMX with respect to CC administration.[30] Borenstein and colleagues[37] reported 14 pregnancies after TMX administration in 12 women who had previously failed to conceive with CC. Overall there were no side effects and fewer treatment cycles were required compared with CC. Ovulation rate and cervical score with TMX therapy were significantly higher compared to CC ($P < 0.005$).

Weseley and Melnick[38] studied 17 CC-resistant patients with hypothalamic anovulation who were prescribed TMX 10 mg/day from cycle day 5 to 9 in two consecutive menstrual cycles. The authors excluded patients with hyperprolactinemia and PCOS. Treatment was monitored by ultrasound for assessment of follicle size and by biochemistry for measurement of serum estradiol levels. Fifteen women failed to ovulate, while of the remaining two women who ovulated, one had hCG on day 16 and conceived. Weseley and Melnick[38] were unable to demonstrate that CC-resistant patients would ovulate with TMX. These researchers subsequently administered the same dose of TMX to 45 patients with hypothalamic anovulation who had not been previously treated. Of interest, the analysis showed that TMX successfully induced ovulation in 84% of the cycles. There was also marked cervical mucus improvement in the TMX cycles as compared with the CC cycles.

In a prospective randomized trial[10] in which 95 anovulatory women without other causes of infertility were enrolled, the overall rate of ovulation in the TMX group was 44.2% and in the CC group was 45.1% (not significant). The ovulation rate per cycle in subjects who received 20 mg TMX was 56.5% and in those who received 50 mg CC was 46% (not significant). Ovulation rates per cycle with 40 mg TMX or 100 mg CC were 27.6% and 39.3% respectively (not significant), while with 60 mg TMX and 150 mg CC were 20.0% and 53.9% respectively (not significant). When trying to correlate the doses of the two compounds with the ovulation rate, there were no statistically significant differences, therefore suggesting that the mechanism was not dose-specific. The cumulative pregnancy rate per ovulatory cycle was 20.0% with TMX and 14.6% with CC (not significant).

In a small (n = 20 subjects) randomized crossover study,[39] CC (100 mg during cycle days 5–9) was compared with CC/TMX combination therapy (50 mg CC and 20 mg TMX during cycle days 5–9). The overall ovulation rate was higher in CC/TMX group compared to the CC group (75.0% versus 43.9%, $P < 0.01$). The pregnancy rate per ovulatory cycle was also higher in the CC/TMX group compared with the CC group (8.6% versus 4.8%, *P value* not reported). It was concluded that CC/TMX was more effective than CC for ovulation induction. Thus, the authors argued that the low pregnancy rate in both groups was due to the antiestrogenic effects of

CC on endometrial development and cervical mucus.

A recent Cochrane review[2] showed no difference between CC and TMX in women with anovulation (fixed OR 1.0, 95% CI 0.5 to 2.1). The use of CC in combination with TMX did not add any positive effect on the pregnancy rate with respect to CC alone (fixed OR 3.3, 95% CI 0.1 to 91.6). There were no trials comparing TMX with placebo, so it is certainly impossible to speculate on this issue at present.

Four prospective clinical trials comparing TMX with CC for induction of ovulation in infertile women with isolated anovulatory infertility were included in a meta-analysis.[40] After pooling the data from all the trials, the use of TMX or CC resulted in similar ovulation rates (OR 0.755, 95% CI 0.513–1.111). There was no benefit of TMX over CC in achievement of pregnancy per treatment cycle (OR 1.056, 95% CI 0.583–1.912) and per ovulatory cycle (OR 1.162, 95% CI 0.632–2.134). Steiner and colleagues concluded that CC and TMX are equally effective in inducing ovulation. Although data about pregnancy rate and treatment response are limited, there does not appear to be a significant benefit of one compound over the other.

We have recently published a controlled observational study[41] comparing the efficacy and safety of TMX versus CC in 102 anovulatory infertile women with PCOS, diagnosed using both biochemical indices and sonographic features. The ovulation rate per cycle of treatment using low dose CC (50 mg) or TMX (20 mg) was 42.8% and 67.2% respectively (OR 0.36, 95% CI 0.17–0.77, $P = 0.009$). The ovulation rate per cycle of treatment using high dose CC (100 mg) or TMX (40 mg) was 56.4% and 54% respectively (not significant). There was a trend towards a higher pregnancy rate per cycle with TMX when compared to CC (22.9% versus 18.3% respectively, not significant). Overall, our results showed that, in a selected population of anovulatory infertile women with PCOS, TMX has better efficacy and similar safety compared to CC.

Recent Advances

As the awareness of adverse effects of chemo- and radiotherapy on reproductive performance increases, more patients seek early referral for assisted reproductive technology in order to preserve their fertility potential. Embryo cryopreservation is a widely established clinical approach to store supernumerary embryos generated from in-vitro fertilization (IVF) treatment. This technique has already been used for fertility preservation in cancer patients.[42]

Since breast cancer cell proliferation and rapid dissemination are promoted by estrogens,[43,44] many would agree that conventional ovarian stimulation regimens are contraindicated in such patients. Although unstimulated (i.e., natural cycle) IVF treatment is an option, however, the chances of obtaining spare embryos for freezing are rather slim.[45] This will inevitably reduce the cumulative reproductive outcome.[46]

Oktay and colleagues[47] used TMX for ovarian stimulation and IVF in 12 women with breast cancer. The authors then compared the outcome with a historical control group of 5 women with breast cancer who had natural cycle IVF. They concluded that TMX stimulation results in a higher number of embryos and may provide a safe method of ovarian stimulation and fertility preservation in breast cancer patients. After a mean follow up of 15 ± 3.6 months (range 3–54), none of the patients had recurrence of cancer.

Conclusion

Clomiphene, rather than TMX, continues to be the first line treatment for induction of ovulation in anovulatory infertile women with PCOS. Although its efficacy is well known in terms of ovulation rate, safety and side effects, the pregnancy outcome remains much lower than expected. There also appears to be a trend toward an increased risk of spontaneous miscarriage.

Current evidence suggests that TMX is equally effective as CC in the induction of ovulation and pregnancy in WHO group 2 anovulatory women.

However, most of the studies in the literature are small and none of them report the live birth rate. Prospective randomized trials (i.e., level I evidence) with adequate statistical power are needed to show whether TMX may play a role in CC-resistant women with PCOS, to assess its correlation with endometrial thickness during the implantation window, and finally, to ensure its efficacy and safety in infertile women with a family history of breast and/or ovarian cancer.

References

1. Fluker MR. Ovulation induction with clomiphene citrate. In: Homburg R, ed. Polycystic Ovary Syndrome. London: Martin Dunitz, 2001.
2. Beck JI, Boothroyd C, Proctor M, Farquhar C, Hughes E. Oral anti-oestrogens and medical adjuncts for subfertility associated with anovulation. The Cochrane Database Systematic Reviews 2005; CD002249.
3. Hull MG, Glazner CM, Kelly NJ, et al. Population study of causes, treatment and outcome of infertility. *Br Med J* 1985; 91: 1693–1697.
4. National Collaborating Centre for Women's, Children's Health/National Institute for Clinical Excellence. Fertility: assessment and treatment for people with fertility problems. London: RCOG Press, 2004.
5. Lobo RA, Carmina E. The importance of diagnosing the polycystic ovary syndrome. *Ann Int Med* 2000; 132: 989–993.
6. Rotterdam ESHRE/ASRM-sponsored PCOS consensus workshop group. *Revised*, 2003 consensus on diagnostic criteria and long-term health risks related to polycystic ovary syndrome (PCOS). *Hum Reprod* 2004; 19: 41–47.
7. Gerhard I, Runnebaum B. Comparison between tamoxifen and clomiphene therapy in women with anovulation. *Arch Gynecol* 1979; 227: 279–288.
8. Ruiz-Velasco V, Rosas-Arceo J, Matute M. Chemical inducers of ovulation: comparative results. *Int J Fertil* 1979; 24: 61–66.
9. Messinis IE, Nillius SJ. Comparison between tamoxifen and clomiphene for induction of ovulation. *Acta Obstet Gynecol Scand* 1982; 61: 377–379.
10. Boostanfar R, Jain JK, Mishell DR, Paulson, RJ. A prospective randomized trial comparing clomiphene citrate with tamoxifen citrate for ovulation induction. *Fertil Steril* 2001; 75: 1024–1026.
11. Butzow TL, Kettel LM, Yen SSC. Clomiphene citrate reduces serum insulin-like growth factor I and increases sex hormone binding globulin levels in women with polycystic ovary syndrome. *Fertil Steril* 1995; 63: 1200–1203.
12. Eden JA, Place J, Carter GD, Jones J, Alaghband-Zadeh J, Pawson ME. The effect of clomiphene citrate on follicular phase increase in endometrial thickness and uterine volume. *Obstet Gynecol* 1989; 73: 187–190.
13. Dehbashi S, Parsanezhad ME, Alborzi S, Zarei A. Effect of clomiphene citrate on endometrium thickness and echogenic patterns. *Int J Gynaecol Obstet* 2003; 80: 49–53.
14. Bonhoff AJ, Naether OG, Johannisson E. Effects of clomiphene citrate stimulation on endometrial structure in infertile women. *Hum Reprod* 1996; 11: 844–849.
15. Sereepapong W, Suwajanakorn S, Triratanachat S, et al. Effects of clomiphene citrate on the endometrium of regularly cycling women. *Fertil Steril* 2000; 73: 287–291.
16. Li TC, Warren MA, Murphy C, Sargeant S, Cooke ID. A prospective, randomised, cross-over study comparing the effects of clomiphene citrate and cyclofenil on endometrial morphology in the luteal phase of normal, fertile women. *Br J Obstet Gynaecol* 1992; 99: 1008–1013.
17. Thomson JL. Effect of two non-steroidal antifertility agents on pregnancy in mice. II. Effects on tubal transport rate and implantation. *J Reprod Fertil* 1968; 16: 363–369.
18. Roumen FJ. Decreased quality of cervix mucus under the influence of clomiphene: a meta-analysis. *Ned Tijdschr Geneeskd* 1997; 141: 2401–2405.
19. Hughes E, Collins J, Vandekerckhove P. Clomiphene citrate for unexplained subfertility in women (Cochrane review). The Cochrane Database Systematic Reviews, 2000; CD000057.
20. Macgregor AH, Johnson JE, Bunde CA. Further clinical experience with clomiphene citrate. *Fertil Steril* 1968; 19: 616–622.
21. Kettel LM, Roseff SJ, Berga SL, Mortola JF, Yen SS. Hypothalamic-pituitary-ovarian response to clomiphene citrate in women with polycystic ovary syndrome. *Fertil Steril* 1993; 59: 532–538.
22. Kousta E, White DM, Franks S. Modern use of clomiphene citrate in induction of ovulation. *Hum Reprod Update* 1997; 3: 359–365.
23. Wolf LJ. Ovulation induction. *Clinical Obstet Gynecol* 2000; 43: 902–915.
24. Pritts EA. Treatment of the infertile patient with

polycystic ovarian syndrome. *Obstet Gynecol Survey* 2002; 57: 587–597.

25. Chosin T, Taito F. Endocrine profiles in tamoxifen-induced ovulatory cycles. *Fertil Steril* 1983; 40: 23–30.

26. Powles TJ, Hickish T, Kanis JA, Tidy A, Ashley S. Effect of tamoxifen on bone mineral density measured by dual-energy x-ray absorptiometry in healthy premenopausal and postmenopausal women. *J Clin Oncol* 1996; 14: 78–84.

27. Osborne CK. Tamoxifen in the treatment of breast cancer. *N Engl J Med* 1998; 339: 1609–1618.

28. Maugeri G, Nardo LG, Campione C, Nardo F. Endometrial lesions after tamoxifen therapy in breast cancer women. *Breast J* 2001; 7: 240–244.

29. Marttunen MB, Cacciatore B, Hietanen P, Pyrhonen S, Tiitinen A, Wahlstrom T, Ylikorkala B. Prospective study on gynaecological effects of two antioestrogens; tamoxifen and toremifene in postmenopausal women. *Br J Cancer* 2001; 84: 897–902.

30. Wu CH. Less miscarriage in pregnancy following Tamoxifen treatment of infertile patients with luteal phase dysfunction as compared to clomiphene treatment. *Early Pregnancy* 1997; 3: 301–305.

31. Furr BJ, Valcaccia B, Challis JR. The effects of Nolvadex (tamoxifen citrate; ICI 46 474) on pregnancy in rabbits. *J Reprod Fertil* 1976; 8: 367–369.

32. Sweet DL, Kinzie J. Consequences of radiotherapy and antineoplastic therapy for the fetus. *J Reprod Med*, 1976; 17: 241–246.

33. Sadek S, Bell SC. The effects of the antihormones RU486 and tamoxifen on fetoplacental development and placental bed vascularisation in the rat: a model for intrauterine fetal growth retardation. *Br J Obstet Gynaecol* 1996; 103: 630–641.

34. Halakivi-Clarke L, Cho E, Onojafe I, Liao DJ, Clarke R. Maternal exposure to tamoxifen during pregnancy increases carcinogen induced mammary tumorigenesis among female rat offspring. *Clin Cancer Res* 2000; 6: 305–308.

35. Rossing MA, Daling JR, Weiss NS, Moore DE, Self SG. Ovarian tumours in a cohort of infertile women. *N Engl J Med* 1994; 331: 771–776.

36. Oates-Whitehead RM, Haas DM, Carrier JAK. Progestogen for preventing miscarriage. The Cochrane Database Systematic Reviews, 2003; CD003511.

37. Borenstein R, Shoham Z, Yemini M, Barash A, Fienstein M, Rozenman D. Tamoxifen treatment in women with failure of clomiphene citrate therapy. *Aust N Z J Obstet Gynaecol* 1989; 29: 173–175.

38. Weseley AC, Melnick H. Tamoxifen in clomiphene-resistant hypothalamic anovulation. *Int J Fertil* 1987; 32: 226–228.

39. Suginami H, Kitagawa H, Nakahashi N, Yano K, Matsubara K. A clomiphene citrate and tamoxifen citrate combination therapy: a novel therapy for ovulation induction. *Fertil Steril* 1993; 59: 976–979.

40. Steiner AZ, Terplan M, Paulson RJ. Comparison of tamoxifen and clomiphene citrate for ovulation induction: a meta-analysis. *Hum Reprod* 2005; 20: 1511–1515.

41. Nardo LG. Management of anovulatory infertility associated with polycystic ovary syndrome: tamoxifen citrate an effective alternative compound to clomiphene citrate. *Gynecol Endocrinol* 2004; 19: 235–238.

42. Meniru, GI, Craft I. In vitro fertilization and embryo cryopreservation prior to hysterectomy for cervical cancer. *Int J Gynaecol Obstet* 1997; 56: 69–70.

43. Allred CD, Allred KF, Ju YH, Virant SM, Helferich WG. Soy diets containing varying amounts of genistein stimulate growth of estrogen-dependent (MCF-7) tumors in a dose-dependent manner. *Cancer Res*, 2001; 61: 5045–5050.

44. Prest SJ, May FE, Westley BR. The estrogen-regulated protein, TFF1, stimulates migration of human breast cancer cells. *FASEB J* 2002; 16: 592–594.

45. Omland AK, Fedorcsak P, Storeng R, Dale PO, Abyholm T, Tanbo T. Natural cycle IVF in unexplained, endometriosis-associated and tubal factor infertility. *Hum Reprod*, 2001; 16: 2587–2592.

46. Davis OK, Rosenwaks Z. Superovulation strategies for assisted reproductive technologies. *Semin Reprod Med* 2001; 19: 207–212.

47. Oktay K, Buyuk E, Davis O, Yermakova I, Veeck L, Rosenwaks Z. Fertility preservation in breast cancer patients: IVF and embryo cryopreservation after ovarian stimulation with tamoxifen. *Hum Reprod* 2003; 18: 90–95.

38

Urinary Gonadotropin Treatment in Patients with Polycystic Ovary Syndrome

Gautam N Allahbadia, Rina Agrawal

Summary

Polycystic Ovary Syndrome (PCOS) is considered to be one of the most common endocrinopathies in women of the reproductive age. Moreover, it is also the most common cause of anovulatory infertility. The main treatments of infertility in PCOS patients are performed by ovarian stimulation with follicle stimulating hormone (FSH), a reduction in insulin concentration and a decrease in luteinizing hormone (LH) levels. These are considered to be the main points of the therapeutic treatment.[1–7] Clomiphene citrate is often used as first-line treatment in PCOS.[8] In case clomiphene citrate treatment is not successful, it is generally preceded by direct FSH stimulation.[9] In order to avoid the occurrence of ovarian hyperstimulation syndrome (OHSS) and multiple pregnancies, FSH stimulation is performed with a low-dose protocol.[7] Human menopausal gonadotropin (hMG) has been used for ovarian stimulation. Unfortunately, hMG has a low specific activity and contains significant amounts of LH. LH was thought to lead to poor oocyte quality, reduced fertilization rates, lower embryonic viability and early pregnancy loss.[10] Elevated LH concentrations frequently, are encountered in patients with PCOS and different studies have linked excessive LH secretion with detrimental effects on reproductive function, such as irregular menstrual cycles, anovulation, infertility and miscarriage.[3,11,12] Elevated LH concentrations may directly or indirectly hasten late follicular phase meiotic maturation and abnormal oocyte maturation may be responsible for the reduced fertility and increased miscarriage rates frequently encountered in women with PCOS.[3,11,12] Therefore, the use of FSH-only products rather than hMG for ovulation induction in PCOS, where endogenous LH is already elevated, seems conceptually better.[13,14] This notwithstanding, it has been questioned whether the above models can be applied to ovulation induction with gonadotropins[12] on the basis that the administration of hMG to patients with PCOS who are not receiving GnRH agonists, does not result in significant increases in serum LH concentrations.[15–17] It is postulated that, during ovulation induction, gonadotropin-stimulated estrogens and inhibins feed back on the hypothalamic–pituitary axis and reduce endogenous gonadotropin secretion and thus, daily LH serum concentrations remain low.[12]

Rationale

Approximately 15% of patients with PCOS remain anovulatory despite treatment with oral antiestrogen medications such as clomiphene citrate. In addition, about half the women with

PCOS ovulating on antiestrogen treatment, fail to conceive. Gonadotropin stimulation is the next step in treatment for women who are "clomiphene resistant", however, results of gonadotropin stimulation in women with PCOS are less successful. In PCOS associated with hypersecretion of LH, purified urinary follicle-stimulating hormone (u-FSH) preparations have theoretical advantages over the use of human menopausal gonadotropin (hMG) preparations (containing both FSH and LH), but whether this claimed advantage extends into clinical practice remains uncertain.

Introduction

Ovulatory disorders are present in approximately 15–25% of couples presenting for an infertility evaluation.[18] The great majority of patients with anovulatory infertility fall into the WHO group II category and most of them have polycystic ovary syndrome (PCOS).[18] In these PCOS infertile patients, clomiphene citrate induction of ovulation is commonly used as the primary mode of therapy. In patients with clomiphene citrate-resistant PCOS, i.e. those who fail to ovulate or conceive, the next step is usually to administer gonadotropins. Human menopausal gonadotropin (hMG), theoretically containing 75 IU of FSH and 75 IU of LH, has been used effectively for ovulation induction, and for years, this has been the only urinary gonadotropin for clinical use. The development and use of other urine- derived FSH preparations (uFSH) containing smaller quantities of LH resulted in higher pregnancy rates compared with the use of hMG in in vitro fertilization (IVF) cycles.[19] The development of a new medicinal product containing human recombinant FSH (r-FSH) was thought to represent the ultimate solution for ovulation induction, given that r-FSH is completely free from LH. Although this presumption was appealing, clinical results in IVF from the use of r-FSH were not outstanding.

Moreover, some recent trials have shown that the addition of exogenous LH to down-regulated r-FSH-stimulated cycles, improved implantation rate,[20] shortened treatment duration, reduced menotropin consumption and may have decreased the occurrence of side-effects.[21]

Clinical Discussion

Multiple pregnancy is one of the most serious complications of fertility treatment. There has been a marked increase in the rate of multiple pregnancies. The increased multiple birth rates since 1975 have been attributed to the higher proportion of patients treated with ovulation-inducing hormones, and since 1985, have been attributed partially to IVF.[22] Thus, the increase in multiple pregnancies is due, mainly to development of multiple follicles in ovulation induction and the transfer of multiple pre-embryos in assisted reproductive technology (ART). Limitation of the number of pre-embryos that are transferred was expected to reduce the rate of multiple pregnancies in ART.[23] However, it is difficult to prevent multiple pregnancy in patients who are receiving gonadotropin therapy because the precise mechanism of monofollicular development is not yet fully known.

Recently, low-dose FSH therapy has been re-evaluated and advocated for women with polycystic ovary syndrome (PCOS).[24] Previous studies[25–27] have demonstrated the efficacy of low-dose FSH treatment in PCOS, particularly with regard to the low rate of multiple pregnancies. This low-dose step-up protocol is based on the concept of the FSH threshold.[28] An FSH-level threshold needs to be reached for ovarian response to occur, and a very narrow range exists between the threshold and ceiling level for mono follicular growth.[29] Recent reports[30–35] have indicated that the rate of mono follicular cycles reached nearly 50%–70% and the incidences of ovarian hyperstimulation syndrome (OHSS) and multiple pregnancy were extremely low in patients who received the low-dose FSH regimen.

On the other hand, Mizunuma et al.[36] previously reported the efficacy of the step-down protocol. This protocol is postulated to mimic the physiologic secretion of endogenous FSH release.[37] In a normal ovulatory cycle, high FSH concentration in the perimenstrual period is essential to cohort growth. After the selection of a dominant follicle, however, the FSH concentration gradually decreases. The number of recruited follicles may be related to the extent and duration of the elevation of serum FSH concentration.[38] The step-down protocol is based on the FSH window concept, and it narrows this FSH window and prevents development of multiple follicles. This protocol has reduced the number of intermediate follicles, compared with the conventional fixed-dose regimen,[36] and the multiple pregnancy rate (PR) has been kept at a low level in normogonadotropic clomiphene citrate–resistant anovulatory patients.[39]

Recently, Aboulghar et al.[40] also demonstrated that low-dose recombinant FSH is as effective as low-dose hMG in producing reasonable ovulation and PRs in women with PCOS and a history of severe OHSS. These results indicate that the gonadotropin stimulation protocol, rather than the preparations of gonadotropin, is a key factor in reducing the incidence of OHSS and multiple pregnancies in ovulation induction in women with PCOS.

Although higher daily hMG doses were needed in cycles with ketoconazole compared with cycles without the drug, the peak E2 levels were substantially lower in the ketoconazole cycles.[41] Although the number of lead follicles did not differ between treatments, the addition of ketoconazole significantly reduced the number of hyperstimulated cycles. Consequently, the cancellation rate dropped dramatically, thus yielding a higher pregnancy rate per patient in the ketoconazole protocols. Use of a very low dose of ketoconazole during ovulation induction effectively attenuates ovarian steroidogenesis in patients with PCOS. This effect may serve as an adjunct to better control the ovarian response in women who are prone to hyperstimulated cycles.[41]

Case studies

The major risks of exogenous gonadotropin therapy for ovulation induction in a patient with polycystic ovaries (PCO) are multiple pregnancies and ovarian hyperstimulation syndrome (OHSS). A recent case report describes a 23-year-old patient, who was referred to the Centre for Reproductive Medicine in Brussels because of a high risk of developing OHSS and rising LH following ovulation induction with a low-dose step-up protocol using urinary gonadotropins.[42] After counseling the patient, the decision was made to perform a rescue IVF cycle. The patient was first coasted with 0.25 mg ganirelix; the serum estradiol concentrations decreased and the LH peak was successfully suppressed. No OHSS occurred. An ongoing twin pregnancy was achieved after the transfer of two embryos. This case report demonstrates the feasibility of coasting with LH-releasing hormone (LHRH) antagonists (0.25 mg ganirelix) and the usefulness of the antagonists for ovulation induction cycles in patients who need rescue IVF.[42]

Recent Advances

Monofollicular development and subsequent mono-ovulation and singleton pregnancy are the aims of ovulation induction therapy. FSH alone is sufficient to stimulate follicular development, even in women with hypogonadotropic hypogonadism,[43] although in these patients, LH activity is required for adequate steroidogenesis, fertilization and implantation.[31,44] It has been hypothesized that LH activity may be of clinical relevance in ovulation induction cycles in anovulatory women as it could promote monofollicular development.[45] Exposure to LH activity during the follicular phase could facilitate selective follicular growth, decrease the number of intermediate-sized follicles and increase the proportion of women who develop one mature follicle. The LH activity in menotropin preparations could be used to promote mono-ovulation in ovulation induction protocols. This could lead to a reduction in the risk of ovarian hyperstimulation syndrome (OHSS) and multiple pregnancies and its associated complications.

There have been some controversies regarding the use of preparations with LH activity in women with polycystic ovary syndrome (PCOS), since these women generally have elevated LH levels. There is, however, extensive clinical documentation with menotropins, supporting their use in clomiphene citrate-resistant women with PCOS.[16,46,47] A meta-analysis of these small studies suggests similar ovulation and pregnancy rates between menotropins and urinary FSH-only preparations in women with PCOS undergoing ovulation induction.[48]

A recent study provides evidence that the ovulation rate with a highly purified hMG (HP-hMG) preparation is at least as good as that achieved with a r-FSH preparation in anovulatory WHO Group II women who failed to ovulate or conceive with clomiphene citrate.[49] However, the data suggest that the follicular dynamics resulting from ovarian stimulation with preparations that contain, or are deprived of LH activity differs. It has been hypothesized that LH activity may be of clinical relevance in ovulation induction cycles in anovulatory women as it could facilitate selective follicular growth, decreasing the number of intermediate-sized follicles and increasing the proportion of women with one single dominant follicle.[45] In the study by Platteau et al.[48] the number of intermediate-sized follicles was reduced with HP-hMG compared with r-FSH, and the proportion of women with bi/multifollicular development tended to be lower.[48] FSH activity will promote the growth of all follicle sizes, while LH activity will affect intermediate-sized follicles which have LH receptors expressed in the granulosa cells. With respect to the treatment efficiency parameters, there were no significant differences between HP-hMG and r-FSH, but because of the differential dynamics of follicular development with HP-hMG, it may take 2–3 days more to reach the human choronic gonadotropin (hCG) criteria.

An important issue to discuss is the perceived risk of OHSS in anovulatory patients receiving preparations with LH activity compared with FSH-only preparations. A meta-analysis of several studies of small sample size found no significant differences in pregnancy rate between urinary FSH preparations and menotropins when used for ovulation induction in women with PCOS;

however, a lower incidence of OHSS was reported in women receiving urinary FSH.[48] The findings from a large recent study indicate that HP-hMG does not increase the risk of OHSS compared with r-FSH preparations.[49] Actually, the higher numbers of OHSS cases, cancellations due to excessive response and multiple pregnancies in the r-FSH group could suggest that the LH activity could result in a safer and more controlled stimulation cycle.

The LH/hCG receptor has an almost ubiquitous distribution in reproductive organs, thus suggesting that the actions of hCG might be more extensive than previously thought.[50,51] Independently of FSH, low-dose hCG can support development and maturation of larger ovarian follicles that have acquired granulosa cells LH/hCG receptors, potentially providing effective and safer ovulation induction regimens. Human chorionic gonadotropin seems to be capable of improving uterine receptivity by enhancing endometrial quality and stromal fibroblast function.[50] Furthermore, through its actions on insulin-like growth factor binding protein-1 and vascular endothelial growth factor, hCG might stimulate endometrial angiogenesis and growth and extend the implantation window, thus making pregnancy more likely.[51]

Filicori et al.[51] recently conducted a study to prove that low-dose hCG alone can be clinically used to replace FSH-containing gonadotropins to complete controlled ovarian hyperstimulation (COH). Patients received [1] recombinant FSH or hMG throughout COH (group A); [2] ovarian priming with recombinant FSH/hMG followed by low-dose hCG (200 IU/day) alone (group B). In group B: [1] the duration and dose of recombinant FSH/hMG administration were reduced, and small but not large preovulatory follicles were reduced with fertilization rates that were higher. The authors concluded that low-dose hCG alone in the late COH stages: [1] reduced recombinant FSH/hMG consumption whereas intracytoplasmic sperm injection (ICSI) outcome was comparable to traditional COH regimens; [2] stimulated follicle growth and maturation independent of FSH administration;

[3] was associated with a reduced number of small preovulatory follicles; [4] did not cause premature luteinization; [5] resulted in a more estrogenic intrafollicular environment.[51]

Patients with polycystic ovary syndrome (PCOS) may need a longer period of pituitary down-regulation to suppress the elevated serum LH and androgen levels effectively during IVF treatment using the gonadotropin releasing hormone (GnRH) agonist long protocol. Hwang et al. proposed a stimulation protocol incorporating Diane-35 and GnRH antagonist (Diane/cetrorelix protocol) and compared it with the GnRH agonist long protocol for PCOS patients.[52] In the Diane/cetrorelix protocol, patients were pre-treated with three cycles of Diane-35, followed by 0.25 mg of cetrorelix on cycle day 3. From day 4, cetrorelix and gonadotropin were administered concomitantly until the day of hCG injection. Serum LH, estradiol and testosterone levels were suppressed comparably in both protocols at the start of gonadotropin administration. Serum LH was suppressed at constant levels without a premature LH surge in the Diane/cetrorelix protocol. The clinical results for both protocols were comparable, with significantly fewer days of injection, lower amounts of gonadotropin used and lower estradiol levels on the day of hCG injection following the Diane/cetrorelix protocol. Furthermore, there was no significant difference in clinical pregnancy outcome between the two stimulation protocols.[52]

Conclusion

LH plays critical roles in the control of folliculogenesis and ovarian function in humans. LH activity administration during gonadotropin ovulation induction can enhance the ovarian response and optimize treatment. More specifically, LH activity (both LH and low-dose hCG) can support growth and stimulate the maturation of larger ovarian follicles as a result of specific granulosa cell receptors that develop after a few days of FSH priming. This action of LH is independent of FSH, and it has been shown

recently that the last stages of follicular development can be supported by sole administration of LH activity in the form of low-dose hCG, without causing premature luteinization.

Reproductively competent oocytes and pregnancy can be obtained with this regimen. Furthermore, LH activity is capable of reducing the development of small ovarian follicles (<10 mm) that may predispose patients to developing complications such as the ovarian hyperstimulation syndrome. Thus, better understanding of the dynamics and mechanisms that control human folliculogenesis and a more rational and selective use of LH activity administration, may allow a reduction in cost and increased safety, while maintaining a high efficacy of the ovulation induction regimens used in PCOS subjects.

References

1. Seibel MM, Kamrava MM, McArdle C, Taymor ML. Treatment of polycystic ovary disease with chronic low-dose follicle stimulating hormone: biochemical changes and ultrasound correlation. *Int J Fertil* 1984; 29: 39–43.
2. Dale PO, Tanbo T, Haug E, Abyholm T. The impact of insulin resistance on the outcome of ovulation induction with low-dose follicle stimulating hormone in women with polycystic ovary syndrome. *Hum Reprod* 1998; 13: 567–570.
3. Homburg R. Adverse effects of luteinizing hormone on fertility: fact or fantasy. *Baillieres Clin Obstet Gynaecol* 1998; 12: 555–563.
4. Jakubowicz DJ, Nestler JE. 17 alpha-Hydroxyprogesterone responses to leuprolide and serum androgens in obese women with and without polycystic ovary syndrome offer dietary weight loss. *J Clin Endocrinol Metab* 1997; 82: 556–560.
5. Nestler JE, Jakubowicz DJ, Evans WS, Pasquali R. Effects of metformin on spontaneous and clomiphene-induced ovulation in the polycystic ovary syndrome. *N Engl J Med* 1998; 338: 1876–1880.
6. Diamanti-Kandarakis E, Kouli RC, Bergiele TA et al. A survey of the polycystic ovary syndrome in the Greek island of Lesbos: hormonal and metabolic profile. *J Clin Endocrinol Metab* 1999; 84: 4006–4011.
7. Yarali H, Zeyneloglu HB. Gonadotrophin treatment

in patients with polycystic ovary syndrome. *Reprod Biomed Online* 2004; 8: 528–537.

8. Sovino H, Sir-Petermann T, Devoto L. Clomiphene citrate and ovulation induction. *Reprod Biomed Online* 2002; 4: 303–310.

9. Homburg R. The management of infertility associated with polycystic ovary syndrome. *Reprod Biol Endocrinol* 2003; 14: 109.

10. Stanger JD and Yovich JL. Reduced in vitro fertilization of human oocytes from patients with raised basal luteinizing hormone levels during the follicular phase. *Br J Obstet Gynaecol* 1985; 92: 385–392.

11. Shoham Z, Jacobs HS, Insler V. Luteinizing hormone: its role, mechanism of action, and detrimental effects when hypersecreted during the follicular phase. *Fertil Steril* 1993; 59: 1153–1161.

12. Filicori M. The role of luteinizing hormone in folliculogenesis and ovulation induction. *Fertil Steril* 1999; 71, 405–414.

13. Hillier SG. Current concepts of the roles of follicle stimulating hormone and luteinizing hormone in folliculogenesis. *Hum Reprod* 1994; 9: 188–191.

14. Simoni M, Nieschlag E. FSH in therapy: physiological basis, new preparations and clinical use. *Reproductive Medicine Review* 1995; 4: 163–177.

15. Anderson RE, Cragun JM, Chang RJ, Stanczyk FZ, Lobo RA. A pharmacodynamic comparison of human urinary follicle-stimulating hormone and human menopausal gonadotropin in normal women and polycystic ovary syndrome. *Fertil Steril* 1989; 52(2): 216–220.

16. Larsen T, Larsen JF, Schioler V, Bostofte E and Felding C. Comparison of urinary human follicle-stimulating hormone and human menopausal gonadotropin for ovarian stimulation in polycystic ovarian syndrome. *Fertil Steril* 1990; 53: 426–431.

17. Sagle MA, Hamilton-Fairley D, Kiddy DS, Franks S. A comparative, randomized study of low-dose human menopausal gonadotropin and follicle-stimulating hormone in women with polycystic ovarian syndrome. *Fertil Steril* 1991; 55: 56–60.

18. ACOG Practice Bulletin. Management of infertility caused by ovulatory dysfunction. *Obstet Gynecol* 2002; 99: 347–358.

19. Daya S, Gunby J, Hughes EG, Collins JA, Sagle MA. Follicle-stimulating hormone versus human menopausal gonadotrophin for in vitro fertilization cycles: a meta-analysis. *Fertil Steril* 1995; 64, 77–86.

20. Gordon UD, Harrison RF, Fawzy M, Hennelly B, Gordon AC. A randomized prospective assessor-blind evaluation of luteinizing hormone dosage and in vitro fertilization outcome. *Fertil Steril* 2001; 75: 324–331.

21. Filicori M, Cognigni GE, Taraborrelli S . Luteinizing hormone activity in menotropins optimizes folliculogenesis and treatment in controlled ovarian stimulation. *J Clin Endocrinol Metab* 2001; 86: 337–343.

22. Imaizumi Y. Recent and long term trends of multiple birth rates and influencing factors in Japan. *Journal of Epidemiology* 1994; 4: 103–109.

23. Jones HW. Twin or more. *Fertil Steril* 1995; 63: 701–702.

24. Meldrum DR. Low-dose follicle-stimulating hormone therapy for polycystic ovarian disease. *Fertil Steril* 1991; 55: 1039–1040.

25. Yen SSC. The polycystic ovary syndrome. *Clin Endocrinol* (Oxf) 1980; 12: 117–207.

26. Kamrava MM, Seibel MM, Berger MJ, Thompson I, Taymor ML. Reversal of persistent anovulation in polycystic ovarian disease by administration of chronic low-dose follicle-stimulating hormone. *Fertil Steril* 1982; 37: 520–523.

27. Polson DW, Mason HD, Kiddy DS, Winston RML, Margara R, Franks S. Low-dose follicle-stimulating hormone in the treatment of polycystic ovary syndrome: a comparison of pulsatile subcutaneous with daily intramuscular therapy. *Br J Obstet Gynaecol* 1989; 96: 746–748.

28. Brown JB. Pituitary control of ovarian function—concepts derived from gonadotrophin therapy. *Aust N Z J Obstet Gynaecol* 1978; 18: 46–54.

29. Ben-Rafael Z, Levy T, Schoemaker J. Pharmacokinetics of follicle stimulating hormone: clinical significance. *Fertil Steril* 1995; 63: 689–700.

30. Buvat-Herbaut M, Marcolin G, Dehaene JL, Verbecq P, Renouard O. Purified follicle-stimulating hormone in polycystic ovary syndrome: slow administration is safer and more effective. *Fertil Steril* 1989; 52: 553–559.

31. Shoham Z, Patel A, Jacobs HS. Polycystic ovarian syndrome: safety and effectiveness of stepwise and low-dose administration of purified follicle-stimulating hormone. *Fertil Steril* 1991; 55: 1051–1056.

32. Hamilton-Fairley D, Kiddy D, Watson H, Sagle M, Franks S. Low-dose gonadotropin therapy for induction of ovulation in 100 women with polycystic ovary syndrome. *Hum Reprod* 1991; 6: 1095–1099.

33. Strowitzki T, Seehaus D, Korell M, Hepp H. Low-dose follicle-stimulating hormone for ovulation induction in polycystic ovary syndrome. *J Reprod Med* 1994; 39: 499–503.

34. Homburg R, Levy T, Ben-Rafael Z. A comparative prospective study of conventional regimen with chronic low-dose administration of follicle stimulating hormone for ovulation induction associated with polycystic ovary syndrome. *Fertil Steril* 1995; 63: 729–733.

35. Grigoriou O, Antoniou G, Antonaki V, Patsouras C, Zioris C, Karakitsos P. Low-dose follicle-stimulating hormone treatment for polycystic ovarian disease. *Int J Gynecol Obstet* 1996; 52: 55–59.

36. Mizunuma H, Takagi T, Yamada K, Andoh K, Ibuki Y, Igarashi M. Ovulation induction by step-down administration of purified urinary follicle-stimulating hormone in patients with polycystic ovarian syndrome. *Fertil Steril* 1991; 55: 1195–1196.

37. Baird DT. A model for follicular selection and ovulation: lessons from superovulation. *J Steroid Biochem* 1987; 27: 15–23.

38. Fauser BCJM, Donderwinkel P, Schoot DC. The step-down principle in gonadotropin treatment and the role of GnRH analogues. *Baillieres Clin Obstet Gynaecol* 1993; 7: 309–330.

39. van Santbrink EJP, Donderwinkel PFJ, van Dessel TJHM, Fauser BCJM. Gonadotropin induction of ovulation using a step-down dose regimen: single-centre clinical experience in 82 patients. *Hum Reprod* 1995; 10: 1048–1053.

40. Aboulghar MA, Mansour RT, Serour GI, Amin YM, Sattar MA, elAttar E. Recombinant follicle-stimulating hormone in the treatment of patients with history of severe ovarian hyperstimulation syndrome. *Fertil Steril* 1996; 66: 757–760.

41. Gal M, Eldar-Geva T, Margalioth EJ, Barr I, Orly J, Diamant YZ. Attenuation of ovarian response by lowdose ketoconazole during superovulation in patients with polycystic ovary syndrome. *Fertil Steril* 1999; 72: 26–31.

42. Fatemi HM, Platteau P, Albano C, Van Steirteghem A, Devroey P. Rescue IVF and coasting with the use of a GnRH antagonist after ovulation induction. *Reprod Biomed Online* 2002; 5(3): 273–275.

43. Shoham Z, Mannaerts B, Insler V and Coelingh-Bennink H. Induction of follicular growth using recombinant human follicle-stimulating hormone in two volunteer women with hypogonadotropic hypogonadism. *Fertil Steril* 1993; 59: 738–742.

44. Balasch J, Miro F, Burzaco I, Casamitjana R, Civico S, Ballesca JL, Puerto B and Vanrell JA. The role of luteinizing hormone in human follicle development and oocyte fertility: evidence from in-vitro fertilization in a woman with long-standing hypogonadotrophic hypogonadism and using recombinant human follicle stimulating hormone. *Hum Reprod* 1995; 10: 1678–1683.

45. Loumaye E, Engrand P, Shoham Z, Hillier SG and Baird DT. Clinical evidence for an LH 'ceiling' effect induced by administration of recombinant human LH during the late follicular phase of stimulated cycles in World Health Organization type I and type II anovulation. *Hum Reprod* 2003; 18: 314–322.

46. Homburg R, Armar NA, Eshel A, Adams J and Jacobs HS. Influence of serum luteinising hormone concentrations on ovulation, conception, and early pregnancy loss in polycystic ovary syndrome. *BMJ* 1988; 297: 1024–1026.

47. McFaul PB, Traub AI and Thompson W. Treatment of clomiphene citrate–resistant polycystic ovarian syndrome with pure follicle-stimulating hormone or human menopausal gonadotropin. *Fertil Steril* 1990; 53: 792–797.

48. Nugent D, Vandekerckhove P, Hughes E, Arnot M and Lilford R. Gonadotrophin therapy for ovulation induction in subfertility associated with polycystic ovary syndrome. *Cochrane Database Syst Rev* CD000410, 2000.

49. Platteau P, Andersen AN, Balen A, Devroey P, Sørensen P, Helmgaard L, Arce JC. Similar ovulation rates, but different follicular development with highly purified menotrophin compared with recombinant FSH in WHO Group II anovulatory infertility: a randomized controlled study. *Hum Reprod* 2006; 21(7): 1798–1804.

50. Filicori M, Fazleabas AT, Huhtaniemi I, Licht P, Rao Ch V, Tesarik J, Zygmunt M. Novel concepts of human chorionic gonadotropin: reproductive system interactions and potential in the management of infertility. *Fertil Steril* 2005; 84(2): 275–84.

51. Filicori M, Cognigni GE, Gamberini E, Parmegiani L, Troilo E, Roset B. Efficacy of low-dose human chorionic gonadotropin alone to complete controlled ovarian stimulation. *Fertil Steril* 2005; 84(2): 394–401.

52. Hwang JL, Seow KM, Lin YH, Huang LW, Hsieh BC, Tsai YL, et al. Ovarian stimulation by concomitant administration of cetrorelix acetate and hMG following Diane-35 pre-treatment for patients with polycystic ovary syndrome: a prospective randomized study. *Hum Reprod* 2004; 19(9): 1993–2000.

39

Recombinant Gonadotropin Use for Ovulation Induction in Polycystic Ovary Syndrome

Lawrence S Amesse, Teresa-Pfaff Amesse

Summary

Many women with polycystic ovary syndrome (PCOS) experience some form of ovulatory dysfunction, thus rendering successful conception unlikely. For these sub-fertile PCOS patients, ovulation induction often plays a vital role in achieving pregnancy. Moreover, a subgroup of PCOS patients demonstrate resistance to the first-line therapeutic agent, clomiphene citrate, hence, the use of recombinant gonadotropins has become an essential second line of therapy for ovulation induction in these women.

Introduction

Polycystic Ovary Syndrome (PCOS) is a common endocrinopathy of the reproductive age woman affecting approximately 5–7% of the female population.[1] The pathophysiology of PCOS is multifactorial and variable clinical and hormonal manifestations have been described. The disorder is characterized by a combination of oligo-ovulation and clinical or biochemical findings of hyperandrogenism, following the exclusion of other etiologies. Outside North America, the characteristic sonographic appearance of polycystic ovaries is also included as a diagnostic criterion.[2] Frequently, insulin resistance is a prominent feature with compensatory hyperinsulinemia associated with hyperandrogenism.[3] Because of ovulatory dysfunction, many of these patients have difficulty conceiving and present for an infertility evaluation. Ovulation induction has become an integral part of the treatment plan for subfertile PCOS patients. A number of induction regimens have been developed and treatment protocols are rapidly advancing. Although weight loss, clomiphene citrate and metformin have been the mainstays for inducing ovulation, the use of urinary and, more recently, recombinant gonadotropins have become a fundamental second line of therapy in clomiphene citrate-resistant PCOS women. Three recombinant gonadotropins are available, recombinant follicle stimulating hormone (r-FSH), recombinant luteinizing hormone (r-LH) and recombinant human chorionic gonadotropin (r-hCG), and each is used to varying capacities in ovulation induction for PCOS. In this chapter, the pathophysiology of the hyperandrogenic ovary and the functions of endogenous gonadotropins are reviewed as a foundation to understanding the roles that recombinant gonadotropins play in inducing ovulation in PCOS patients.

Clinical Discussion

Pathophysiology of anovulation in PCOS

One of the biochemical hallmarks of PCOS is

inappropriate gonadotropin secretion, particularly luteinizing hormone (LH), by the hypothalamic-pituitary unit. High concentrations of LH stimulate theca cells to increase their production of intra-ovarian androgens that in turn, inhibit ovulation, resulting in oligo-ovulation or anovulation.[4] The elevation in serum LH levels is due to increases in LH pulse frequency and LH amplitude.[5,6] In obese PCOS patients, elevated LH levels are associated with an increased LH pulse amplitude, while in non-obese PCOS patients LH elevation is associated with increases in LH pulse frequency.[5,6] Although the mechanism underlying these differences is poorly understood, it appears to reflect abnormal variations of the hypothalamic gonadotropin stimulating hormone (GnRH) pulse generator, and may represent a fundamental difference between obese and non-obese PCOS patients.[5,6] Because the LH levels are markedly elevated and there is little change in follicle stimulating hormone (FSH) levels, PCOS patients often have a characteristic LH: FSH ratio that is > 2:1, instead of the usual 1:1 ratio found in normal ovulating women. Interestingly, the LH in PCOS patients also demonstrates greater bioactivity, and this finding may also account for excess ovarian androgen production.[5,6]

The ovaries of PCOS patients demonstrate normal recruitment of primordial follicles and the follicles develop properly to the early antral stage. However, their growth becomes arrested at the antral stage and they fail to develop into dominant follicles. The exact mechanism involved in the failure of follicles to advance is unknown, but it is thought that intra-ovarian inhibitors block the action of FSH or insulin-like growth factor-1 (IGF-1) required for follicular development.[7]

Role of gonadotropins in ovulation

The gonadotropins FSH and LH are glycoprotein hormones that are synthesized and released by the anterior lobe of the pituitary through a complex balance of positive and negative feedback mechanisms.[8,9] They play distinct, yet complementary roles in regulating ovulation and

their synergistic actions are responsible for stimulating follicle growth and oocyte maturation. A threshold FSH level must be reached for appropriate ovarian response, and the follicle requires stimulation by LH for final oocyte maturation and release.[10,11] Requirements for FSH vary as the follicle grows with the predominant role of FSH occurring during the early follicular phase of the menstrual cycle where it regulates steriodogenesis and induces synthesis of LH receptors.

Our knowledge of the role LH plays in the follicular phase of the menstrual cycle and its influence in follicular development is evolving.[12,13] Genes involved in the biochemical pathways that regulate ovulation respond to LH stimulation. During the late follicular phase granulosa cells of the dominant follicle become receptive to LH. Under LH stimulation, follicles measuring >10–12 mm in diameter continue to develop. Simultaneously, smaller follicles that do not express LH receptors undergo atresia due to increasing levels of ovarian androgens and diminishing FSH levels.[14,15] Ovulation is the decisive step of this process, representing the final stage of folliculogenesis. FSH and LH both activate the aromatase system, which enables the follicle to produce estradiol, spontaneously rupture (ovulate) and luteinize the granulosa cells. Disintegration of the follicular wall and subsequent release of an oocyte are triggered by the LH surge.[14] The LH surge also promotes luteinization that supports the corpus luteum during early pregnancy, before the placenta takes over this role.

A delicate physiological balance between FSH and LH concentrations must be maintained in order for folliculogenesis and ovulation to be achieved. Both gonadotropins appear to have "threshold" levels. Threshold FSH levels are required for early follicular development and threshold levels of LH facilitate follicular development by enhancing steriodogenesis.[10,11] Concentrations of LH beyond the threshold level suppress aromatase activity, promote androgen excess and inhibit cell growth. Subsequently, development ceases. LH levels that disrupt folliculogenesis are considered the "ceiling" response by the ovary.[10,16,17] Both threshold and ceiling levels are crucial for normal ovulation to occur, but defining these precise levels becomes more significant during pharmacologically induced ovulation.

Human chorionic gonadotropin (hCG) is used in ovulation induction as a surrogate for the LH surge. Endogenous hCG is synthesized and secreted by the placental syncytiotrophoblasts and is responsible for maintaining the corpus luteum during the first trimester of pregnancy.

Structure and pharmacokinetics of gonadotropins

The amino acid sequences and structures of FSH, LH and the human placental hCG are quite similar. Both, FSH and LH have a molecular weight of approximately 30 kDaltons, while the molecular weight of hCG is 43 kDaltons. Gonadotropins are heterodimeric glycoproteins composed of two non-covalently linked polypeptide chains, subunits α and β.[18] The α subunits of LH, FSH and hCG consist of identical amino acid sequences. The amino acid sequences of their respective β subunits have minor variations, helping to distinguish FSH from LH as well as from hCG. As an example, the β subunit of hCG differs from the LH β subunit by only an additional 31 amino acids located at the C-terminus of the hCG molecule.[18] Both, FSH and LH are released in a pulsatile manner from the anterior lobe of pituitary in response to gonadotropin releasing hormone (GnRH) secreted from the hypothalamus. In contrast, hCG is predominately produced by placental trophoblast cells.

The biological activity and potency of gonadotropins are influenced by a number of intrinsic and extrinsic factors. One of the more widely examined factors includes the composition of the carbohydrate moieties, which are a result of post-translation modification. The carbohydrate chains are composed of monosaccharides, one of the most important being sialic acid. Terminal sialylation of the protein backbone of the hormone varies with steroid levels and is an important regulator of hormone bioactivity. Indeed, it is sialic acid that determines the molecule's isoelectric properties that in turn, influence receptor binding affinity, bioactivity, and rates of absorption and clearance.[19–21] Gonadotropins with a lower number of sialic side chains have a more basic charge, higher receptor binding affinity and intrinsic bioactivity than their acidic isoforms, but are more rapidly cleared. In contrast, the more acidic gonadotropins that have a greater number of sialic acid determinants show lesser intrinsic receptor binding activity. However, their overall activity is 20-fold higher than the basic isoforms due to higher absorption rates, lower rates of clearance and longer elimination half-lives.[20,21]

Recombinant gonadotropins for ovulation induction in PCOS

The primary objective of pharmacologic induced ovulation in PCOS is the selection of a single or very few mature follicles that develop to pre-ovulatory size and spontaneously rupture. This contrasts with the multifollicular approach used in other areas of assisted reproduction. Important factors affecting the clinical effectiveness and safety of ovulation induction in PCOS need to be considered. These factors include the following parameters: rate of single follicle development, number of multiple pregnancies, incidence of ovarian hyperstimulation syndrome (OHSS), ovulation rate per cycle, number of miscarriages, rate of singleton live births per cycle and the cumulative singleton live birth rate.[22]

There is no consensus on the definitive ovulation induction treatment protocol for PCOS. Various treatment regimes have been used with varying levels of success, reflecting in part the multifactorial nature of the syndrome. The first line of therapy has been clomiphene citrate. If clomiphene citrate fails to induce ovulation, which is experienced in approximately 20% of the cases, or if pregnancy is not achieved, gonadotropins are then indicated.[23] Some clomiphene citrate resistant patients may represent PCOS subgroups that exhibit variations in their response to exogenous FSH threshold levels. Some PCOS women who fail to ovulate after clomiphene citrate may have greater ovarian dysfunction that is associated with a requirement for higher threshold dosages of exogenous FSH.[24] There are PCOS women who ovulate in response to clomiphene citrate, but fail to conceive and they may have lower FSH thresholds, requiring lower dosages of exogenous FSH to achieve appropriate ovarian stimulation.[24]

The use of gonadotropins in ovulation induction and other infertility treatments has evolved steadily over the last 50 years. Through the technologies of genetic engineering, recombinant gonadotropins have been developed and are replacing the less pure urinary-derived preparations. Indeed, they are becoming an integral part of the therapeutic armamentarium of infertility practices worldwide. Recombinant FSH is becoming the standard therapeutic agent used for ovulation induction in PCOS patients who are refractory to clomiphene citrate therapy. Recombinant hCG is becoming more widely used in ovulation induction as well. In contrast, recombinant LH is less widely used for reasons that will be discussed later.

Development of recombinant gonadotropins: historical perspective

The first gonadotropins used for stimulating ovulation were derived from human pituitary extracts. This method was almost entirely replaced by gonadotropins retrieved from human menopausal urine. Indeed, the first gonadotropin preparation, developed by Donini and Montezemolo in 1949, involved a process that retrieved gonadotropins from human menopausal urine. The purification technique required > 5 liters of urine to produce 75 units of human menopausal gonadotropins.[25] Human menopausal gonadotropin (hMG) was, for the first time, used in ovulation induction in 1958, and three years later, the first pregnancy using these agents was reported.[26]

Early preparations of hMG contained equal amounts of FSH and LH. Concerns over the high levels of LH found in the hMG preparations and the potential deleterious effects of LH on folliculogenesis led to the development of purification techniques that separated the two gonadotropins. Immunopurification with polyclonal antibodies was initially used to separate FSH from LH. Similar purification techniques were later developed utilizing monoclonal antibodies, and it was this purification scheme that resulted in highly purified urinary FSH (u-FSH) preparations. The extracted hormone preparations were 95% pure and had several hundred-fold enhancement of specific gonadotropin activity with only negligible LH activity. The amount of urinary proteins was significantly reduced, thus diminishing the levels of irritants. As a result, urinary FSH extracts from menopausal urine became the first preparations recommended for subcutaneous injection.[27]

Attempts to obtain even purer gonadotropin preparations were made possible with recombinant DNA technologies. Eukaryotic systems were developed in 1980's for cloning gonadotropin genes. Transfection of the Chinese hamster ovary (CHO) cell lines with genes for both the α and ß subunits of FSH, LH or hCG resulted in the production of biologically active recombinant FSH (r-FSH), recombinant LH (r-LH) and recombinant hCG (r-hCG).[27] The first recombinant gonadotropin to be used for assisted reproduction was r-FSH. The first birth following treatment with recombinant gonadotropins occurred in 1992, and shortly thereafter, r-FSH became widely available.[28] Recombinant LH and recombinant hCG were also developed and are now available for therapeutic use.

Recombinant FSH preparations

Recombinant FSH has been available since the mid-1990's. van Dessel and colleagues[29] reported in 1991, the first successful pregnancy after ovulation induction with r-FSH in PCOS. It has been widely used by fertility experts throughout the world, replacing urinary-derived products to become the primary source of gonadotropins used in assisted reproduction technologies. Although more expensive than its urinary-derived counterpart, r-FSH is superior with respect to product purity and specificity and there is no risk of transferring infectious agents. A number of studies have shown r-FSH to be as efficacious as urinary FSH in inducing ovulation in PCOS patients.[22,30–33]

There are currently, two injectable forms of recombinant FSH that have been synthesized and purified, follistim α and follistim β. Follistim α is produced by Serono Laboratories (Geneva, Switzerland) under the trade name of Gonal F®, while Follistim β is produced by Organon (Oss, the Netherlands) and is sold as Follistim® or Puregon®. Both preparations are similar to endogenous FSH and urinary FSH (u FSH) with minor differences found in the carbohydrate moieties. Their carbohydrate side chains are more basic and less acidic than pituitary FSH.[34] Follistim α and follistim β are very similar in their isohormone profiles. Their carbohydrate moieties and isoelectric charge distributions are comparable and they share similar levels of clinical efficacy. How these two recombinant gonadotropins differ is in the methods used in their purification.

Follistim α is produced in genetically engineered Chinese hamster ovary (CHO) cell lines and is purified by ultrafiltration. The purification procedure involves five normal chromatography separations and a reverse-phase high performance liquid chromatography (HPLC) separation.[27] The final procedure, immunoaffinity chromatography, is the mainstay for removing contaminants and product purification.[35] Follistim β like follistim α is derived from the culture supernatant media of CHO cell lines. The purification process involves anion and cation exchange chromatography, hydrophobic interaction extraction and a size exclusion chromatography step.[36]

FSH isoforms

Although all FSH molecules contain the same amino acid sequence, commercially available FSH products, all contain different amounts of FSH isoforms. Each isoform exhibits differences in their bioavailability, clearance rates and binding affinities. The differences in glycosylation between endogenous FSH, u-FSH and r-FSH, have a profound effect on the clearance rate and hence, the bioactivity and hormone potency of these preparations.[37] FSH isoforms that are highly glycosylated correlate with diminished clearance rates and longer half-lives when contrasted with less glycosylated isoforms. The addition of sialic acid results in an attenuated ability of FSH to bind its native receptor, and this results in diminished *in vitro* activity.[20]

Degrees of glycosylation and changes in isoelectric charge on the FSH molecule in serum will vary depending on the stage of the menstrual cycle due to the cyclic fluctuations in FSH and estrogen concentrations. The pre-ovulatory phase of the menstrual cycle is associated with the synthesis of FSH molecules containing lower sialic acid and sulphate content when compared with the postmenopausal FSH molecules that are highly sialylated. Analysis of the sialic acid composition of r-FSH indicates that it is more similar to mid-cycle, endogenous FSH than to post-menopausal u-FSH.[35,37,38]

Pharmacokinetics of r-FSH preparations: follistim α and follistim β

In an analysis of the two r-FSH preparations, follistim α and follistim β exhibited an identical *in vitro* immunopotency of 0.35 ± 0.01, and the biopotency of the two preparations was very similar. The isoelectric charge distribution between follistim α and follistim β differed slightly with a pI in both groups between 4.26–4.50, reflecting their similar carbohydrate complexity. It was the conclusion of the authors that follistim α and follistim β are quite similar in their properties, and from that they extrapolated that no differences in clinical effectiveness would be expected.[39] When administered subcutaneously, the half-life of r-FSH is similar to the 37-hour half-life of u-FSH, but contrasts with the 4-hour half-life of endogenous FSH.[37–39]

Recombinant FSH versus urinary FSH

Until the arrival of r-FSH, urinary FSH was the standard gonadotropin used in assisted reproduction and it is to this standard that the efficacy and safety of r-FSH must be compared. A number of comparative clinical studies with r-FSH and u-FSH have been conducted in women with PCOS who underwent ovulation induction. All have reported that both gonadotropin preparations are equally efficacious in ovulation induction.[22,30–33] In one study, patients randomized to the r-FSH group experienced significantly higher rates of ovulation and pregnancies and experienced shorter treatment durations and lower dosages of gonadotropin.[32] No significant differences were identified between r-FSH and u-FSH with respect to development of ovarian hyperstimulation syndrome (OHSS) and miscarriage rates.[31]

The clinical effectiveness and safety of r-FSH and u-FSH was analysed in an open, randomized, comparative study using the low-dose step-up protocol for ovulation induction. A total of 20 women with PCOS who were clomiphene citrate-resistant were enrolled.[40] A total of six pregnancies resulted in four live births, all belonging to the r-FSH group. Four patients developed OHSS. No differences were identified between the two groups with respect to the number of vials used and stimulation days.[40] Although it was the author's assertion that r-FSH was superior to u-FSH with respect to pregnancy rates, the small study size precludes universal acceptance of their conclusion. The data indicates that r-FSH is as effective as u-FSH when a low-dose protocol is used for ovulation induction in PCOS. It also reveals a trend towards a higher pregnancy rate in the examined patient population for r-FSH.

Gerli and colleagues[30] examined the efficacy and cost-effectiveness of r-FSH and u-FSH in a prospective, randomized, comparison study of ovulation induction in 170 women with PCOS.[30] No significant differences were identified between the r-FSH and u-FSH groups with respect following outcomes: follicular maturation, length of stimulation, pregnancy and delivery rates and multiple pregnancies. The cost per cycle of u-FSH was significantly lesser than that for r-FSH, although a significantly higher amount of u-FSH had to be administered. The data indicated that u-FSH was more cost-effective.[30]

Comparative studies of r-FSH and u-FSH analyzing embryo quality in *in* vitro fertilization embryo transfer (IVF-ET) cycles have been conducted. Controlled ovarian stimulation (COS) protocols for in vitro fertilization (IVF) produce a greater number of follicles and oocytes than those achieved by ovarian stimulation protocols without IVF. The following studies may provide some insight into this parameter. In a retrospective study of 811 r-FSH and 555 u-FSH IVF cycles, Racowsky and associates[41] analyzed whether any differences in embryo quality existed between r-FSH and u-FSH.[41] Factors used in assessing embryo quality included embryo cell number and degree of fragmentation. Rates of implantation and pregnancies were also considered. The data indicated that r-FSH resulted in a higher percentage of mature oocytes, improved embryo cleavages, more embryos available for freezing and higher implantation rates than u-FSH.[41] These findings were supported by an earlier study by Cheon et al.[42] In their prospective, randomized, double-blind study of 241 women undergoing controlled ovarian hyperstimulation for IVF-ET, the total FSH dosage and dosage per oocyte retrieval were significantly lower in the r-FSH group than in the u-FSH cohort. No significant differences were detected in the fertilization rate, quality of embryos transferred and pregnancy rates.[42]

Role of recombinant FSH in ovulation induction for PCOS

Treatment protocols that administer heading r-FSH for inducing ovulation in PCOS have varied and are continuously evolving. Superovulation protocols for normal ovulating women that use 150IU FSH are not recommended for women with PCOS. PCOS patients are highly sensitive to gonadotropins and are at a high risk of developing ovarian hyperstimulation. Thus, extensive monitoring and modifications of standard protocols are necessary. Many clinicians prefer starting at 75IU and adjusting the dosage according the patient response. There are variations of this treatment modality with the chronic low-dose protocols being the most commonly used regimens. There are two categories of chronic low-dose protocols: the low-dose step-up regimen and the low-dose step-down regimen. These protocols were designed to reduce the risk of developing multiple follicles and thus, diminish the likelihood of developing OHSS and/or multiple pregnancies.[43,44] Indeed, the chronic low-dose approach has been effective in reducing OHSS particularly when r-FSH is used.

Stimulation protocols

Low-Dose Step-up Protocols using r-FSH

The low-dose step-up protocols are widely used at many centers. The major advantage of this approach is that the hypothalamus-pituitary-ovarian axis remains intact, helping to prevent the development of multiple follicles.[45] Provided strict adherence to criteria used for hCG administration is observed, multiple pregnancies are avoided. The protocol was first developed for urinary FSH, but is now also used with r-FSH at many centers. After spontaneous or progesterone-induced withdrawal bleeding, a starting dose of 75IU of FSH is given and maintained over the next 14 days. When follicle maturity is achieved, hCG is administered. Ultrasound monitoring of the ovarian response and biochemical evaluation of serum estradiol levels is performed every 2-3 days. In cases where no ovarian response is detected after 14 days, the dose is increased by 37.5IU at weekly intervals up to a maximum dose of 225IU per day. When a dominant follicle is identified, the threshold FSH dose is maintained until the follicle measures 17 mm in diameter, and it is at this time that hCG is administered. Cycle cancellation occurs under one of the two following conditions:

presence of three or more follicles, measuring ≥15 mm, on ultrasound, or no follicular response after 35 days of treatment. Fourteen days after hCG administration, a serum pregnancy test is performed. In cases where ovulation has occurred, but there is no pregnancy, r-FSH is reintroduced at a subthreshold dose. This dose is determined by subtracting 37.5IU from the preceding threshold dose. Strict adherence to the stepwise increments must be observed. When multiple follicles develop, the regimen must be modified by either reducing the initial r-FSH dose, or decreasing the increments.[22]

Clinical studies have evaluated the low-dose step-up approach.[46,47] In a prospective, randomized, crossover study, follicular response to two different doses of r-FSH was investigated in 15 clomiphene citrate-resistant PCOS women.[46] Each subject was given a starting dose of 37.5IU or 50IU of r-FSH respectively on day 3 of the menstrual cycle with the dosage maintained for the subsequent 14 days. The step-up portion of the protocol involved respective incremental increases of r-FSH of 37.5IU or 50IU after 14 days of stimulation if no follicular response was noted. A second adjustment was performed 7 days later if no follicle formation was detected. The mean duration of treatment was 13 days with both the dosages. No significant differences in monofollicular development were found between the two dosages. As expected, the authors observed that the total amount of hormone used was significantly lesser when the initial starting dose was 37.5IU.[46]

In another study that was a variation of the above protocol, PCOS patients were administered a starting dose of 50IU or 100IU r FSH alone and this gonadotropin was administered on alternate days.[47] The dosage was increased stepwise at weekly intervals in the absence of follicular development. Using this regimen, the authors reported that 22 of 27 cycles were ovulatory and six pregnancies were achieved. The authors concluded that alternate day follistim β is a suitable stimulation protocol for many PCOS patients.[47]

Low-dose Step-down Protocols using r-FSH

The step-down protocols represent another category of the chronic low-dose regimens. When this stimulation protocol was first developed, it was designed to reproduce the PCOS physiology. This was achieved by administering a higher initial dose of FSH than that adhered to in the step-up protocol and then gradually, the FSH dose was decreased during the period of follicular development.[48,49]

A popular step-down protocol was first developed for urinary FSH, but now r-FSH is used in its place at many centers. In this protocol, a starting dose of 150IU of FSH is administered after spontaneous or progesterone-induced withdrawal bleeding and this dose is maintained until a dominant follicle, measuring ≥ 10 mm diameter on transvaginal ultrasound, is identified. At this point the FSH dose is reduced by defined intervals until hCG is given to induce ovulation. The reported monofollicular development was 88% in the cycles managed in this manner.[48] At our center, we have followed a similar protocol using r -FSH and observed comparable ovarian responses to that reported with urinary FSH.

Christin-Maitre and colleagues,[50] in a recent prospective, randomized multicenter study of 83 women with PCOS compared the step-up to the step-down protocol.[50] In the step-up arm of the study, patients were given a starting a dose of 50IU follistim β and the amount was increased to 75IU after 14 days if no dominant follicle was identified. One week later the dosage was increased to 100IU if there was still no follicular development. In the step-down protocol, stimulation was initiated with 100IU of follistim β followed by incremental decreases of 25IU for 3 days when follicular development > 9 mm was noted. This was followed by a second incremental decrease to 50IU that was maintained until hCG was administered. The pregnancy rates for each group were comparable. The study concluded that monofollicular development and ovulation were achieved more effectively with the step-up protocol than with the step-down protocol.[50]

Balasch and colleagues[51] conducted a crossover study that compared the low-dose step-up protocol with a modified step-down protocol in 26 clomiphene citrate-resistant PCOS women.[51] Patients were administered a one-time dose of 300 IU of r-FSH on day 3 of the menstrual cycle followed by three days without therapy, corresponding to days 4 through 6 of the menstrual cycle. On menstrual cycle day 7, daily doses of 75IU r-FSH were reinstated and maintained over the subsequent three days. The dosage was then adjusted depending on the ovarian response to the initial stimulation. Fewer multifollicular cycles and lower cycle cancellation rates were reported for the step-down protocol than in the step-up approach. Although no significant differences were identified in the amount of gonadotropins used or the length of stimulation and pregnancy rates, the authors concluded that the step-down protocol might be more appropriate than the step-up method in terms of avoiding multifollicular development.[51]

Comparative clinical trials using r FSH in step-up and step-down protocols have demonstrated comparable results. These approaches should be considered in PCOS patients for whom ovarian hyperstimulation is a concern. As in normal physiology, a delicate balance of FSH, LH, inhibin and other factors must be maintained in order to achieve folliculogenesis and ovulation and this same balance must be replicated in pharmacologically induced ovulation. Indeed, the treatment protocol must prevent multifollicular development, reduce the time-span of low-dose regimens and at the same time, create a pharmacologically induced physiology that enhances monofollicular development and ovulation.

Recombinant luteinizing hormone preparations

Recombinant LH (r-LH) has been used in clinical trials for a number of years. Prior to its development, the only available source of exogenous LH was from urinary-derived hMG. A disadvantage of hMG preparations is that highly variable levels of LH and FSH are present. Quite often, hMG has to be augmented with hCG, which can accumulate and potentially exert detrimental effects on follicular development and oocyte quality.[52]

The European Medicines Evaluation Agency (EMEA) approved recombinant LH for use in 2000. In the United States of America, it has been approved for use by the Food and Drug Administration (FDA) for infertile women with marked LH and FSH deficiencies, such as hypogonadotrophic hypogonadism. In this setting, r-LH is indicated in managing their anovulation and is used as a supplement to FSH-only treatment.[15] Recombinant LH has been used successfully to trigger ovulation following controlled ovarian hyperstimulation cycles. It is thought by some experts that r-LH is an optimal way of adding "pure" LH to ovulation induction cycles since there is no hCG activity in these preparations. However, concerns over its cost, which is nearly double that of both r-FSH and r-hCG, may significantly limit its use at most fertility centers.[53]

Pharmacokinetics of recombinant LH
Lutropin alfa is marked by Serono Laboratories as Luveris® and is dispensed in 75IU vials. This recombinant glycoprotein has a molecular weight of 29.4 kD, which is similar to endogenous LH and it also contains two glycosylation sites.[15] When administered subcutaneously, maximum serum concentrations are achieved in 4–16 hours. The measured half-life of r-LH is 14 hours and it has a bioavailability of 56%.[14,15,54] This finding is similar to the hMG preparation, which has a half-life of 18 hours when administered via the subcutaneous route.[20, 21,55]

Role of recombinant LH in ovulation induction for PCOS
The role of endogenous LH in PCOS is incompletely understood. Patients with PCOS often have elevated LH serum levels, and this appears to be detrimental to reproductive function. A recent report suggests that the compromised reproduction observed in women with PCOS is more closely related to insulin resistance than to LH elevation.[56] Other studies have indicated that the ovaries of PCOS patients are inherently different and that the response is not related to the LH elevation.[5,6]

Clinical trials have evaluated LH in ovulation induction. Two recent meta-analyses of 14 randomized, controlled, comparative trials of hMG and pure FSH in ovulation induction for PCOS women were conducted. There were no significant differences in treatment outcomes between the two preparations with respect to ovulation and achieved pregnancies.[57,58] In a small, double-blind study, r-LH was used in ovulation induction protocols for women with PCOS who hyper-responded to FSH stimulation. Patients in the r-LH group demonstrated significant follicular growth arrest, suggesting that there is an LH ceiling during late follicular maturation that prevents follicle development.[15] However, since this study has been critically evaluated for inherent flaws, the information it provided about r-LH may not be adequate.

Another clinical study reported that r-LH was associated with a reduction in the prevalence of OHSS when compared with r-hCG.[59] This work was conducted in IVF-ET trials, so the observed effect may not apply to ovulation induction. Most controlled super-ovulation protocols avoid the use of exogenous LH. It appears that the role of r-LH in ovulation induction for PCOS may be limited until further studies addressing its behavior are undertaken.

Role of recombinant LH in triggering ovulation for PCOS
Although r-LH supplementation of r-FSH in ovulation induction is not usually indicated in PCOS, some experts have advocated its use as a trigger for ovulation in these patients. This is because of the theoretical decreased risk of r-LH in developing OHSS compared with conventional hCG preparations. The shorter half-life of r-LH as opposed to that of the urinary hCG preparations has led to the speculation that r-LH may promote periovulatory maturation in a more selected cohort

of follicles. This hypothesis was supported by a report from the European Study Group that indicated that the incidence of ovarian hyperstimulation was decreased when r-LH (15,000-30,000IU) was used in place of hCG to trigger the final steps in oocyte maturation in IVF cycles.[59] Because of the large amount of LH needed for triggering ovulation, i.e. r-LH is produced in 75IU vials, this investigation has not been extended to studies involving ovulation induction. In his commentary, "Time to revolutionize the triggering of ovulation", Emperaire nevertheless recommends that research be devoted to improving the properties of r-LH. In the interest of patients' safety and to improve the luteal phase of the menstrual cycle, he suggests that the surges induced by r-LH be refined to simulate that of endogenous LH.[60]

Recombinant hCG preparations

Recombinant hCG preparations are derived through DNA technologies from genetically engineered CHO cells lines. After growth and cell expression, hCG is secreted into the culture media and banked over 30 days. It undergoes purification by repeated chromatography.[61,62] The main advantage of recombinant hCG is that it is free of contaminants and can be administered subcutaneously, thus avoiding an intramuscular injection. Another advantage is that there is a controlled source with little variation in preparations. Both urinary hCG and r-hCG appear equivalent with respect to ongoing pregnancies, pregnancy rate, miscarriages and the incidence of ovarian hyperstimulation.

Pharmacokinetics of recombinant hCG

Commercially available products of r-hCG were first available in 2001 and are marketed under the trade name Ovidrel® (Serono Laboratories, Randolph, MA). Choriogonadotropin alfa contains 257.5 μg of r-hCG that delivers 250 μg of r-hCG. A subcutaneous dose of 250 μg r-hCG is equivalent to 5000 units of urinary hCG (u-hCG) delivered intramuscularly. Maximum serum concentration is achieved after approximately

12–24 hours and the mean bioavailability is approximately 40%. The half- life of recombinant hCG is 38.2 hours when administered subcutaneously, which is similar to the 34-hour half-life of endogenous hCG. The elimination half-life is 29.2 hours with a median clearance of 0.51 liters per hour.[21,63] There are no indications that choriogonadotropin alfa is metabolized and excreted differently than endogenous hCG.

Role of r-hCG in ovulation induction for PCOS

Recombinant hCG (r-hCG) has the promise becoming the drug of choice for initiating ovulation. It is used in various areas of assisted reproduction, but for PCOS, it is used as an LH surrogate to mimic the LH surge and induce ovulation. During late follicular maturation, the mid-cycle LH surge is responsible for oocyte meiosis and follicle rupture. In the absence of the endogenous LH surge, choriogonadotrophin alfa acts an analogue of LH and binds to the LH/hCG receptors of ovarian granulosa and theca cells. The single 250 μg dose is administered when appropriate follicle development is detected by monitoring estradiol levels and vaginal ultrasound. It is given one day following the last dose of FSH. One dose of r-hCG appears to be equally effective in achieving final follicular maturation as the old-line urinary hCG, and the use of this formulation reduces the total dose of hCG. As a precaution, this exogenous gonadotropin may cause OHSS and multiple pregnancies.

A number of randomized, clinical, comparative studies, most of which involve IVF-ET, have examined the efficacy and safety of r-hCG and urinary hCG. Nearly all have reported similar findings regarding oocyte number and pregnancy rates with the overall consensus that there are no significant differences between the two preparations in terms of the above stated outcomes. A few clinical studies have reported on the use of r-hCG in ovulation induction for anovulatory women. In a prospective, randomized, double blind, comparative study, r-hCG and u-hCG were analyzed in 177 anovulatory or oligo-ovulatory women undergoing ovarian stimulation. Using the r-FSH low-dose step-up protocol, the subjects were randomized to receive either 250 µg r-hCG or 5000IU u-hCG. The results from this study indicated that r-hCG and u-hCG were equivalent with respect to ovulation rates and number of pregnancies. As expected, fewer adverse events, such as injection site reactions, were reported with the r-hCG preparation than with u-hCG.[64]

Conclusions

The monofollicular approach to ovulation induction in PCOS represents a challenge to the clinician. Not only does it require great skill and experience on the part of the specialist, but there are multiple patient factors that must be overcome. These patients are often clomiphene citrate-resistant and are inclined to develop multiple follicles along with the consequent complications of ovarian hyperstimulation syndrome and multiple pregnancies. They also experience a high rate of early pregnancy losses. Urinary-derived gonadotropins have been successfully used in ovarian stimulation and for decades, they have been the mainstay of infertility practices. The development and availability of r-FSH and r-hCG have provided an excellent alternative to the older-line products. Indeed, r-FSH and r-hCG are widely used in assisted conception throughout the world. In contrast, the role of r-LH in ovarian stimulation has been limited, although it may well have a role in triggering ovulation in PCOS. Recombinant FSH and r-hCG have been shown by multiple clinical studies to be as effective and safe as the urinary-derived preparations, and they have successfully been used in treating infertility. By nature of their production, they are pure, maintain a high degree of product consistency, and their subcutaneous route of delivery renders them more tolerable. These properties enable better dose titration for individual patients and this, together with more refinements in stimulation protocols, will enhance their future role in ovulation induction for women with polycystic ovary disease.

References

1. Franks S. Polycystic ovary syndrome. *NEJM* 1995; 333: 853–861.
2. Homburg R. What is polycystic ovarian syndrome? A proposal for a consensus on the definition and diagnosis of polycystic ovarian syndrome. *Hum Reprod* 2002; 17: 2495–2499.
3. Dunaif A, Segal KR, Futterweit W, et al. Profound peripheral insulin resistance, independent of obesity, in polycystic ovary syndrome. *Diabetes* 1989; 38: 1165–1174.
4. De Ziegler D, Steingold K, Cedars M, et al. Recovery of hormone secretion after chronic gonadotropin-releasing hormone agonist administration in women and polycystic ovarian disease. *J Clin Endocrinology Metab* 1989; 68: 1111–1117.
5. Yen SSC, Vela P, Rankin J. Inappropriate secretion of follicle stimulating hormone and luteinizing hormone in polycystic ovary syndrome. *J Clin Endocrinol Metab* 1970; 30: 435–442.
6. Rebar R, Judd HL, Yen SSC, et al. Characterization of the inappropriate gonadotropin secretion in polycystic ovary syndrome. *J Clin Invest* 1976; 57: 1320–1329.
7. Lara HE, Dissen GA, Leyton V, et al. An increased intraovarian synthesis of nerve growth factor and its low affinity receptor is a principal component of steroid-induced polycystic ovary in the rat. *Endocrinology* 2000; 14: 1059–1072.
8. Hay DL. Placental histology and the production of human choriogonadotrophin and its subunits in pregnancy. *Br J Obstet Gyneecol* 1988; 95: 1268–1275.
9. Ooi GT, Tawadros N, Escalona RM. Pituitary cell lines and their endocrine applications. *Mol Cell Endocrinol* 2004; 228: 1–21.
10. Hillier SG. Ovarian stimulation with recombinant gonadotropins: LH as adjunct to FSH. In: Jacobs HS, ed. The new frontier in ovulation induction. Carnforth, UK.; *Parthenon* 1993: 39–47.
11. Brown JB. Pituitary control of ovarian function–concepts derived from gonadotrophin therapy. *Aust N Z J Obstet Gynaecol* 1978; 18: 45–46.
12. Shoham Z, Jacobs HS, Insler V. Luteinizing hormone: its role in the selection of the preovulatory follicle. *Clin Obstet Gynecol* 1984; 27: 927–940.
13. Chappel SC, Howes, C. Reevaluation of the roles of luteinizing hormone and follicle-stimulating hormone in the ovulatory process. *Hum Reprod* 1991; 61: 206–212.
14. Caglar GS, Asimakopoulos B, Nikolettos N, et al.

Recombinant LH in ovarian stimulation. *Reprod Biomed Online* 2005; 10: 774–785.

15. The European Recombinant LH Study Group. Loumaye E, et al. Recombinant human luteinizing hormone to support human recombinant follicle stimulating hormone induced follicular development in LH and FSH deficient anovulatory women: a dose finding study. *J Clin Endocrinol Metab* 1998; 83: 1507–1514.

16. Loumaye E, Engrand P, Shoham Z, et al. Clinical evidence for an LH 'ceiling' effect induced by administration of recombinant human LH during the late follicular phase of stimulated cycles in World Health Organization type I and type II anovulation. *Hum Reprod* 2003; 18: 314–322.

17. Filicori M, Cognigni GE, Ciampaglia W. What clinical evidence for an LH ceiling? *Hum Reprod* 2003; 18: 1556–1557.

18. Pierce JG, Parsons TF. Glycoprotein hormones: structure and function. *Annu Rev Biochem* 1981; 50: 449–465.

19. Bishop LA, Robertson DM, Cahir N, et al. Specific roles for the asparagine-linked carbohydrate residues of recombinant human follicle stimulating hormone in receptor binding and signal transduction. *Mol Endocrinol* 1994; 8: 722–731.

20. Ulloa-Aguirre A, Timossi T, Mendez JP. Is there any physiological role for gonadotrophin oligosaccharide heterogeneity in humans. *Hum Reprod* 2001; 16: 599–604.

21. Lathi RB, Milki AA. Recombinant gonadotropins. *Curr Women's Health Rep* 2001; 1: 157–163.

22. Yarali H, Zeyneloglu HB. Gonadotropin treatment in patients with polycystic ovary syndrome. *Reproductive Biomed Online* 2004; 8: 528–537.

23. Imani B, Eijkemans MH, te Velde ER, et al. Predictors of patients remaining anovulatory during clomiphene citrate induction of ovulation in normogonadotropic oligoamenorrheic infertility. *J Clin Endocrinol Metab* 1998; 83: 2361–2365.

24. Imani B, Eijkemans MJ, Faessen GH, et al. Prediction of the individual follicle-stimulating hormone threshold for gonadotropin induction of ovulation in normogonadotropic anovulatory infertility: an approach to increase safety and efficiency. *Fertil Steril* 2002; 77: 83–90.

25. Donini P. and Montezemolo R. Rassegna di Clinica, Terapia e Scienze Affini. Biologic Laboratories, *Institute Serono* 1949; 48: 3–28.

26. Borth R, Lunedfeld B, Menzi A. Human pituitary gonadotropins: a workshop conference. Proceedings of the 1959 Gatlinburg, Tennessee meeting of the G-Club and the NIH. Thomas C. Charles (Springfield, IL) 1961; 255–257.

27. Howles CM. Genetic engineering of human FSH (Gonal-F). *Hum Repro Update* 1996; 2: 172–191.

28. Kousta E, White DM, Piazzi A, et al. Successful induction of ovulation and completed pregnancy using recombinant human luteinizing hormone and follicle-stimulating hormone in a woman with Kallman's syndrome. *Hum Reprod* 1996; 11: 70–71.

29. van Dessel HJ, Donderwinkel PF, Coelingh Bennink HJ, et al. First established pregnancy and birth after induction of ovulation with recombinant human follicle-stimulating hormone in polycystic ovary syndrome. *Hum Reprod* 1994; 9: 55–56.

30. Gerli S, Casini ML, Unfer V, et al. Ovulation induction with urinary FSH or recombinant FSH in polycystic ovary syndrome patients: a prospective randomized analysis of cost-effectiveness. *Reprod Biomed Online* 2004; 9: 494–499.

31. Bayram N, van Wely M, van der Veen F. Recombinant FSH versus urinary gonadotrophins or recombinant FSH for ovulation induction in subfertility associated with polycystic ovary syndrome. *Cochrane Database Syst Rev* 2001; 2: CD002121.

32. Coelingh Bennink HJ, Fauser BC, Out HJ. Recombinant follicle-stimulating hormone (FSH; Puregon) is more efficient than urinary FSH (Metrodin) in women with clomiphene citrate-resistant, normogonadotropic, chronic anovulation: a prospective, multicenter, assessor-blind, randomized, clinical trial. European Puregon Collaborative Anovulation Study Group. *Fertil Steril* 1998; 69: 19–25.

33. Loumaye E, Martineau I, Piazzi A, et al. Clinical assessment of human gonadotrophins produced by recombinant DNA technology. *Hum Reprod* 1996; 1 Suppl 1: 95–107.

34. Hard K, Mekking A, Damm JB, et al. Isolation and structure determination of the intact sialylated N-linked carbohydrate chains of recombinant human follitropin expressed in Chinese hamster ovary cells. *Eur J Biochem* 1990; 193: 263–271.

35. Recombinant human FSH Product Development Group: Recombinant follicle stimulating hormone: development of the first biotechnology product for the treatment of infertility. *Hum Reprod Update* 1998; 4: 862–881.

36. Olijve W, de Boer W, Mulders JW. Molecular biology of human recombinant follicle stimulating hormone (Puregon). *Mol Hum Reprod* 1996; 2: 371–382.

37. le Cotonnec JY, Porchet HC, Beltrami V, et al.

Clinical pharmacology of recombinant follicle stimulating hormone (rFSH). I. Comparative pharmacokinetics with urinary human follicle stimulating hormone. *Fertil Steril* 1994; 61: 669–678.

38. le Cotonnec JY, Porchet HC, Beltrami V, et al. Clinical pharmacology of recombinant follicle stimulating hormone (rFSH). II. Single does and steady state pharmacokinetics. *Fertil Steril* 1994; 61: 679–686.

39. Horsman G, Talbot JA, McLoughlin JD, et al. A biological, immunological and physico-chemical comparison of the current clinical batches of the recombinant FSH preparations Gonal-F and Puregon. *Hum Reprod* 2000; 15: 1898–1902.

40. Szilagyi A, Bartfai G, Manfai A, et al. Low-dose ovulation induction with urinary gonadotropins or recombinant follicle stimulating hormone in patients with polycystic ovary syndrome. *Gynecol Endocrinol* 2004; 18: 17–22.

41. Racowsky C, Orasanu B, Hinrichsen MJ, et al. Embryo quality based on ovulation induction: defining the differences. *Reprod Biomed Online* 2005; 11: 22–25.

42. Cheon KW, Byun HK, Yang KM, et al. Efficacy of recombinant human follicle-stimulating hormone in improving oocyte quality in assisted reproductive techniques. *J Reprod Med* 2004; 49: 733–738.

43. Homburg R, Levy T, Ben-Rafael Z. A comparative prospective study of conventional regimen with chronic low-dose administration of follicle-stimulating hormone for anovulation associated with polycystic ovary syndrome. *Fertil Steril* 1995; 63: 729–733.

44. Stowitzki T, Seehaus D, Korell M, et al. Low-dose FSH stimulation in polycystic ovary syndrome: comparison of 3 FSH-preparations. *Exp Clin Endocrinology Diabetes* 1998; 106: 435–439.

45. van der Meer M, Hompes PG, Scheele F, et al. The importance of endogenous feedback for monofollicular growth in low-dose step-up ovulation induction with follicle-stimulating hormone in polycystic ovary syndrome: a randomized study. *Fertil Steril* 1996; 66: 571–576.

46. Balasch J, Fabregues F, Creus M, et al. Recombinant human follicle-stimulating hormone for ovulation induction in polycystic ovary syndrome: a prospective, randomized trial of low starting doses in a chronic low-dose step-up protocol. *J Assist Reprod Genet* 2000; 17: 561–565.

47. Buckler H, Robertson WR, Anderson A. Ovulation induction with low dose alternate day recombinant follicle stimulating hormone (Puregon). *Hum Reprod* 1999; 14: 2969–2973.

48. van Santbrink EJ, Fauser BC Urinary follicle-stimulating hormone for normogonadotropic clomiphene-resistant anovulatory infertility: prospective, randomized comparison between low dose step-up and step-down regimens. *J Clin Endocr and Metab* 1997; 82: 3597–3602.

49. van Santbrink EJ, Donderwinkel PF, van Dessel TJ, et al. Gonadotrophin induction of ovulation using a step-down dose regimen: single-centre clinical experience in 82 patients. *Hum Reprod* 1995; 10: 1048–1053.

50. Christin-Maitre S, Hugues JN; Group. A comparative randomized multicenter study comparing the step-up versus step-down protocol in polycystic ovary syndrome. *Human Reprod* 2003; 18: 1626–1631.

51. Balasch J, Vidal E, Penarrubia J, et al. Suppression of LH during ovarian stimulation: analyzing threshold values and effects on ovarian response and the outcome of assisted reproduction in down-regulated women stimulated with recombinant FSH. *Hum Reprod* 2001; 16: 1636–1643.

52. Baer G, Loumaye E. Comparison of recombinant human luteinising hormone (r-hLH) and human menopausal gonadotropin (hMG) in assisted reproductive technology. *Curr Med Res Opin* 2003; 19: 83–88.

53. Filocori M, Cognigni GE, Samara A, et al. The use of LH activity to drive folliculogenesis: exploring uncharted territories in ovulation induction. *Hum Reprod Update* 2002; 8: 543–557.

54. Talbot JA, Mtichell R, Hoy AM. Recombinant human luteinizing hormone: a partial physiochemical, biological and immunological characterization. *Mol Hum Reprod* 1996; 2: 799–806.

55. le Cotonnec JY, Loumaye E, Porchet HC, et al. Pharmacokinetic and pharmacodynamic interactions between recombinant human luteinizing hormone and recombinant human follicle-stimulating hormone. *Fertil Steril* 1998; 69: 201–209.

56. Nestler JE, Stovall D, Akhter N, et al. Strategies for the use of insulin-sensitizing drugs to treat infertily in women with polycystic ovary syndrome. *Fertil Steril* 2002; 77: 209–215.

57. Nugent D, Vandekerckhove P, Hughes E, et al. Gonadotrophin therapy for ovulation induction in subfertility associated with polycystic ovary syndrome. *Cochrane Database Syst Rev* 2000; 4: CD000410.

58. Larsen T, Bostofte E, Larsen JF, et al. Comparison

of urinary human follicle stimulating hormone and human menopausal gonadotropin for ovarian stimulation in polycystic ovary syndrome. *Fert Steril* 1990; 53: 426–431.

59. European Recombinant LH Study Group. Human recombinant luteinizing hormone is as effective as, but safer than, urinary human chorionic gonadotropin in inducing final follicular maturation and ovulation in in vitro fertilization procedures: results of a multicenter double-blind study. *Hum Reprod* 2000; 15: 1446–1451.

60. Emperaire JC, RG Edwards Time to revolutionize the triggering of ovulation. Reproductive Biomed Online 2004; 9: 480–483.

61. Chang P, Kenley S, Burns T, et al. Recombinant human chorionic gonadotropin (rhCG) in assisted reproductive technology: results of a clinical trial comparing two doses of rhCG (Ovidrel) to urinary hCG (Profasi) for induction of final follicular maturation in in vitro fertilization-embryo transfer. *Fertil Steril* 2001; 76: 67–74.

62. Al-Inany HG, Aboulghar M, Mansour RT, et al. Recombinant versus urinary gonadotrophins for triggering ovulation in assisted conception. *Hum Reprod* 2005; 20: 2061–2073.

63. Trinchard-Lugan I, Khan A, Porchet HC, et al. Pharmacokinetics and pharmacodynamics of recombinant human chorionic gonadotrophin in healthy male and female volunteers. *Repro Biomed Online* 2002; 4: 106–115.

64. International Recombinant Human Chorionic Gonadotropin Study Group. Induction of ovulation in World Health Organization group II anovulatory women undergoing follicular stimulation with recombinant human follicle-stimulating hormone: a comparison of recombinant human chorionic gonadotropin (rhCG) and urinary hCG. *Fertil Steril* 2001; 75: 1111–1118.

40

Ovarian Hyperstimulation Syndrome: Strategies for Prevention in Women with Polycystic Ovary Syndrome

Laurel Stadtmauer, Patricia Tambucho, Sergio Oehninger

Summary

Ovarian hyperstimulation syndrome (OHSS) is a serious, iatrogenic complication of superovulation. The following is a review of strategies to prevent or minimize the development of OHSS, including individualization of gonadotropin dosing for ovarian stimulation, coasting, and embryo cryopreservation. Other recent advances are also addressed, including *in vitro* maturation of immature oocytes, and the use of gonadotropin releasing hormone (GnRH) agonists or recombinant luteinizing hormone (r-LH) to trigger ovulation in a GnRH antagonist treated cycle. Also discussed are therapeutic applications of colloid volume expanders such as albumin and hydroxyethyl starch. A review of our experience with OHSS-prevention at the Jones Institute for Reproductive Medicine, as well as case studies, is presented. All approaches are largely based on our current understanding of the underlying pathophysiology of OHSS.

Rationale

Ovarian hyperstimulation syndrome (OHSS) is a serious and potentially life-threatening complication of ovarian stimulation and ovulation induction, and is very common in women with PCOS. It is important to identify strategies to reduce the risk in this population and continue to strive for methods to prevent or eliminate this syndrome.

Introduction

Ovarian hyperstimulation syndrome is most often seen in women undergoing ovulation induction with exogenous gonadotropins, but it can also rarely occur following administration of clomiphene citrate, or after a spontaneous pregnancy.[1] Because women with PCOS have many small to mid-sized antral follicles, they are sensitive to gonadotropin stimulation, leading to increased estradiol levels. Risk factors predisposing to OHSS include polycystic ovary syndrome (PCOS), young age, history of previous OHSS and low body weight. The incidence of OHSS has been reported to be as high as 33%, with severe OHSS occurring in about 5% of gonadotropin treated cycles.[1]

Generally, OHSS is preceded by the development of multiple ovarian follicles in conjunction with a high serum estradiol (E_2) level. Luteinization following administration of human chorionic gonadotropin (hCG) is mandatory for the development of OHSS. hCG in an estrogen environment will bind to the endothelial cells in the uterus and to the granulosa cells in the ovary, leading to an increase in vascular endothelial growth factor (VEGF) and inflammatory cytokines such as interleukin-6. This leads to vascular leakage and follicle wall breakdown.[3] The early form of OHSS occurs 3–7 days after human chorionic gonadotropin (hCG) administration, while the late form of OHSS occurs about 14 days following hCG administration in a conception cycle, most often from endogenous trophoblast production of hCG. Multiple gestation is a further risk factor for the late form of OHSS.[1] OHSS is self-limited and recovery generally occurs in the late luteal phase of non-conception cycles. If pregnancy occurs, however, the time course of the disease may be extended to several weeks.[4]

OHSS is characterized by abdominal distension due to ovarian enlargement and increased capillary permeability leading to loss of fluid, protein and electrolytes into the peritoneal cavity. There is third spacing of intravascular fluid and ovarian enlargement. Severe cases are associated with a rapid weight gain from fluid, ascites, with pleural effusion and oliguria. There is a decreased intravascular volume leading to hemoconcentration, and thromboembolism may result from the hypercoagulability.[5,6] Symptoms of severe OHSS include abdominal distension and ascites, abdominal pain and decreased urine output. In addition, death following OHSS due to cerebral infarction and pulmonary edema has been reported in the literature.[7]

Treatment is supportive with replacement of intravascular fluids and paracentesis. Clinical parameters such as, weight gain, changes in abdominal girth and hemoconcentration, are useful for monitoring clinical progression. Severe OHSS often requires hospitalization and medical intervention. Intravenous fluids (normal saline) and plasma expanders, such as albumin or hydroxyethyl starch, may be useful in maintaining intravascular volume, and an anticoagulant may be necessary to prevent thrombosis. Periodic paracentesis may be performed to relieve physical discomfort, as well as to alleviate renal and respiratory compromise. There are multiple reviews on the strategies for management of OHSS.

Prevention of OHSS relies principally on identifying patients at risk and individualization of stimulation protocols.[8] Patterns of response to ovarian stimulation may also provide clues regarding susceptibility to OHSS. For example, the development of a large cohort of mid-size antral follicles (>20 visualized on ultrasound) associated with high and rapidly increasing estradiol levels, $E_2 > 3000$ pg/mL on the day of hCG administration, and use of GnRH agonists with more than 15 oocytes retrieved during in vitro fertilization (IVF), are all potential risk factors.[2]

Clinical Discussion

Ovarian stimulation with gonadotropins

Women with PCOS have an exaggerated responses to gonadotropins. It is useful, in this highly susceptible group, to begin stimulation with low gonadotropin doses and then carefully increase or decrease with small changes in the dosage. In ovulation induction, the goal is to achieve monofollicular ovulation. Administration of low dose gonadotropins in a slow protocol has been shown to be successful in achieving monofollicular ovulation in the majority of the cases.[9] The low dose step-up protocol consists of starting with a dose of gonadotropins (50–75 IU/day) for 7 to 14 days and increasing the dose by 25 to 37.5 IU/day if no response is observed. A recent study compared a conventional step-up treatment with chronic low-dose administration of follicle stimulating hormone (FSH). The step-up protocol consisted of incremental dose rises of 75 IU every 5–7 days according to the response. The conventional dose protocol led to a 24% pregnancy rate with 11% OHSS and 33% multiple pregnancies, while the chronic low dose regimen led to 70% mono-ovulatory cycles and a pregnancy rate of 40% per patient (20% per cycle) with a multiple pregnancy rate of < 6% and a 1% OHSS rate.[10] A comparison of the step-down protocol (starting with a dose of 150 IU but decreasing the dose by 37.5 IU when a follicle of 10 mm was seen, and decreasing by this amount every 3 days) and the step-up procedure, in a randomized study, showed that the step-up protocol yielded higher rates of monofollicular development than the step-down protocol with decreased OHSS.

Use of metformin with gonadotropins

Co-treatment with metformin has been shown to improve the ovarian response to exogenous gonadotropins in clomiphene-resistant PCOS women, and may be a strategy to reduce OHSS.[12] In this study, metformin was used in conjunction with FSH therapy among PCOS patients resistant to clomiphene citrate. Metformin co-treatment showed a more orderly growth of follicles and a reduction in the multifollicular development.

We also found a more orderly ovarian stimulation in women with PCOS undergoing IVF who had undergone metformin pre-treatment.[13] There appeared to be a shift in follicle size in the metformin group with a reduction of the number of small follicles in the recruited cohort. However, Yarali et al.[14] in a prospective randomized trial, did not find an effect of metformin pre-treatment on ovarian response when co-administered with FSH in clomiphene citrate-resistant PCOS women. Although this study, using the low-dose step-up protocol, did not show significant improvements in insulin sensitivity, this was in an obese group of patients and the trends were still towards lower duration of stimulation, fewer total numbers of vials and lower estradiol levels on the day of hCG in the metformin group. Based on these studies, it is possible that metformin use may lower the risk of OHSS by lowering estradiol levels and the number of small antral follicles in the cohort, although further studies are still needed to confirm this hypothesis.

Ovarian stimulation in IVF

The two most popular ovarian stimulation regimens with gonadotropins for in vitro fertilization (IVF) include the oral contraceptives overlapping with GnRH agonists[15] and a low gonadotropin regimen, or oral contraceptives plus GnRH antagonists.[16] Careful monitoring of serum estradiol levels with ultrasonographic assessment of follicle size and number helps to identify patients at risk for OHSS. When possible, after establishing a given gonadotropin dosage, one should try to step down gonadotropin dosages when the leading follicles are ≥ 13 mm. This approach provides the milieu necessary for the larger follicles to continue development while shrinking the smaller follicles. The net impact of such an approach results in fewer intermediate and small follicles on the day of hCG, thus theoretically reducing the risk of OHSS.

There may be a benefit to the use of GnRH antagonist cycles in reducing OHSS. In a controlled paired study of the agonist vs. antagonist cycles, the antagonist cycles led to decreased estradiol levels and OHSS rates.[17] As hCG is a risk factor for OHSS, other strategies have involved reducing the ovulatory dose of hCG. The customary dose of hCG is 10000 IU; however, the dosage can be reduced by 1/2 to trigger ovulation when women have high estradiol levels (over 3000 pg/ml).[18] Lowering the dose of hCG to these levels does not appear to affect oocyte quality or pregnancy rates.

Coasting

Coasting refers to the withholding of gonadotropins in women who exhibit extremely high estradiol levels (> 3000 pg/mL) and delaying hCG administration until estradiol levels decrease, usually below 3000 pg/ml. This has been effective in reducing the risk of OHSS without lowering pregnancy rates and avoiding cycle cancellation. Coasting reduces the number of intermediate and small follicles by removing the FSH stimulus, while maintaining the growth of the larger follicles Although coasting is associated with good pregnancy rates, there may be a reduced number of mature oocytes retrieved and reduced oocyte quality if prolonged, or if the estradiol levels are high.[20,21,22] Cancellation of oocyte retrieval should be considered if estradiol levels increase over 7000 pg/ml, or drop by more than 20% after hCG administration in coasted cycles, as oocyte quality, and pregnancy rates are generally poor when such a pattern is observed.[23,24]

Coasting is effective for ≤ 3 days before a significant reduction in implantation and pregnancy rates is seen.[24,25] There is a significant reduction in implantation and pregnancy rates in patients who are coasted 4 days or longer when compared to those coasted for fewer days without a difference in oocyte quality. However, Isaza et al.[26] found lower pregnancy and implantation rates in oocytes recipients whose donors were coasted for > 4 days consistent with a reduction in embryo quality. Our experience is in agreement with these studies showing a reduction in implantation and pregnancy rates in patients who were coasted for a higher number of days and whose embryos were transferred in a fresh cycle. When the embryos were cryopreserved and thawed and transferred in a subsequent cycle, the deleterious effect of coasting was not seen. This is consistent with an effect of high estradiol levels and coasting on the endometrium rather than an oocyte quality effect.[27]

Cryopreservation – should all embryos be cryopreserved?

Cryopreservation of all embryos following oocyte retrieval is another strategy to reduce the risk of OHSS and avoid cycle cancellation as a pregnancy in the stimulated cycle increases the risk for developing OHSS. Cryopreservation can be done at the 1-cell stage (2PN), at the 4-cell embryo stage, or at the blastocyst stage. The decision whether to cryopreserve all embryos vs. proceeding with a fresh embryo transfer can be made based on the patient's clinical progression and transfer can be delayed to the day 5 blastocyst stage if there is a question. Fresh embryo transfer can be performed if no overt signs or symptoms of moderate-severe OHSS are observed. Strategies to freeze all embryos or transfer in a subsequent cycle are usually based on the institution's experience and success rates with freezing, at various stages of in vitro embryonic development. Our experience is to cryopreserve at the pronuclear stage if possible, otherwise to transfer a maximum of 2 embryos and cryopreserve the remaining on day 3. Cryopreservation should be considered in

cases where prolonged coasting is performed or where the peak estradiol levels are > 7000 pg/ml. In this group, there are few pregnancies and better results with cryopreserved embryos.[24,27] There have been several reports confirming our experience that subsequent cryopreserved-thawed embryo transfers in such cycles yield reasonable pregnancy rates.[28,29]

In a Cochrane Review, Angelo et al.[30] recently examined the published experience regarding cryopreservation of embryos as a means of preventing OHSS. The included studies compared cryopreservation of all embryos versus embryo transfer after 48 hours; however, all study participants received intravenous albumin, a potential prophylactic agent, at oocyte retrieval, for the prevention of OHSS thus, potentially confounding the results. The other study compared cryopreservation versus fresh embryo transfer but here, the fresh embryo transfer group also received albumin, thus also confounding the results. The review of the two studies found no difference in all outcomes examined between the two groups and thus, concluded that there is insufficient evidence to support routine cryopreservation, and insufficient evidence for the relative merits of intravenous (IV) albumin versus cryopreservation.

Intravenous albumin administration

Prophylactic treatment with volume expanders such as albumin, hydroxyethyl starch (HES) and saline in high-risk patients may reduce the risk of OHSS.[31–34] Albumin or HES, given at the time of oocyte retrieval, may diminish the risk of OHSS by increasing the intravascular volume and decreasing third space fluid loss.

Aboulghar et al.[35] performed a search of the literature from 1966 through 2001, and published a meta-analysis of five single-center parallel randomized controlled studies that compared the use of human albumin with placebo or no treatment in the prevention of severe ovarian hyperstimulation syndrome. From those 5 studies, a significant reduction in severe OHSS was demonstrated in the albumin group, with an odds ratio of 0.28 (95% CI 0.11 to 0.73). They concluded that those trials showed a clear benefit from administration of intravenous albumin near the time of oocyte retrieval in the prevention of severe OHSS in high-risk patients.

The prophylactic use of intravenous volume expanders at retrieval is controversial, as other investigators have not been able to confirm the efficacy of albumin.[36,37] In addition, albumin has some side effects including nausea, vomiting, febrile reactions, allergic reactions, the potential risk of viral and prion transmission. Therefore, HES may be preferable as studies comparing HES with IV albumin have shown an equivalent reduction in the incidence of moderate, severe, and overall OHSS.[34]

In summary, the prophylactic use of intravenous albumin near oocyte retrieval remains controversial, and its benefit may, in fact be practice-specific or patient population-specific. The best way is to avoid gonadotropins altogether and use other strategies as will be discussed.

Ovarian drilling

One way to reduce the risk of OHSS and avoid gonadotropins is by ovarian drilling. In the initial report from Stein and Leventhal, women with PCOS were treated with bilateral ovarian wedge resection leading to the resumption of menstrual cycles and 85% pregnancies. Subsequent reports have shown poor success, and the concern with this procedure was the invasiveness and risk of periovarian adhesions.

The advances in laparoscopic techniques have resulted in renewed interest in ovarian drilling with the hopes that there is a decreased likelihood of adhesions and morbidity using this technique. Multiple studies have looked at the success using methods including electrocautery, laser and the harmonic scalpel. All have shown equivalent success with resumption of ovulation and menstrual cyclicity in approximately 80% of the patients.[38] The techniques involve thermal damage and necrosis of the ovarian stroma by drilling holes in each ovary, destroying the androgen-producing stroma. The result is a long-term

reduction in the intraovarian androgen production and reduction in the LH pulse amplitude and an effect on the pituitary-ovarian axis. However, there does not seem to be an improvement in insulin sensitivity.

One of the largest studies that followed patients long-term, found that 84% of women were still ovulating after 20 years of surgery and the androgen levels stayed normal.[39] Donesky and Adashi[40] reviewed 29 reports of laparoscopic ovarian diathermy and calculated an aggregate ovulation rate of 84% from the group of studies with a pregnancy rate of 55% in a total of 729 patients.[40] The conception interval was approximately 68% pregnancy rates within 12 months and 73% within 24 months. The majority of pregnancies were seen within the first year of surgery. A meta-analysis comparing patients undergoing ovarian drilling or gonadotropin therapy, concluded that there was insufficient evidence to determine a difference in pregnancy or ovulation rates in clomiphene resistant patients.[41] In this study, there was no evidence of a difference in the live birth rates or ongoing pregnancy rates and miscarriage rates in women with clomiphene resistant PCOS undergoing laparoscopic ovarian drilling compared with gonadotropin treatment. Therefore, the reduction in the multiple pregnancy rate and rate of OHSS, makes this option attractive. However, there are ongoing concerns about long-term effects of laparoscopic ovarian drilling (LOD) on ovarian function and adhesions. This conclusion was supported by a recent study comparing, in a randomized, double blind, placebo-controlled fashion, the effectiveness of laparoscopic ovarian drilling with metformin administration in the treatment of clomiphene resistant women with PCOS.[42] The authors found equivalent ovulation rates, but an improvement in the pregnancy, abortion and live-birth rates in patients on metformin treatment.

Case studies

We undertook a retrospective review of the incidence of OHSS in IVF and intrauterine insemination (IUI) cycles at our institution for the last 3 years (2003–2005). We treated over 300 women with PCOS with gonadotropins during this period of time. The overall rate of degree of severe OHSS in our PCOS patients who underwent ovulation induction and IVF, was less than 1.0%. We had only 8 women requiring paracentesis, but 2 required hospital admission with serious complications: one with pulmonary embolism and the other with pleural effusion. 7 of the 8 patients conceived, and 6 patients went on to deliver children (4 singletons, 2 twins, 1 spontaneous abortion). We will present 3 sample cases showing our strategy and treatment:

Case 1

As shown in Table 40.1, this patient (patient 1), a 32 year old with a body mass index (BMI) of 28 kg/m^2 was stimulated for ovulation induction. She was stimulated with 75IU of r-FSH daily from day 3 after a progesterone withdrawal induced period to day 11, with increased growth of follicles and increased estradiol levels. On day 12, the estradiol level was 745 pg/mL and she had 4 follicles measuring 13–15 mm in average diameter with multiple follicles less than 10 mm. Her r-FSH dosage was dropped to 50 units and Ganirelix, a GnRH antagonist was started to suppress the luteinizing hormone (LH) and prevent premature luteinization of the follicles. On day 14, her estradiol level increased to 1990 pg/mL and she had 4 follicles that increased in size to 16–17 mm. She was coasted for 2 days and Ganirelex was continued. Ovidrel (r-hCG) was given on day 16, with 4 follicles at >19 mm. and the estradiol level had decreased to 1500 pg/mL. She was counseled as to the risk of multiple pregnancies. IUI was performed 36 hours after the hCG injection. Sixteen days after the r-hCG injection, she was complaining of nausea, vomiting and abdominal bloating. An ultrasound revealed a small amount of ascites and moderate OHSS was diagnosed. Her serum level of beta hCG was positive at 495 IU and her hemogolobin was 12.5 g/dl. One week later, she presented to the emergency room with severe

shortness of breath. A chest x-ray showed a large, left pleural effusion and she had massive ascites. Her hemoglobin had increased to 16.0 g/dl. She was admitted to the hospital with a diagnosis of severe OHSS. She was treated with IV normal saline, albumin and furosemide for diuresis and prophylactic sq heparin (5000 units, b.i.d.). Her hemoglobin dropped to 12.5 g/dl and her symptoms improved. Paracentesis was performed with 2500cc of ascites removed. After 24 hrs, she was discharged and followed in the office where a paracentesis was performed 2 additional times. Her pleural effusion and ascites improved over the next 2 weeks. At 7 weeks, ultrasound showed a single intrauterine pregnancy with a positive fetal heart. However, she lost the pregnancy at 9 weeks. Within 4 weeks her pregnancy test was negative and her pleural effusion had resolved.

Case 2

Patient 2 was a 31-year old female with PCOS undergoing ovarian stimulation for IVF. As shown in Table 40.2, patient 2 was stimulated after oral contraceptive pills (OCP)/lupron downregulation of the ovaries. She had a step-down protocol. She was started on r-FSH with a dose of 225IU from day 3–5, decreased to 200 IU from day 6–7, decreased to185IU on days 8–9, and to 112 IU on days 10–11. Recombinant hCG was given on day 12 with a peak estradiol level of 4100 pg/mL. Oocyte retrieval was performed on cycle day 14 and 23 oocytes were retrieved.

On the second day after retrieval, she felt bloated and complained of some shortness of breath. Transvaginal ultrasound showed enlarged ovaries and mild ascites, and her hemoglobin was 11.0 g/dl. On the 3rd day post-retrieval she felt slightly better and 2 embryos were transferred. Her symptoms improved and then worsened about 11 days after transfer. She had a weight gain of 8 lbs, increased abdominal distension and her hemoglobin increased to 14.5 g/dl with a positive β-hCG of 249 IU.

Paracentesis was performed using a vaginal approach in the office with 1100cc of ascites

Table 40.1 Ovulation induction protocol and characteristics of Patient 1

Day	2	3	4	5	6	7	8	9	10	11	12	13	14	15	16	16
r-FSH		75	75	75	75	75	75	75	75	75	50	50	–	–		
Ganirelix											0.25 mg	0.25 mg	0.25 mg	0.25 mg	r-hCG	
E2 (pg/mL)		37					199				785		1990		1500	
LH IU		2.7					2.1				3.8		1.6		1.3	
FSH IU		5.1														
Ultrasound R		small					10<10 mm				10<10 mm		15 10<10 mm		18	
Follicles L.		small					10<10 mm				15/14/ 14/13 10<10 mm		17/17/ 16/16 10<10 mm		25/22/ 2/1/21	
Total follicles > 10 mm		3										4		5	5	
Endometruim		3					6B				7B		8B		7B	

Table 40.2 Ovulation induction protocol and characteristics of Patient 2

Day	2	3	4	5	6	7	8	9	10	11	12	13	14	15	16
r-FSH		225	225	225	200	200	185	185	112	112	r-hCG				
Lupron (mg)		0.5	0.5	0.5	0.5	0.5	0.5	0.5	0.5	0.5					
E2 (pg/mL)		<25			478		935		3180	3685	4100	6435			
LH IU															
FSH IU															
Ultrasound	r	small			8/8/8/ 8/8/8/ 8/8/7/ 7/7/7		13/12/ 9/8/ 8/8/8/ 7/7/7		15/14/ 14/13/ 12/12/ 12	18/18/ 17/15/ 14/14/13	19,19, 18,18, 17,15, 14,14,13	19,19, 2018/17/ 17/16/16/ 16/16			
Follicles	1	small			8/8/8/ 8/8/8/7 7/7/7/7		10/10/ 9/9/9/ 9/9/9/9/ 8/8		15/13/12/ 12/11/ 11/11	17/17/16/ 15/15/ 14/14	18,18,18, 17,17,16, 16,16,	19,18,18, 17,17/16/ 16/16/ 15/15			
Total follicles >16										25	25	25			
Endometrium					8B		10B			11B	11B	11B			

fluid removed. She improved and then 3 days later, symptoms worsened with nausea, vomiting, and abdominal distension, requiring a repeat culdocentesis. Beta hCG increased to 3183 IU. Her symptoms slowly improved and she delivered a twin pregnancy at term.

Case 3

A 27 year-old female with a history of OHSS, who wanted to avoid gonadotropins went through a cycle of IVF with in vitro maturation (Table 40.3). She had polycystic appearing ovaries on baseline ultrasound (cycle day 3). A repeat transvaginal ultrasound on cycle day 10 revealed polycystic ovaries with no dominant follicle >10 mm, endometrial thickness of 7 mm and an estradiol level of 75 pg/mL. An injection of hCG was given followed by oocyte retrieval 35 hours later. Oocyte retrieval was performed using low aspiration pressure and a single lumen needle and 21 immature (GV) oocytes were retrieved. Maturation of the oocytes was done using IVM culture techniques (human serum FSH and hCG added to the media) and 60% of the oocytes matured. Intracytoplasmic sperm injection (ICSI) was performed 32 hours after retrieval of the mature oocytes. We transferred 3 embryos on day 4 after retrieval and cryopreserved the remaining embryos. The patient did not conceive in this cycle but subsequently conceived in a frozen-thawed cycle and delivered a healthy singleton.

Recent Advances

Gonadotropin releasing hormone (GnRH) agonists/antagonists

Typically, human chorionic gonadotropin (hCG) is used to trigger the luteinizing hormone (LH) surge, and is necessary for oocyte maturation and ovulation induction in women undergoing ovarian stimulation. Because of its longer half-life (>24 hours versus 60 min for LH), hCG administration results in a prolonged stimulation of the corpus luteum.[43] This sustained effect may further exacerbate the risk for developing OHSS. An alternative to hCG-induced ovulation is the use of GnRH agonists. GnRH agonists can induce a prolonged release of endogenous LH that can effectively induce oocyte maturation and ovulation.[44] GnRH agonists can only be used in women who have not had previous pituitary down regulation with GnRH agonists such as in GnRH antagonist cycles.[45] Therefore, the use of GnRH agonists to trigger oocyte maturation and ovulation is an effective way of stimulating ovulation in the high-responder PCOS patient with a potential prevention of the development of OHSS. However, studies show that the use of a GnRH agonist to trigger oocyte maturation, alters the luteal phase steroidogenic profile that may affect implantation if the appropriate supplementation with estrogen and progesterone are not used.[44]

Recent prospective randomized controlled trials with over 300 patients showed that even with luteal supplementation, we should proceed with caution before using the GnRH agonist in IVF to avoid OHSS.[46,47] These studies showed a significantly lower ongoing pregnancy in the group receiving GnRH agonist to trigger oocyte maturation. The argument that may be used in the first study[46] is that the duration and type of luteal support may not have been sufficient, although both 90 mg of micronized progesterone vaginally and 4 mg estradiol per day were used, because it was discontinued with a positive pregnancy test. However, the second study[47] showed a significantly lower ongoing pregnancy rate after GnRH agonist triggering with luteal support continued to 7 weeks of gestation.

GnRH antagonists may be the preferential stimulation protocol in PCOS patients with the use of hCG for ovulation. This protocol may alleviate the development of OHSS in patients at high risk, by blocking endogenous LH stimulation of the ovary. In a prospective, randomized study comparing the long protocol using the GnRH agonist Buserelin to a GnRH antagonist protocol using Cetrorelix, Ludwig et al.[48] found a statistically significant reduction in the incidence of OHSS with the antagonist protocol with no difference in pregnancy rates.[48] Further trials will however, be needed to confirm these observations.

Table 40.3 Ovulation induction protocol followed by in vitro maturation in Patient 3

Day	2	3	4	5	6	7	8	9	10	11	12	13	14	15	16
r-FSH												r-hCG			
E2		29									75	79			
LH		6.4									11.7	9			
FSH		6.1									0.9	1			
P4															
Ultrasound (right)		small									10/s small				
Follicles (left)		small									small				
Total follicles															
Endometriuim		A1									7.4B				

In our current randomized, controlled trial exploring the role of Ganirelix in addition to gonadotropins to suppress the premature LH surge in ovulation induction, we have found high pregnancy rates with low rates of OHSS.[49]

Recombinant human luteinizing hormone

A third alternative to hCG or GnRH agonist is recombinant human luteinizing hormone (r-hLH). r-hLH also has a shorter half life than hCG (a few hours for r-hLH versus 24h for hCG) and it is not necessary to have an intact hypothalamic pituitary axis. The European Recombinant LH Study Group found that a single dose of r-hLH (15,000 or 30,000 IU) resulted in a highly significant reduction in OHSS compared with a single injection of hCG (5,000 IU).[50] However, because of its relatively short half-life, the cost of the increased dosage and the possibility of requiring multiple dosages due to the possibility of inadequate luteal function, we need to proceed cautiously with this alternative as well.

In vitro maturation of immature oocytes

For PCOS patients who are at high risk of OHSS and who may have had a history of OHSS in the past, avoiding gonadotropin stimulation altogether should be the most effective strategy to avoid OHSS. This involves IVF with in vitro maturation (IVM) of immature oocytes retrieved from non-stimulated ovaries. Reasonable pregnancy rates can be achieved in women with PCOS following IVM.[51,52] Recent studies show clinical pregnancy rates of 20–30%.

Parameters as age (<35 years) and baseline antral follicular count (>10 immature oocytes following retrieval) are predictive of good outcomes and should be used as selection criteria for IVM treatment. Women with PCOS and normo-ovulatory patients at risk of developing OHSS might also benefit from early retrieval of immature oocytes or "minimally" stimulated ovaries, followed by IVM and embryo transfer or cryopreservation of immature oocytes. IVM is an alternative treatment for patients at risk of

OHSS instead of canceling the cycle. hCG priming before oocyte retrieval seems beneficial in terms of oocyte yield and maturational competence, and increases the harvest of mature oocytes, leading to better endometrial synchronization with the developing embryo. It also increases the pregnancy rates.[53] hCG can be given when the follicle size reaches 12–14 mm (when the potential of the granulosa cell for producing vasoactive factors might be decreased). This led to a 47.1% clinical pregnancy rate in one study.[54] Current practice suggests oocyte retrieval timing in a follicular range between 8–12 mm.

Although the pregnancy rate was lower, the abortion rate, gestational age, birth weight at delivery, and obstetric complications of pregnancies conceived by IVM-ET in women with PCOS were comparable with those of other women with PCOS treated by conventional IVF-ET. IVM followed by IVF-ET seems to be a useful treatment option for women with PCOS, thus avoiding the risk of OHSS.

The concerns about in-vitro maturation include inadequate cytoplasmic maturation and concerns about epigenetics and adequate preparation of the endometrium. Also, the oocyte granulosa cell communication may be affected by early hCG. This is a current area of research and with improved pregnancy rates, is a viable alternative to avoid OHSS and simplify IVF.

Conclusion

Can we eliminate severe OHSS? We do not believe that OHSS can be completely eliminated without avoiding gonadotropins. Our approach to minimize the incidence and severity of ovarian hyperstimulation syndrome is based on identifying those patients at risk and avoiding gonadotropins if possible. With gonadotropin stimulation, individualization of the protocol and the use of the lowest dosage possible are indicated. In IVF, reducing the number of embryos transferred and reducing the incidence of multiple births is also an important strategy. Other strategies, such as reducing or avoiding hCG, are aimed at reducing the vascular permeability factors that are produced. Our strategies for treatment of PCOS with reduction of OHSS are outlined as follows:

Sequence of interventions used to treat patients with PCOS interested in fertility

First

- Lifestyle modification with weight loss
  - Low carbohydrate diet and exercise
- Insulin Sensitizing agents
  - Metformin (Glucophage®)
  - Rosiglitazone (Avandia®)

Second

- Ovulation induction
  - Clomiphene citrate (Clomid®)
  - Gonadotropins (Gonal F® or Follistim®) – low dose step-up protocol

Third

- In vitro fertilization
  - GnRH agonist (Lupron®)-low dose step-down protocol (Table 40.1)
  - GnRH antagonist (Ganirelix®)-favored (Table 40.2)
- Ovarian surgery
- In vitro maturation of immature oocytes (Table 40.3)

References

1. Delbaere A, Smits G, Olatunbosun O, Pierson R, Vassart G, Costagliola S. New insights into the pathophysiology of ovarian hyperstimulation syndrome. What makes the difference between spontaneous and iatragenic syndrome? *Hum Reprod* 2004; 19: 486–498.
2. Whelan JG, Vlahos NF. The Ovarian hyperstimulation syndrome. *Fertil Steril* 2000; 73: 883–895.
3. Geva E, Jaffe RB. Role of vascular endothelial growth factor in ovarian physiology and pathology. *Fertil Steril* 2000; 74: 429–438.
4. Grudzinskas JG, Egbase PE. Prevention of ovarian hyperstimulation syndrome: novel strategies. *Human Reprod* 1998; 13: 2051–2053.
5. Worrell G, Wijdicks E, Eggars S, Phan T, Demario M, Mullany C. Ovarian hyperstimulation syndrome with ischemic stroke due to an intracardiac thrombus. *Neurology* 2001; 57: 1342–1344.
6. Hignett M, Spence J, Claman P. Internal jugular vein thrombosis: a late complication of ovarian hyperstimulation syndrome despite mini-dose heparin prophylaxis. *Hum Reprod* 1995; 10: 3121–3123.
7. Cluroe A, Synek B. A fatal case of ovarian hyperstimulation syndrome with cerebral infarction. *Pathology* 1995; 27: 344–346.
8. Arslan M, Bocca S, Mirkin S, Barroso G, Stadtmauer L, Oehninger S. Controlled ovarian hyperstimulation protocols for in vitro fertilization: two decades of experience after the birth of Elizabeth Carr. *Fertil Steril* 2005; 84: 555–569.
9. White DM, Polson DW, Kiddy DS, et al. Induction of ovulation with low dose gonadotropins in polycystic ovary syndrome: slow administration is safer and more effective. *Fertil Steril* 1989; 52: 553–559.
10. Homburg R, Levy T and Ben-Rafael Z. A comparative prospective study of conventional regimen with chronic low-dose administration of follicle-stimulating hormone for anovulation associated with polycystic ovary syndrome. *Fertil Steril* 1995; 63: 729–733.
11. Christin_Maitre S and Hugues JN. A comparative randomized multicentric study comparing the step-up verses the step-down protocol in polycystic ovary syndrome. *Hum Reprod* 2003;18: 1621–1631.
12. De Leo V, la Marca A, Ditto A, Morgante G, Cianci A. Effects of metformin on gonadotropin-induced ovulation in women with polycystic ovary syndrome. *Fertil Steril* 1999; 72: 282–285.
13. Stadtmauer LA, Toma SK, Riehl RM, Talbert LM Metformin treatment of patients with polycystic ovary syndrome undergoing in vitro fertilization improves outcomes and is associated with modulation of the insulin like growth factors. *Fertil Steril* 2001; 75: 505–509.
14. Yarali H, Yildiz BO, Demirol A, Zeyneloglu HB, Yigit N, Bukulmez O, Koray Z Co-administration of metformin during rFSH treatment in patients with clomiphene citrate-resistant polycystic ovarian syndrome: a prospective randomized trial. *Hum Reprod* 2002; 17: 289–294.
15. Damario MA, Barmat L, Liu H, Davis OK, Rosenwaks Z. Dual suppression with oral contraceptives and gonadotropin releasing-hormone agonists improves in-vitro fertilization outcome in high responder patients. *Hum Reprod* 1997; 12: 2359–2365.

16. Huang J-L. Seow K-M, Lin Y-H et al. Ovarian stimulation by comcomitant adminstration of cetrorelix acetate and hMG following Diane-35 pre-treatment for patients with polycystic ovary syndrome: a prospective randomized study. *Hum Reprod* 2004; 19: 1993–2000.

17. Ragni G, Vegetti W, Riccaboni A, Engl B, Brigante C, Crosignani RG. Comparison of GnRH agonists and antagonists in assisted reproduction cycles of patients at high risk of ovarian hyperstimulation syndrome. *Hum Reprod* 2005; 20: 2421–2425.

18. Abdalla HI, Ah- Moye, Brinsden P et al. The effect of the dose of hCG and the typed gonadotropin stimulation on oocyte recovery rates in an IVF program. *Fertil Steril* 1997; 48: 958–963.

19. Grochowski D, Wolczynski S, Kucxynski W, Domitrz J, Szamatowicz J, Szamatowicz M. Correctly timed coasting reduces the risk of ovarian hyperstimulation and gives good cycle outcome in an in vitro fertilization program. *Gynecol Endocrinol* 2001; 15: 234–238.

20. Tortoriello DV, McGovern PG, Colon JM. "Coasting" does not adversely affect outcome in a subset of highly responsive in vitro fertilization patients. *Fertil Steril* 1998; 69: 454–460.

21. Fluker, M, Hooper WM, Yuzpe AA. Withholding gonadotropins ("coasting") to minimize the risk of ovarian hyperstimulation during superovulation and in vitro fertilization – embryo transfer cycles. *Fertil Steril* 1999; 71: 294–301.

22. Dhont M, Van der Streten F, De Sutter P. Prevention of severe ovarian hyperstimulation by coasting. *Fertil Steril* 1998; 70: 847–850.

23. Benadiva C, Davis O, Kligman I, et al. Withholding gonadotropin administration is an effective alternative for the prevention of ovarian hyperstimulation syndrome. *Fertil Steril* 1997; 67: 721–724.

24. Stadtmauer LA, Toma SK, Riehl RM, Talbert LM. The impact of metformin therapy on ovarian stimulation and outcome in "coasted" patients with polycystic ovary syndrome undergoing in-vitro fertilization. *Reprod Bio Online* 2002; 5: 112–116.

25. Ulug U, Bahceci M, Erden HF, Shalev E, Ben-Shlomo I. The significance of coasting duration during ovarian stimulation for conception in assisted fertilization cycles. *Hum Reprod* 2002; 17: 310–317.

26. Isaza V, Garcia-Velasko J, Aragones M, Remohi J, Simon C, Pellicer A. Oocyte and embryo quality after coasting: the experience from oocyte donation. *Hum Reprod* 2002; 17: 1777–1782.

27. Arslan M, Bocca, S, Jones E, Mayer J, Stadtmauer L, and Oehninger O. Effect of coasting on the implantation potential of embryos transferred after cryopreservation and thawing. *Fertil Steril* 2005; 84: 867–873.

28. Pattinson HA, Highett M, Dunphy BC, et al. Outcome of thaw embryo transfer after cryopreservation of all embryos in patients at risk of ovarian hyperstimulation syndrome. *Fertil Steril* 1994; 6: 1192.

29. Queenan JT Jr, Veeck LL, Toner JP, et al. Cryopreservation of all prezygotes in patients at risk of severe hyperstimulation does not eliminate the syndrome, but the chances of pregnancy are excellent with subsequent frozen-thaw transfers. *Hum Reprod* 1997; 12: 1573.

30. Angelo A, Amso N. Embryo freezing for preventing ovarian hyperstimulation syndrome: a Cochrane review. *Hum Reprod* 2002; 17(11): 2787–2794.

31. Abramov Y, Fatum M, Abrahamov D, Schenker J. Hydroxyethylstarch versus human albumin for the treatment of severe ovarian hyperstimulation syndrome: a preliminary report. *Fertil Steril* 2001; 75(6): 1228–1230.

32. Asch RH, Ivery G, Goldsman M, Frederick JL, Stone SC, Balmaceda JP. The use of intravenous albumin in patients at high risk for severe ovarian hyperstimulation syndrome [see comments]. *Hum Reprod* 1993; 8: 1015–1020.

33. Shoham Z, Weissman A, Barash A, Borenstein R, Schachter M, Insler V. Intravenous albumin for the prevention of severe ovarian hyperstimulation syndrome in an in vitro fertilization program: a prospective, randomized, placebo-controlled study. *Fertil Steril* 1994; 62: 137–142.

34. Gokmen O, Ugur M, Ekin M, Keles G, Turan C, Oral H. Intravenous albumin versus hydroxyethyl starch for the prevention of ovarian hyperstimulation in an in-vitro fertilization programme: a prospective randomized placebo controlled study. *Eur J Obstet Gynecol Reprod Bio* 2001; 96: 187–192.

35. Aboulghar M, Evers JH, Al-Inany H. Intra-venous albumin for preventing severe ovarian hyperstimulation syndrome. Cochrane Database of Systematic Reviews, 2002; 2: CD001302.

36. Ben-Chetrit A, Eldar-Geva T, Gal M, et al. The questionable use of albumin for the prevention of ovarian hyperstimulation syndrome in an IVF programme: a randomized placebo-controlled trial. *Hum Reprod* 2001; 16: 1880–1884.

37. Ng E, Leader A, Claman P, et al. Intravenous albumin does not prevent the development of severe ovarian hyperstimulation syndrome in an in-vitro fertilization programme. *Human Reprod* 1995; 10: 807–810.

38. Gjonnaess H. Polycystic ovarian syndrome treated by ovarian electrocautery through the laparoscope. *Fertil Steril* 1984; 41: 20–25.

39. Amer SAKS, Banu Z, Li TC, Cooke ID. Long-term follow-up of patients with polycystic ovary syndrome after laparoscopic ovarian drilling: endocrine and ultrasonographic outcomes. *Hum Reprod* 2002; 17: 2851–2857.

40. Donesky BW, Adashi EY. Surgically induced ovulation in the polycystic ovary syndrome: wedge resection revisited in the age of laparoscopy. *Fertil Steril* 1995; 63: 439–463.

41. Farquhar C, Vandekerckhove P, Arnot M Lilford R. Laparoscopic "drilling' by diathermy or laser for ovulation induction in anovulatory polycystic ovary syndrome. *Cochrane Database syst Rev* 2000; CD001122.

42. Palomba S, Orio F Jr, Falbo A, Russo T, Tolino A, Zullo F. Plasminogen activator inhibitor 1 and miscarriage alter metformin treatment and laparoscopic ovarian drilling in patients with polycystic ovary síndrome. *Fertil Steril* 2005; 84: 761–765.

43. Fauser BC, de Jong D, Olivennes F, et al. Endocrine profiles after triggering of final oocyte maturation with GnRH agonist after cotreatment with the GnRH antagonist ganirelix during ovarian hyperstimulation for *in vitro* fertilization. *J Clin Endocrin Metabol* 2002; 87: 709–715.

44. Lewit N, Kol S, Manor D, Itskovitz-Eldor J Comparison of gonadotropin-releasing hormone analogues and human chorionic gonadotrophin for the induction of ovulation and prevention of ovarian hyperstimulation syndrome: a case-control study. *Hum Reprod* 1996; 11: 1399–1402.

45. Itskovitz-Eldor J, Kol S, Mannaerts B. Use of a single bolus of GnRH agonist triptorelin to trigger ovulation after GnRH antagonist ganirelix treatment in women undergoing ovarian stimulation for assisted reproduction with special reference to the prevention of ovarian hyperstimulation syndrome: a preliminary report. *Hum Reprod* 2000; 15 9: 1965–1968.

46. Humaidan P, Bredkjaer HE, Bungum L et al. GnRH agonist (buserelin) or hCG for ovulation induction in GnRH antagonist IVF/ICSI cycles: a prospective randomized study. *Hum Reprod* 2005; 20: 1213–1220.

47. Kolibianakis EN, Schultz-Mosgau A, Schroer A van Steirteghem A, Devroey P, Diedrich K, Griesinger G. A lower ongoing pregnancy rate can be expected when GnRH agonist is used for triggering final oocytes maturation instead of hCG in patients undergoing IVF with GnRH antagonists. *Hum Reprod* 2005; 20: 2887–2892.

48. Ludwig M, Felberbaum, Devroey et al. Significant reduction of the incidence of ovarian hyperstimulation syndrome (OHSS) by using the LHRH antagonist Cetrorelix in controlled ovarian stimulation for assisted reproduction. *Arch Gynecol Obstet* 2000; 264: 29–32.

49. Stadtmauer LA, Kariya K, Arslan M, Oehninger S. Impact of GnRH antagonist (Ganirelix) on the outcome of controlled ovarian hyperstimulation (COH) in PCOS patients: a prospective and randomized study. *Fertil Steril* 2005; 84: S314.

50. The European Recombinant LH Study Group. Recombinant Human Luteinizing Hormone Is as Effective as, But Safer Than, Urinary Human Chorionic Gonadotropin in Inducing Final Follicular Maturation and Ovulation in In Vitro Fertilization Procedures: Results of a Multicenter Double-Blind Study. *J Clin Endocrin & Metab* 2001; 86: 2607–2618.

51. Cha K-Y, Chian R-C. Maturation *in vitro* of immature human oocytes for clinical use. *Human Reprod Update* 1998; 4(2): 103–120.

52. Child TJ, Abdul-Jalil AK, Gulekli B, Tan SL. In vitro maturation and fertilization of oocytes from unstimulated normal ovaries, polycystic ovaries, and women with polycystic ovary syndrome. *Fertil Steril* 2001; 76(5): 936–942.

53. Chian RC, Buckett WM Tulandi T and Tan SL Prospective randomized study of human chorionic gonadotrophin priming before immature oocyte retrieval from unstimulated women with polycystic ovarian syndrome. *Hum Reprod* 2000; 15: 165–170.

54. El-Sheikh MM, Hussein M, Fouad S, El-Sheikh R, Bauer O, Al-Hasani S. Limited ovarian stimulation (LOS), prevents the recurrence of severe forms of ovarian hyperstimulation syndrome in polycystic ovarian disease. *Eur J Obstet Gynecol Reprod Biol* 2001; 94: 245–249.

Frequently Asked Question:

1. Is coasting harmful?

A-Based on our personal experience and the experience of many studies, embryo quality is usually not affected, but reduced implantation and pregnancy rates are observed in patients with high peak estradiol levels >7000 pg/ml who required coasting for >3 days. In addition, low pregnancy rates are found if the estradiol levels drop precipitously and drop after the hCG.

Embryo cryopreservation should always be undertaken when the risk of OHSS is excessive. In our experience, the deleterious effects of coasting (i.e. the effect of the high levels of estrogen on the endometrium) could be overcome by cryopreservation. Prolonged coasting has a minimally deleterious effect on embryo survival after the thaw, but it does not affect implantation as the pregnancy rates in such cycles are similar to the fresh cycles.

41

Gonadotropin Regimens and Oocyte Quality in Women with Polycystic Ovaries

Mohamed Aboulghar, Hesham Al-Inany

Summary

Polycystic Ovary Syndrome (PCOS) is a common cause of female infertility due to endocrine disorders mainly high tonic luteinizing hormone (LH) concentrations. Exogenous gonadotropins offer an opportunity to correct the abnormal systemic endocrine environment, characteristic of women with PCOS, helping them to ovulate and achieve conception. Gonadotropins are particularly important for maturation of oocytes, but the type and dose required is still not clear. In assisted reproductive technology (ART) programs, it seems that there is little, or no difference in the effect of various gonadotropins on the quality of oocytes. In vitro maturation of oocytes is emerging as an alternative technique in women with PCOS to avoid ovarian hyperstimulation syndrome (OHSS).

Introduction

Polycystic Ovary Syndrome (PCOS) is defined by chronic anovulation, clinical or biochemical signs of hyperandrogenism, following the exclusion of other etiologies. The Rotterdam revised diagnostic criteria for PCOS include 2 out of 3 symptoms, oligo and/or anovulation, clinical and/or biochemical signs of hyperandrogenism, polycystic ovaries (PCO)

following exclusion of other etiologies (congenital adrenal hyperplasia, androgen secreting tumor, Cushing's syndrome).[1] Polycystic ovary syndrome is a very common endocrine disorder. Among women who present with oligomenorrhea, 87% have PCO, and of women with regular menstrual cycles who present with hirsutism, 92% have PCO.[2] Over 50% of patients who present with recurrent miscarriage have PCO.[3] Despite large numbers of epidemiological, clinical, laboratory and experimental studies, the etiology and pathophysiology of the syndrome still remains fragmentary, obscure and probably multifactorial.[4]

Polycystic ovary syndrome may result from disturbances in various endocrine systems, but there is increasing evidence that PCOS is an oligogenic disorder, that ensues from the interaction of a small number of key genes with environmental factors determining the clinical and biochemical manifestations.[5,6] There is a wide spectrum of clinical and biochemical features associated with polycystic ovary syndrome that spans from the presence of PCO only, to the syndrome (Stein-Leventhal syndrome) characterized by obesity, hyperandrogenism, menstrual disturbance, and anovulatory subfertility. Menstrual disturbances in PCOS include oligomenorrhea (40 days or longer between the menstrual periods), amenorrhea (absence of menstruation for > 3 months without evidence of pregnancy), or erratic bleeding (loss of the cyclic menstrual pattern).[7,8]

Clinical Discussion

Oocyte quality in PCOS

High tonic luteinizing hormone (LH) concentrations are one of the hallmarks of PCOS.[9] High LH has been claimed to decrease oocyte quality and cause a higher miscarriage rate.[10,11] Oocyte quality, or developmental competence, is acquired during folliculogenesis and affects early embryonic survival. Although the spermatozoon provides an essential contribution to the generation of a new individual, the developmental fate of the embryo is principally dictated by the oocyte. As an oocyte grows, it acquires the ability to resume and complete meiosis, successfully undergo the fertilization process, and initiate and sustain embryonic development. It is known that these changes involve the nuclear and cytoplasmic compartments respectively, but the underlying cellular and molecular mechanisms are still poorly understood.[12]

The quality of oocytes obtained from polycystic ovaries as judged by rates of fertilization and embryo cleavage, with or without ovarian stimulation by gonadotropins, is similar to that of oocytes obtained from normal ovaries.[13,14] Women with polycystic ovaries have normal rates of fertilization and embryo cleavage after ovulation induction for in vitro fertilization (IVF).[15,16] Indeed, blastocyst cell numbers were found to be significantly higher, following a titrated gonadotropin regimen, in women with polycystic ovaries compared to those with tubal infertility.

Assisted reproduction and oocyte quality

The quality of embryos obtained in IVF is dependent upon the quality of oocytes, fertilization and the laboratory conditions for in vitro culture.[17] Serhal et al.[18] found that the outcome of intracytoplasmic sperm injection (ICSI) is directly related to oocyte quality and the woman's age is the most important factor affecting oocyte quality, the chance of having a live birth, and risk of miscarriage when her own oocytes are used.[19]

Morphological assessment of oocytes and embryos remains the gold standard to determine oocyte and embryo quality in clinical practice. The concentrations of hormones in the follicular fluid may reflect oocyte maturity and quality but cannot be applied practically in every case.

Intracytoplasmic sperm injection gives a unique opportunity to validate the rate of metaphase II oocytes after removal of the cumulus and corona cells. Thus, it can be determined whether oocyte quality in PCOS women is reduced or not. Ludwig et al.[20] retrospectively studied oocyte quality and treatment outcome in ICSI cycles of PCOS patients and they found that the rate of metaphase II oocytes (53.48% versus 62.66%), the rate of germinal vesicle oocytes (4.63% versus 7.45%) and the fertilization rate of metaphase II oocytes (62.66% versus 56.42%) were not different between PCOS and non-PCOS patients respectively. However, the mean absolute number of normally fertilized oocytes was significantly higher in PCOS patients (5.00 versus 3.56, $P < 0.01$), due to a higher number of oocytes retrieved. The cumulative embryo score was higher in the PCOS group (2.69 versus 2.17, $P < 0.05$) and a greater number of embryos were transferred per cycle. Despite a higher mean number of embryos transferred and a higher cumulative embryo score, the pregnancy rate/ cycle and multiple pregnancy rate was similar, with a significantly higher clinical abortion rate in PCOS patients. This demonstrates that despite a given nuclear maturity of oocytes, cytoplasmic factors might negatively influence the developmental potential of embryos and the outcome of pregnancies in PCOS patients.[20]

The hypothesis of a cytoplasmic factor is supported by data from Sengoku et al.[21] They performed a cytogenetic analysis on oocytes from PCOS and non-PCOS patients, but could not find a higher incidence of numerical chromosomal abnormalities in unfertilized oocytes retrieved from PCOS patients after hormonal stimulation according to a long protocol. Interestingly, the only differences between the two groups were a higher number of oocytes retrieved and a lower fertilization rate in the PCOS group. There was no difference between the groups in the clinical pregnancy and miscarriage rates.

Oocyte developmental competence is also affected by follicle size.[22] It seems that oocytes from small follicles have not yet completed maturation. However, oocytes can be collected in an immature state without stimulation regimens during human assisted reproduction and matured in vitro. The minimum size of follicle required for developmental competence in humans is 5–7 mm in diameter. Maturation in vitro can be accomplished in humans, but is associated with a loss of developmental competence unless the oocyte is near completion of its preovulatory growth phase. This loss of developmental competence is associated with the absence of specific proteins in oocytes cultured to metaphase II in vitro.[23]

Oocyte and embryo quality can be adversely affected by a number of factors, including advanced maternal age,[24] raised basal follicle stimulating hormone (FSH) concentration and smoking.[25] However, the effect of gonadotropin regimens is still unclear. The response of PCOS women to gonadotropins has been described as exaggerated or explosive in nature, often resulting in higher E2 levels on the day of human chorionic gonadotropin (hCG) administration, associated with the harvest of an increased number of immature oocytes. The higher percentage of poor-quality oocytes in polycystic ovaries (PCO) would explain the lower fertilization rates that have been reported in some,[17,26] but not all studies,[27] in patients with PCOS compared with control women undergoing assisted reproductive technology (ART). Therefore, factors involving individual susceptibility and the PCO state itself may be important considerations. This notwithstanding, it has been suggested that high ovarian response in women without PCO is also associated with compromised oocyte quality.[28,29] Raziel et al.[30] reported that the clinical pregnancy rate of IVF patients who developed severe ovarian hyperstimulation syndrome (OHSS), but not

having PCOS, was significantly higher than that in patients without OHSS. Nevertheless, their abortion rate was also significantly higher.[30] It has been hypothesized that OHSS might have a possible detrimental effect on the quality of the oocytes and thus, detrimental effects on the quality of the embryos.[31]

Type of gonadotropins and oocyte quality

In assisted reproductive technologies, multiple follicular growth via gonadotropin administration is still an integral part of the IVF/ICSI procedure.[32] To assess the effect of gonadotropins on oocyte quality, there should be no statistically significant difference in age and other demographic characteristics, culture conditions and technique between the groups except the stimulation protocol. Thus, it can be assumed that the fertilization rate, quality of embryos and implantation rate depend upon the quality of oocytes. If there is a difference in oocyte quality, this difference may then be attributed to the gonadotropins used.

There are very few studies examining the effects of different gonadotropin preparations on oocyte quality in patients with PCOS. This is of special importance if we consider that superovulation could have a detrimental effect on oocyte quality. However, evidence from the literature is unclear. Imthurn et al.[33] in a prospective study, examined the nuclear maturity of oocytes in two groups of women receiving urinary FSH (Metrodin HP; Serono) and human menopausal gonadotropin [hMG (Pergonal; Serono)] in a short protocol of pituitary down-regulation prior to ICSI. The urinary FSH group had a significantly higher proportion of metaphase II oocytes (88.8% versus 80.6% respectively) and morphologically normal oocytes (85.6% versus 77.6% respectively) compared with the hMG group. This study suffered from the use of a short protocol associated with very high follicular phase LH concentrations, exclusion of cycles with fewer than three oocytes from the analysis and crossover design in 10 subjects. In a retrospective analysis[34] of conventional IVF cycles, in a long protocol of down-regulation, urinary FSH (Metrodin; Serono) stimulation resulted in a significantly higher percentage of mature oocytes than the urinary FSH/hMG (Metrodin/Pergonal) combination (57% versus 34% respectively). The drawbacks of this study were the retrospective nature and examination of conventional IVF cycles. The removal of the corona-cumulus complex before the ICSI procedure allows a more precise determination of nuclear maturity of the oocyte.[35]

Contrary to the above two studies, Jacob et al.[36] retrospectively demonstrated a similar percentage of metaphase II oocytes in women receiving hMG (Humegon; Organon, Oss, The Netherlands) and recombinant human follicle stimulating hormone [r-hFSH (Puregon; Organon)] in down-regulated cycles for ICSI.[36] Similarly, another retrospective study[37] found a comparable percentage of metaphase II oocytes retrieved after a long protocol of pituitary down-regulation and ovarian stimulation with hMG (Humegon or Pergonal) or urinary FSH (Metrodin HP) in women undergoing ICSI. Because of the conflicting evidence, it remains uncertain whether the use of FSH (especially r-hFSH) will increase the percentage of nuclear mature oocytes after ovarian stimulation, resulting in better oocyte and embryo quality.

Another study included one group of 21 and one group of 22 anovulatory women with PCOS who underwent ovulation induction with human urinary follicle stimulating hormone (hU-FSH)/human chorionic gonadotropin (hCG) and human menopausal gonadotrophin (hMG)/hCG, respectively. No statistically significant differences in ovulation rate were found between patients treated with hU-FSH (95.2%) and those treated with hMG (100%). The numbers of patients who conceived, delivered, and aborted respectively following the use hU-FSH and hMG, respectively were 8 (38.1%) vs 11 (50.0%), 6 (28.5%) vs 8 (36.3%), and 2 (9.5%) vs 3 (13.6%). There were no multiple pregnancies. Serum 17 beta-estradiol levels and the number of maturing follicles prior to hCG injection were significantly higher with hU-FSH than hMG, while there were

no differences in the diameter of the dominant follicle prior to hCG administration. Ovarian hyperstimulation was discovered more frequently after hU-FSH/hCG (40%) than hMG/hCG treatments (22.2%). These data do not confirm an effective advantage of the use of hU-FSH for ovulation induction in cases of PCOS.[38]

In a randomized controlled trial (RCT) by Ng et al.[39] 40 women undergoing ovarian stimulation for intracytoplasmic sperm injection were randomized to receive a standard protocol of either hMG or r-hFSH in down-regulated cycles. Prior to microinjection, each denuded oocyte was videotaped to assess nuclear maturity, morphology of the zona pellucida, oocyte and polar body and the zona thickness, and diameters of oocyte and ooplasm. Fertilization and subsequent embryo development of each oocyte were followed. The embryologists were blind to the type of gonadotropin each patient had received for stimulation. No significant differences were found between the two groups with regard to the demographic data, the ovarian responses and pregnancy/implantation rates. The percentages of metaphase II oocytes in the hMG and rhFSH groups were similar (86.9% versus 87.4% respectively). All other parameters assessing oocyte and embryo quality were also comparable between the two groups.[39]

Conclusion

Thus, it seems that there is no difference in the quality of oocytes received and outcomes of IVF/ICSI following the administration of different gonadotropins. Moreover, it seems that analogues of gonadotropin releasing hormones (GnRH) administered during late follicular development offer an opportunity to correct, *in vivo*, the abnormal systemic endocrine environment (notably normalization of serum LH levels) characteristic of women with PCOS. Consequently, the metabolism of eggs and embryos, fertilization and embryo development are similar in women with PCOS treated on a titrated gonadotropin regimen to those of women with tubal disease.

It has been shown in vitro, that the morphological appearance and metabolic activity of embryos from PCOS women are similar to those observed in embryos of women with tubal disease.[15] On the other hand, it seems that there is a particular subgroup of PCO patients with lower fertilization rates and embryos unable to implant. These patients are obese and nonhyperandrogenic and show derangements in insulin secretion.[40]

Based on the limited data available in the medical literature, it appears that gonadotrophins have little or no effect on oocyte quality. However, more studies are required to address this specific issue especially in view of in vitro maturation of oocytes.

References

1. The Rotterdam ESHRE/ASRM- sponsored PCOS consensus workshop group. Revised 2003 consensus on diagnostic criteria and long term health risks related to polycystic ovary syndrome (PCOS). *Hum Reprod* 2004; 19(1): 41–47.

2. Hull MG. Epidemiology of infertility and polycystic ovarian disease: endocrinological and demographic studies. *Gynecol Endocrinol* 1987; 1(3): 235–245.

3. Sagle M, Bishop K, Ridley N. Recurrent early miscarriage and polycystic ovaries. *BMJ* 1988; 297: 1027–1028.

4. Kurjak A. An atlas of transvaginal color Doppler. The Parthenon publishing Group. London, Casterton, New York, 1994.

5. Harrington DJ, Balen AH. Polycystic ovary syndrome: aetiology and management. *Br J Hosp Med* 1996; 56: 17–20.

6. Franks S, Gharani N, Waterworth D. The genetic basis of polycystic ovary syndrome. *Hum Reprod* 1997; 12: 2641–2648.

7. Leventhal ML. The Stein-Leventhal syndrome. *Am J Obstet Gynecol* 1958; 76: 825–838.

8. Stein IF, Leventhal ML. Amenorrhea associated with bilateral polycystic ovaries. *Am J Obstet Gynecol* 1935; 29: 181–191.

9. MacDougall MJ, Tan SL, Balen A, Jacobs HS. A controlled study comparing patients with and without polycystic ovaries undergoing in-vitro fertilization. *Hum Reprod* 1993 Feb; 8(2): 233–237.

10. Homburg R, Armar NA, Eshel A, Adams J, Jacobs HS. Influence of serum luteinising hormone concentrations on ovulation, conception, and early pregnancy loss in polycystic ovary syndrome. *BMJ* 1988; 297(6655): 1024–1026.

11. Homburg R, Jacobs HS. Etiology of miscarriage in polycystic ovary syndrome. *Fertil Steril* 1989; 51(1): 196–197.

12. Coticchio G, Bonu MA, Borini A, Flamigni C. Oocyte cryopreservation: a biological perspective. *Eur J Obstet Gynecol Reprod Biol* 2004; 115 (Suppl 1): S2–7.

13. Barnes FL, Kausche A, Tiglias J, Wood C, Wilton L, Trounson A. Production of embryos from in vitro-matured primary human oocytes. *Fertil Steril* 1996; 65: 1151–1156.

14. Child TJ, Abdul-Jalil AK, Gulekli B, Tan SL. In vitro maturation and fertilization of oocytes from unstimulated normal ovaries, polycystic ovaries, and women with polycystic ovary syndrome. *Fertil Steril* 2001; 76: 936–942.

15. Hardy K, Robinson FM, Paraschos T, Wicks R, Franks S, Winston RM. Normal development and metabolic activity of preimplantation embryos in vitro from patients with polycystic ovaries. *Hum Reprod* 1995; 10(8): 2125–2135.

16. Hardy K, Wright CS, Franks S, Winston RM. In vitro maturation of oocyte. *Br Med Bull* 2000; 65: 588–602.

17. Aboulghar MA, Mansour RT, Serour GI, Ramzy AM, Amin YM. Oocyte quality in patients with severe ovarian hyperstimulation syndrome. *Fertil Steril* 1997; 68(6): 1017–1021.

18. Serhal PF, Ranieri DM, Kinis A, Marchant S, Davies M, Khadum IM. Oocyte morphology predicts outcome of intracytoplasmic sperm injection. *Hum Reprod* 1997; 12: 1267–1270.

19. Krisher RL. The effect of oocyte quality on development. *J Anim Sci* 2004; 82 E-Suppl: E14-23.

20. Ludwig M, Finas DF, Al-Hasani A, Diedrich K, Ortmann O. Oocyte quality and treatment outcome in intracytoplasmic sperm injection cycles of polycystic ovarian syndrome patients. *Hum Reprod* 1999; 14: 354–358.

21. Sengoku K, Tamate K, Takuma N, Yoshida T, Goishi K, Ishikawa M. The chromosomal normality of unfertilized oocytes from patients with polycystic ovarian syndrome. *Hum Reprod* 1997; 12(3): 474–477.

22. Marchal R, Vigneron C, Perreau C, Bali-Papp A, Mermillod P. Effect of follicular size on meiotic and developmental competence of porcine oocytes. *Theriogenology* 2002; 57(5): 1523–1532.

23. Trounson A, Anderiesz C, Jones G. Maturation of human oocytes in vitro and their developmental competence. *Reproduction* 2001; 121(1): 51–75.

24. Sherins RJ, Thorsell LP, Dorfmann A, Dennison-Lagos L, Calvo LP, et al. Intracytoplasmic sperm injection facilitates fertilization even in the most severe forms of male infertility: pregnancy outcome correlates with maternal age and number of eggs available. *Fertil Steril* 1995; 64(2): 369–375.

25. Zenzes MT, Reed TE, Casper RF. Effects of cigarette smoking and age on the maturation of human oocytes. *Hum Reprod* 1997; 12(8): 1736–1741.

26. Dor J, Shulman A, Levran D, Ben-Rafael Z, Rudak E, Mashiach S. The treatment of patients with polycystic ovarian syndrome by in-vitro fertilization and embryo transfer: a comparison of results with those of patients with tubal infertility. *Hum Reprod* 1990; 5: 816–818.

27. Ashkenazi J, Farhi J, Orvieto R, Homburg R, Dekel A, Feldberg D, et al. Polycystic ovary syndrome patients as oocyte donors: the effect of ovarian stimulation protocol on the implantation rate of the recipient. *Fertil Steril* 1995; 64: 564–567.

28. Tarín JJ, Pellicer A. Consequences of high ovarian response to gonadotropins: a cytogenetic analysis of unfertilized human oocytes. *Fertil Steril* 1990; 54: 665–670.

29. Reis-Soares S, Rubio C, Rodrigo L, Simón C, Remohí J, Pellicer A. High frequency of chromosomal abnormalities in embryos obtained from oocyte donation cycles. *Fertil Steril* 2003; 80: 656–657.

30. Raziel A, Friedler S, Schachter M, Strassburger D, Mordechai E, Ron-El R. Increased early pregnancy loss in IVF patients with severe ovarian hyperstimulation syndrome. *Hum Reprod* 2002; 17: 107–110.

31. Fabregues F, Pearrubia J, Vidal E, Casals G, Vanrell JA, Balasch J. Oocyte quality in patients with severe ovarian hyperstimulation syndrome: A self-controlled clinical study. *Fertil Steril* 2004; 82: 827–833.

32. Al-Inany H, Aboulghar MA, Mansour RT, Serour GI. Ovulation induction in the new millennium: recombinant follicle-stimulating hormone versus human menopausal gonadotropin. *Gynecol Endocrinol* 2005; 20(3): 161–169.

33. Imthurn B, Macas E, Rosselli M, Keller PJ. Nuclear maturity and oocyte morphology after stimulation with highly purified follicle stimulating hormone compared to human menopausal gonadotrophin. *Hum Reprod* 1996; 11(11): 2387–2391.

34. Mercan R, Mayer JF, Walker D, Jones S, Oehninger S, Toner JP, Muasher SJ. Improved oocyte quality is obtained with follicle stimulating hormone alone than with follicle stimulating hormone/human menopausal gonadotrophin combination. *Hum Reprod* 1997; 12: 1886–1889.

35. Rattanachaiyanont M, Leader A, Leveille MC. Lack of correlation between oocyte-corona-cumulus complex morphology and nuclear maturity of oocytes collected in stimulated cycles for intracytoplasmic sperm injection. *Fertil Steril* 1999; 71: 937–40.

36. Jacob S, Drudy L, Conroy R, Harrison RF. Outcome from consecutive in-vitro fertilization/intracytoplasmic sperm injection attempts in the final group treated with urinary gonadotrophins and the first group treated with recombinant follicle stimulating hormone. *Hum Reprod* 1998; 13(7): 1783–1787.

37. Weissman A, Meriano J, Ward S, Gotlieb L, Casper RF. Intracytoplasmic sperm injection after follicle stimulation with highly purified human follicle-stimulating hormone compared with human menopausal gonadotropin. *J Assist Reprod Genet* 1999; 16(2): 63–68.

38. Venturoli S, Paradisi R, Fabbri R, Porcu E, Orsini LF, Flamigni C. Induction of ovulation in polycystic ovary: human menopausal gonadotropin or human urinary follicle stimulating hormone? *Int J Fertil* 1987; 32(1): 66–70.

39. Ng, EYL Lau, WSB Yeung, PC. Ho hMG is as good as recombinant human FSH in terms of oocyte and embryo quality: a prospective randomized trial. *Hum Reprod* 2001; 16(2): 319–325.

40. Cano F, Garcia-Velasco JA, Millet A, Remohi J, Simon C, Pellicer A. Oocyte quality in polycystic ovaries revisited: identification of a particular subgroup of women. *J Assist Reprod Genet* 1997; 14(5): 254–261.

Surgical Treatment

42

Surgical Treatment of Polycystic Ovary Syndrome Associated with Infertility

Stephen Gordts, Sylvie Gordts, Patrick Puttemans, Rudi Campo

Summary

Polycystic Ovary Syndrome (PCOS) is one of the most common reasons of anovulation. In clomiphene resistant patients, ovulation induction with gonadotropins, even with careful and meticulous monitoring, often results in cycle cancellation because of the risk of ovarian hyperstimulation and the risk of multiple pregnancies. As an alternative treatment to ovulation induction with gonadotropins, laparoscopic cautery of the ovaries has been reported to be effective with resumption of normal ovulatory cycles. In contrast to standard laparoscopy, a less invasive way for exploration of the female pelvis is offered by the transvaginal approach. Instead of a CO_2 pneumoperitoneum pre-warmed Ringer lactate is used as the distension medium in transvaginal laparoscopy, to keep the organs afloat. As the endoscope is in the same axis as the tubo-ovarian structures, it offers direct access to the tubes and ovaries, without supplementary manipulation. This way, drilling of the ovarian capsule can easily be performed using a bipolar needle. A very low morbidity, high patient compliance and comparable results as at standard laparoscopy, are in favor of this technique.

Introduction

Polycystic Ovary Syndrome (PCOS) is reported to affect ~7% of women.[1] Infertility due to chronic anovulation is the most common reason for women to seek medical assistance. Clomiphene citrate is a first choice drug for inducing ovulation, but approximately 20% of the women are resistant.[2]

Ovulation induction with gonadotropins, although routinely performed in clomiphene resistant patients, requires careful and extensive monitoring to exclude the risk of ovarian hyperstimulation. Several dose regimens have been used, the low dose step-up regimen being considered as the safest and most efficient.[3] Despite these precautions, the risk for ovarian hyper stimulation and the risk for multiple pregnancies, remains a real burden.

Laparoscopic electrocautery of the ovaries was shown to be effective in women with clomiphene resistant PCOS, resulting in a resumption of normal ovulatory cycles,[4–6] and was introduced as an alternative treatment to ovulation induction with gonadotropins. The cumulative pregnancy rate after ovarian surgery for PCOS is about 55%.[4,7,8] Patients without resumption of spontaneous ovulation after electrocautery may become sensitive to clomiphene citrate after treatment and/or easier to stimulate with gonadotropins. Postoperative adhesion formation is one of the possible complications after surgery upon the ovary. These adhesions, however, are more common after laparotomy than after laparoscopy. Standard laparoscopy, however, requires general anesthesia and hospitalization without resumption of work for several days. The procedure is not innocuous and severe complications such as injuries to the major blood vessels, visceral perforation and cardiac arrest have been reported. One third of the major complications are caused by the instillation of pneumoperitoneum and insertion of trocar.[9]

We reported the possibility of a less invasive way of exploring the female pelvis by the technique of transvaginal laparoscopy.[10] The technique is based on vaginal access and the use of a watery medium for distension. It also offers the possibility of limited indications for minimal invasive operative procedures.

Materials and Methods

Surgical procedure

The procedure is performed under general anesthesia with the patient in a dorsal decubitus position. Access to the pouch of Douglas is obtained through a needle puncture of the posterior fornix. For this purpose, a special access trocar was developed, enabling entry into the pouch of Douglas with a simple needle and consecutively dilating the point of entry up to the diameter of

the outer trocar (4 mm). The instrument is equipped with a spring load needle (Fig. 42.1), making access through the vaginal wall quicker and easier. The length of the loaded needle entering the pouch of Douglas can be preset between 1 cm and 2.5 cm. A preset depth of 1.5 cm is normally used except in obese patients. The spring load needle also reduces the risk of failure of entry by avoiding peritoneal tenting.

The use of pre-warmed Ringer lactate, as a distension medium, keeps the organs afloat and provides remarkable and accurate visualization. For the operative procedure, a 2.9 mm endoscope is used with an optical angle of 30°. This endoscope fits in an outer operative sheath of 5 mm or 7 mm diameter (Fig. 42.2), respectively with one or two working channels. Through these channels, 5 Fr instruments like scissors, biopsy and grasping forceps, a bipolar needle and bipolar coagulation probe can be introduced. For the operative procedures, the same access trocar is used as for the diagnostic ones. A special developed obturator allows easy exchange between the diagnostic and the operative outer sheaths. Since pre-warmed Ringer lactate is used as a watery distension medium throughout the procedure, the use of bipolar current is mandatory.

An advantage of the vaginal approach is the

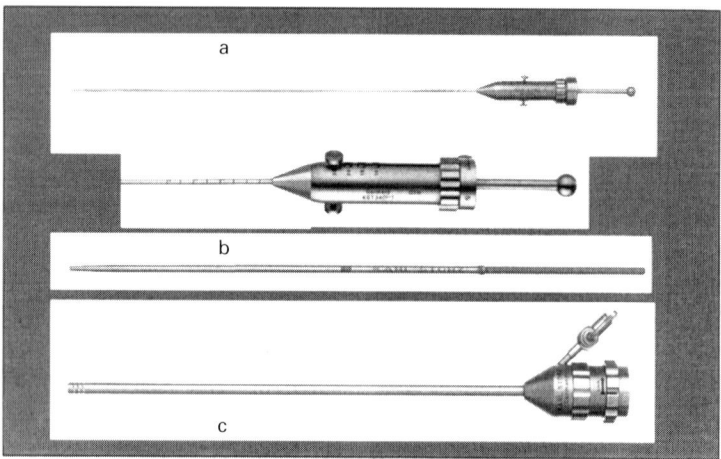

Figure 42.1   A specially developed needle – trocar system consists in three parts: a spring load needle (a) with close up of the needle, dilating trocar (b) and outer trocar (c). The spring load system allows quick access to the pouch of Douglas. (K. Storz, Tuttlingen, Germany).

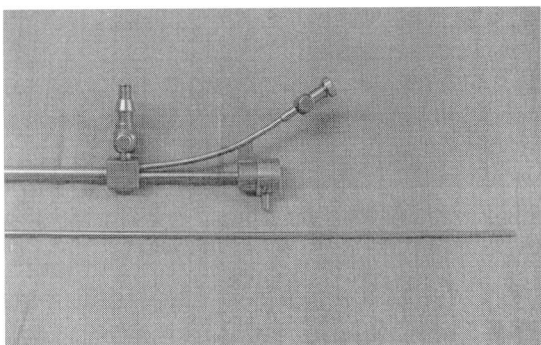

Figure 42.2 Operative sheath with one working channel and obturator.

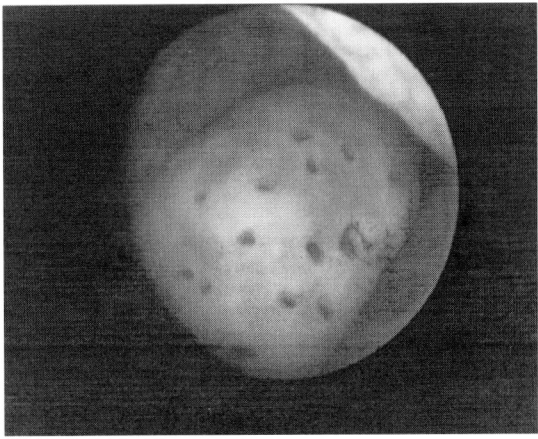

Figure 42.4 Final view after the electrosurgery: 10–15 holes are randomly made upon the ovarian surface.

direct access to the tubo-ovarian organs and fossa ovarica without the use of any additional manipulation. Therefore, the transvaginal route for drilling of the ovarian capsule is of particular interest in the treatment of clomiphene resistant PCO cases.

For the purpose of drilling of the ovarian capsule, a 5 Fr bipolar needle (Storz, Tuttlingen) is used (Fig. 42.3). The needle is insulated with a free length of 8 mm. After instillation of enough warm Ringer lactate (± 300cc), the total ovarian surface can easily be identified and inspected. Because of the distension and floating of organs, the intestines are kept at a distance. The 5 Fr bipolar needle is gently pushed against the ovarian surface and current with an energy output of 70 Watts is activated. To obtain a maximal effect following energy delivery, the inflow of Ringer lactate is stopped during activation of the current. This enables easy insertion of the needle in the ovarian tissue with a depth of 0.8 cm up till the insulated part. A small needle diameter minimizes superficial damage and reduces the risk of postoperative adhesion formation. In total, between 10–15 small holes of ±1.5 mm are made, preferentially on the antero-lateral side of each ovary (Fig. 42.4). The procedure is easy to perform, with low morbidity, and at the same time, allows a complete exploration of the female

pelvis with dye test, salpingoscopy and diagnostic hysteroscopy. As prophylaxis, patients are administered 1000 mg of amoxicillin preoperatively.

Results

Transvaginal drilling of the ovarian capsule was performed in our unit in 39 patients. No conversion to standard laparoscopy was necessary and no complications occurred. The mean age of the patients at the time of surgery was 30.38 y (SD ± 3.8), mean body mass index (BMI) 29.4 kg/m (SD ± 9.7) with mean infertility duration of 26.5 months (SD ± 2.6). As a complete exploration including hysteroscopy was performed at the time of intervention, additional female pathology was detected in 12 patients (31%) of whom 10 patients presented with a congenital uterine pathology (6 with a T-shaped uterus and 4 with a septate uterus), one with an intra-uterine polyp, and one with tubal pathology. Additional male pathology was present in 15 (38%) of the couples. Six patients were lost to follow-up.

Of the remaining 33 patients, spontaneous ovulatory cycles were resumed in 9 (27%) patients following drilling, 6 of whom did not receive any additional treatment, 1 was referred for intrauterine insemination and 2 were referred for in vitro fertilization (IVF). Ovulation induction,

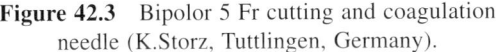

Figure 42.3 Bipolor 5 Fr cutting and coagulation needle (K.Storz, Tuttlingen, Germany).

using a combined regime of 100 mg clomiphene citrate and human menopausal gonadotropin (hMG) 75 IU/day, starting on day 6 of the treatment cycle was necessary in 10 (30%) patients. In 7 of these patients, ovulation induction was combined with intrauterine insemination. In vitro fertilization (IVF) was performed in 17 (51%) patients, mostly due to aberrant semen parameters (n = 10), or previous failed IVF attempts.

In total 25 patients (76%) became pregnant after the procedure with a mean duration between procedure and onset of pregnancy of 7.2 months (SD ± 5.4). A spontaneous pregnancy occurred in 6 of the 9 patients resuming a normal ovulatory cycle after drilling; of those patients requiring controlled ovarian hyperstimulation (COH), or COH with IUI, 7 conceived; of the 17 patients referred to our IVF program, 12 conceived. There were no multiple pregnancies and none of the pregnancies ended in an abortion. (Table 42.1)

Table 42.1 Ovarian drilling and pregnancy outcome

	No.	Pregnant	
No treatment	6	6	100%
ovulation induction	3	1	33%
ovulation induction +IUI	7	6	86%
IVF	17	12	71%
Total	33	25	75.80%

Clinical Discussion

Our own experience confirms the results of Fernandez et al.[11] and Casa et al.[12] showing the feasibility of the transvaginal approach for drilling of the ovarian surface by electrocautery. These results are comparable with those obtained after standard laparoscopic procedures.

In our experience, the morbidity after the operative transvaginal procedure was very low, and in contrast with the experience after operative standard laparoscopy. At the most, patients complained of a slight tenderness in the lower abdomen and all the patients were able to return home the same day with resumption of full activity one or two days later. Therefore, this approach

is indicated in the following patients: (i) CC-resistant patients who fail to react to a daily dose of 150 mg, (ii) as an alternative to medical treatment with a prolonged low dose step-up protocol with gonadotropins, (iii) patients who respond to clomiphene citrate but fail to conceive, and (iv) patients with an exaggerated response to gonadotropins, instead of a liberal referral to an IVF program.

The exact number of drillings is arbitrarily set to 10–15 holes on each ovarian surface. As there is no spreading of current, the bipolar technique offers maximum safety with precisely localized tissue destruction.

The use of a fine bipolar needle minimizes the trauma on the ovarian surface and reduces the risk of postoperative adhesion formation. Recent data show that apart from the surgical trauma, the high and prolonged intra-abdominal pressure caused by the CO_2 pneumoperitoneum, is known to be the major reason for adhesion formation by hypoxemia of the mesothelial layer.[13] The use of a watery distension medium reduces the risk of postoperative adhesion formation.

Recently, two complications have been reported after transvaginal drilling due to the wrong interpretation of the intestinal surface as the ovarian surface.[14] They occurred during the initial experience of the authors with the transvaginal technique, underlining the necessity of training and a learning period before attempting surgery by transvaginal laparoscopy (TVL). As for each operative procedure, anatomical identification of the different structures is mandatory and by filling up the abdomen with enough Ringer lactate (at least 300cc) intestines will be kept at a distance.

In the transvaginal approach, direct access to the fossa ovarica and the ovaries, the use of hydrofloatation and close inspection are of major benefit, excluding the need for supplementary manipulations.

In PCOS patients, obesity is frequently present often causing problems and failure of entry at standard laparoscopy. Certainly, in these patients, the transvaginal access offers a major advantage. The spring load needle reduces the risks of peritoneal tenting, offering an easier and safer way of access in these patients. In contrast to standard laparoscopy, there is no need for the extreme Trendelenberg position and the use of a high CO_2 intrabdominal pressure.

In a recently published study of 1000 TVL procedures, Verhoeven et al.[15] reported 32 failures (3.2%) with failed access in 11 patients (1.1%) and absent or poor visualization in 21 patients (2.1%). Bowel perforation occurred in 5 patients (0.5%). Rectal perforation is a potentially serious complication of transvaginal access. In a survey of 3,667 procedures, the incidence of bowel perforation was 0.65%, which decreased after initial experience to 0.25%. There was no delayed diagnosis and sepsis, and all but one case was managed conservatively with antibiotics.[16] An analysis of the complications in function of experience, confirmed the importance of the learning curve, with a clear decline in complications and failed access after 50 procedures. Routine vaginal examination and vaginal ultrasound to exclude pathology of the pouch of Douglas is strongly recommended to avoid complications. Acute clinical conditions such as bleeding, infection, obliterated cul de sac or large ovarian cysts are strict contraindications for the transvaginal approach.

The high incidence of additional uterine pathology was remarkable in our group of patients. This has also been reported in previous studies,[17,18] indicating the need of an ultrasonographic and/or hysteroscopic exploration of the uterine cavity in PCOS patients.

Restoration of monofollicular cycles, reduction of multiple pregnancies and lower rate of miscarriages are factors in favor of this surgical treatment for PCOS. If a supplementary treatment with gonadotropins is necessary after drilling, an easier ovarian response is obtained with a lower dose of medication and with a reduction of cancelled cycles.

Recently, in a multicentric randomized clinical trial, the total treatment cost up to an ongoing pregnancy has been reported to be the same for electrocautery and ovulation induction with r-FSH, but due to a lower incidence of multiple pregnancies, the electrocautery strategy results in a lower cost.[19]

Conclusion

The transvaginal approach for performing electrocautery of the ovarian capsule offers a valuable and less invasive alternative to the standard laparoscopic procedure in patients with clomiphene resistant PCOS. In contrast to a long-lasting and sometimes difficult ovulation induction with gonadotropins with its risks of hyperstimulation and multiple pregnancies, electrocautery of the ovarian capsule, due to its low morbidity and high patient compliance is, in our experience, the treatment of choice. Offering the possibility of resumption of normal ovulatory cycles and as such, the possibility of spontaneous conception for these couples, there is certainly no place for a liberal referral to a more costly and more complicated treatment with in vitro fertilization.

References

1. Balen A, Michelmore K. What is polycystic ovary syndrome? Are national views important? *Hum Reprod* 2002; 17: 2219–2227.
2. Imani B, Eijkemans MJ, te Velde ER, Habbema JD, Fauser BC. Predictors of patients remaining anovulatory during clomiphene citrate induction of ovulation in normogonadotrophic oligomenorrheic infertility. *J. Clin. Endocrinol. Metab* 1998; 83: 2361–2365.
3. Christin-Maitre S, Hugues JN. A comparative randomized multicentric study comparing the step-up versus step-down protocol in polycystic ovary syndrome. *Hum Reprod* 2003; 18: 1626–1631.
4. Donesky BW, Adashi EY. Surgically induced ovulation in the polycystic ovary syndrome: wedge resection revisited in the age of laparoscopy. *Ferti Steril* 1995; 63: 439–463.
5. Gjonnaess H. Polycystic ovarian syndrome treated by ovarian electrocautery through the laparoscope. *Fertil Steril* 1984; 41: 20–25.
6. Greenblatt E, Casper RF. Endocrine changes after laparoscopic ovarian cautery in polycystic ovarian syndrome. *Am J Obstet Gynecol* 1987; 156: 279–285.
7. Campo S. Ovulatory cycles, pregnancy outcome and

complications after surgical treatment of polycystic ovary syndrome. *Obstet Gynecol Surv* 1998; 53: 297–308.

8. Felemban A, Tan SL, Tulandi T. Laparoscopic treatment of polycystic ovaries with insulated needle cautery: a reappraisal. *Fertil Steril* 2000; 73: 266–269.

9. Brosens I, Gordon A, Campo R, Gordts S. Bowel injury in gynecologic laparoscopy. *J Am Assoc Gynecol Laparosc* 2003; 10: 9–13.

10. Gordts S, Campo R, Rombauts L, Brosens I. Transvaginal hydrolaparoscopy as an outpatient procedure for infertility investigation. *Hum Reprod* 1998; 13: 99–103.

11. Fernandez H. Two complications of ovarian drilling by fertiloscopy *Gynecol Obstet Fertil* 2003; 31: 844–846]. *Gynecol Obstet Fertil* 2004; 32: 265–266.

12. Casa A, Sesti F, Marziali M, Gulemi L, Piccione E. Transvaginal hydrolaparoscopic ovarian drilling using bipolar electrosurgery to treat anovulatory women with polycystic ovary syndrome. *J Am Assoc Gynecol Laparosc* 2003; 10: 219–222.

13. Molinas CR, Koninckx PR. Hypoxaemia induced by CO(2) or helium pneumoperitoneum is a co-factor in adhesion formation in rabbits. *Hum Reprod* 2000; 15: 1758–1763.

14. Chiesa-Montadou S, Rongieres C, Garbin O, Nisand I. About two complications of ovarian drilling by fertiloscopy. *Gynecol Obstet Fertil* 2003; 31: 844–846.

15. Verhoeven H, Gordts S, Campo R, Puttemans P, Brosens I. Role of transvaginal laparoscopy in the investigation of female infertility: a review of 1000 procedures. *Gynecol Surgery* 2004; 1: 191–193.

16. Gordts S, Watrelot A, Campo R, Brosens I. Risk and outcome of bowel injury during transvaginal pelvic endoscopy. *Fertil Steril* 2001; 76: 1238–1241.

17. Appelman Z, Hazan Y, Hagay Z. High prevalence of mullerian anomalies diagnosed by ultrasound in women with polycystic ovaries. *J Reprod Med* 2003; 48: 362–364.

18. Ugur M, Karakaya S, Zorlu G, Arslan S, Gulerman C, Kukner S et al. Polycystic ovaries in association with mullerian anomalies. *Eur J Obstet Gynecol Reprod Biol* 1995; 62: 57–59.

19. van Wely M, Bayram N, van d, V, Bossuyt PM. An economic comparison of a laparoscopic electrocautery strategy and ovulation induction with recombinant FSH in women with clomiphene citrate-resistant polycystic ovary syndrome. *Hum Reprod* 2004; 19: 1741–1745.

43

Reproductive Outcome Following Laparoscopic Ovarian Drilling for the Treatment of PCOS

Yashodhara Mhatre, Pritesh Naik, Gautam N Allahbadia

Summary

Polycystic Ovary Syndrome (PCOS) is characterized by anovulation (irregular or absent menstrual periods) and hyperandrogenism (elevated serum testosterone and androstenedione). Patients with this syndrome may complain of abnormal bleeding, infertility, obesity, excess hair growth, hair loss and acne. In addition to the clinical and hormonal changes associated with this condition, vaginal ultrasound shows enlarged ovaries with an increased number of small (6–10 mm) follicles around the periphery (Polycystic Appearing Ovaries or PAO). While ultrasound reveals that polycystic appearing ovaries are commonly seen in upto 20% of women in the reproductive age range, PCOS is estimated to affect about half as many or approximately 6–10% of women. The condition appears to have a genetic component, and those affected, often have both male and female relatives with adult-onset diabetes, obesity, elevated blood triglycerides, high blood pressure and female relatives with infertility, hirsutism and menstrual problems. Infertility treatments include weight loss, diet management, ovulation medications (clomiphene, letrozole, Follistim, Gonal-F), ovarian drilling surgery and in vitro fertilization (IVF). Other symptoms have been managed by oral contraceptive pills (OCPs), and antiandrogen medication such as, spironolactone, flutamide or finasteride. With the availability of laparoscopic ovarian cautery, there has been resurgence in interest in the surgical treatment of clomiphene citrate-resistant polycystic ovary syndrome (PCOS). A comparison of ovulation and pregnancy rates between ovarian cautery and gonadotropin ovulation induction in such women has revealed no difference in success rates and little difference in the cost. Laparoscopic Ovarian Drilling (LOD) can resolve infertility within 4-6 months in 50-60% of couples Owing to the potential advantages of ovarian cautery, this surgery has been recommended as the next line of treatment if clomiphene citrate fails to induce ovulation in PCOS patients, before gonadotropins are introduced.[1]

Rationale

Polycystic Ovary Syndrome (PCOS) accounts for 90% of women with oligomenorrhea (infrequent periods), 30% of women with amenorrhea (absent of periods), and over 70% of women with anovulation. There is little agreement when it comes to how PCOS is diagnosed. Traditional treatments have been difficult, expensive and have limited success when used alone. Patients with PCOS treated with gonadotropins often have a polyfollicular response and are exposed to the risks of ovarian hyperstimulation syndrome (OHSS) and multiple pregnancies. LOD may avoid or reduce the risk of OHSS and multiple pregnancies associated with gonadotropins with the same success rate of conception. The high pregnancy rate, and economic aspect of the procedure make it an attractive management approach for patients with PCOS.[2] Though studies report that LOD may reduce the need for medical ovulation induction and enable diagnosis of those women with anatomic infertility who can achieve pregnancy only by in vitro fertilization treatment,[3] in lieu of the risks attributed to the procedure, the extent to which this procedure can be used as a viable option in anovulatory patients with PCOS, is still debated. There is an uncertainty about the impact of laparoscopic ovarian drilling (LOD) on the natural history of PCOS.[4]

Introduction

Most physicians will consider the diagnosis of polycystic ovary syndrome (PCOS) after making sure that the patients do not have other conditions such as Cushing's disease (*overactive adrenal gland*), thyroid problems, congenital adrenal hyperplasia or increased prolactin production by the pituitary gland. Thyroid stimulating hormone (TSH), 17-hydroxyprogesterone, prolactin and a dexamethasone suppression test may be advisable. After reviewing the medical history, the physicians will determine which tests are necessary. Estimation of the patient's height and weight with any increase in facial or body hair or loss of scalp hair, acne and acanthosis nigricans (a discoloration of the skin under the arms, breasts and in the groin), elevated androgen levels (male hormones), dehydroepiandrosterone sulfate (DHEAS) or testosterone(T), a two hour insulin and glucose tolerance test, help make the diagnosis. Many physicians tell their patients that insulin values are normal, when in fact, the value indicates that insulin may be playing a role in stimulating the development of PCOS. Most laboratories report levels less than 25–30 mIU/ml as normal, while in fact, levels over 10 mIU/ml on a fasting blood

sample suggest that PCOS may be related to hyperinsulinism. As women with polycystic ovary syndrome may be at a greater risk for other medical conditions, testing for cardiovascular risk factors such as, blood lipids, homocysteine, C-reactive protein (CRP) and plasminogen activator inhibitor (PAI-1)-(a blood factor that promotes abnormal clotting), should also be carried out.

Weight loss if she is over-weight

This simple measure may restore menstruation and ovulation in patients with polycystic ovary syndrome. Exercise and weight control also reduce the likelihood of developing type 2 diabetes in later life.

Ovulation induction with clomiphene citrate (clomid) tablets

Induction of ovulation with clomiphene citrate tablets is the first choice and is an effective treatment of women with PCOS. It restores menstruation and ovulation in about 70% of women and some 30% will conceive within three months of treatment. Clomiphene tablets maybe combined with steroid tablets to suppress androgen production. If this fails after a six month trial, then controlled ovarian stimulation (COS) with follicle stimulating hormone (FSH) or human menopausal gonadotropin (hMG) combined with human chorionic gonadotropin (hCG) is used. Because polycystic ovaries are usually sensitive to stimulation by hormones, it is important to start with a low dose and adjust the dose according to the response. Monitoring of treatment is essential because these patients are susceptible to develop ovarian hyperstimulation syndrome (OHSS) and multiple pregnancies.

Laparoscopic ovarian drilling

Advances in laparoscopic techniques have resulted in a resurgence of interest in surgical induction of ovulation. Laparoscopic ovarian drilling (LOD) is an effective surgical procedure in clomiphene-resistant women with PCOS. It may be used as a first line of treatment, or as a second line of treatment after patients have proved resistant to clomiphene, or as a third line of treatment after failed ovulation induction with gonadotropins.[5] This laparoscopic procedure is a less invasive modification of ovarian wedge resection, involving the formation of multiple holes on the surface of the ovary by using laser or electrocautery.[6] Using a unipolar electrode, 8 to 15 craters, 2 to 4 mm deep, are created in the capsule of each ovary (Figure 43.1). Using this technique, ovulation was restored in 92% of the patients with a pregnancy rate of 80%.[7]

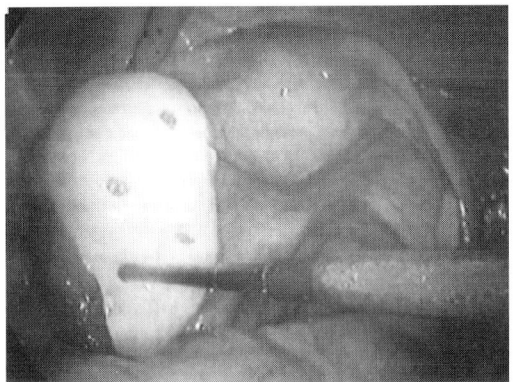

Figure 43.1 The ovarian capsule following LOD

Other names that have been used to describe the procedure are laparoscopic ovarian electrocautery, laparoscopic ovarian diathermy, and laparoscopic electro-coagulation. The term laparoscopic ovarian drilling has gained popularity and is in widespread clinical use. Lasers, including CO_2, argon, KTP, and Nd-YAG, have also been used. The technique is similar to that of electrocautery, and success rates have been similar.[6] With few exceptions,[8–13] most observational studies have involved a small number of women. In general, the results indicate that laparoscopic ovarian drilling restores menstrual cyclicity and ovulation in approximately 80% of women.[7,9–11,13–15] The beneficial effect of laparoscopic ovarian drilling on ovulatory function appears to be maintained over a long period.[7,10,15]

Metformin vs. LOD

Malkawi et al.[16] evaluated the efficacy of metformin compared with ovarian drilling in the treatment of clomiphene citrate (CC)-resistant women with polycystic ovary syndrome in a prospective trial. Patients were allocated into two groups; group 1 included 64 women who received metformin, 850 mg twice daily throughout the cycle, and group 2 included 97 women who underwent laparoscopic ovarian drilling. Failure to achieve spontaneous ovulation or pregnancy within 3 months after treatment was followed by the administration of CC with increments of 50 mg (up to 150 mg/day) for both the groups. There were no significant differences in rates of ovulation (79.7% vs. 83.5%) and pregnancy (64.1% vs. 59.8%) between the metformin group and the drilling group respectively. Hence, CC-resistant patients with polycystic ovary syndrome can be treated effectively, either by metformin, or by laparoscopic ovarian drilling. The efficacy of LOD may be attributed to a significant improvement in menstrual cycle pattern and the rates of ovulation and pregnancy, probably due to the significant decrease in the levels of androgens and luteinizing hormone.

Clinical Discussion

Effects of laparoscopic ovarian drilling on ART outcome

Clinical data on women conceived in comparison to those who did not, reveals no difference between women who had pre- and/or postoperative medical ovulation treatment and those who had none.[5] Malkawi and Qublan[17] evaluated the biochemical, clinical and reproductive results after LOD in 63 clomiphene-citrate-resistant women with polycystic ovary syndrome (PCOS). Patients were allocated to two groups: group I (n = 26) had five punctures per ovary, and group II (n = 37) had 10 punctures per ovary. There were no significant differences in terms of body mass index, and insulin and glucose levels before and after the procedure between the two groups. Androgen levels and luteinizing hormone concentrations showed a statistically significant decrease after the treatment. The clinical and reproductive outcome, including menstrual cyclicity, ovulation, and pregnancy rates were similar in both groups. The authors concluded that laparoscopic ovarian drilling is an effective treatment in clomiphene-citrate-resistant women with PCOS. Five, instead of ≥10, punctures per ovary are sufficient to ameliorate the hyperandrogenic status in these women, improving their clinical and reproductive outcome.[17]

Tulandi et al.[18] evaluated the changes in ovarian volume and the reproductive outcome after laparoscopic ovarian drilling of polycystic ovaries (PCO) in clomiphene-resistant anovulatory women in a prospective study. They reported an ovulation rate of 88.2% and a cumulative pregnancy rate of 70% at 12 months, and concluded that laparoscopic ovarian drilling may result in a transient increase, with a subsequent significant reduction in ovarian volume.[18] Kriplani et al.[19] in a similar study, reported a spontaneous ovulation rate of 81.8%, cumulative ovulation rate of 93.9%, and a pregnancy rate of 54.5%. However, they additionally pointed out that successful pregnancies were commonly complicated by gestational diabetes mellitus and pregnancy-induced hypertension. Pregnancy rates were low (23.5%) in women with tuboperitoneal disease and those whose partners had subfertile male factors. A short duration of infertility (<3 yrs), and absence of pre-existing tubal disease were associated with better outcomes.[19] In yet another long-term follow up study on PCOS patients who underwent LOD, the proportion of women with regular menstrual cycles was reported to have increased significantly from 8% before LOD to 67% post-operatively [relative risk (RR) = 1.6, 95% confidence interval (CI) = 1.4-1.9, P < 0.05]. After LOD, 49% women conceived spontaneously during the first year and 38% during medium- and long-term follow-up. Among women with hirsutism and acne, 23% and 40% respectively experienced long-term improvement after LOD.[20]

Mechanism of action of LOD and effect on physiological parameters

The mechanism of action of LOD is unclear. It appears to exert its beneficial effect by destroying the androgen-producing ovarian stroma. This results in a reduction in intraovarian androgen production and decreased circulating androgen concentrations.[21,22] The reduction in total and free testosterone is approximately 40–50%.

The serum LH concentration increases immediately after surgery[10,19,23] and then decreases.[14,21,24] Although the LH pulse frequencies do not change, the LH pulse amplitudes are markedly reduced. Pituitary responsiveness to gonadotropin releasing hormone (GnRH) stimulation also decreases concomitantly with a decline in serum testosterone concentration,[25,26] suggesting that destruction of ovarian stroma has an indirect modulating effect on the pituitary–ovarian axis.[21] Serum LH concentrations appear to be the best determinant of response to treatment.[11,14] Women with serum LH concentrations > 10 IU/L have a significantly better response to laparoscopic ovarian drilling than do those with lower preoperative levels, and they experience a higher reduction in LH and testosterone concentrations.

Whereas LH concentrations decrease after laparoscopic ovarian drilling, the effect of this procedure on FSH is variable and less pronounced. The FSH concentration generally increases rapidly and thereafter, demonstrates a cyclical rise, in keeping with the restoration of ovulatory function. Normal inhibin pulsatility is restored, in association with the onset of regular ovulatory cycles, indicating the resumption of normal intraovarian paracrine signaling. Kucuk and Kilic-Okman[27] reported a significant decrease in serum T, LH, homocysteine levels and LH-FSH ratio after LOD, than at baseline (0.93 ± 0.15 vs. 0.67 ± 0.11 ng/ml, p < 0.001; 12.72 ± 1.13 vs. 7.36 ± 0.57 mIU/ml, p < 0.001; 9.77 ± 1.06 vs. 7.13 ± 0.99 micromol/L, p < 0.001; 2.16 ± 0.22 vs. 1.29 ± 0.13, p < 0.001, respectively) and a significant increase in sex hormone binding globulin (SHBG) levels compared to their baseline values (370.7 ± 19.08 vs. 404.7 ± 16.71 nmol/L, p < 0.001) respectively. However, there were no differences between E2, FSH, DHEAS, and PRL concentrations (p = 0.255, p = 0.140, p = 0.250, p = 0.137, respectively) following LOD in comparison to their baseline measurements. The spontaneous ovulation rate was 77% with a 54% chance of conception at 12 months after surgery.[27] Api et al.[2] additionally reported a significant reduction in Ferriman Gallwey (FG) scores after LOD with a restoration of regular menses in 93.3% of the subjects and a 64.4% spontaneous pregnancy rate.

The increase in FSH secretion would be expected to result in a normal ratio of LH to FSH,[22] recruitment of a new cohort of follicles, and resumption of ovarian function. These endocrine changes occur rapidly and are sustained for several years.

With regard to the vascular endothelial growth factor (VEGF), Tulandi et al.[28] reported significantly lower VEGF concentrations in women with normal ovaries (4.5 ± 1.7 ng/mL) than in women with PCOS, but no difference in VEGF levels in women with PCOS before (6.0 ± 1.2 ng/mL) and after ovarian drilling (5.5 ± 1.2 ng/mL). They observed no difference in glucose and insulin responses to oral glucose tolerance test (OGTT) before and after ovarian drilling.[28] Api et al[2] reported no changes in the glucose levels and glucose/insulin ratio following LOD.

On the contrary, Amin et al.[29] reported that LOD reduced serum VEGF in addition to insulin-like growth factor (IGF-1), T, and LH in clomiphene-resistant patients with polycystic ovary syndrome, and reduced ovarian blood flow velocities, evident by the significantly increased Doppler indices (pulsatility index and resistance index) of ovarian stromal blood flow.[29] The reduced vascularization index and vascularization flow index of the intraovarian stroma following treatment,[4,29] may explain the reduction of ovarian hyperstimulation syndrome in women with PCOS after LOD.

However, PCOS women with hyperinsulinemia respond differently to LOD than do those with normoinsulinemia. Among women with hyperinsulinemia, while LOD decreases glucose and insulin responses to OGTT, regardless of the insulin level, surgery does not influence adrenal steroid dynamics.[30]

No reduction has been reported in high-density lipoprotein cholesterol (HDL-C) in CC-resistant oligomenorrheic women with polycystic ovaries after LOD.[27]

Determinants of treatment outcome

Body mass index also appears to influence the response to treatment. Women with body mass index (BMI) ≥35 kg/m^2, serum testosterone concentration ≥4.5 nmol/l, free androgen index (FAI) ≥ 15 and/or with a duration of infertility > 3 years seem to be poor responders to LOD. In LOD responders, serum LH levels > 10 IU/l appeared to be associated with higher pregnancy rates.[3] Levels of BMI, fasting blood sugar, and leptin were higher and LH, LH/FSH, and the sugar/insulin ratio were reported to be lower in obese anovulatory young women with PCOS who were resistant to clomiphene citrate. Logistic multiple regression analysis has shown that the duration of infertility, modality used in treatment (laser or diathermy) and the pre-operative LH levels were the main determinants of the outcome. The success rate in women with infertility duration of less than three years, treated with diathermy, in whom the pre-operative LH level was more than 10 IU/L, reached 79%.[31]

Grossly obese women tend to respond less well than non-obese women. However, because of the heterogeneity of the population studied, the influence of obesity on ovarian response and pregnancy rates is unclear.[4] As expected, pre-existing tubal disease and duration of infertility of more than 3 years' lead to a low pregnancy rate after laparoscopic ovarian drilling.[13]

Benefits and risks of laparoscopic ovarian drilling

Laparoscopic ovarian drilling may be beneficial both, to endocrine profiles and to intraovarian stromal flow in patients with PCOS.[4] LOD produces long-term improvement in menstrual regularity and reproductive performance in about one-third of the cases. A modest and sustained improvement in acne and hirsutism can be expected in approximately 40% and 25% of patients respectively.[20] These surgical techniques can be performed as outpatient procedures and may be combined with a diagnostic laparoscopy. Knowledge of the long-term effects of these techniques is still limited, but results appear promising, with spontaneous ovulation being initiated in 70 to 90% of women. Of the patients who remain anovulatory or oligo-ovulatory after these procedures, most will have been rendered sensitive to clomiphene citrate with conception rates approximating 60%. The mechanism of action remains uncertain, but is likely to involve alteration of the intraovarian steroid environment and, in turn, the feedback to the hypothalamic-pituitary axis. The overall result is normalization of gonadotropin drive and follicular microenvironment, allowing follicular recruitment and development to proceed to ovulation.[32]

However, LOD carries the usual risks of laparoscopy and general anesthesia. Two other potential complications are periadnexal adhesion formation and premature ovarian failure. The incidence of postoperative adhesion formation is estimated to be 19% to 43%, and may be as high as 82%. This complication seems to be more frequent with laser treatment than with electrocoagulation, and the use of adhesion barriers does not reduce its incidence. However, abdominal lavage and use of an insulated needle cautery may help to prevent its occurrence. Because laparoscopic ovarian drilling may result in ovarian failure, excessive ovarian drilling and electrocoagulation of the ovarian hilum should be avoided. Ovarian atrophy has been observed after ovarian wedge resection, but there has been no report of premature ovarian failure after laparoscopic ovarian drilling. Adhesion formation and the theoretical risk of ovarian failure, emphasize the need to reserve laparoscopic ovarian drilling as a second-line treatment for clomiphene citrate–resistant anovulatory women.

Recent Advances

Laparoscopic ovarian drilling (LOD) is the accepted second-line treatment for clomiphene citrate-resistant anovulatory infertility in polycystic ovary syndrome (PCOS). Although multiple pregnancy rates are reduced with ovarian drilling procedures, postoperative adhesion formation is a potential complication in up to 85% of the women subjected to laparoscopic destructive ovarian procedures.[33] Laparoscopic ovarian multi-needle intervention (LOMNI) is a new surgical approach for the treatment of clomiphene citrate-resistant infertility in polycystic ovary syndrome, resulting in a significant improvement in cycle regularity (p <0.01) and cumulative pregnancy rates (35.3%) compared to ovulation induction (33.3%). The absence of adverse events such as post-operative adhesion formation and the significantly (p <.001) lower cost of LOMNI compared to ovulation induction treatment make it a safe, inexpensive, and effective procedure for the treatment of CC-resistant infertility in patients with PCOS. LOMNI seems to preserve the beneficial effects and probably omits unwanted effects (such as adhesion formation) of LOD.[33]

Transvaginal ovarian drilling (TVOD) is less invasive and less expensive when compared with laparoscopic ovarian diathermy and effective in improving IVF results in difficult to treat patients (repeated poor performance in > or = 2 previous IVF cycles) with PCOS.[34]

This technique yields significantly higher fertilization and cleavage rates (66% vs. 27% respectively and 72% vs. 54%, respectively) compared to cycles prior to surgery, and pregnancy and implantation rates similar to those for normovulatory patients undergoing IVF for tubal factor infertility.

Conclusions

Although laparoscopic ovarian drilling (LOD) has been widely used to induce ovulation in women with polycystic ovary syndrome, predicting the clinical response to this treatment, remains to be elucidated further.[3] Laparoscopic ovarian drilling improves menstrual disturbances and ovulatory dysfunction to some extent. However, the pregnancy rates after the treatment are not significantly increased. Marked obesity, marked hyperandrogenism, pre-existing tubal disease and/or long duration of infertility in women with PCOS, seem to predict resistance to LOD. High LH levels in LOD responders appear to predict higher probability of pregnancy.

Laparoscopic ovarian drilling in the management of patients with PCOS, should be re-examined in the context of a randomized controlled trial and should be used only sparingly. Future clinical studies with long-term follow-up will be required to determine the relapse rate and fecundity rates following these procedures. The risk of postoperative adhesion formation and the role of second-look laparoscopy in the prevention of this undesirable complication remain uncertain. Until more complete, long-term information is known, caution must be exercised and complete information provided to the patient with respect to the possible adverse affects.

References

1. Kovacs GT, Clarke S, Burger HG, Healy DL, Vollenhoven B. Surgical or medical treatment of polycystic ovary syndrome: a cost-benefit analysis. *Gynecol Endocrinol* 2002; 16(1): 53–55.
2. Api M, Gorgen H, Cetin A. Laparoscopic ovarian drilling in polycystic ovary syndrome. *Eur J Obstet Gynecol Reprod Biol* 2005; 119(1): 76–81.
3. Amer SA, Li TC, Ledger WL. Ovulation induction using laparoscopic ovarian drilling in women with polycystic ovarian syndrome: predictors of success. *Hum Reprod* 2004(8): 1719–1724.
4. Wu MH, Huang MF, Tsai SJ, Pan HA, Cheng YC, Lin YS. Effects of laparoscopic ovarian drilling on young adult women with polycystic ovarian syndrome. *J Am Assoc Gynecol Laparosc* 2004; 11(2): 184–190.
5. Cleemann L, Lauszus FF, Trolle B.Laparoscopic ovarian drilling as first line of treatment in infertile women with polycystic ovary syndrome. *Gynecol Endocrinol* 2004; 18(3): 138–143.
6. Tulandi T, al Took S. Surgical management of polycystic ovarian syndrome. *Baillieres Clin Obstet Gynaecol* 1998; 12: 541–553.
7. Gjönnaess H. Polycystic ovarian syndrome treated by ovarian electrocautery through the laparoscope. *Fertil Steril* 1984; 41: 20–25.
8. Farquhar C, Vandekerckhove P, Arnot M, Lilford R. Laparoscopic "drilling" by diathermy or laser for ovulation induction in anovulatory polycystic ovary syndrome. *Cochrane Database Syst Rev* 2000; CD001122.
9. Naether OG, Fischer R. Adhesion formation after laparoscopic electrocoagulation of the ovarian surface in polycystic ovary patients. *Fertil Steril* 1993; 60: 95–98.
10. Naether OG, Baukloh V, Fischer R, Kowalczyk T. Long-term follow-up in 206 infertility patients with polycystic ovarian syndrome after laparoscopic electrocautery of the ovarian surface. *Hum Reprod* 1994; 9: 2342–2849.
11. Liguori G, Tolino A, Moccia G, Scognamiglio G, Nappi C. Laparoscopic ovarian treatment in infertile patients with polycystic ovarian syndrome (PCOS). Endocrine changes and clinical outcome. *Gynecol Endocrinol* 1996; 10: 257–264.
12. Li TC, Saravelos H, Chow MS, Chisabingo R, Cooke ID. Factors affecting the outcome of laparoscopic ovarian drilling for polycystic ovarian syndrome in women with anovulatory infertility. *Br J Obstet Gynaecol* 1998; 105: 338–344.
13. Felemban A, Tan SL, Tulandi T. Laparoscopic treatment of polycystic ovaries with insulated needle cautery: a reappraisal. *Fertil Steril* 2000; 73: 266–269.
14. Farhi J, Soule S, Jacobs HS. Effect of laparoscopic ovarian electrocautery on ovarian response and outcome of treatment with gonadotropins in clomiphene citrate-resistant patients with polycystic ovary syndrome. *Fertil Steril*, 1995; 64: 930–935.
15. Merchant RN. Treatment of polycystic ovary disease with laparoscopic low-watt bipolar electrocoagulation of the ovaries. *J Am Assoc Gynecol Laparosc* 1996; 3: 503–508.
16. Malkawi HY, Qublan HS, Hamaideh AH. Medical vs. surgical treatment for clomiphene citrate-resistant women with polycystic ovary syndrome. *J Obstet Gynaecol* 2003; 23(3): 289–293.
17. Malkawi HY, Qublan HS. Laparoscopic ovarian drilling in the treatment of polycystic ovary syndrome: how many punctures per ovary are needed to improve the reproductive outcome? *J Obstet Gynaecol Res* 2005; 31(2): 115–119.
18. Tulandi T, Watkin K, Tan SL. Reproductive

performance and three-dimensional ultrasound volume determination of polycystic ovaries following laparoscopic ovarian drilling. *Int J Fertil Womens Med* 1997; 42(6): 436–440.

19. Kriplani A, Manchanda R, Agarwal N, Nayar B.Laparoscopic ovarian drilling in clomiphene citrate-resistant women with polycystic ovary syndrome. *J Am Assoc Gynecol Laparosc* 2001; 8(4): 511–518.

20. Amer SA, Gopalan V, Li TC, Ledger WL, Cooke ID. Long term follow-up of patients with polycystic ovarian syndrome after laparoscopic ovarian drilling: clinical outcome. *Hum Reprod* 2002; 17(8): 2035–2042.

21. Keckstein J. Laparoscopic treatment of polycystic ovarian syndrome. *Baillieres Clin Obstet Gynaecol* 1989; 3: 63–81.

22. Aakvaag A, Gjönnaess H. Hormonal response to electrocautery of the ovary in patients with polycystic ovarian disease. *Br J Obstet Gynaecol* 1985; 92: 258–264.

23. Sakata M, Tasaka K, Kurachi H, Terakawa N, Miyake A, Tanizawa O. Changes of bioactive luteinizing hormone after laparoscopic ovarian cautery in patients with polycystic ovarian syndrome. *Fertil Steril* 1990; 53: 10–13.

24. Amer SA, Banu Z, Li TC, Cooke ID. Long-term follow-up of patients with polycystic ovary syndrome after laparoscopic ovarian drilling. Endocrine and ultrasonographic outcomes. *Hum Reprod* 2002; 17: 851–857.

25. Pirwany I, Tulandi T. Laparoscopic treatment of polycystic ovaries: is it time to relinquish the procedure? *Fertil Steril* 2003; 80(2): 241–251.

26. Balen AH, Jacobs HS. A prospective study comparing unilateral and bilateral laparoscopic ovarian diathermy in women with the polycystic ovary syndrome. *Fertil Steril* 1994; 62: 921–925.

27. Kucuk M, Kilic-Okman T. Hormone profiles and clinical outcome after laparoscopic ovarian drilling in women with polycystic ovary syndrome. *Med Sci Monit* 2005; 11(1): CR29–34.

28. Tulandi T, Saleh A, Morris D, Jacobs HS, Payne NN, Tan SL. Effects of laparoscopic ovarian drilling on serum vascular endothelial growth factor and on insulin responses to the oral glucose tolerance test in women with polycystic ovary syndrome. *Fertil Steril* 2000; 74(3): 585–588.

29. Amin AF, Abd el-Aal DE, Darwish AM, Meki AR. Evaluation of the impact of laparoscopic ovarian drilling on Doppler indices of ovarian stromal blood flow, serum vascular endothelial growth factor, and insulin-like growth factor-1 in women with polycystic ovary syndrome. *Fertil Steril* 2003; 79(4): 938–941.

30. Saleh A, Morris D, Tan SL, Tulandi T. Effects of laparoscopic ovarian drilling on adrenal steroids in polycystic ovary syndrome patients with and without hyperinsulinemia. *Fertil Steril* 2001; 75(3): 501–504.

31. Li TC, Saravelos H, Chow MS, Chisabingo R, Cooke ID. Factors affecting the outcome of laparoscopic ovarian drilling for polycystic ovarian syndrome in women with anovulatory infertility. *Br J Obstet Gynaecol* 1998; 105(3): 338–344.

32. Greenblatt E. Surgical options in polycystic ovary syndrome patients who do not respond to medical ovulation induction. *Baillieres Clin Obstet Gynaecol* 1993; 7(2): 421–433.

33. Kaya H, Sezik M, Ozkaya O. Evaluation of a new surgical approach for the treatment of clomiphene citrate-resistant infertility in polycystic ovary syndrome: laparoscopic ovarian multi-needle intervention. *J Minim Invasive Gynecol* 2005; 12(4): 355–358.

34. Ferraretti AP, Gianaroli L, Magli MC, Iammarrone E, Feliciani E, Fortini D. Transvaginal ovarian drilling: a new surgical treatment for improving the clinical outcome of assisted reproductive technologies in patients with polycystic ovary syndrome. *Fertil Steril* 2001; 76(4): 812–816.

Pregnancy and PCOS

44

Are Women with Polycystic Ovary Syndrome at an Increased Risk of Pregnancy-Induced Hypertension and/or Pre-eclampsia?

Socorro Benavides, Alfonso Nájar Gutiérrez, Alfonso Javier Gutiérrez

Summary

Polycystic Ovary Syndrome (PCOS) is a common condition characterized by menstrual abnormalities and clinical or biochemical features of hyperandrogenism. Features of PCOS may manifest at any age, ranging from childhood (premature puberty), teenage years (hirsutism, menstrual abnormalities), middle life (infertility, glucose intolerance) to later life (diabetes mellitus and cardiovascular diseases). Androgen excess and insulin resistance are common in women with PCOS. Insulin resistance (IR) and compensatory hyperinsulinemia appear to impart an increased risk of glucose intolerance, and lipid abnormalities that are recognized not only in patients with type 2 diabetes mellitus, but also in patients with essential hypertension, hyperlipidemia, and obesity. These risks are known as the components of metabolic syndrome and their accumulation, increases the risk of developing macrovascular disease, and cardiovascular diseases that are present in some patients with PCOS.[1]

On the other hand, hypertensive disorders of pregnancy affect approximately 3–8% of pregnancies and are a major cause of maternal, fetal and neonatal morbidity and mortality. Despite the frequency of these disorders, their cause is unknown. In the present chapter, we review the risk factors present in PCOS, that increase the risk of developing pregnancy-induced hypertension and/or pre-eclampsia.

Rationale

Although the literature directly linking PCOS with pre-eclampsia or pregnancy induced hypertension is scarce, there is a clear correlation between PCOS and several conditions, such as obesity and insulin resistance, which are known to increase the risk of cardiovascular disease, particularly during pregnancy. In this chapter, we will cover the subject of these conditions as they relate to PCOS and pre-eclampsia.

Introduction

The first recognition of an association between glucose intolerance and hyperandrogenism was made by Achard and Thiers in 1921 and was called the 'diabetes of bearded women'. The association between increased insulin resistance and PCOS is now well recognized.

Polycystic ovary syndrome remains one of the most common hormonal disorders in women, with an estimated prevalence between 5–10%.[2,3]

The polycystic ovary syndrome, has multiple components: reproductive, metabolic, and cardiovascular, with health implications in women affected with it.[4] The consequences of PCOS extend beyond the reproductive axis; women with the disorder are at a substantial risk for developing metabolic and cardiovascular abnormalities similar to those that make up the metabolic syndrome.[5]

The metabolic syndrome is one of the major public-health challenges worldwide,[6] and is closely related with both, type 2 diabetes and cardiovascular disease (CVD). These factors have been known for more than 80 years. In 1988, Reaven described 'Syndrome X': insulin resistance, hyperglycemia, hypertension, low high density lipoprotein (HDL)-cholesterol, and raised VLDL-triglycerides.[7] Surprisingly, he omitted obesity, now seen by many as an essential component (visceral obesity).[6] Reaven proposed that insulin resistance played a causative role. Both, PCOS and the metabolic syndrome share insulin resistance as a central pathogenic feature, and are viewed as a sex-specific form of the metabolic syndrome, called "Syndrome XX".[8] There is a considerable overlap between PCOS and the metabolic syndrome; 46% of women with PCOS also have metabolic syndrome, compared with 23% in the general female population above the age of 20 years.[5]

The idea of fetal programming has been linked to the development of CVD.[9] Interestingly, a link between low birth weight and PCOS has been found in precocious puberty. Young girls with precocious puberty are at an increased risk of developing PCOS, particularly if they had low birth weight. It has been proposed that this is the result of *in utero* fetal adaptation to undernutrition, resulting in permanent metabolic changes. The malnourished newborn is prone to develop obesity, IR, and type-2 diabetes. Weight gains can be rapid during adrenarche at 8-9 years of age associated with premature pubarche. An early biochemical lesion is low in HDL levels with a rise in triglyceride levels when approaching puberty, after which hypertension becomes more common.

Young women with PCOS generally have blood pressure within the normal range.[10] However, they have an increased prevalence of labile day-time blood pressure, which might predispose them to sustained hypertension later in life.[11] Adolescents with PCOS fail to exhibit the fall in blood pressure that usually occurs at night, which is regarded as an early risk factor for developing hypertension.[12]

Hypertension develops in some women with PCOS during their reproductive years,[5,10] and sustained hypertension may develop in later life in women with the disorder.[13] Reduced vascular compliance[14] and vascular endothelial dysfunction were noted in most,[13,14] but not all,[15] studies of women with PCOS. Furthermore, the degree of impairment in vascular reactivity is significantly greater than can be explained by obesity alone.[13]

The association of essential hypertension with insulin resistance and hyperinsulinemia has been well described.[16,17] However, it was not until recent years that more widespread interest developed in the possible role of insulin resistance in the pathogenesis of pregnancy-induced hypertension (PIH).

Around the time of the menopause, women with PCOS are 2.5 times more likely to have hypertension than their age-matched controls, which has been attributed to their associated obesity.[18]

Clinical Discussion

As different etiologies may lead to the same phenotype in different women, we focus on the potential role of insulin resistance and associated abnormalities as pathogenic factors for the development of PIH. Insulin resistance and elevated androgens provide a plausible link between PIH and PCOS.

Insulin is the most potent anabolic hormone known and is essential for appropriate tissue development, growth, and maintenance of whole-body glucose homeostasis. This hormone is secreted by the β cells of the pancreatic islets of Langerhans in response to increased circulating levels of glucose and amino acids after a meal.

Insulin regulates glucose homeostasis at many sites, reducing hepatic glucose output (via decreased gluconeogenesis and glycogenolysis) and increasing the rate of glucose uptake, primarily into striated muscle and adipose tissue. In muscle and fat cells, the clearance of circulating glucose depends on the insulin-stimulated translocation of glucose transporter GLUT 4 isoform to the cell surface[19] and the essential phosphoinositol 3-kinase (PI3) activation. Insulin also profoundly affects lipid metabolism, increasing lipid synthesis in liver and fat cells, and attenuating fatty acid release from triglycerides in fat and muscle. Insulin resistance occurs when normal circulating concentrations of the hormone are insufficient to regulate these processes appropriately. Thus by definition, insulin resistance is a defect in signal transduction.

It must be considered that there may be no single or common defect that underlies peripheral insulin resistance. Insulin resistance is most likely, a complex phenomenon with several genetic defects combined with environmental stresses, such as obesity and infections, to generate the phenotype.

The cause (s) of PIH are uncertain and include immune, genetic, and placental abnormalities. All may contribute to endothelial dysfunction characteristic of pre-eclampsia.

Insulin resistance and normal pregnancy

In normal pregnancy, plasma volume increases by 40%,[20] associated with a reduction in peripheral vascular resistance (40 to 80%), and a rise in cardiac output, renal blood flow, and glomerular filtration rate.[21] The renin-angiotensin-aldosterone system is activated despite the increase in plasma volume.[22] This activation is believed to be related to prostanoids, for example, prostacyclin and prostaglandin E_2, direct effects of estrogen, or an antinatruretic action of progesterone.

Blood pressure generally falls in the first and second trimesters therefore, women with high blood pressure before the 20th week of gestation are assumed to have pre-existing hypertension.

The frequency of superimposed pre-eclampsia is between 15 and 25%, increasing maternal and fetal risk.

Insulin resistance and hyperinsulinemia are characteristic of normal pregnancies, are maximal in the third trimester, and rapidly return to normal after delivery. This is probably mediated by several hormonal changes, including elevation in levels of human placental lactogen, progesterone, cortisol, and estradiol. The basis of the insulin resistance seen in normal pregnancy is not well understood. Increased risk for pre-eclampsia and/or gestational hypertension has been reported in several conditions associated with insulin resistance. These include gestational diabetes, polycystic ovary syndrome, obesity and increased weight gain.[3] Both, PCOS and metabolic syndrome have been associated with an increased risk of cardiovascular disease.[23,24] and both have hypertension, dyslipidemia, elevated serum glucose and central obesity in common. Insulin resistance is secondary to abnormalities in the insulin receptor, which may then result in a breakdown in the glucose homeostasis mechanism.

Etiology

The cause(s) of PIH are uncertain and include immune, genetic, and placental abnormalities. All may contribute to endothelial dysfunction characteristic of pre-eclampsia. Hypertension during pregnancy can be classified into two main groups: women who are hypertensive when they become pregnant, and those who are hypertensive for the first time in the second half of pregnancy. (Table 44.1)

Current hypotheses include: inflammatory disease, vascular-mediated factors, placental ischemia, genetic predisposition, immunologic derangements (a maternal immune reaction to a paternal antigen in the placenta), increased insulin resistance (associated elevations in the levels of insulin, free fatty acids, and triglycerides), dietary calcium deficiency, increased oxidative stress, and prostaglandin imbalance (an increased ratio of thromboxane to prostacyclin levels).

Table 44.1 Classification is based on the National High Blood Pressure Education Working Group Report on High Blood Pressure in Pregnancy.

New onset in pregnancy (after 20 week of gestation in a previously normotensive woman):

1. Preeclampsia: blood pressure of at least 140 mm Hg systolic or 90 mm Hg diastolic, with urine protein al least 300 mg in 24 hrs.
2. Gestational hypertension: Blood pressure at least 140 mm Hg systolic or 90 mm Hg diastolic, without proteinuria or other signs of pre-eclampsia.
3. Pre-existing hypertension:
   a Without exacerbation
   b with superimposed pre-eclampsia.

Pre-eclampsia is likely to be multifactorial in origin, and characteristics of the mother and the placenta may interact to lead to its development.

Pathophysiology

Pre-eclampsia typically manifests in the third trimester of a first pregnancy and resolves in the immediate puerperium. Rarely do "early" (< 20 weeks gestation) forms of the disorder occur. It is multisystemic, primarily affecting the vasculature, kidneys, liver and brain. Pre-eclampsia is diagnosed in a woman with new onset of hypertension (> 140/90 mmHg), usually after gestational week 20 accompanied by proteinuria 300 mg/dL. Other common clinical and laboratory manifestations include facial and distal extremity edema, hemoconcentration, thrombocytopenia, hypoalbuminemia, elevated uric acid levels, liver enzyme abnormalities and hypocalciuria. The diagnosis is more difficult in women with preexisting chronic hypertension, but it is prudent to consider "superimposed pre-eclampsia" when systolic or diastolic blood pressure (BP) levels increase more than 30 and 15 mmHg respectively, proteinuria > 300 mg/dL appears and protein excretion increases dramatically. Pre-eclampsia may progress to a life-threatening convulsive phase called *eclampsia*, when there is evidence of "HELLP" syndrome (hemolysis, elevated liver function test and low platelets).[25]

Polycystic ovary syndrome, which is associated with insulin resistance, elevated testosterone, and low SHBG levels, has been linked to an increased risk for pregnancy-induced hypertension even in the absence of associated obesity. Elevated androgen levels may be explained, at least in part, by increases in inhibin A,[26] which have also been described in women with pre-eclampsia. Elevated testosterone levels were found 17 years after pre-eclamptic pregnancy, suggesting that endothelial dysfunction in pre-eclampsia is an underlying characteristic of affected women.[27]

Evaluation of long likelihood ratios in multivariable modeling indicates that first trimester SHBG has the strongest association with future gestational diabetes. Owing to its sensitivity and positive predictive value, SHBG may be a useful marker in the evaluation for the prediction of gestational diabetes mellitus (GDM).

The presence of hyperinsulinemia in non-pregnant women, years after a diagnosis of pre-eclampsia, indicates that these women may be at increased risk, although the observed association between insulin resistance and PIH *does not prove a causal relation*. This observation nonetheless, raises the possibility of potential preventive strategies before and during pregnancy. Management of obesity and excessive weight gain before pregnancy (risk of GDM and macrosomia), are among potential measures to decrease the risk of PIH. Excessive weight gain during pregnancy is another risk factor for pregnancy-induced hypertension. The recommendations we make in the diagnosis of patients with PCOS before pregnancy are presented in Table 44.2.

Lipids

Abnormal lipid profiles have been demonstrated in adolecents with PCOS.[28] In these teenagers, elevated triglycerides and low high density lipoproteins (HDL) are more consistently observed in obese PCOS patients.[28] Often, the only abnormality in lean PCOS women is a reduced HDL-2 a sub-fraction of HDL.

Although, low density lipoprotein (LDL) levels are often only modestly elevated in PCOS, the

Table 44.2 Mnemonic Table listing the steps that can be carried out in order to avoid pregnancy complications in women with PCOS.

PCOS is confirmed with any 2 of the following 3 disorders: Oligomenorrhea or amenorrhea, hyperandrogenism (hirsutism, acne, alopecia) or hyperandrogenemia (elevated levels of total or free testosterone). PCOS on ultrasonography.

Risk factors are: increased body weight, (particularly if body fat is distributed in an android pattern), history of gestational diabetes type 2 diabetes in a first-degree relative, and Caribbean-Hispanic, Mexican American or African-American heritage.

Early recognition of insulin resistance provides a unique opportunity to prevent or delay development of type 2 diabetes and the sequelae of CVDs.

Vascular disease in PCOS is higher if hypertriglyceridemia, increased levels of VLDL, LDL-C, cholesterol and decreased levels of HDL-C are present, with predisposition to macrovascular disease and thrombosis. PCOS and metabolic syndrome share insulin resistance as a central pathogenetic feature.

Exercise or physical activity, changes in diet, changes in life style, attenuate insulin resistance, ameliorate (but not necessarily normalize) many of the metabolic aberrations in women with PCOS.

Normal BMI (Body mass index): If women with PCOS are overweight and need fertility treatment such as, ovulation induction, this need must be deferred until the BMI is preferably less than 30 kg/m^2.

Treatment with metformin has been reported to improve miscarriage rates and reduce the incidence of gestational diabetes, SHBG and LH concentrations.

Increased adiposity, increased particularly visceral adiposity reflected by an increased waist circumference (> 35 inches or 88 cm) or waist-to-hip ratio has been associated with hyperandrogenemia, insulin resistance, glucose intolerance and dyslipidemia.

Obesity is a key factor in determining cardiovascular risk particularly in older PCOS women.

No smoking, in the Lipid Research Clinics Prevalence Study. Smoking ≤ 20 cigarettes/day was shown to decrease HDL-C levels by 11–14% in a dose-dependent manner.[47]

---

percentage of the more atherogenic small, dense LDL component (LDL III) is higher.[29] Insulin

and body fat distribution play an important role in regulating lipid levels.[30]

In women with established pre-eclampsia, cholesterol, triglycerides,[28] and free fatty acid levels have been reported to be higher and HDL-C levels lower.[24] A potential mechanism through which hyperlipidemia may predispose to hypertension is by altering the prostaglandin balance and causing vasoconstriction.

Alterations in blood vessel function

Decreased antioxidant capacity has been demonstrated in women with PCOS and oxidative stress has been implicated in the pathogenesis of atherosclerosis.[31]

Coagulopathy is a feature of the metabolic syndrome with reduced fibrinolysis, increased plasma viscosity and platelet dysfunction being observed in women with PCOS. The long term increase in risk of CVD with PCOS may arise as a result of changes in blood vessel physiology or abnormal coagulation.[32]

Obesity

Obesity is defined as a body mass index (BMI) ≥ 30.4 kg/m^2, but we must also consider the body fat distribution. Visceral fat deposition is associated more closely with dyslipidemia and hyperinsulinemia than subcutaneous fat. Around 50% of patients with PCOS are obese. 70% of lean PCOS women have this pattern of fat deposition, and have been found to be hyperinsulinemic with reduced serum HDL levels compared to normal women,[33] the obese patient being at a higher risk.

Weight loss in obese or overweight women with PCOS prior to conception, may be the most effective primary intervention for short and long term health (reduced risk of diabetes and impaired glucose tolerance, increased regularity of ovulatory cycles and spontaneous conception, improved hirsutism and reduced early pregnancy loss).

The Metabolic Syndrome and PCOS

The metabolic syndrome is diagnosed when three

or more of the following criteria according to the National Institutes for Health (NIH) are present: (a) fasting serum triglycerides ≥ 1.70 mmol/l; (b) high-density lipoprotein (HDL)-cholesterol < 1.30 mmol/l; blood pressure ≥ 130/85 mmHg; (c) serum glucose ≥ 6.0 mmol/l or (d) waist circumference > 88 cm.[34]

Recently, the International Diabetes Federation has redefined the concept of metabolic syndrome (MS). The new concept will help identify people at increased risk (for more information see reference.[35]) The consensus group also recommended additional criteria including, tomographic assessment of visceral adiposity and liver fat, biomarkers for adipose tissue (adiponectin, leptin), apolipoprotein B, LDL particle size, formal measurement of insulin resistance and an oral glucose-tolerance test, endothelial dysfunction, urinary albumin, inflammatory markers (C-reactive protein, tumour necrosis α, interleukin 6), and thrombotic markers (plasminogen activator-inhibitor type 1, fibirinogen), that should be a part of further research into the metabolic syndrome. These factors should be combined with assessment of CVD outcome and development of diabetes (Table 44.3). Researchers and clinicians should use the new criteria for the identification of high- risk individuals and for research studies.

Treatment

It is not clear if PCOS represents an independent risk factor for CVD other than that of the metabolic syndrome. The identification and treatment of the features that these two conditions have in common (hypertension, dyslipidemia, elevated serum glucose, hyperinsulinemia and central obesity), have been shown to reduce the risk. The diagnosis of PCOS during adolescence provides an excellent opportunity to begin the primary intervention. (See Questions and Table 44.2)

Strategies to improve sensitivity to insulin are required, for example diet, exercise and the use of insulin-sensitizing drugs, such as metformin and the thiazolidinediones.

Table 44.3   Features metabolic syndrome and PCOS, associated with Pre-eclampsia

Biomarkers	Metabolic syndrome	PCOS
1. Hypertension	+	+ or −
2. Hyperinsulinemia	+	+ or −
3. Glucose Intolerance	+	+ or −
4. Central Obesity	+	+ or −
5. Lipid abnormalities		
a ↑ tryglycerides	+	+ or −
b ↓ HDL	+	+ or −
c ↑ LDL	+	+ or −
6. ↑ Leptin	+ or −	+ or −
7. ↑ TNF α	+ or −	+ or −
8. ↑ PAI-1 and ↑ TPA Ag	+ or −	+ or −
9. ↑ testosterone	+ or −	+
10. ↓ SHBG	+ or −	+
11. Family history of DM.	+ or −	+ or−

Abbreviations: HDL = High density lipoprotein; LDL = low density lipoprotein; TNF α = Tumor necrosis factor α; TPA Ag = tissue plasminogen activator antigen; PAI-1 = plasminogen activator-inhibitor-1 SHBG = sex hormone binding globulin. DM = Diabetes Mellitus
PAI-1 = plasminogen activator-inhibitor-1 may reflect impaired fibrinolysis, which might predispose to the coagulopathy associated with pre-eclampsia; PAI − 2, primarily produced by the placenta, is increased before the development of disease. TPA Ag: higher levels and elevations are proportional to the magnitude of proteinuria. TNF α levels, in the early third trimester, may predict the development of pre-eclampsia. CRP is not predictive of pre-eclampsia. SHBG: lower levels are predictive of the development of pre-eclampsia.

Case studies

Due to the heterogeneity of the clinical manifestations of PCOS, the diagnosis of this condition is carried out when the patient seeks help in achieving a pregnancy. Frequently, the patient is treated with low complexity schemes for induction of ovulation, without being studied thoroughly. The following is a sample case study.

Case Study 1

A 32-year old patient presented with a maternal family history of diabetes mellitus type 2, positive tobacco use, and a diagnosis of PCOS. Pregnancy was achieved by a private practice physician with the use of clomiphene citrate. The patient's BMI was 30 kg/m^2 prior to conception, with an irregular follow up during the pregnancy.

The first visit to the emergency ward was made at 33 weeks of pregnancy according to a reliable last menstrual period (LMP), and a syndrome characterized by cephalea, scotomata and edema of inferior extremities. During the examination, the patient had a BP of 150/120 mmHg, was conscious, well hydrated but disoriented. Her fundal height was 28 cm and fetal heart rate (FHR) was 148 beats/min. There was no uterine activity. Vaginal examination revealed a formed posterior cervix with a 2 cm dilation, intact membranes, with cephalic presentation. Edema level of the lower extremities was +++ and deep tendon reflexes (DTR) were +++.

The emergency lab results were as follows: Hb 15.8 g/dl, haematocrit 44.7%, platelets 118 000 prothrombin time (PT):14.3/12 sec, partial thromboplastin time: (PTT) 36/33sec, creatinine: 1.07 mg/dl, uric acid: 8.9 mg /dl, total bilirubin: 0.65 mg /dl (indirect 0.4 mg /dl, direct 0.23 mg / dl), lactate dehydrogenase (LDH): 485 U/L, aspartate aminotransferase (AST): 90 U/L, alanine aminotransferase (ALT): 37U/L, electrolytes: (Na: 138 mEq/L; Cl mEq/L: 107; K: 4.6 mEq/L; Ca: 10.20 mEq/L; Mg: 3.29 mEq/L).

Urine dipstier was diagnosed with more than 30 mg of protein. At the emergency room, she was diagnosed with severe PIH-HELLP. The recommended treatment was parenteral hydration and single dose of 30 mg oral hydrazine, and transfer to the intensive care unit (ICU).

At the ICU, an antihypertensive treatment was recommended with oral alfamethyldopa (AMD), 500 mg every 8 hours, and hydralazine 50 mg every 6 hours, Magnesium sulfate (MgSO4) 4 g, I. V. loading dose followed by 1 g/h for 24 hrs. Dexamethasone 16 mg I.V. and 40% dextran 300 ml was given every three hours. Monitoring for the BP curve, hourly diuresis (by a Foley probe) and CVP was performed.

Evolution: At 12 hours, the patient was drowsy, with intermittent cephalea without other signs of vasospasms. BP was 130/80 to 85 mmHg, normal PCV, 80 ml/h diuresis, FHR 142 beats/min, exalted DTR +. It was decided to end the pregnancy by cesarean section.

A female baby weighing 2,175 gms with an APGAR score 7 and 8 was delivered and transferred to intermediate care nursery. Her subsequent evolution was satisfactory.

The patient was returned to the ICU with an estimated blood loss of 500 ml and the double hypertensive treatment with MgSO4 and dexamethasone was continued. Her evolution was satisfactory; she was discharged from the ICU after 2 days, and stayed in a regular room.

Recently, the Norway group, conducted a prospective cohort study comprising of 29 non-insulin-resistant PCOS women, 23 insulin resistant PCOS women and a control group of 355 women who had conceived after assisted reproduction. The frequency of hypertension was significantly elevated in PCOS women (11.5%) compared to controls (0.3%), P< 0.01. However, the frequency of pre-eclampsia was significantly elevated only in the insulin resistant PCOS women (13.5%) compared to controls (7.0%), p < 0.02, and GDM was significantly more frequent in PCOS women than controls.[34]

Fridstrom et al.[37] reported a trend for higher blood pressure in PCOS women in the third trimester and during labor. However, the PCOS women did not have their insulin sensitivity tested.

Endothelial dysfunction is an early abnormality in insulin-resistant states that might contribute to premature atherosclerosis. Sub-clinical chronic low-grade inflammation might be an important factor in the pathogenesis of insulin resistance and type 2 diabetes.[38] C-reactive protein (CRP) promotes atherosclerotic processes and endothelial cell inflammation. Population studies show a strong correlation between proinflammatory biomarkers (such as CRP, interleukin 6, and TNF α) and perturbations in glucose homeostasis, obesity and atherosclerosis.

CRP levels may be independently related to the degree of insulin resistance, independent of obesity.

Several prospective epidemiological studies have tested the hypothesis that the circulating insulin concentrations are a cardiovascular risk factor.[39] None of these studies, however, distinguished between insulin and insulin resistance as the possible atherogenic factor. It might be the other way around – that the insulin resistance itself, by the production of pro-inflammatory cytokines, induces atherogenesis, and that, hyperinsulinemia could be the body's compensatory attempt to suppress the inflammation and overcome insulin resistance.[40] Eventually, however, the total amount of insulin secreted by the pancreas is also decreased after several years of insulin resistance-i.e., beta cells become exhausted implying that, the eventually prevailing insulin concentration will not be sufficient to counter the overwhelmingly strong insulin resistance.

Recent Advances

The protein product of the ob gene (obesity mice) named Leptine ("leptos" meaning thin), is produced by differentiated adipocytes, although production has been demonstrated in other tissues, such as the fundus of stomach, the skeletal muscle, the liver, and the placenta.[41] Leptin acts on the central nervous system, in particular, the hypothalamus, suppressing food intake and stimulating energy expenditure.[42]

Leptin, a satiety hormone, regulates appetite and energy balance of the body. Adiponectin could suppress the development of atherosclerosis and liver fibrosis, and might play a role as an anti-inflammatory hormone. Increased resistin concentrations might cause insulin resistance and thus, could link obesity with type 2 diabetes. These hormones have important roles in energy homeostasis, glucose and lipid metabolism, reproduction, cardiovascular function, and immunity. They directly influence other organ systems, including the brain, liver and skeletal muscle, and are significantly regulated by the nutritional status. This newly discovered secretory function has extended the biological relevance of adipose tissue, which is no longer considered as only an energy storage site. The pathophysiology that links maternal obesity and pregnancy-induced hypertension is a subject of intensive research.[43,44] The main hypothesis involves an endothelial dysfunction caused by obesity, which predisposes the patient to pre-eclampsia. However, obesity is associated with increased insulin resistance, which is thought to play a critical role in the predisposition for pre-eclampsia as well.[45]

Non-pregnant obese adults have an increased secretion of leptin and resistin, as well as decreased secretion of adiponectin.[46] The changes in these hormone levels, are known to increase insulin resistance and atherosclerosis. Leptin is heavily secreted by the placenta during pregnancy, and increased leptin is thought to play a role in the pathophysiology of pre-eclampsia.[47]

In very recent study, Hendler and colleagues[48] compared adipokine levels between women with and without pre-eclampsia based on maternal BMI, normal weight, overweight and obese women. They concluded that the increase in adiponectin in normal weight women with pre-eclampsia may represent the normal physiologic feedback response. This mechanism may not function properly in the overweight and obese gravida with pre-eclampsia because of increased adiponectin and IR.[48]

Conclusions

The possibility that a young woman with PCOS who is asymptomatic, may progress to a PCOS patient with obesity, hyperandrogenism, hyperinsulinemia, altered menstrual cycle, and infertility, may be a function of time. It is important that PCOS patients be treated as soon as the diagnosis for PCOS is made.

Metabolic abnormalities and obesity have long been associated with the development of cardiovascular disease in the general population. These same outcomes are also associated with PCOS. An increased prevalence of hypertension, dyslipidemia, obesity and hyperinsulinemia, as well as changes in coagulation and blood vessel function, provide an explanation as to why women with PCOS are at an increased risk of developing cardiovascular disease over the years. The risk of CVD is uncertain at present, but two factors need to be borne in mind: the young age of the cohorts studied so far (~55 years) and the possibility that unknown factor(s) may be present in PCOS, which protect the heart in the face of other risk factors.

Although current practice does not recommend aggressive treatment of individuals who exhibit impaired fasting glucose (IFG), impaired glucose tolerance (IGT), or both, these high risk individuals represent an attractive target for slowing or reversing the progression to diabetes and reducing CVD too.

Lack of knowledge regarding the etiology of pre-eclampsia limits the understanding of the disorder, however, if the risk factors present in PCOS like impaired fasting glucose (IFG) or IGT are decreased, insulin resistance, obesity and lipid abnormalities, the morbidity and mortality of this disease may be decreased. With the application of modern technologies in molecular and cell biology, the cause of pre-eclampsia may be discovered in the first decade of this millennium.

References

1. Anand SS, Yi Q, Gerstein H, et al. Relationship of Metabolic syndrome and fibrinolytic dysfunction to cardiovascular disease. *Circulation* 2003; 108(4): 420–425.

2. Asuncion M, Calvo RM, San Millan JL, Sancho J, Avila S, Escobar-Monrreale HF. A prospective study of the prevalence of the polycystic ovary syndrome in unselected Caucasian women from Spain. *J Clin Endocrinol Metab* 2000; 85: 2434–2438.

3. Kauffman RP, Baker VM, DiMarino P, Gimpel T, Castracane VD. Polycystic ovarian syndrome an insulin resistance in white and Mexican American Women: a comparison of two distinct populations. *Am J Obstet Gynecol* 2002; 187: 1362–1369.

4. Radon PA, McMahon MJ, Meyer WR. Impaired glucose tolerance in pregnant women with polycystic ovary syndrome. *Obstet Gynecol Reprod Biol* 1999; 94: 194–197.

5. Gluek CJ, Papanna R, Wang P, Goldenberg N, Sieve-

Smith L. Incidence and treatment of metabolic syndrome in newly referred women with confirmed polycystic ovarian syndrome. *Metabolism* 2003; 52: 908–915.

6. Eckel RH, Grundy SM, Zimmet PZ. The metabolic syndrome. *Lancet* 2005; 365: 1415–1428.

7. Reaven G. Role of insulin resistance in human disease. *Diabetes* 1988; 37: 1595–1607.

8. Sam S, Dunaif A. Polycystic ovary syndrome: Syndrome XX? *Trends Endocrinol Metab* 2003; 14: 365–370.

9. Barker DJ, Clark PM. Fetal undernutrition and disease in later life. *Rev Reprod* 1997; 2(2): 105–112.

10. Zimmermann S, Phillips RA, Dunaif A, et al. Polycystic ovary syndrome lack of hypertension despite profound insulin resistance. *J Clin Endocrinol Metab* 1992; 75: 508–513.

11. Holte J, Gennarelli G, Berne C, Bergh T, Lithell H. Elevated ambulatory day-time blood pressure in women with polycystic ovary syndrome: a sign of a pre-hypertensive state? *Hum Reprod* 1996; 11(1): 23–28.

12. Arslanian SA, Lewy VD, Danadian K. Glucose intolerance in obese adolescents with polycystic ovary syndrome: role of insulin resistance and Beta-cell dysfunction and risk of cardiovascular disease. *J Clin Endocrinol Metab* 2001; 86: 66–71.

13 Kelly CJG, Speirs A, Gould GW, Petrie JR, Lyall H, Connell JMC. Altered vascular function in young women with polycystic ovary syndrome. *J Clin Endocrinol Metab* 2002; 87: 742–746.

14. Orio F Jr, Palomba S, Cascella T, et al. Early impairment of endothelial structure and function in young normal-weight women with polycystic ovary syndrome *J Clin Endocrinol Metab* 2004; 89: 4588–4593.

15. Mather KJ, Verma S, Corenblum B, Anderson TJ, Normal endothelial structure and function despite insulin resistance in healthy women with the polycystic ovary syndrome. *J Clin Endocrinol Metab* 2002; 87: 3871–3875.

16. The Rotterdam ESHRE/ASRM-sponsored PCOS consensus workshop group. Revised 2003 consensus on diagnostic criteria and long-therm health risks related to polycystic ovary syndrome (PCOS). *Human Reproduction* 2004; 19(1): 41–47.

17. American Diabetes Association: Position statement: Screening for diabetes. *Diabetes Care* 2005; 25 (suppl): S21–S24.

18. Elting MW, Karsen TJM, Bezemer PD, Shoemaker J. Prevalence of diabetes mellitus, hypertension and

cardiac complaints in a follow-up study of a Dutch PCOS population. *Hum Reprod* 2001; 16: 556–560.

19. Shulman, GI. Cellular mechanism of insulin resistance. *J Clin Invest* 2000; 106: 171–176.

20. De Swiet DS, Klein VR, Tyson JE, et al. Risk factors for the occurrence of pregnancy-induced hypertension, *Clin Exp Hypertens* 1987; B6: 281–287.

21. Chesley LC, Lindheimer MD. Renal hemodynamics and intravascular volume in normal and hypertensive pregnancy. Handbook of Hypertension, Amsterdam, *Elsevier* 1988; 10: 38–65.

22. Graves Sw, Moore TJ, Seely EW. Increased platelet angiotensin II receptor numbers in pregnancy-induced hypertension, *Hypertension* 1992; 20: 627–632.

23. National High Blood Pressure Education Program. Working group report on high blood pressure in pregnancy. 2000; Bethesda: NIH; NIH publication 00–3029.

24. Wild S, Pierpoint T, Mckeigue P, Jacobs H. Cardiovascular disease in women with polycystic ovary syndrome at long-term follow-up: a retrospective cohort study. *Clin Endocrinol* 2000; 52: 595–600.

25. Seely EW, Solomon CG. Insulin resistance and its potential role in pregnancy-induced hypertension. *J Clin Endocrinol Metab* 2003; 88: 2393–2398.

26. Muttukrishna S, Knight PG, Groome NP, Redman CW, Ledger WL. Activin A and inhibin A as a possible endocrine markers for preeclampsia *Lancet* 1997; 349: 1285–1288.

27. Urman B, Sarac E, Dogan L, Gurgan T. Pregnancy in infertile PCOS patients: complications and outcome. *J Reprod Med* 1997; 42: 501–505.

28. Silfen ME, Denburg MR, Manibo AM, et al. Early endocrine, metabolic and sonographic characteristics of polycystic ovary syndrome: comparison between nonobese an obese adolescents. *J Clin Endocrinol Metab* 2003; 88: 4682–4688.

29. Pirwany IR, Fleming R, Greer IA, Packard CJ, Sattar N. Lipids and lipoprotein subfractions in women with PCOS: relationship to metabolic and endocrine parameters. *Clin Endocrinol (Oxf)* 2001; 54(4): 447–453.

30. Ciampelli M, Fulghesu AM, Cucinelli F, Pavone V, Ronsisvalle E, Guido M, Caruso A, Lanzone A. Impact of insulin and body mass index on metabolic and endocrine variables in polycystic ovary syndrome. *Metabolism* 1999; 48(2): 167–172.

31. Fenkci V, Fenkci S, Yilmazer M, Serteser M. Decreased total antioxidant status and increased oxidative stress in women with polycystic ovary syndrome may contribute to the risk of cardiovascular disease. *Fert and Ster* 2003; 80: 123–127.

32. Paradisi G, Steinberg HO, Hempfling A, Cronin J, Hook G, Shepard MK, Baron AD. Polycystic ovary syndrome is associated with endothelial dysfunction. *Circulation* 2001; 103(10): 1410–1415.

33. Kirchengast S, Huber J. Body composition characteristics and body fat distribution in lean women with polycystic ovary syndrome. *Hum Reprod* 2001; 16: 1255–1260.

34. National Institute of Health, Third report of the national cholesterol education program export panel on detection, evaluation and treatment of high blood cholesterol in adults (adult treatment Panel III). Washington DC:NIH Publication, 2001; 01–3670.

35. International Diabetes Federation. The IDF consensus worldwide definition of the metabolic syndrome. 2005 april 14: http://www.idf.org/webdata/docs/Metab_syndrome_def. Pdf (accessed November 4, 2005.

36. Bjercke S, Dale PO, Tanbo T, Storeng R, Ertzeid G, Abyholm T. Impact of insulin resistance on pregnancy complications and outcome in women with polycystic ovary syndrome. *Gynecol Obstet Invest* 2002; 54(2): 94–98.

37. Fridstrom M, Nissell H, Sj´øblom P, Hillensj´ø T. Are women with polycystic ovary syndrome at an increased risk of pregnancy-induced hypertension and/or preeclampsia? *Hypert Pregn* 1999; 18: 73–80.

38. Fernandez-Real JM, Ricart W. Insulin resistance and chronic cardiovascular inflammatory syndrome. *Endoc Rev* 2003; 24: 278–301.

39. De Vries MJ, Dekker DA, Schoemaker J. Higher risk of pre-eclampsia in the polycystic ovary syndrome. A case control study. *Eur J Obstet Gynecol Reprod Biol* 1988; 76: 91–95.

40. Danona P, Aljada A, Bandyopadhyay A. Inflammation: the link between insulin resistance, obesity and diabetes. *Trends Immunol* 2004; 25: 4–7.

41. Baratta M. Leptin-from a signal of adiposity to a hormone mediator in peripheral tissues. *Med Sci Monit* 2002; 8: RA282–292.

42. Webber J. Energy balance in obesity. *Proc Nutr Soc* 2003; 62: 539–543.

43. Solomon CG, Seely EW. Hypertension in pregnancy: a manifestation of the insulin resistance syndrome? *Hypertension* 2001; 37: 147–152.

44. Engeli S, Negrel R, Sharma AM. Physiology and pathophysiology of the adipose tissue renin-

angiotensin system. *Hypertension* 2002; 40: 609–611.

45. Kaaja R, Laivuori H, Pulkki P, Tikkanen MJ, Hiilesmaa V, Ylikorkala O. Is there any link between insulin resistance and inflammation in established preeclampsia? *Metabolism* 2004; 53(11): 1433–1435.

46. Moller DE, Kaufman KD. Metabolic syndrome: a clinical and molecular perspective, *Annu Rev Med* 2005; 56: 45–62.

47. Poston L, Leptin and pre-eclampsia. *Semin Reprod Med* 2002; 20: 131–138.

48. Hendler I, Blackwell SC, Mehta SH, Whitty JE, Russell E, Sorokin Y, Cotton DB. The levels of leptin, adiponectin, and resistin in normal weight, overweight, and obese pregnant women with and without preeclampsia. *Am J Obstet Gynecol* 2005; 193(3 Pt 2): 9799–9783.

49. Criqui MH, Wallace RB, Heiss G, Mishkel M, Schonfeld G, Jones GT. Cigarette smoking and plasma high-density lipoprotein cholesterol. The Lipid Research Clinics Program Prevalence Study. *Circulation* 1980; 62 (4 Pt 2): IV70–6.

Frequently Asked Questions

1. Do therapeutic lifestyle changes improve the risk of coronary heart disease (CHD) in patients with PCOS?

Lifestyle changes include smoking cessation, weight loss, exercise and diet. The Lipid Research Clinics Prevalence Study[49] reported an inverse relationship between body mass index and HDL-C, and an increase in HDL-C of approximately 2 mg/dl for every 4.5 Kg weight reduction, and a direct relationship between exercise and HDL-C. Smoking was shown to decrease HDL-C.

2. What is the contraceptive of choice in a woman with PCOS in her reproductive age?

The best pharmacological treatment of proven effectiveness is a combination of the synthetic progestogen, cyproterone acetate with ethinyl estradiol. Cyproterone acetate is antigonadotropic and antiandrogenic, while estrogen increases the hepatic production of SHBG, resulting in lower free testosterone.

3. Weight loss in obese women with PCOS may be difficult. What are the treatments other than metformin that are useful?

The FDA-approved obesity drugs like Xenical (gastrointestinal lipase inhibitor) and Meridia, may soon be joined by a promising canabinoid receptor blocker named Accomplia (Rimonabat in Europe)

4. Should metformin be stopped immediately after pregnancy is diagnosed?

There is presently no evidence to suggest that metformin is teratogenic. On the contrary, metformin has been reported to reduce miscarriage rates and reduce the incidence of gestational diabetes.

5. Should a patient with eclampsia, with blood pressure at 200/120 mm Hg with evidence of a generalized seizure, first be given diazepam or MgSO₄?

The Eclampsia Trial established $MgSO_4$ as the most effective therapy for eclampsia, both to treat active seizures and to prevent further seizures. The regimen should be 4 g IV loading dose followed by 1g/h for 24 hours.

6. Compared to singleton pregnancies, what can be expected for women with twin gestations and hypertension?

Compared to singleton pregnancies, women with twin gestations have higher rates of gestational hypertension and pre-eclampsia.

7. A 34 year old G3 P2 at 6 weeks gestation presents for evaluation. She has a history of chronic hypertension that developed two years after her last pregnancy. She has been taking Enelapril 10 mg, PO daily. Her pre-pregnancy blood pressure measurements were 120–130/70–80 mmHg. She is otherwise, completely healthy. What would you advise be done about her antihypertensive medication

The Enalapril should be stopped and blood pressure followed to see whether or nor it rises.

8. How should hypertension in pregnancy be managed?

The initial aim of treatment should be to reduce the systolic blood pressure by approximately 10 mmHg in a controlled manner. This can be effectively achieved with oral Labetalol or Nifedipine. There is now some evidence to suggest that early treatment reduces the incidence of respiratory distress syndrome as well as hypertensive crisis in the mother. The use of ACE-inhibitors is not indicated during pregnancy.

9. In the assessment of severe pre-eclampsia, we recommend in the following considerations.

Uric acid is a better indicator of fetal morbidity than blood pressure. If the platelet count is greater than 100,000/mm³, there is no need to carryout coagulation screening, since it is unlikely to be abnormal. The urine stick testing tends to over-estimate the presence of proteinuria and this should be quantified by a 24-hour urine collection.

45

Long-term Consequences of Polycystic Ovary Syndrome

Alfonso Javier Nájar Gutiérrez, Landaverde Molina María Mercedes

Summary

Polycystic Ovary Syndrome (PCOS) is the most common endocrine disturbance affecting women of reproductive age and it is characterized by a broad complex spectrum of metabolic alterations, which include hypersecretion of luteinizing hormone (LH), elevated androgens, lack of progesterone (P) production, chronic hyperinsulinemia, decreased sex hormone-binding globulin (SHBG) and low insulin-like growth factor-binding protein-1 (IGFBP-1).

Increased risks for long-term events, including gynecological cancers, have been described for PCOS. Even though the mechanisms are not completely understood, hormones appear to play an important role in the development or promotion of some female malignancies. The principal mechanism by which hormones influence cancer risk is by their regulatory effects in maintaining the balance among cell proliferation, differentiation and apoptosis. Although PCOS combines most, if not all of the endocrine risks for endometrial cancer, the available scientific evidence does not support this association. Furthermore, epidemiological and clinical observations have implicated a variety of factors linking breast cancer or ovarian cancer to endocrine function. The few available data appear to exclude a strong association with PCOS. Further investigation is needed to clarify these possible relations. Genetic alterations in estrogen (E) metabolism must be evaluated as a risk factor for hormone-dependent malignant disorders.

Rationale

Cancer is a major public health problem in developed countries, because of a high incidence of death rates. In 2005, 211, 240 cases of breast cancer were diagnosed in the United States.[1] Breast cancer, which has the highest incidence among the different types of female cancers in the United States, alone is expected to account for 32% of all new cancer cases among women. Statistical estimates in 2005 have shown that breast cancer contributes to 15% of all deaths, ovarian cancer 6% and uterine corpus 3%, with a cumulative rate of 24% due to the reproductive tract.[1] In Mexico and Latin America, breast cancer is the second cause of the total cancer deaths, with a mortality rate of 11.7 per 100,000 women between 25 and 64 years.[2,3]

Polycystic ovary syndrome (PCOS) is a condition marked by chronic anovulation, hyperandrogenemia and infertility, and affects approximately 4–7% of women of reproductive age.[4] PCOS is a heterogeneous entity with variations in its clinical and endocrine presentation. It is characterized by aberrations in gonadotropin secretion, increased ovarian androgen biosynthesis, abnormalities in estrogen

(E) secretion and frequently insulin resistance. The presence of an abnormal hormonal milieu in women with PCOS may contribute to the increased risk for some tumors in this group of patients. Obesity, anovulation, infertility, and hormonal treatment for infertility are so frequent in PCOS that these conditions are difficult to isolate as an independent risk factor for developing some types of cancer. Because of hyperandrogenemia and chronic anovulation, women with PCOS may be followed more closely than women without them.

The use of fertility drugs (FDs) in women with ovulation disorders has held an important place in infertility treatment for 40 years. However, the use of drugs for ovulation induction in assisted conception is a different concept. Concerns about the long-term effects of FDs used with or without assisted reproduction regarding breast, ovarian and endometrial cancer, have been raised in both situations.

Introduction

During the last 30 years, it has become apparent that sex hormones can be linked to the development and promotion of genital cancers, hence the possible relationship between sex hormones and such malignancies has been studied.[4–6]

Originally described by Stein Leventhal in 1934, PCOS is nowadays a clinical entity recognized worldwide with variability in prevalence rates in women of reproductive age. This may be due to the use of different criteria for its diagnosis. It is well known that women with PCOS are at an increased risk for a number of adverse gynecological and reproductive outcomes.[7] These women suffer from hormonal disturbances and because of their infertility, most of them receive hormonal treatments, which alter their endogenous hormonal condition and receptors status. Hence, the possibility of an increased cancer risk among PCOS women, the possible link between cancer and infertility and the contribution of fertility treatments to an increased risk of tumors, or acceleration in the progression of the malignancy has been questioned.[4–6,8–11]

Despite several efforts to investigate the etiology of female reproductive cancer, it is not well understood. Clinical evidence shows that reproductive performance and hormones are believed to play a fundamentals role. According to several epidemiological studies, nulliparity has been demonstrated as a risk factor for carcinoma of the breast,[5] endometrium[4,5] and ovaries.[5] Additionally, an exogenous administration of E without opposed progesterone (P) promotes endometrial cancer development.[4,5,10,12] In the same way, a promoting role for E,[5] especially in conjunction with P,[4] has been proposed in the etiology of the breast cancer. Reports of ovarian cancer in women who have a undergone fertility treatments, question the potential neoplastic effects of ovulation-inducing drugs.[5,13,14] However, in PCOS women or infertile women, endogenous hormonal disturbances are already present prior to the use of fertility medications.

Clinical Discussion

Endometrial cancer

The risk factors for type I endometrial carcinoma, related to E exposure, include early menarche, late age at menopause, nulliparity, infertility, chronic anovulation, diabetes, hypertension, unopposed E replacement therapy, tamoxifen use, obesity and hirsutism.[4,6,8–10,12,14,15]

Polycystic ovary syndrome is the most common cause of anovulatory infertility, oligoamenorrhea, amenorrhea and hirsutism.[14,15] Most women are chronically amenorrheic or oligomenorrheic because of the lack of P effect to mediate ovulation. These prolonged anovulatory women are not E deficient, otherwise, the ovarian function necessary to transform androgens into estrogens (Es) and the peripheral conversion, would place them in a "state of mild hyperestrogenism",[7] which is a cause of constant stimulation of the uterine lining leading to endometrial hyperplasia or cancer. Hence, it is not surprising that a number of researchers have found that PCOS patients have a higher incidence of endometrial cancer.[15] This risk may be influenced by the presence of diabetes and obesity, both of which have been traditionally considered as independent risk factors for cancer of the endometrium.[4,6,9,10,12]

Since the first association between prolonged anovulation, chronic hyperestrogenism and endometrial cancer,[16] the mechanism has been elucidated. It has been described that the agonist-bound P receptor-A in human reproductive tissues, inhibits E-receptor mediated transcription activity by the E receptor. Exposure to unopposed E leads to increased mitotic activity of endometrial cells and increased number of DNA replication errors, thus enhancing the onset of a malignant phenotype.[4,5,10,12] Hypersecretion of LH, a characteristic feature of PCOS, has also been implicated. Receptors of LH and human chorionic gonadotropin (hCG) are over expressed in endometrial carcinomas.[15] There is also evidence that insulin and the insulin-like growth factor (IGF) system play a major role in the regulation of endometrial proliferation and in the pathogenesis of endometrial cancer.[4,10,12] Specific receptors for insulin and IGF as well as high affinity IGF-binding proteins (IGFBPs) have been detected in normal and carcinomatous endometrial tissue. Because insulin upregulates aromatase activity in endometrial glands and stroma, intrinsic E production is enhanced in PCOS patients with high circulating insulin levels.[4]

Polycystic ovary syndrome combines most, if not all of the endocrine risk factors for endometrial cancer: mild hyperestrogenism, chronic hyperinsulinemia,[12] increased IGF-1, low IGFBP-1, decreased sex-hormone binding globulin (SHBG), elevated androgens and lack of P production, among others.[4] The predominant theory describing the relationship between endogenous steroid hormones and endometrial malignancy risk is known as the *unopposed E hypothesis*. It is proposed that endometrial cancer risk is increased in women who have high bioavailable plasma levels of Es and/or low circulating P, such that the mitogenic effects of Es are insufficiently counterbalanced by P. Increased proliferation rates increase the probability that mutations accumulate in proto-oncogenes and tumor repressor genes. Proliferative stimuli may also enhance the established tumor growth.[4,6,10,12]

Chronic hyperinsulinemia is clearly another major risk factor for endometrial cancer. This could be explained by the action of insulin on at least two sites: first, on the endometrium, where it may stimulate tumor development by reducing levels of IGFBP-1 and consequently, increasing IGF-1 activity and may also promote tumor development through its own endometrial receptors, and second, in the ovary; chronic hyperinsulinemia contributes to the characteristic ovarian hyperandrogenism, associated with anovulation and P deficiency.[4,6,10,12]

The association between PCOS and endometrial cancer was first suggested in 1949,[16] but an early important study done by Dockerty and Jackson,[18] highlighted this association in 1957, showing a 37% prevalence of endometrial cancer in women with PCOS.[18] Available scientific evidence suggesting that PCOS significantly increases the risk of future endometrial cancer is not qualitative enough to support the link. Case reports and epidemiological reports have identified an association between endometrial malignancy and infertility, but when these infertile women are grouped according to the cause of infertility, anovulation is shown to be the main cause of increased endometrial malignancy risk in infertile patients.[5]

The differences in diagnostic criteria used in several studies for PCOS should be taken into account. Majority of the available evidence of an increased risk of endometrial cancer in PCOS women does not compare with general population, which seriously limits the application of these studies. The limited available evidence is based on case series, retrospective cohorts, cross sectional and case control studies as is shown in Table 45.1.[16–32] Unfortunately, because of the variable diagnostic criteria and studies with no suitable controls, it is impossible to do a meta-analysis to calculate a relative risk of endometrial cancer in women with PCOS.[4,15] Hence, the evidence for an increased risk of endometrial cancer in PCOS is incomplete and contradictory.[4,15]

Table 45.1   Studies reporting the possible association between polycystic ovary syndrome and endometrial carcinoma

Authors	Study Design	Description
Speert (1949)[16]	Case series	14 women < 40 years with EC 8 with cystic ovaries and 1 with sclerotic ovaries
Dockerty et al, (1951)[17]	Case series	36 women < 40 years with EC 14 had cystic ovaries
Dockerty and Jackson, (1957)[18]	Case series	Many thousand of endometrial cancer cases: 16 women with PCOS.
	Cross sectional	27 women with PCOS on biopsy: None had EC
Jafari et al, (1978)[19]	Case series	6 women with PCOS and EC (Average age 27.8 years)
Ramzy and Nisker (1979)[20]	Case-Control	15 ovaries from patients of EC, 25 from women with PCOS and 21 from controls. 11.1% of the ovaries from women with EC had features suggestive of PCOS
Coulam et al, (1983)[21]	Cohort	1270 women with chronic anovulation RR of EC 3.1 (95% CI 1.1–7.3)
Gallup and Stock, (1984)[22]	Case series	111 patients with EC. PCOS was present in 31.2% of women under 40 years old and 2.3% of older women
Dennefos et al, (1985)[23]	Case Report	A young woman with moderately differentiated EC and PCOS
Escobedo et al, (1991)[24]	Case-control	399 with EC and 3040 controls. OR for EC 4.2 for "ovarian factor" (95% CI 1.7–10.4)
Smyczek-Gargya and Geppert, (1992)[25]	Case Report	2 women with PCOS and EC (17 and 36 years old)
Chadli-Debbiche et al, (1993)[26]	Case Report	A 38 years old woman with PCOS and EC
Goluda and Andrzejewski, (1995)[27]	Case Report	A 40 years old woman with superficial, well-differentiated EC and PCOS
Gregorini (1997)[4]	Case Report	2 women < 40 years with EC and PCOS
Salha et al, (1997)[28]	Case Report	A young woman with PCOS and EC
Ho et al, (1997)[29]	Retrospective Cohort	116 women with endometrial hyperplasia with no increased prevalence of endometrial carcinoma in cases of PCOS
Pierpoint et al, (1998)[30]	Retrospective Cohort	786 women with PCOS Mortality from "miscellaneous cancers" not increased
Wild et al, (2000)[31]	Retrospective Cohort	319 women with PCOS and 3040 controls OR for EC 5.3
Kurabayashi et al, (2003)[32]	Case series	4 infertile women with PCOS associated with EC

EC, endometrial cancer; PCOS, polycystic ovary syndrome; RR, relative risk;CI, confidence interval; OR, odds ratio.

Breast cancer

Epidemiological and experimental evidence have demonstrated that the etiology of breast cancer is related to the lifetime cumulative exposure of the breast epithelium to Es and especially P. The observation that early menarche, late menopause and shorter time interval between age at menarche and age at which menstruation becomes regular, which are predictors of breast cancer, has suggested that chronic anovulation might be protective against breast cancer. Nevertheless, the association between PCOS and breast cancer has been variably reported. Studies consistent with a positive association between these conditions include reports of an increased prevalence of anovulatory endometrial hyperplasia and ovarian stromal hyperplasia, as well as increased testosterone levels among some, but not all series of women with breast cancer.[4,10]

Obesity, including central obesity, seems to increase the risk for postmenopausal breast cancer but not the premenopausal risk. This contrasting situation may be influenced by the differences in E synthesis and metabolism in both groups. The association between breast cancer risk and insulin resistance has not been well studied, but it has been suggested that obesity, elevated androgen levels and the increased levels of insulin and IGF-1, characteristic features of the PCOS, could promote the development of breast cancer through different mechanisms: decreased levels of SHBG and increased levels of free Es in hyperandrogenic women, direct mitogenic stimulation of cancer cells by insulin and IGF-I, aromatization of testosterone to estradiol with stimulation of E receptor-positive cells, and direct stimulation by binding of androgen to androgen-receptor-positive cancer cells.[4]

The overwhelming evidence from epidemiological data regarding the association between PCOS and breast cancer results is contradictory. These studies are summarized in Table 45.2. Further information and long- term prospective studies are needed to better establish the facts about this association.[4,6,10,21,30,31,33–35]

Table 45.2 Studies reporting the possible association between polycystic ovary syndrome and breast carcinoma

Authors	Study Design	Description
Coulam et al, (1983)[21]	Retrospective Cohort	1270 women with chronic anovulation versus population incidence rates RR associated with PCOS: Premenopausal: 1.3 (95% CI 0.3–3.2) Perimenopausal: 0.9 (95% CI 0.2–2.5) Postmenopausal 3.6 (95% CI 1.2–8.3)
Gammon and Thompson, (1991)[33]	Case-control	4730 breast cancer cases (23 PCOS) and 4688 controls (44 PCOS). 20–54 years old. OR (associated with PCOS): Age adjusted, 0.52 (95% CI 0.32–0.87) Multivariate, 0.47 (95% CI 0.26–0.85)
Anderson et al, (1997)[34]	Prospective Cohort (Iowa Women's health study)	472 women with PCOS, 55–69 years old at the study entry. RR (associated with PCOS): Age adjusted, 1.2 (95% CI 0.7–2.0) Multivariate, 1.0 (95% CI 0.6–1.9)
Pierpoint et al, (1998)[30]	Retrospective Cohort	SMR (calculated versus national rates) for 786 cases of PCOS. Mean 30 years for follow-up SMR (associated with PCOS): 1.48 (95% CI 0.79–2.54)
Wild et al, (2000)[31]	Retrospective Cohort	319 women with PCOS and 3040 controls Women with PCOS were not at significantly increased risk of mortality or morbidity from breast cancer
Atiomo et al, (2003)[35]	Case-control	41 women with PCOS and 66 controls Statistically significant positive family history of breast cancer in women with PCOS

RR, relative risk; PCOS, polycystic ovary syndrome; OR, odds ratio; CI, confidence interval; SMR, standardized mortality ratio.

Ovarian cancer

The actual etiology of ovarian cancer is still unknown. Most studies have established risk factors according to the reproductive performance. Parity and a long duration of oral contraceptive use have been described as protective. Several hypotheses have been proposed to explain the epidemiology of epithelial ovarian cancer. Firstly, according to the "incessant ovulation" hypothesis, ovarian cancer might be promoted by repeated ovulations disrupting the ovarian epithelium, leading to malignant transformation of the epithelial cells. Secondly, persistent stimulation of the ovary by gonadotropins increases the risk of malignant changes. Thirdly, exposure of the ovarian epithelium to environmental agents may have possible carcinogenic effect. Fourthly, according to the "endometriosis hypothesis", endometriosis implants may act to promote irritation, inflammatory reaction and development of ovarian cancer. Finally, the ovarian cancer risk may be increased by factors associated with excessive androgenic stimulation of ovarian epithelial cells and may be decreased by factors related to greater P stimulation.[8]

Though, the etiology of ovarian cancers is not clear, the abnormal hormonal milieu of PCOS might predispose towards ovarian malignancies.

Gonadotropins, Es and androgens have been demonstrated, *in vitro*, to promote the proliferation of normal and malignant human ovarian cells. Receptors for LH have been found in tumor epithelial cells, suggesting that serum LH may have direct influence on tumor growth. Es may participate in promoting ovarian malignancies by the prevention of apoptosis through Bcl-2 up-regulation. Androgens might also be related to ovarian carcinogenesis. *In vitro*, proliferation of normal human ovarian epithelial cells is more effective with 5α- dihydrotestosterone than with testosterone; in animal models, both androgens promote growth in ovarian cancer cell lines. Androgens may promote carcinogenesis by decreasing the transforming growth factor-β (TGF-β) levels, thus leading to an escape in the growth inhibition mediated by TGF-β_1.[4,8]

Although the epidemiological findings have been considered in the context of the proposed etiological hypotheses, there are methodological problems in the available scientific evidence. Some studies have suggested increased ovarian cancer risk in PCOS patients and others have found no increase in such risk. Few studies have been done to evaluate this association and the available ones are summarized in Table 45.3.[4,21,30,35–37]

Table 45.3   Studies reporting possible association between Polycystic Ovarian Syndrome and ovarian carcinoma

Authors	Study Design	Description
Coulam et al, (1983)[21]	Retrospective Cohort	1270 women with chronic anovulation versus population incidence rates No increased risk. Only one case in 14,499 women-years of follow up
Resta et al, (1993)[36]	Cross sectional	200 hysterectomy and bilateral salpingo-oophorectomy specimens High frequency of hyperplastic and metaplastic changes in the surface epithelium or in the inclusion cysts of patients with polycystic ovary disease
Schildkraut et al, (1996)[37]	Case-control	PCOS patients: 7 cases with ovarian cancer and 24 patients controls OR 2.5 (95% CI 1.1–5.9) Multivariate, OR 2.4 (95% CI1.0–5.9)
Pierpoint et al, (1998)[30]	Retrospective Cohort	786 women with PCOS SMR (associated with PCOS): 0.39 (95% 0.01–2.17)
Atiomo et al, (2003)[35]	Case-control	41 women with PCOS and 66 controls

Statistically no significant positive family history of ovarian cancer in women with PCOS
PCOS, polycystic ovary syndrome; OR, odds ratio; SMR, standardized mortality ratio.

Fertility drugs and cancer

The use of ovulation–inducing drugs in the treatment of infertility is increasing according to the absolute number of women who report some form of infertility. Attention has been focused on the possible association between the use of fertility drugs (FDs) and the development or promotion of cancer of the ovaries, endometrium, and breast. It is surprising that though assisted reproductive technology has advanced with a higher use of FDs, the long-term effects of FDs on the female reproductive system have not been studied properly.[8,10,11]

Since hormonal and reproductive factors are known to be involved in the etiology of female reproductive cancers, an effect of the ovulation-inducing drugs on the risks of these cancers is theoretically possible. There are presently three lines of evidence concerning the potential effects of ovulation-inducing drugs on cancer risk. First, the most commonly used drugs are effective for stimulating ovulation and the elevated levels of estradiol related to the doses of these drugs, that are not observed in a regular cycle, is a factor implicated in the etiology of both, breast and ovarian cancer. Second, these drugs increase both E and P levels, hormones which are recognized for their roles in the development or growth of gynecologic cancers. Finally, the clinical and epidemiological evidence have linked the use of FDs with an increased number of various cancers.[11]

Fertility drugs are used primarily during the follicular phase of the menstrual cycle to increase the serum concentrations of gonadotropins to promote follicle maturation and ovulation. The most commonly used FDs include: (a) anti-estrogens, such as clomiphene citrate (CC), a selective E receptor modulator; (b) human menopausal gonadotropins (hMG), a combination of follicle stimulating hormone (FSH) and luteinizing hormone (LH); (c) human chorionic gonadotropin (hCG); (d) gonadotrophin releasing hormone analogues (GnRH-a) and (e) progestogens for luteal support.[8]

The available scientific evidence suggests a link between FDs and the risk of gynecologic cancers, but the absence of comparison groups (control groups) in clinical studies, limits the application of the possible conclusions. The better existing evidence is based on analytic studies that rely on both retrospective and prospective cohorts. In most studies, the standardized incidence ratio (SIR) is used to compare the disease experience of infertile women with that in the general population. SIR compares the number of observed cancers in the cohort of interest to the number expected, based on incidence rates in the general population. Several authors have presented excellent reviews of all the previous evidence but no clinical trials which have been done to evaluate the possible effects of the FDs on cancer risks.[8,11]

Ovarian cancer

Parity and oral contraceptives use have been reported to decrease ovarian cancer risk; nulliparity and infertility have been reported to increase this risk. However, the available evidence regarding the association between FDs and ovarian cancer risk is contradictory.[8,11,13,38]

Each hypothesis, before being proposed, should broadly focus on the clinical evidence that supports it. It is not clear which one of the above theories offers the best explanation for the observed association between ovarian cancer and reproductive risk factors. The association between the risk of ovarian cancer and fertility drugs has been examined in numerous case-control and cohort studies, but only two epidemiological studies have demonstrated an increased risk following the use of fertility medication.[11,39,40]

In a metanalysis of 12 case-control studies (Table 45.3), addressing the etiology of ovarian cancer, only three studies considered the use of FDs drugs without specific information about the type of drug and its duration of use. Prior use of fertility drugs was compared with women who had no infertility history with an odds ratio of 2.8 (95% CI 1.3–6.1). The ovarian risk was limited to nulligravid women with a 27-fold increase in risk, but the estimate was made with just 12 exposed cases and 1 exposed control. The other study was a retrospective cohort of 3,837 infertile women who were followed for cancer incidence. The authors estimated that clomiphene citrate (CC) use, was associated with an adjusted 2.3-fold increased risk (95% CI, 0.5–11.4), based on nine ovarian cancers. It also pointed out the importance of the duration of drug use, with an increased risk of ovarian cancer following CC use for longer than twelve months (RR 11.1 95% CI, 1.5–82.3).[39,40]

Despite these results, several recent cohort studies have failed to find confirmatory evidence for a large increment in ovarian cancer risk associated with FDs, even when dose, formulation and number of treatment cycles were considered. While the results of most recent studies may seem convincing when compared with previous studies, several observations indicate a need for further studies. On the basis of the available evidence, it is not appropriate to conclude an association between ovarian cancer and the use of FDs.[11]

Breast cancer

Breast cancer is the most frequently seen cancer in women. Its multifactorial etiology and epidemiology have been extensively studied, supporting an important role for endogenous and exogenous hormones. Estradiol promotes some breast cancer cell lines in culture and stimulates duct tissue of the breast; oophorectomy palliates some breast cancers, and combined hormone replacement therapy appears to increase the risk of breast cancer. Hence, the persistent E level in PCOS patients might be expected to increase the risk of breast cancer in this group of women.[8,10,11,41]

The association between FDs and breast cancer risk might be considered a public health issue, given the large number of women being medicated with these drugs and the high incidence of breast cancer. Only few studies have assessed breast cancer risk in relation to FDs, despite the proven effects of these drugs on ovulation and hormone patterns suggesting an association.[41]

The available data is based on cohort and case-control studies, but most of them have not found any important association. The methodological limitations of these studies should be noted: small numbers of cancers, imprecise information (patterns or indications of drug use), inadequate controls, among others.[11]

On the other hand, several studies have suggested an association between FD use and breast cancer risk, but the results are inconsistent, with some reporting potential increases in risk, and others a decrease. Given the hormonal etiology of breast cancer, some authors have found a risk elevation among women with long term use of menopausal gonadotropins. Use for at least 6 or more months for six cycles was associated with an odds ratio (OR) ranging from 2.7 to 3.8. A possible explanation of their findings has been proposed based on the effects of gonadotropin therapy on E and P levels. However, other authors have found no link between the use of CC and cancer risk, and yet others have described a reduced risk of invasive and *in situ* breast cancer associated with it. CC is a non-steroidal antiestrogen that is structurally related to tamoxifen, which has been reported to exert anti-proliferative effects on human breast cancer cells. On the contrary, a recent multicenter study did not demonstrate either a decreased risk associated with clomiphene, or an increased risk associated with gonadotropins.[11]

Considering this contradictory and limited available information, future studies should be performed in order to clarify the association between breast cancer and FD use.

Endometrial cancer

The role of endogenous gonadal hormones in the etiology of endometrial carcinoma is much better understood than that of breast and ovarian cancer. Some clinical reports endorse the presence of adenomatous hyperplasia of the endometrium in women exposed to FDs. Just one existent case-control study with only seven exposed cases, has found no association. The evidence available from cohort studies is contradictory. Most of them did not observe an association, but two large cohort studies have reported an increased risk of endometrial cancer. One of these studies described a two-fold increase in risk of uterine cancers in association with FDs, in 21 women during an average 20 years follow-up period. The other study, found a non-significant increase in risk associated with CC (relative risk 1.8; 95% CI, 0.9–3.3) in 39 cases of endometrial cancer, but with higher drug dosages or longer follow-up periods, increases in risk were observed. It must be noted that the investigations had limited power to detect effects because of the small number of cases. Further studies are needed to show this possible relationship.[11]

Some other authors have considered the association between FDs and non-gynecologic cancers, such as melanoma, thyroid and colon cancer, but the scant available data does not substantiate any conclusions.

Recent Advances

Estradiol is a pleiotropic hormone, due to its property as a nuclear transcription factor for a number of different genes involved in the etiology of several diseases. The individual genetic variability of the estradiol metabolism has been noted as an important contributor to disease susceptibility with some variations according to the ethnic background. According to this, genetic variations in genes encoding cytochrome (CYP) 450 enzymes play an important role. CYP P450 enzymes are important for the production, bioavailability, and degradation of estradiol.[42]

Cytochrome P450c17 (CYP 17) is an important enzyme in the synthesis of estradiol that facilitates hydroxylation of pregnenolone to P. Mutant CYP 17 alleles are associated with elevated serum levels of steroid hormones, endometrial and breast cancer. Among women with PCOS, mutant CYP 17alleles are sufficient to aggravate the clinical presentation of the disease.[42]

Also, genetic alterations such as microsatellite instability, PTEN mutations, K-ras mutations and β-catenin mutations, have been described for type I endometrial carcinomas. Recently, a pentanucleotide repeat polymorphism

[(TAAAA)n] in the CYP11A gene, which encodes the cholesterol side-chain cleavage enzyme, has also been identified that might represent a linkage between PCOS and carcinoma of the breast.[42–44]

Further studies are needed to identify common genetic predisposition factors that interact with lifestyle conditions and contribute to the development of PCOS and to examine whether these factors predispose to gynecologic cancers.

Conclusion

PCOS is the most common endocrinopathy in women of reproductive age. Although the mechanisms are not well understood, endogenous hormones appear to play an important role in the development and/or promotion of long-term consequences, such as gynecologic cancers. PCOS shares the major endocrine risk factors considered for some female malignancies. It is a risk factor of primary interest because its etiology appears to be strongly related to obesity, elevated androgens and hyperinsulinemia. Long-term exposure to E has been known to cause and increase cancer risk. The association between PCOS and endometrial malignancy has been recognized for many years, but the available evidence is not strong enough to clarify the degree of risk. Hence, no strong association between PCOS and female cancers can be concluded according to the available data. An understanding of hormonal functions in gynecological cancers may result in the development of more successful strategies for adequate detection and primary prevention. Further studies are required to assess the significance of genetic variations of E metabolism as a risk factor for hormone – dependant disorders.

References

1. Jemal A, Murray T, Ward E, Samuels A, Tiwari RC, Ghafoor A, Feuer EJ, Thun MJ. Cancer statistics, 2005. *CA Cancer J Clin* 2005; 55(1): 10–30.
2. Anonymous Reproductive health mortality statistics. Mexico, 2002. *Salud Publica Mex* 2004; 46: 75–88.

3. Anonymous. Mexico's mortality statistics: deaths registered in 2002. *Salud Publica Mex* 2004; 46: 85–169.

4. Gregorini SD, Lespi PJ, Alvarez GR. Endometrial carcinoma with polycystic ovaries. Report of two cases in women younger than 40 years old. *Medicina (B Aires)* 1997; 57(2): 209–212.

5. Meirow D, Schenker JG. The link between female infertility and cancer: epidemiology and possible aetiologies. *Hum Reprod Update* 1996; 2: 63–75.

6. Solomon CG. The epidemiology of polycystic ovary syndrome. Prevalence and associated disease risk. *Endocrinol Metab Clin North Am* 1999; 28: 247–263.

7. Bucccola JM, Reynols EE. Polycystic ovary syndrome: a review for primary providers. *Prim Care Office Pract* 2003; 30: 697–710.

8. Klip H, Burger CW, Kenemans P, van Leeuwen FE. Cancer risk associated with subfertility and ovulation induction: a review. *Cancer Causes Control* 2000; 11: 319–344.

9. Balem A. Polycystic ovary syndrome and cancer. *Hum Reprod Update* 2001; 7: 522–525.

10. Kaaks R, Lukanova A, Kurzer MS. Obesity, endogenous hormones, and endometrial cancer risk: a synthetic review. *Cancer Epidemiol Biomarkers Prev* 2002; 11(12): 1531–1543.

11. Brinton LA, Moghissi KS, Scoccia B, Westhoff C, Lamb EJ. Ovulation induction and cancer risk. *Fertil Steril* 2005; 83: 261–274.

12. Akhmedkhanov KA, Zeleniuch-Jacquotte A, Toniolo P. Role of exogenous and endogenous hormones in endometrial cancer. *Ann N Y Acad Sci* 2001; 943: 296–315.

13. Brinton LA, Lamb EJ, Moghissi KS et al. Ovarian Cancer Risk after the Use of Ovulation-Stimulating Drugs. *Obstet Gynecol* 2004; 103: 1194–1203.

14. Ayhan A, Salman MC, Celik H, Dursun P, Ozyuncu O, Gultekin M. Association between fertility drugs and gynecology cancer, breast cancer, and childhood cancers. *Acta Obstet Gynecol Scand* 2004; 83: 1104–1111.

15. Hardiman P, Pillays OS, Atiomo W. Polycystic ovary syndrome and endometrial carcinoma. *Lancet* 2003; 361: 1810–1812.

16. Speert H. Carcinoma of the endometrium in young women. *Surg Gynecol Obstet* 1949; 88: 332–336.

17. Dockerty MB, Lovelady B, Foust GT. Carcinoma of corpus uteri in young women. *Am J Obstet Gynecol* 1951; 61: 966–981.

18. Dockerty MB, Jackson RL. The Stein-Leventhal syndrome: analysis of 43 cases with special reference to association with endometrial carcinoma. *Am J Obstet Gynecol* 1957; 73: 161–173.

19. Jafari K, Javaheri G, Ruiz G. Endometrial adenocarcinoma and the Stein-Leventhal syndrome. *Obstet Gynecol* 1978; 51: 97–100.

20. Ramzy I, Nisker JA. Histologic study of ovaries from young women with . endometrial adenocarcinoma. *Am J Clin Pathol* 1979; 71: 253–256.

21. Coulam CB, Annegers JF, Kranz JS. Chronic anovulation syndrome and associated neoplasia. *Obstet Gyencol* 1983; 61: 403–407.

22. Gallup DG, Stock RJ. Adenocarcinoma of the endometrium in women 40 years of age or younger. *Obstet Gyencol* 1984; 64: 417–420.

23. Dennefors BL, Knutson F, Janson PO, Jansson I, Hamberger L. Ovarian steroid production in a woman with polycystic ovary syndrome associated with endometrial cancer. *Acta Obstet Gynecol Scand* 1985; 64(5): 387–392.

24. Escobedo LG, Lee NC, Peterson HB, Wingo PA. Infertility associated endometrial cancer risk may be limited to specific subgroups of infertile women. *Obstet Gynecol* 1991: 77: 124–128.

25. Smyczek-Gargya B, Geppert M. Endometrial cancer associated with polycystic ovaries in young women. *Pathol Res Pract* 1992; 188: 946–948.

26. Chadli-Debbiche A, Dellembach P, Philippe E, Hummel M. Endometrioid adenocarcinoma of the uteris isthmus associated with atypical endometrial hyperplasia an polycystic ovaries. Apropos of a case with bicornuate uterus in a 38 year old woman. *Arch Anat Cytol Pathol* 1993; 41: 171–174.

27. Goluda M, Andrzejewski L. A rare case of concurrent endometrial carcinoma and PCO syndrome. *Ginekol Pol* 1995; 66: 484–485.

28. Salha O, Martín-Hirsch P, Lane G, Sharma V. Endometrial carcinoma in a young patient with polycystic ovary syndrome: First suspected at time of embryo transfer. *Human Reprod* 1997; 12: 959–962.

29. Ho SP, Tan KT, Pang MW, Ho TH. Endometrial hyperplasia and the risk of endometrial carcinoma. *Singapore Med J* 1997; 38: 11–15.

30. Pierpoint T, McKeigue PM, Isaacs AJ, Wild SH, Jacobs HS. Mortality of women with polycystic ovary syndrome at long-term follow-up. *J Clin Epidemiol* 1998; 51: 581–586.

31. Wild S, Pierpoint T, Jacobs HS, McKeigue PM. Long-term consequences of polycystic ovary syndrome: results of a 31 year follow-up study. *Hum Fertil* 2000; 3: 101–105.

32. Kurabayashi T, Kase H, Susuki M, Sugaya S, Fujita K, Tanaka K. Endometrial abnormalities in infertile women. *J Reprod Med* 2003; 48: 455–459.

33. Gammon MD, Thompson WD. Polycystic ovaries and the risk of breast cancer. *Am J Epidemiol* 1991; 134: 818–824.

34. Anderson KE, Sellers TA, Chen PL, Rich SS, Hong CP, Folsom AR. Association of Stein-Leventhal syndrome with the incidence of postmenopausal breast carcinoma in a large prospective study of women in Iowa. *Cancer* 1997; 79(3): 494–499.

35. Atiomo WU, El-Mahdi E, Hardiman P. Familial associations in women with polycystic ovary syndrome. *Fertil Steril* 2003; 80: 143–145.

36. Resta L, Russo S, Clucci GA, Prat J. Morphologic precursors of ovarian epithelial tumors. *Obstet Gynecol* 1993; 82: 181–186.

37. Schildkraut JM, Schwingl PJ, Bastos E, Evanoff A, Hughes C. Epithelial ovarian cancer risk among women with polycystic ovary syndrome. *Obstet Gynecol* 1996; 88: 554–559.

38. Kashyap S, Moher D, Fung MF, Rosenwaks Z. Assisted reproductive technology and the incidence of ovarian cancer: a meta-analysis. *Obstet Gynecol* 2004; 103(4): 785–794.

39. Whittemore AS, Harris R, Itnyre J, the Collaborative Ovarian Cancer Group. Characteristics relating to ovarian cancer risks: collaborative analysis of 12-US case-control studies. II. Invasive epithelial ovarian cancers in white women. *Am J Epidemiol* 1992; 136: 1184–1203.

40. Rossing MA, Daling JR, Weiss NS, Moore DE, Self SG. Ovarian tumours in a cohort of infertile women. *N Engl J Med* 1994; 331: 771–776.

41. Brinton L, Scoccia B, Moghissi KS et al. Breast cancer risk associated with ovulation-stimulating drugs. *Hum Reprod* 2004; 19: 2005–2013.

42. Huber JC, Schneeberger, Tempfer CB. Genetic modeling of estrogen metabolism as a risk factor of hormone-dependent disorders. *Maturitas* 2002; 41: s55–s64.

43. Zheng W, Gao YT, Shu XO, Wen W, Cai Q, Dai Q, Smith JR. Population-based case-control study of CYP11A gene polymorphism and breast cancer risk. *Cancer Epidemiol Biomarkers Prev* 2004; 13(5): 709–714.

44. Ogawa K, Sun C, Horii A. Exploration of genetic alterations in human endometrial cancer and melanoma: distinct tumorigenic pathways that share a frequent abnormal PI3K/AKT cascade. *Oncol Rep* 2005; 14(6): 1481–1485.

46

The Role of Lifestyle Modifications in Polycystic Ovary Syndrome

Andrea Riccardo Genazzani, Francesca Cristello, Patrizia Monteleone, Maria Rosaria Parisen Toldin, Paolo Giovanni Artini

Summary

Polycystic Ovary Syndrome (PCOS) is a common endocrine condition, now recognised as a metabolic syndrome, which may include hyperinsulinemia, hyperlipidemia, diabetes mellitus and, possibly, vulnerability to heart diseases, as well as the more conventionally recognised clinical and/or biochemical hyperandrogenism, anovulation, infertility, endometrial cancer risk and obesity.

In the last ten years, several studies have recommended lifestyle interventions with weight loss, diet and exercise in obese or overweight women with PCOS, as the first therapeutic approach to improve clinical, metabolic and endocrinological features of these patients. When these measures prove to be unsuccessful and insulin resistance remains elevated, insulin-sensitizing agents are indicated.

Recent studies predict that the future therapeutic strategy in obese patients with PCOS appears to be a combination of lifestyle modifications that include a hypocaloric diet, and the use of insulin-sensitizing agents, particularly metformin.

Rationale

To evaluate the efficacy of behavioural modifications on future well-being as a first line treatment for women with polycystic ovary syndrome.

Introduction

Polycystic ovary syndrome (PCOS) is one of the most common endocrinopathies in women, affecting 5% to 10% of fertile age women. The syndrome not only interferes with reproduction, but is in many ways, a systemic disease.[1] Women with PCOS present at least two of the following features: polycystic ovaries (PCO), hyperandrogenism and anovulation. However, because of the abnormal hormonal profile, women with this syndrome may also complain of abnormal bleeding, infertility, obesity, excess hair growth, hair loss and acne.

The etiology of PCOS is uncertain, but it is thought to result from an interaction of familiar and environmental components. Precisely, although the insulin regulatory molecules on the theca cells are responsive to insulin, those in the muscle and liver are resistant.

In the ovary, the cardinal feature is functional hyperandrogenism. Circulating concentrations of insulin and luteinizing hormone (LH) are generally high. The theca cells, which envelop the follicle and produce androgens for conversion to estrogens, are over-responsive to this stimulation. They increase in size and overproduce androgens. The rise in LH levels is thought to be caused by the relatively high and unchanging concentrations of estrogens that may alter the feedback on the hypothalamic-pituitary axis.

The high levels of androgens, estrogens, insulin and LH combined, lead to the classic PCOS presentation of hirsutism, anovulation, dysfunctional bleeding, and altered glucose metabolism.

The pathogenesis of PCOS is poorly understood, but the primary defect may be insulin resistance. In fact, interest in PCOS has recently increased with the discovery that this syndrome involves far more than the reproductive system. PCOS is now recognised as a metabolic syndrome which may include hyperinsulinemia, hyperlipidemia, diabetes mellitus and, possibly, vulnerability to heart diseases, as well as the more conventionally recognized clinical and/or biochemical hyperandrogenism, anovulation, infertility, endometrial cancer risk and obesity.[2,3]

Some authors have recently suggested that the condition may begin during fetal life, with either intrauterine growth retardation or post-term birth. Researchers have claimed that these children are more prone to hyperinsulinism, premature pubarche and signs of PCOS early in reproductive life.[1,4]

Hyperinsulinemia and dyslipidemia are detectable before and during pubertal development, and are commonly accompanied by low serum levels of insulin-like growth factor binding-protein 1 (IGFBP-1) and sex hormone-binding globulin (SHBG), and by an increased prevalence of anovulation from late adolescence onwards, even without any clinical signs of androgen excess.[4]

The criteria used for the diagnosis and definition of PCOS are as heterogeneous as is the disorder itself. There is an ongoing debate about the blood tests needed, if any. In these women, the pituitary axis is hyperactive (higher LH pulses), leading to overproduction of ovarian (androstenedione, testosterone) and adrenal dehydroepiandrosterone sulfate (DHEA-S) androgens. Androgenic bioactivity is also increased due to the lower SHBG levels and higher P450c17 (17-α hydroxylase, 17, 20-lyase) activity. Every one of these hormonal dysfunctions could be minimal and not so valuable if considered alone.

Some authors found that the LH/FSH ratio correlates with both, the number of small follicles and the stromal artery pulsatility index. The combined assessment of ovarian morphology by transvaginal ultrasound and colour Doppler may provide insight into the etiopathogenesis of PCOS.[5]

Because PCOS is now considered a metabolic syndrome, it is suggested that patients have a thorough clinical evaluation. It is essential to exclude glucose intolerance. Insulin measurement, alone, has limited value; its interpretation may not be accurate in obese patients. Some investigators have recommended calculating an index of insulin resistance from glucose and insulin levels (eg, the homeostasis model assessment [HOMA] or quantitative insulin sensitivity check index [QUICKI].[6]

The incidence of obesity in women with PCOS varies between countries and ethnic groups. In the United States, about 50% of women with PCOS are overweight or obese, but this prevalence differs little from that in the general community. In other countries, PCOS appears to be associated with obesity, but at a lower rate than in the USA. Obesity tends to be central (abdominal) in its distribution, and even lean women with PCOS may have a fat distribution favouring central omental and visceral fat.

In a study of women with PCOS, performed about twenty years ago, most women were found to be hyperinsulinemic and to have a glucose metabolism that was resistant to the stimulatory effects of insulin.[7] Insulin resistance is aggravated by physical inactivity, upper abdominal obesity, hyperandrogenism, pregnancy, the ageing process, and by medications such as thiazide diuretics, corticosteroids and certain hormonal steroid preparations.

PCOS patients fall under four main categories: obese non insulin-resistant, obese insulin-resistant, non-obese non insulin-resistant, non-obese insulin-resistant. Treatment of these patients must be individualized accordingly.

Clinical Discussion

Conditions of excess weight and obesity are increasingly prevalent in developed and developing countries that have adopted a Western lifestyle and diet. Obesity, defined as a state of excessive adipose tissue, is frequently associated with PCOS: approximately 50% of these patients are obese or overweight. Women with PCOS tend to have a body mass index (BMI) outside the acceptable range (19–25 kg/m^2) and a central distribution of adiposity. This pathological condition contributes to menstrual disorders, with chronic anovulation and infertility, and to hyperinsulinemia. Moreover, it has major adverse medical consequences, largely due to its association with non insulin-dependent diabetes, hyperlipidemia, hypertension and cardiovascular disease.[8] The determining factor seems to be the "central-type" body fat distribution [9], or the presence of androgenic-type obesity, with prevailing fat deposition in the trunk, identifiable from a waist-hip ratio greater than 0.85. Even lean women with PCOS may have a fat distribution favouring central omental and visceral fat.

Although obesity is considered responsible for the onset of insulin resistance, recent studies have demonstrated that hyperinsulinemia is independent of obesity as it is also present in many lean patients, and that, insulin resistance is more severe in PCOS patients than in obese women.[10] Many investigators have shown that lean women with PCOS have insulin resistance and that overweight PCOS subjects are more severely affected than unaffected patients with the same BMI without the syndrome.[11]

Sometimes women with PCOS are not really overweight, but they have a history of difficulty in losing weight even under hypocaloric regimens.

Subjects with PCOS who are overweight are less likely to achieve a pregnancy spontaneously, or with medical assistance, are more likely to miscarry, have a higher prevalence of fetal abnormality and suffer more pregnancy complications.[12]

Therefore, the first-line therapeutic approach to adopt in obese and overweight PCOS patients is a hypocaloric diet, low in saturated and trans fat and high in fibre. Regular physical activity is also necessary to normalize the body weight of patients. Indeed, several studies have shown that a reduction in body fat increases insulin sensitivity, with a consequent decrease in plasma concentrations of insulin, both in obese and overweight PCOS patients.[13–15]

Weight loss also significantly improves clinical, metabolic and endocrinological features of PCOS:[16] changes in plasma androgen levels, improvement in hirsutism and resumption of ovulation.[17,18] Proper eating habits are essential to control hyperinsulinemia, even in cases where weight loss is not significant. According to some authors, a reduction in body weight of even 5%, seems to restore regular ovulatory cycles in 90% of women with PCOS.[18,19]

An epidemiological study in the UK that followed up women with a histological diagnosis of PCOS after wedge resection of the ovaries, found clear evidence of an increase in the rate of diabetes among these patients.[20] This confirmed the results of many other studies from the USA and Europe: in obese women with PCOS, progression from normal glucose function to impaired glucose tolerance or diabetes mellitus is more rapid than in women without PCOS.[21]

Insulin resistance is independently related to PCOS as PCOS women with normal weight may show a degree of hyperinsulinemia and impaired glucose disposal after meals and during glucose tolerance tests.[22] It is uncertain whether this insulin resistance results from a specific genetic post-receptor defect, such as a defect in serine phosphorylation,[23] or whether it is due to a decrease in insulin receptor substrate 1 (IRS-1) and insulin receptor substrate-2 (IRS-2) associated phosphoinositol-3 kinase (Pl3K) activators, as seen in type 2 diabetes.

Insulin-resistance in PCOS is not due primarily to obesity (as lean women with PCOS could also be insulin-resistant) or to hyperandrogenism[24] (as androgen blockade reduces insulin resistance by only 10%–15%).[25] However determined, insulin resistance leads to hyperinsulinemia as pancreatic insulin secretion rises to maintain normoglycemia. Hyperinsulinemia can then stimulate lipid storage, altered lipoprotein and cholesterol metabolism and possibly, altered steroid hormone metabolism. Hyperinsulinemia increases ovarian androgen production by stimulating an ovarian enzyme complex cytochrome P450c17, either directly, and/or by stimulating pituitary LH secretion.[26]

Moreover, in the past decade, studies have shown that women with PCOS have a high prevalence of hyperlipidemia,[27] hypertension,[28] and progression to type 2 diabetes mellitus,[29] which are similar to the features of the so-called "metabolic syndrome" or "Syndrome X".

Women with PCOS are nearly twice as likely to have the metabolic syndrome in comparison to the general female population. Women demonstrating characteristics of both PCOS and the metabolic syndrome are found to have more severe insulin resistance.

Although the mechanisms interlinking premature pubarche, hyperinsulinism and ovarian hyperandrogenism remain unknown, this triad may result, at least in part, from a common early origin rather than from a direct relationship later on in life.[30]

Among girls with precocious pubarche (defined as the appearance of pubic hair before the age of 8 years), those with low birth weight are at risk for progression to PCOS, hyperinsulinemia, hyperandrogenemia, dyslipidemia, dysadipocytokinemia, and central fat excess.[31]

Another study group investigated twenty-seven girls with premature pubarche by ultrasonographic and colour Doppler analyses to determine the incidence of PCO, to longitudinally assess their evolution, and to search for any hormonal correlation. They found that, among girls with premature pubarche, the prevalence of PCO was 41%. Moreover, advanced skeletal maturation, tall stature, and increased hair distribution were constant in these patients. They concluded that polycystic ovaries are often present among girls with premature pubarche and progressively evolve.[32]

A recent study examined the influence of birth weight and early postnatal weight gain on overnight fasting adrenal androgen and cortisol levels in 770, 8-year old children from a large normal United Kingdom birth cohort. They found that adrenal androgen levels were highest in small infants who gained weight rapidly during early childhood. Based on these considerations, they suggested that greater adrenal androgen secretion could be one link between early growth retardation and risk for adult diseases, possibly by enhancing insulin resistance and central fat deposition.[33]

Before and during pubertal development, it is possible to find the hyperinsulinemia and dyslipidemia generally associated with low serum levels of IGFBP-1 and SHBG, and to an increased prevalence of anovulation from late adolescence onwards, even without any clinical signs of androgen excess. In girls, premature pubarche, hyperinsulinism, low IGFBP-1, dyslipidemia, anovulation and hyperandrogenism have been related to reduced fetal growth, with a hypothetical prenatal origin of this heterogeneous syndrome.[34]

Early metformin therapy seems to prevent progression from precocious pubarche to PCOS in a high-risk group of formerly low birth-weight girls. This confirms the key role of hyperinsulinemic insulin resistance in the ontogeny of PCOS. Furthermore, normalization of body composition, lipid profiles, and growth hormone (GH) secretion, could reduce the long-term cardiovascular risk.[35]

Unfortunately, in adolescence, the normalizing effects of metformin are reversed as soon as metformin therapy is discontinued.[31] It is certainly more useful to educate adolescents to adopt a "healthy" lifestyle.

Attempts to reduce weight, increase exercise and stop smoking will fail if the woman with PCOS is not educated about the long term adverse health implications of this condition. Too often, these women are told only about the cosmetic nuisances of hirsutism or acne. However, though lifestyle changes are difficult to maintain, overweight women with PCOS seeking a pregnancy, are highly motivated, making this a first-line intervention.[2,36] Long-term changes in weight are more difficult to maintain. Obesity should be treated with a structured diet and exercise program.[37] Simply telling a patient to "lose weight" or "eat less" is unlikely to result in a significant reduction in weight, judging from experience in the management of type 2 diabetes. Consultation with dieticians working in type 2 diabetes or commercial weight reduction programs may be useful in refractory obesity; in fact, changes in diet and exercise habits can delay the onset of diabetes.

Some studies have found that women with PCOS exhibit an adverse cardiovascular risk profile.[38,39] In this way, they have a greater risk for developing hypertension compared to women of the same age, because they develop stiff arteries that may increase their risk of cardiovascular disease and stroke. In the first study of its kind, researchers compared the elasticity of arteries in women with normal ovaries, those with PCO, and those with PCOS.[39] On average, women with PCOS had arteries nearly twice as stiff as the arteries in women with normal ovaries. Artery stiffness in women with PCOS lay roughly midway between the other two groups. Stiff arteries are an indication of atherosclerosis; as fatty plaques form and builds in artery walls, the vessels lose some of their elasticity.

There is evidence for an association between metabolic cardiovascular syndrome and coronary and aortic calcification among women with PCOS. To prevent the risk of early-onset cardiovascular disease, women with PCOS should automatically be screened for the metabolic syndrome and insulin resistance. Given the large number of women with PCOS and the long incubation period for sub-clinical atherosclerosis, early and aggressive intervention through lifestyle modification and/or pharmacological therapies (*i.e.* metformin and insulin sensitizers) may significantly reduce the morbidity and mortality from coronary heart disease in the female population.[38]

To prevent cardiovascular disease, it is important to lose weight, decrease the amount of total dietary fat, exercise at least 30 minutes four times a week, check blood pressure every six months for values higher than 140/90 mm Hg and check high density lipoprotein (HDL) and total cholesterol profile.

As for the reproductive potential, PCOS is frequently associated with infertility due to the lack of ovulation because of a failure of the follicles to develop beyond 10 mm in diameter. Most cycles are anovulatory, and induction of ovulation is needed. The risk of ovulatory infertility is highest in obese women but is also slightly increased in moderately overweight and underweight women.[40] Body fat distribution in women of reproductive age seems to have more impact on fertility than age or obesity.[9] Several studies have shown that weight loss can significantly improve clinical and metabolic parameters and lead to resumption of ovulation within weeks.[15,19]

Clark and colleagues[37] demonstrated that even a 5% reduction in body mass restores ovulation and fertility. These authors devised a program of exercise and sensible eating that has become a model across the world for treating PCOS.[37]

Women with PCOS, who have irregular periods or amenorrhea, are at an increased risk for developing endometrial carcinoma, related chronic anovulation with consequent continued secretion of estrogens unopposed by progesterone. However, the evidence is incomplete and contradictory. It is more likely that this risk applies only to obese women.

Chronically elevated insulin and insulin-like growth factors have been implicated as contributors to a variety of cancers and degenerative conditions. However, at this time, there is no clear evidence to suggest that women with PCOS are at any increased risk for ovarian or breast cancer.[41]

Case studies

The analysis of clinical studies of the last 10 years shows that, in women with PCOS, whether overweight or obese, weight loss attained by modifications in lifestyle, is an important factor in restoring reproductive function.

Ten years ago, Holte and colleagues underlined the impact of weight reduction on metabolic, endocrine, and anthropometric variables in PCOS patients. Thirteen obese insulin-resistant (IR) women with PCOS were compared to two groups of weight stable (no diet) women, 21 IR and non-IR PCOS women and 23 normal control subjects. The patients were matched to the BMI the diet group reached after weight loss. Insulin resistance in obese women with PCOS was reduced by weight loss to levels similar to BMI-matched control subjects, suggesting that insulin resistance in PCOS is not a feature of PCOS per se. The findings of this study underline the strong association in PCOS between insulin-resistance and truncal-abdominal fat mass. Reduced levels of free fatty acids and testosterone may contribute to improved insulin sensitivity. After weight loss, persistently increased insulin secretion seems to be a feature of this syndrome and may favor weight gain.[14]

In 1999, a study by Huber-Bucholz et al.[36] confirmed that lifestyle modifications in patients with PCOS is the best initial management for obese women seeking to improve their reproductive function: weight reduction and exercise were shown to help overcome menstrual disturbance and infertility. This study evaluated the relationship between changes in insulin sensitivity, LH, and ovulation patterns before and after a 6 month diet and exercise program in 18 infertile anovulatory obese PCOS women aged 22–39 years with normal glucose tolerance, and a BMI of 27–45 kg/m^2, compared to 10 age- and weight-matched PCOS women with regular monthly ovulation. The program proposed in this study promoted healthy lifestyle factors without rapid weight loss and led to a reduction of central fat and improved insulin sensitivity. These changes occurred with minimal weight loss, which is encouraging for women who have constantly failed to achieve reproductive success on a variety of short term low calorie diets. Changes in insulin sensitivity and falling serum insulin values may be the metabolic mediator of these results.[36]

More recently, Hoeger and colleagues[42] carried out an interesting prospective, randomized,

placebo-controlled pilot trial. The aim of the study was to observe the effect of intensive lifestyle modifications and/or metformin therapy on ovulation and androgen concentrations in overweight women with polycystic ovary syndrome. They recruited 38 overweight or obese women with PCOS. All the subjects were randomized to one of four 48-week interventions: metformin 850 mg twice a day, lifestyle modifications plus metformin 850 mg twice a day, lifestyle modifications plus placebo, or placebo alone. Preliminary estimates of treatment effect on ovulation were measured by weekly urinary pregnanediol glucuronide, and on total testosterone and free androgen index. Modest weight reduction was found in all treatment groups, with the most significant reduction occurring in the group treated with a combination of metformin and lifestyle intervention. Significant androgen reduction occurred in the combination group only. Ovulation rates did not differ significantly between groups.

Recent Advances and Conclusions

In several recent studies, the future therapeutic strategy in obese patients with PCOS appears to be a combination of lifestyle modifications that include a hypocaloric diet, and the use of insulin sensitizing agents, particularly metformin.[19,43,44]

In women with PCOS with an abdominal obesity phenotype, long-term treatment with metformin added to a low-calorie diet, induced a greater reduction of body weight and abdominal fat, particularly the visceral depots, and a more consistent decrease in serum insulin, testosterone, and leptin concentrations. Moreover, these changes were associated with a more significant improvement of hirsutism and menstrual abnormalities.[43]

On the contrary, recent randomized, placebo-controlled, double-blind studies in very obese patients with anovulatory PCOS (BMI>30 Kg/m^2) showed that metformin alone, at a dose of 850 mg twice daily, has no effect on menstrual frequency, body weight or insulin sensitivity, despite a fall in total testosterone and waist circumference, while a modest weight loss alone, through lifestyle changes, is able to improve menstrual cyclicity.[44]

Insulin-sensitizing agents, particularly metformin, are a relatively recent therapeutic strategy used in the management of infertility in PCOS women with insulin resistance and also for its observed potential effect in early pregancy loss reduction.

In fact, it has very recently been demonstrated that an effective reduction of insulin resistance induces regular menstrual cycles and fertility.[45] Drugs with insulin-sensitizing properties should not be recommended indiscriminately in PCOS women, but only in those with insulin resistance and/or obesity. New insulin-sensitizing agents such as thiazolidinediones (rosiglitazone and pioglitazone) are being proposed for the treatment of the insulin resistance. In the light of their potential hepatotoxic effects, clinical studies are needed to introduce these compounds in daily clinical practice.

The rationale for continuing metformin treatment in women who conceive is to prevent miscarriage during the first trimester and the development of gestational diabetes in the second and third trimesters.[46] However, its safety has not been established for use during gestation.

Several investigators have shown that subjects with PCOS have higher levels of stress and a more negative self-image than controls. Any lifestyle modifications should address behaviour therapy and a better understanding of the psychological background of subjects with PCOS. Moderate exercise, reduction of smoking, dietary modifications and reduction of psychosocial stressors would probably be of greatest benefit. Support groups could make it easier for patients to implement these lifestyle changes. Insulin-sensitizing agents may be helpful in selected cases.

References

1. Diamanti-Kandarakis E, Kouli CR, Bergiele AT, Filandra FA, Tsianateli TC, Spina GG, et al A survey of the polycystic ovary syndrome in the Greek island of Lesbos: hormonal and metabolic profile. *J Clin Endocrinol Metab* 1999; 84: 4006–4011.

2. Norman RJ, Davies MJ, Lord J, Moran LJ. The role of lifestyle modification in polycystic ovary syndrome. *Trends Endocrinol Metab* 2002; 13: 251–257.

3. Lobo RA, Carmina E. The importance of diagnosing the polycystic ovary syndrome. *Ann Intern Med* 2000; 132: 989–993.

4. Ibanez L, Potau N, Ferrer A, Rodriguez-Hierro F, Marcos MV, De Zegher F. Anovulation in eumenorrheic, nonobese adolescent girls born small for gestational age: insulin sensitization induces ovulation, increases lean body mass, and reduces abdominal fat excess, dyslipidemia, and subclinical hyperandrogenism. *J Clin Endocrinol Metab* 2002; 87: 5702–5705.

5. Battaglia C, Genazzani AD, Salvatori M, Giulini S, Artini PG, Genazzani AR, et al. Doppler, ultrasonographic and endocrinological environment with regard to the number of small subcapsular follicles in polycystic ovary syndrome. *Gynecol Endocrinol* 1999 Apr; 13(2): 123–129.

6. Abassi F, Reaver GM. Evaluation of the quantitative insulin sensitivity index as an estimate of insulin sensitivity in humans. *Metabolism* 2002; 51: 235–237.

7. Burghen GA, Givens JR, Kitabchi AE. Correlation of hyperandrogenism with hyperinsulinism in polycystic ovary disease. *J Clin Endocrinol Metab* 1980; 50: 113–116.

8. Norman RJ, Clark AM. Obesity and reproductive disorders: a review. *Reprod Fertil Dev* 1998; 10(1): 55–63.

9. Zaadstra BM, Seidell JC, Van Noord PA, te Velde ER, Habbema JD, Vrieswijk B, Karbaat J. Fat and female fecundity: prospective study of effect of body fat distribution on conception rates. *BMJ* 1993; 306(6876): 484–487.

10. Dunaif A. Insulin resistance and the polycystic ovary syndrome: mechanism and implications for pathogenesis. *Endocr Rev* 1997; 18(6): 774–800.

11. Legro RS, Kunselman AR, Dodson WC, Dunaif A. Prevalence and predictors of risk for type 2 diabetes mellitus and impaired glucose tolerance in polycystic ovary syndrome: a prospective, controlled study in 254 affected women. *J Clin Endocrinol Metab* 1999; 84(1): 165–169.

12. Wang JX, Davies M, Norman RJ. Body mass and probability of pregnancy during assisted reproduction treatment: retrospective study. *BMJ* 2000; 321(7272): 1320–1321.

13. Andersen P, Seljeflot I, Abdelnoor M, Arnesen H,

Dale PO, Lovik A, Birkeland K. Increased insulin sensitivity and fibrinolytic capacity after dietary intervention in obese women with polycystic ovary syndrome. *Metabolism* 1995; 44(5): 611–616.

14. Holte J, Bergh T, Berne C, Wide L, Lithell H. Restored insulin sensitivity but persistently increased early insulin secretion after weight loss in obese women with polycystic ovary syndrome. *J Clin Endocrinol Metab* 1995; 80(9): 2586–2593.

15. Pasquali R, Antenucci D, Casimirri F, Venturoli S, Paradisi R, Fabbri R, et al. Clinical and hormonal characteristics of obese amenorrheic hyperandrogenic women before and after weight loss. *J Clin Endocrinol Metab* 1989; 68: 173–179.

16. Pasquali R, Pelusi C, Genghini S, Cacciari M, Gambineri A. Obesity and reproductive disorders in women. *Hum Reprod Update* 2003; 9: 359–372.

17. Guzick DS, Wing R, Smith D, Berga SL, Winters SJ. Endocrine consequences of weight loss in obese, hyperandrogenic, anovulatory women. *Fertil Steril* 1994; 61(4): 598–604.

18. Kiddy DS, Hamilton-Fairley D, Bush A, Short F, Anyaoku V, Reed MJ, Franks S. Improvement in endocrine and ovarian function during dietary treatment of obese women with polycystic ovary syndrome. *Clin Endocrinol* (Oxf) 1992; 36(1): 105–111.

19. Ciampelli M, Lanzone A. Insulin and polycystic ovary syndrome: a new look at an old subject. *Gynecol Endocrinol* 1998; 12(4): 277–292.

20. Pierpoint T, McKeigue PM, Isaacs AJ, Wild SH, Jacobs HS. Mortality of women with polycystic ovary syndrome at long-term follow-up. *J Clin Epidemiol* 1998; 51: 581–586.

21. Norman RJ, Masters L, Milner CR, Wang JX, Davies MJ. Relative risk of conversion from normoglycaemia to impaired glucose tolerance or non-insulin dependent diabetes mellitus in polycystic ovarian syndrome. *Hum Reprod* 2001; 16: 1995–1998.

22. Dunaif A, Segal KR, Futterweit W, Dobrjansky A. Profound peripheral insulin resistance, independent of obesity, in polycystic ovary syndrome. *Diabetes* 1989; 38: 1165–1174.

23. Dunaif A. Molecular mechanisms of insulin resistance in the polycystic ovary syndrome. *Semin Reprod Endocrinol* 1994; 12: 15–20.

24. Barbieri RL, Hornstein MD. Hyperinsulinemia and ovarian hyperandrogenism: cause and effect. *Endocrinol Metab Clin North Am* 1988; 17: 685–703.

25. Moghetti P, Tosi F, Castello R, Magnani CM, Negri C, Brun E, et al. The insulin resistance in women with hyperandrogenism is partially reversed by antiandrogen treatment: evidence that androgens impair insulin action in women. *J Clin Endocrinol Metab* 1996; 81: 952–960.

26. Legro R, Finegood D, Dunaif A. A fasting glucose to insulin ratio is a useful measure of insulin sensitivity in women with polycystic ovary syndrome. *J Clin Endocrinol Metabol* 1998; 83: 2694–2698.

27. Robinson S, Henderson AD, Gelding SV, Kiddy D, Niththyananthan R, Bush A, et al. Dyslipidaemia is associated with insulin resistance in women with polycystic ovaries. *Clin Endocrinol* 1996; 44: 277–284.

28. Wild RA. Obesity, lipids, cardiovascular risk, and androgen excess. *Am J Med* 1995; 98(1A): 27S–32S. Review.

29. Birdsall MA, Farquhar CM, White HD. Association between polycystic ovaries and extent of coronary artery disease in women having cardiac catherization. *Ann Int Med* 1997; 126: 32–35.

30. Ibanez L, de Zegher F, Potau N. Premature pubarche, ovarian hyperandrogenism, hyperinsulinism and the polycystic ovary syndrome: from a complex constellation to a simple sequence of prenatal onset. *J Endocrinol Invest* 1998; 21(9): 558–566.

31. Ibanez L, Valls C, Marcos MV, Ong K, Dunger DB, De Zegher F. Insulin sensitization for girls with precocious pubarche and with risk for polycystic ovary syndrome: effects of prepubertal initiation and postpubertal discontinuation of metformin treatment. *J Clin Endocrinol Metab* 2004; 89(9): 4331–4337.

32. Battaglia C, Regnani G, Mancini F, Iughetti L, Bernasconi S, Volpe A, et al. Isolated premature pubarche: ultrasonographic and color Doppler analysis: a longitudinal study. *J Clin Endocrinol Metab* 2002; 87(7): 3148–3154.

33. Ong KK, Potau N, Petry CJ, Jones R, Ness AR, Honour JW, et al. Avon Longitudinal Study of Parents and Children Study Team Opposing influences of prenatal and postnatal weight gain on adrenarche in normal boys and girls. *J Clin Endocrinol Metab* 2004; 89(6): 2647–2651.

34. Ibanez L, Potau N, Dunger D, de Zegher F. Precocious pubarche in girls and the development of androgen excess. *J Pediatr Endocrinol Metab* 2000; 13 Suppl 5: 1261–1263.

35. Ibanez L, Ferrer A, Ong K, Amin R, Dunger D, de Zegher F. Insulin sensitization early after menarche prevents progression from precocious pubarche to polycystic ovary syndrome. *J Pediatr* 2004; 144(1): 23–29.

36. Huber-Buchholz MM, Carey DG, Norman RJ. Restoration of reproductive potential by lifestyle modification in obese polycystic ovary syndrome: role of insulin sensitivity and luteinizing hormone. *J Clin Endocrinol Metab* 1999; 84: 1470–1474.

37. Clark AM, Ledger W, Galletly C, Tomlinson L, Blaney F, Wang X, Norman RJ. Weight loss results in significant improvement in pregnancy and ovulation rates in anovulatory obese women. *Hum Reprod* 1995; 10: 2705–2712.

38. Talbott EO, Zborowski JV, Rager JR, Boudreaux MY, Edmundowicz DA, Guzick DS. Evidence for an association between metabolic cardiovascular syndrome and coronary and aortic calcification among women with polycystic ovary syndrome. *J Clin Endocrinol Metab* 2004; 89(11): 5454–5461.

39. Lakhani K, Seifalian AM, Hardiman P. Impaired carotid viscoelastic properties in women with polycystic ovaries. *Circulation* 2002; 106(1): 81–85.

40. Grodstein F, Goldman MB, Cramer DW. Body mass index and ovulatory infertility. *Epidemiology* 1994; 5(2): 247–250.

41. Hardiman P, Pillay OC, Atiomo W. Polycystic ovary syndrome and endometrial carcinoma. *Lancet* 2003; 361(9371): 1810–1812.

42. Hoeger KM, Kochman L, Wixom N, Craig K, Miller RK, Guzick DS. A randomized 48-week, placebo-controlled trial of intensive lifestyle modification and/or metformin therapy in overweight women with polycystic ovary syndrome: a pilot study. *Fertil Steril* 2004; 82(2): 421–429.

43. Pasquali R, Gambineri A, Biscotti D, Vicennati V, Gagliardi L, Colitta D, et al. Effect of long-term treatment with metformin added to hypocaloric diet on body composition, fat distribution, and androgen and insulin levels in abdominally obese women with and without the polycystic ovary syndrome. *J Clin Endocrinol Metab* 2000; 85(8): 2767–2774.

44. Tang T, Glanville J, Hayden CJ, White D, Barth JH, Balen AH. Combined lifestyle modification and metformin in obese patients with polycystic ovary syndrome. A randomized, placebo-controlled, double-blind multicentre study. *Hum Reprod* 2005 Sep 30; [Epub ahead of print].

45. Genazzani AD, Battaglia C, Malavasi B, Strucchi C, Tortolani F, Gamba O. Metformin administration modulates and restores luteinizing hormone spontaneous episodic secretion and ovarian function in nonobese patients with polycystic ovary syndrome. *Fertil Steril* 2004; 81(1): 114–119.

46. Checa MA, Requena A, Salvador C, Tur R, Callejo J, Espinos JJ, et al. Reproductive Endocrinology Interest Group of the Spanish Society of Fertility. Insulin-sensitizing agents: use in pregnancy and as therapy in polycystic ovary syndrome. *Hum Reprod Update* 2005; 11(4): 375–390.

Frequently Asked Questions

1. How should PCOS be diagnosed?

PCOS should be diagnosed based on a physical exam, ultrasound of the ovaries, and the results of blood tests. During the physical examination, one should evaluate the presence of hirsutism and virilization of external genitalia.Ultrasound features of PCO are an increase in ovarian volume and the presence of numerous follicles distributed as a "string of pearls" around the stroma. Usually, ultrasound diagnosis is made if there are at least 10-12 cysts that are less than 10 mm in size in each ovary. The PCO tends to be enlarged to 1.5–3 times the size of a normal ovary, and often presents an increase in the stromal tissue at the center of the ovary and around the follicles.

As for blood tests, a good basic screening would include:

- fasting comprehensive biochemical and lipid panel;
- 2-hour OGTT with insulin levels (also called IGTT);
- basal hormone testing (LH/FSH ratio; total testosterone; DHEAS; SHBG; androstenedione; prolactin; TSH)

2. What are the long-term health risks associated with PCOS?

Irregular menstrual periods and the absence of ovulation cause women to produce estrogen, but not progesterone. Hence, women with PCOS have an increased risk of endometrial hyperplasia or cancer in addition to an increased risk for insulin-resistance, type 2 diabetes, high cholesterol, high blood pressure. Getting the symptoms under control at an early age may help to reduce this risk.

3. Does PCOS get worse over time?

Polycystic ovary syndrome may worsen during the reproductive years (ages 20–40), especially if associated with weight gain. A healthy lifestyle is probably the best prevention. It seems that as women reach menopause, ovarian function changes and the menstrual cycle may become more normal. But even with falling male hormone levels, excessive hair growth continues, and male pattern baldness or thinning hair gets worse after menopause. Currently, the best recommendation is to monitor cholesterol, triglycerides, blood pressure, and glucose/insulin levels as one might for 'Syndrome X', and treat any minor abnormalities with diet and exercise, and more substantial alterations with medication.

4. What is the connection between insulin resistance and PCOS?

At least 30% of women with PCOS are insulin-resistant. Hyperinsulinemia produces hyperandrogenism by stimulating ovarian androgen production and by reducing serum SHBG. This can heighten PCOS symptoms. Reducing insulin resistance through the use of insulin-sensitizing medications can restore ovulatory function in many women with PCOS. It appears that even some patients who do not test as being insulin-resistant may benefit from these medications.

5. Is a diet modification needed in addition to taking insulin-sensitizing medications?

The medications themselves may help, but lifestyle changes are fundamental. It is generally recommended that patients taking metformin or one of the glitazones, reduce carbohydrate intake and increase exercise to improve glucose metabolism and help possible weight loss if overweight. Seeking a consultation with a registered dietician and beginning a structured exercise program are central to an effective therapeutic plan.

6. What testing should be done before prescribing insulin-sensitizing medications and what kind of monitoring should be done afterwards?

Before metformin is prescribed, a comprehensive biochemical panel should be performed that includes liver enzymes and alanine transaminase

(ALT). If there are liver or kidney abnormalities, caution should be used and the benefits weighed before choosing to use these medications.

During therapy with metformin, estimation of fasting blood sugar should be performed periodically, along with insulin and HbA1c measurements to monitor glycemic control and the therapeutic response to medication; it is also recommended that kidney function tests be repeated periodically.

Liver function tests should also be obtained if one has symptoms suggestive of hepatic dysfunction, such as jaundice, nausea, vomiting, abdominal pain, fatigue, anorexia, or dark urine.

7. How is PCOS treated?

Because there is no cure for PCOS, it needs to be managed to prevent problems. Treatment is based on the symptoms of each patient and depending on her anxiety to conceive, or requirement for contraception.

8. How does PCOS affect a woman during pregnancy?

In women with PCOS, there appears to be a higher rate of miscarriage (45% or more), gestational diabetes, pregnancy-induced high blood pressure, and premature delivery. The exact reason of the elevated risk of miscarriage is still under investigation. Miscarriage may be associated with elevated levels of LH, or insulin, or glucose, which may impede implantation or cause problems with early embryonic development. There is a possibility that insulin resistance reduces egg quality, or that late ovulation (after cycle day 16) may be associated with poor follicle development and decreased egg quality.

9. Will losing weight jumpstart fertility in overweight patients with PCOS?

Weight loss may help reduce insulin resistance, resulting in spontaneous or improved ovulation. Quick weight loss may cause more harm than good, so slow weight loss is best. Losing 10% of one's body weight should be enough to show some improvement in symptoms.

10. Is someone with PCOS more likely to have gestational diabetes?

Many women with PCOS are insulin resistant, and pregnancy tends to be a time of increased glucose intolerance as well. Considering the two associations, there is an increased incidence of gestational diabetes.

Index